D1582698

PEDIATRIC ONCOLOGY

Deborah Tomlinson
Nancy E. Kline
(Eds.)

Pediatric Oncology Nursing

Advanced Clinical Handbook

Second Edition

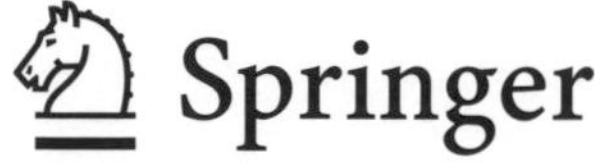

Library of Congress
Control Number 2009934491
ISBN 978-3-540-87983-1
e-ISBN 978-3-540-87984-8
Springer Heidelberg Dordrecht London New York
ISSN 1613-5318
DOI: 10.1007/978-3-540-87984-8

Deborah Tomlinson MN, RN
Dip Cancer Nursing
Child Health Evaluative Sciences
Hospital for Sick Children
Child Health Evaluative
Toronto ON
Canada

Nancy E.Kline PhD, RN, CPNP, FAAN,
Director, Research and Evidence-Based Practice
Department of Nursing
Memorial Sloan-Kettering Cancer Center
New York, NY
USA
Cover design: eStudio Calamar, Figueres Berlin

Springer is a part of Springer Science+Business Media

springeronline.com

Printed on acid-free paper

9 8 7 6 5 4 3 2 1

Springer.com

Dedication

To all pediatric nurses. Your contribution to our world's future is beyond words.

To Chris and our children, Vivian, Sam, Suzanne and Angus – for giving me reason.
Deborah Tomlinson

To my parents, and my husband Michael. Thank you for your unwavering support throughout this endeavor.
Nancy E. Kline

Preface

Pediatric Oncology Nursing: Advanced Clinical Handbook is a joint effort between nurses in Canada, the United Kingdom, and the United States. This is the second edition, and has been another wonderful opportunity to bring together the expertise of hematology and oncology nurses from two continents. The book is designed to be a comprehensive clinical handbook for nurses in advanced practice working with pediatric hematology/oncology patients. Specific issues related to young children and adolescents with cancer and hematologic disorders are discussed.

Thirty-one contributors and two editors participated in the writing of this text. Individuals in advanced practice and academic roles – nurse practitioners, clinical nurse specialists, nutritionists, clinical instructors, lecturers, academicians, and educators – were involved. One of the most appealing features of this text is the vast experience represented by our authors from different countries and different educational backgrounds.

The book is divided into 5 sections: pediatric cancers, hematologic disorders, treatment of childhood cancer, side effects of treatment and disease, and supportive and palliative care. Many tables and illustrations are included for quick reference in the clinical setting. Future perspectives and opportunities for new treatment options and research are discussed.

Part I focuses on pediatric cancers – the leukemias, lymphomas, and solid tumors. The most common pediatric tumors as well as some rare tumors are discussed in regards to epidemiology, etiology, molecular genetics, symptoms and clinical signs, diagnostic and laboratory testing, staging and classification, treatment, prognosis, and follow up care.

Part II focuses on pediatric hematology. The anemias, bleeding disorders, neutropenia, thrombocytopenia, and bleeding disorders are discussed in detail. Epidemiology, etiology, symptoms and clinical signs, diagnostic and laboratory procedures, treatment, prognosis, and follow up care are included for each of the disorders.

Part III covers cancer treatment, including chemotherapy, radiation therapy, hematopoetic stem cell transplantation, surgery, gene therapy, biotherapy, complimentary and alternative medicine, and clinical trials. The principles and description of treatment, method of treatment delivery, potential side effects, and special considerations for each type of treatment are discussed.

Part IV focuses on the side effects of cancer treatment in relation to metabolic processes and gastrointestinal, hematologic, respiratory, renal, cardiovascular, neurologic, musculoskeletal, integumentary, endocrine, and auditory systems. The incidence, etiology, treatment, prevention, and prognosis are included for each side effect reviewed.

Part V includes the essential information regarding supportive and palliative care of pediatric cancer patients. Nutrition, hydration, pain, blood transfusion therapy, growth factors, and care of the dying child and the family are covered. The principles of treatment for these conditions, method of delivery, and special considerations for certain conditions are included.

The Editors of Pediatric Oncology Nursing: Advanced Clinical Handbook want to recognize, thank, and acknowledge everyone who participated in the development of this text. We are profoundly aware of the personal time and commitment that was devoted to make this an outstanding resource and we are grateful. It is our hope that nurses in advanced clinical practice will find this publication useful, and that it will enrich knowledge and improve care for children and adolescents with cancer and hematologic disorders.

ON, Canada — Deborah Tomlinson
NY, USA — Nancy E. Kline

Contributors

Linda D'Andrea MSN, RN, CS, CPON®, CCRN
Memorial Sloan Kettering Cancer Center,
New York, NY, USA

Jane Belmore RSCN, RGN, Dip. Palliative Care
Schiehallion Day Care Unit, Yorkhill NHS Trust,
Glasgow, Scotland, UK

Joan O'Brien Shea MSN, RN
Children's Hospital Boston,
Boston, MA, USA

Karyn Brundige MSN, RN, CPNP, ARNP
Children's Hospital and Regional Medical Center,
Seattle, WA, USA

Rosalind Bryant MN, APRN-BC, PNP
Baylor College of Medicine,
Pediatric Nurse Practitioner,
Texas Children's Hospital,
Houston, TX, USA

Christine Chordas MSN, RN, CPNP
Dana Farber Cancer Institute,
Boston, MA, USA

Sandra Doyle MN, RN
Division of Haematology/Oncology,
Hospital for Sick Children,
Toronto, ON, Canada

Biljana Dzolganovski MMedSc, CCRP
Child Health Evaluative Services,
Hospital for Sick Children,
Toronto, ON, Canada

Angela M. Ethier PhD, RN, CNS, CPN, CT
Houston, TX, USA

Lindsay Gainer MSN, RN
Hematopoetic Stem Cell Transplant Unit,
Children's Hospital Boston,
Boston, MA, USA

Sara Gonzalez MS, RD, LD
Texas Children's Hospital,
Houston, TX, USA

Kristen Graham BSN, RN, CPON®
Dana Farber Cancer Institute,
Boston, MA, USA

Ali Hall RSCN, RGN, BA, M.Phil.,
Adv.Dip. Child Development,
Schiehallion Day Care Unit, Yorkhill NHS Trust,
Glasgow, Scotland, UK

Joan O'Hanlon-Curry MS, RN, CPNP, CPON®
Pediatric Hematology Oncology,
The Children's Hospital at Montefiore,
Bronx, NY, USA

Eleanor Hendershot RN, BScN, MN
Division of Hematology/Oncology,
Hospital for Sick Children,
Toronto, ON, Canada

Jane Khorrami SRN
Beatson West of Scotland Cancer Centre,
Gartnavel General Hospital,
Glasgow, Scotland

Nancy E. Kline PhD, RN, CPNP, FAAN
Memorial Sloan Kettering Cancer Center,
New York, NY, USA

Elena Ladas MS, RD
Columbia University,
New York, NY, USA

Irene Loch RN, Dip Cancer Nursing
Beatson West of Scotland Cancer Centre,
Gartnavel General Hospital,
Glasgow, Scotland

Anne-Marie Maloney RN, BSc, MSc
Division of Haematology/Oncology,
Hospital for Sick Children,
Toronto, ON, Canada

Martina Nathan RSCN, RGN, BSc, PGCE (M level),
ENB 240, ENB 998, Cardiff University,
Eastgate House, Cardiff,
Wales, UK

Colleen Nixon MSN, RN, CPON®
Children's Hospital Boston,
Boston, MA, USA

Robbie Norville MSN, RN, CPON®
Texas Children's Cancer Center,
Houston, TX, USA

Margaret Parr RGN, RSCN, ENB240
Children's Services,
Queen's Medical Centre,
Derby Road, Nottingham, UK

Janice Post-White PhD, RN, FAAN
University of Minnesota School of Nursing,
Minneapolis, MN, USA

Fiona Reid RSCN, RN
Morven House Raigmore Hospital,
Inverness, UK

Cheryl Rodgers MSN, RN, CPNP, CPON®
Texas Children's Cancer Center,
Houston, TX, USA

Carol Rossetto MSN, RN, CPNP, CPON®
Memorial Sloan-Kettering Cancer Center,
New York, NY, USA

Cara Simon PhD, RN, CPNP
Texas Children's Cancer Center,
Houston, TX, USA

Deborah Tomlinson MN, RN,
Dip Cancer Nursing,
Child Health Evaluative Services,
Hospital for Sick Children,
Toronto, ON, Canada

Julie Watson RN, MSN, CPNP
Complex Care Service, Paediatric Medicine,
The Hospital for Sick Children,
Toronto, ON, Canada

Sue Zupanec RN, MN
Division of Hematology/Oncology,
Hospital for Sick Children,
Toronto, ON, Canada

Contents

PART I

1 Leukemia
Sue Zupanec • Deborah Tomlinson

1.1 Introduction 2
1.2 Acute Lymphoblastic Leukemia 3
1.2.1 Epidemiology 3
1.2.2 Etiology 4
1.2.3 Molecular Genetics 6
1.2.4 Symptoms and Clinical Signs 7
1.2.5 Diagnostics 8
1.2.6 Staging and Classification 9
1.2.7 Treatment 12
1.2.8 Prognosis 16
1.2.9 Follow-Up 16
1.2.10 Future Perspectives 17
1.2.11 Relapsed ALL 17
1.3 Acute Myeloid Leukemia 19
1.3.1 Epidemiology 19
1.3.2 Etiology 19
1.3.3 Molecular Genetics 20
1.3.4 Symptoms and Clinical Signs 20
1.3.5 Diagnostics 21
1.3.6 Staging and Classification 21
1.3.7 Treatment 22
1.3.8 Prognosis 24
1.3.9 Follow-Up 24
1.3.10 Future Perspectives 24
1.4 Chronic Myeloid Leukemia 25
1.4.1 Epidemiology and Etiology 25
1.4.2 Molecular Genetics 25
1.4.3 Symptoms and Clinical Signs 25
1.4.4 Diagnostics 26
1.4.5 Treatment 26
1.4.6 Prognosis 26
1.4.7 Future Perspectives 26
1.5 Juvenile Myelomonocytic Leukemia 26
1.6 Langerhans Cell Histiocytosis 27
1.6.1 Epidemiology and Etiology 27
1.6.2 Diagnostics 28
1.6.3 Symptoms and Clinical Signs 28
1.6.4 Treatment 29
1.6.5 Prognosis 29
References 29

2 Lymphoma
Sue Zupanec

2.1 Lymphoma 33
2.2 Hodgkin Lymphoma 33
2.2.1 Epidemiology 34
2.2.2 Etiology 34
2.2.3 Molecular Genetics 34
2.2.4 Symptoms and Clinical Signs 34
2.2.5 Diagnostics 36
2.2.6 Staging and Classification 38
2.2.7 Treatment 39
2.2.8 Prognosis 42
2.2.9 Follow-Up 43
2.2.10 Relapsed/Refractory HL 43
2.2.11 Future Perspectives 44
2.3 Non-Hodgkin Lymphomas 44
2.3.1 Epidemiology 44
2.3.2 Etiology 45
2.3.3 Molecular Genetics 45
2.3.4 Symptoms and Clinical Signs 46
2.3.5 Diagnostics 48
2.3.6 Staging and Classification 50
2.3.7 Treatment 50
2.3.8 Prognosis 54
2.3.9 Follow-Up 54
2.3.10 Treatment of Relapsed/Refractory NHL . . 55
2.3.11 Future Perspectives 55
References 56

3 Solid Tumor
Eleanor Hendershot

3.1 Ewing's Sarcoma Family of Tumors 60
3.1.1 Epidemiology 60
3.1.2 Etiology 60
3.1.3 Molecular Genetics 60
3.1.4 Symptoms and Clinical Signs 61
3.1.5 Diagnosis 61
3.1.6 Staging and Classification 63
3.1.7 Treatment 63
3.1.8 Prognosis 64

3.1.9 Follow-Up 65
3.1.10 Future Perspectives 65
3.2 Osteosarcoma 65
3.2.1 Epidemiology 66
3.2.2 Etiology 66
3.2.3 Molecular Genetics 66
3.2.4 Signs and Symptoms 67
3.2.5 Diagnostics 67
3.2.6 Staging and Classification 68
3.2.7 Treatment 68
3.2.8 Prognosis 71
3.2.9 Follow-Up 71
3.2.10 Future Perspectives 71
3.3 Liver Tumors 72
3.3.1 Epidemiology 72
3.3.2 Etiology 72
3.3.3 Molecular Genetics 72
3.3.4 Symptoms and Clinical Signs 72
3.3.5 Diagnostics 73
3.3.6 Staging and Classification 74
3.3.7 Treatment 75
3.3.8 Prognosis 76
3.3.9 Follow-Up 76
3.3.10 Future Perspectives 77
3.4 Neuroblastoma 77
3.4.1 Epidemiology 77
3.4.2 Etiology 77
3.4.3 Molecular Genetics 77
3.4.4 Symptoms and Clinical Signs 79
3.4.5 Diagnostics 80
3.4.6 Staging and Classification 81
3.4.7 Treatment 82
3.4.8 Prognosis 85
3.4.9 Follow-Up 85
3.4.10 Future Perspectives 86
3.5 Renal Tumors 86
3.5.1 Epidemiology 86
3.5.2 Etiology 87
3.5.3 Molecular Genetics 87
3.5.4 Symptoms and Clinical Signs 87
3.5.5 Diagnostics 88
3.5.6 Staging and Classification 89
3.5.7 Treatment 89
3.5.8 Prognosis 92
3.5.9 Follow-Up 93
3.5.10 Future Perspectives 93
3.6 Retinoblastoma 93
3.6.1 Epidemiology 93
3.6.2 Etiology 94
3.6.3 Molecular Genetics 94
3.6.4 Signs and Symptoms 94
3.6.5 Diagnostics 95
3.6.6 Staging and Classification 96
3.6.7 Treatment 96
3.6.8 Prognosis 99
3.6.9 Follow-Up 100
3.6.10 Future Directions 100
3.7 Rhabdomyosarcoma 100
3.7.1 Epidemiology 100
3.7.2 Etiology 101
3.7.3 Molecular Genetics 101
3.7.4 Symptoms and Clinical Signs 101
3.7.5 Diagnostics 101
3.7.6 Staging and Classification 103
3.7.7 Treatment 103
3.7.8 Prognosis 106
3.7.9 Follow-Up 106
3.7.10 Future Perspectives 106
3.8 Non-Rhabdomyosarcomatous Soft-Tissue Sarcomas 107
3.8.1 Alveolar Soft-Part Sarcoma 108
3.8.2 Desmoid Tumor (Aggressive Fibromatosis) 108
3.8.3 Desmoplastic Small Round Cell Tumor . . 108
3.8.4 Infantile Fibrosarcoma 109
3.8.5 Infantile Hemangiopericytoma 109
3.8.6 Infantile Myofibromatosis 109
3.8.7 Leiomyosarcoma 109
3.8.8 Liposarcoma 109
3.8.9 Malignant Peripheral Nerve Sheath Tumor 110
3.8.10 Synovial Sarcoma 110
3.9 Germ Cell Tumors 110
3.9.1 Epidemiology 111
3.9.2 Etiology 111
3.9.3 Molecular Genetics 112
3.9.4 Symptoms and Clinical Signs 112
3.9.5 Diagnostics 112
3.9.6 Staging and Classification 113
3.9.7 Treatment 113
3.9.8 Prognosis 115
3.9.9 Follow-Up 115
3.9.10 Future Perspectives 116
3.10 Rare Tumors 116
3.10.1 Adrenocortical Carcinoma 116
3.10.2 Melanoma 117
3.10.3 Nasopharyngeal Carcinoma 118
3.10.4 Pleuropulmonary Blastoma 118
3.10.5 Thyroid Carcinoma 119
References 119

4 Central Nervous System Tumors

Nancy E. Kline • Joan O'Hanlon-Curry

4.1 Causes/Epidemiology 129
4.2 Distribution/Classification 129
4.3 Staging 130
4.4 Molecular Genetics of Brain Tumors 130

4.5 Diagnosis . . . 130
4.6 Specialist Referral . . . 130
4.7 Hydrocephalus . . . 130
4.8 Treatment . . . 131
4.8.1 Surgery . . . 131
4.8.2 Radiotherapy . . . 131
4.8.3 Chemotherapy . . . 132
4.9 Prognosis . . . 132
4.10 Specific Tumors . . . 132
4.10.1 PNETs/Medulloblastomas . . . 132
4.10.2 Astrocytomas/Glial Tumors . . . 133
4.10.3 Malignant Gliomas . . . 134
4.10.4 Other High-Grade Gliomas . . . 134
4.11 Follow-Up . . . 138
4.11.1 The Late Effects and Rehabilitation of Survivors . . . 138
4.11.2 Palliative Care . . . 139
4.11.3 Future Perspectives/New Innovations . . . 139
References . . . 140

PART II

5 Anemias
Rosalind Bryant

5.1 Anemia . . . 142
5.2 Iron-Deficiency Anemia . . . 146
5.2.1 Epidemiology . . . 146
5.2.2 Etiology . . . 146
5.2.3 Molecular Genetics . . . 146
5.2.4 Symptoms/Clinical Signs . . . 146
5.2.5 Diagnostic Testing . . . 147
5.2.6 Treatment . . . 148
5.2.7 Transfusion . . . 148
5.2.8 Erythropoietin (Epogen) . . . 148
5.2.9 Prognosis . . . 149
5.3 Sickle Cell Disease . . . 149
5.3.1 Epidemiology . . . 149
5.3.2 Etiology . . . 149
5.3.3 Molecular Genetics . . . 149
5.3.4 Symptoms/Clinical Signs . . . 149
5.3.5 Diagnostic Testing . . . 150
5.3.6 Complications of SCD . . . 151
5.3.7 Prognosis . . . 158
5.3.8 Future Perspectives . . . 158
5.4 Thalassemia . . . 158
5.4.1 Alpha (α)-Thalassemia . . . 158
5.4.2 Beta Thalassemia (Cooley Anemia) . . . 159
5.4.3 Diagnostic Testing . . . 160
5.4.4 Treatment . . . 160
5.4.5 Treatment of Hemosiderosis (Iron Overload) . . . 160
5.4.6 Chelation Therapy . . . 161
5.4.7 Clinical Advances (Hemosiderosis) . . . 161
5.4.8 Prognosis . . . 161
5.4.9 Follow-Up . . . 162
5.4.10 Future Perspectives . . . 162
5.5. Hemolytic Anemia . . . 162
5.5.1 Hereditary Spherocytosis . . . 162
5.5.2 Autoimmune Hemolytic Anemia . . . 164
5.5.3 Glucose-6-Phosphate Dehydrogenase Deficiency . . . 165
5.6 Bone Marrow Failure Syndromes . . . 167
5.6.1 Aplastic Anemia . . . 167
References . . . 170

6 Neutropenia
Karyn Brundige

6.1 Epidemiology . . . 173
6.2 Etiology . . . 174
6.3 Symptoms and Clinical Signs . . . 175
6.4 Diagnostic Testing . . . 175
6.5 Treatment . . . 176
6.6 Prognosis . . . 177
6.7 Follow-Up . . . 178
References . . . 178

7 Thrombocytopenia
Karyn Brundige

7.1 Epidemiology . . . 179
7.2 Etiology . . . 180
7.3 Symptoms and Clinical Signs . . . 180
7.4 Diagnostic Testing . . . 182
7.5 Treatment . . . 182
7.6 Prognosis . . . 184
7.7 Follow-Up . . . 184
7.8 Future Perspectives . . . 184
References . . . 184

8 Bleeding Disorders
Joan O'Brien-Shea

8.1 Hemophilia . . . 187
8.1.1 Epidemiology . . . 187
8.1.2 Etiology . . . 187
8.1.3 Genetics . . . 188
8.1.4 Symptoms and Clinical Signs . . . 188
8.1.5 Diagnostic Testing . . . 190
8.1.6 Treatment . . . 191
8.1.7 Prognosis . . . 194
8.1.8 Follow-Up . . . 194

8.1.9 Future Perspectives 194
8.2 von Willebrand Disease 194
8.2.1 Epidemiology 194
8.2.2 Etiology 195
8.2.3 Genetics 195
8.2.4 Symptoms and Clinical Signs 195
8.2.5 Diagnostic Testing 196
8.2.6 Treatment 199
8.2.7 Prognosis 200
8.2.8 Follow-Up 200
References 201

PART III

9 Chemotherapy
Christine Chordas • Kristen Graham

9.1 Introduction 204
9.2 Cancer Cell Characteristics 204
9.2.1 The Cell Cycle 204
9.2.2 Cell Cycle Control 205
9.3 Chemotherapy 206
9.3.1 Principles 206
9.3.2 Resistance 206
9.3.3 The Principles of Pharmacokinetics, Pharmacodynamics, and Pharmacogenomics 206
9.3.4 Chemotherapy Techniques 207
9.4 Clinical Trials 207
9.4.1 Phase I Clinical Trials 208
9.4.2 Phase II Clinical Trials 208
9.4.3 Phase III Clinical Trials 208
9.4.4 Phase IV Clinical Trials 208
9.5 Chemotherapy Agents 208
9.5.1 Antimetabolites 211
9.5.2 Alkylating Agents 216
9.5.3 Antitumor Antibiotics 217
9.5.4 Anthracycline Antibiotics 218
9.5.5 Plant Derivatives 218
9.5.6 Antiangiogenic Agents 219
9.5.7 Miscellaneous Agents 220
9.6 Chemotherapy Protectants 221
9.6.1 Allopurinol (Zyloprim) 221
9.6.2 Amifostine (Ethyol) 221
9.6.3 Dexrazoxane (Zinecard) 221
9.6.4 Leucovorin Calcium (LCV, Wellcovorin, Citovorum Factor, Folic Acid) 221
9.6.5 Mesna (Mesnex) 221
9.6.6 Palifermin 222
9.7 Administration of Chemotherapy Agents 222
9.7.1 Preparation 222
9.7.2 Administration and Practice Considerations 223
9.8 Professional Guidelines to Minimize the Risk of Medication Errors 224
9.8.1 Prescribing Errors 224
9.9 Safe Practice Considerations 224
9.9.1 Mixing Chemotherapeutic Agents 225
9.9.2 Transporting Cytotoxic Agents 225
9.9.3 Safe Handling After Chemotherapy 225
9.9.4 Disposal of Cytotoxic Materials 225
9.9.5 Spill Management 226
9.9.6 Procedures Following Accidental Exposure 226
9.9.7 Storage 226
9.9.8 Medical Management 226
9.10 Administration of Chemotherapy in the Home 226
9.11 Immediate Complications of Chemotherapy Administration 226
9.11.1 Extravasation 227
9.11.2 Acute Hypersensitivity Reactions (HSRs) to Chemotherapy 230
9.11.3 Risk Factors for Hypersensitivity, Flare Reactions, or Anaphylaxis 230
9.11.4 Recommended Steps to Prevent HSRs 230
9.11.5 Emergency Management of HSR/Anaphylaxis 230
9.12 Summary 231
References 231

10 Radiotherapy
Irene Loch • Jane Khorrami

10.1 Introduction 233
10.2 Radiation 233
10.3 Principles of Treatment 234
10.4 Treatment Planning 234
10.4.1 CT Simulation 234
10.4.2 Simulation 234
10.5 Treatment Methods 235
10.5.1 External Beam Radiotherapy (Teletherapy) 235
10.5.2 Fractionation 237
10.5.3 Total Body Irradiation (TBI) 237
10.5.4 Brachytherapy 237
10.5.5 Sealed Sources 237
10.5.6 Unsealed Sources 237
10.6 Side Effects of Radiotherapy 238
10.6.1 Acute Effects 238
10.7 Special Considerations 240
10.7.1 Preparation of Children and Young People 240
10.8 Future Perspectives 240
10.8.1 Image-Guided Radiotherapy 240

10.8.2 Intra-Operative Radiotherapy 240
10.8.3 Proton Radiotherapy (PRT) 240
References 241

11 Hematopoietic Stem Cell Transplantation
Robbie Norville • Deborah Tomlinson

11.1 Principles of Treatment 243
11.2 Stem Cell Collection (Harvest) 244
11.2.1 Bone Marrow Stem Cells 244
11.2.2 Peripheral Blood Stem Cells 246
11.2.3 Umbilical Cord Blood Stem Cells 246
11.3 Donor Stem Cell Typing/ Tissue Typing 247
11.4 Donor Stem Cell Sources 248
11.5 Stem Cell Processing and Infusion 249
11.5.1 ABO Mismatch 249
11.5.2 Graft vs. Leukemia 251
11.6 Description of Treatment 251
11.7 Potential Side Effects 253
11.7.1 Early Side Effects 253
11.7.2 Intermediate Side Effects 257
11.7.3 Late Side Effects 261
11.8 Special Considerations 263
11.9 Future Perspectives 264
References 265

12 Surgical Approaches to Childhood Cancer
Carol L. Rossetto

12.1 Principles of Treatment 269
12.2 Method of Delivery 270
12.2.1 Preoperative Evaluation 270
12.2.2 Postoperative Nursing Care 271
12.3 Potential Side Effects 271
12.3.1 Complications of Medical Therapy Requiring Surgical Evaluation 271
12.3.2 Complications Arising from Surgical Management of Solid Tumors 272
12.4 Special Considerations 273
12.4.1 Vascular Access Devices 273
12.5 Future Perspectives 274
12.5.1 New Surgical Techniques and Directions for Future Research 274
References 275

13 Cell and Gene Therapy
Robbie Norville

13.1 Introduction 277
13.2 Principles of Treatment 278
13.2.1 Genetic Deficit Repair 278
13.2.2 Viral-Mediated Gene Transfer 278
13.2.3 Drug-Resistant Genes 278
13.2.4 Angiogenetics Inhibitors 279
13.2.5 Gene Marking 279
13.2.6 Cell Therapy 279
13.3 Method of Delivery 279
13.3.1 Viral Vectors 280
13.3.2 Plasmid Vectors 280
13.4 Potential Side Effects 280
13.5 Special Considerations 281
13.6 Future Perspectives 281
References 281

14 Biological and Targeted Therapies
Lindsay Gainer

14.1 Introduction 283
14.2 Principles of Treatment 284
14.3 Description of Treatment 285
14.3.1 Cytokines 285
14.3.2 Interferons 285
14.3.3 Interleukins 286
14.3.4 Colony-stimulating Factors 286
14.3.5 Fusion Proteins 286
14.3.6 Monoclonal Antibodies 287
14.4 Cancer Vaccines 288
14.5 Other Immunomodulating Agents 288
14.5.1 Nonspecific Immunomodulating Agents 288
14.5.2 Retinoids 289
14.5.3 Thalidomide 289
14.6 Adoptive Immunotherapy 289
14.7 Molecular Targeted Therapy 289
14.8 Method of Delivery 290
14.9 Potential Side Effects 291
14.10 Future Perspectives 292
References 293

15 Complementary and Alternative Medicine
Janice Post-White • Elena Ladas

15.1 Introduction 295
15.2 CAM Modalities 296

15.2.1 Acupuncture . . . 296
15.2.2 Biological Therapies . . . 297
15.2.3 Mind–Body Therapies . . . 299
15.2.4 Movement Therapies . . . 300
15.2.5 Aromatherapy . . . 301
15.2.6 Massage . . . 302
15.2.7 Energy Therapies . . . 303
15.3 Future Perspectives . . . 303
References . . . 304

16 Clinical Trials
Biljana Dzolganovski

16.1 The Role of Clinical Trials . . . 307
16.1.1 The Need for Research . . . 307
16.1.2 Phases of Clinical Trials . . . 308
16.1.3 Study Types . . . 308
16.1.4 Research Ethics: Principles, Policies, and Guidelines . . . 308
16.1.5 Legal and Ethical Issues Regarding Participation of Children in Research . . . 310
16.1.6 Research in Pediatrics . . . 312
16.2 Research Networks . . . 312
16.2.1 Cooperative Group Research . . . 312
16.2.2 Importance of Participation in Clinical Trials . . . 314
16.3 Progress Made Through Clinical Trials . . . 315
16.3.1 Treatments and Therapy Delivery . . . 315
16.3.2 Quality of Life Measures and Supportive Care . . . 319
16.3.3 Complementary and Alternative Medicine . . . 320
16.3.4 Late Effects . . . 321
16.3.5 Palliative Care . . . 321
16.4 Perception of Clinical Trials . . . 322
16.5 Future of Clinical Trials . . . 324
16.6 The Role of the Clinical Research Associate . . . 324
16.6.1 Introduction . . . 324
16.6.2 Clinical Research Associate . . . 325
16.6.3 The Role of the CRA . . . 326
16.6.4 The Role of the Clinical Research Nurse . . . 328
References . . . 329

PART IV

17 Metabolic System
Deborah Tomlinson

17.1 Cancer Cachexia . . . 337
17.1.1 Incidence . . . 337
17.1.2 Etiology . . . 338
17.1.3 Treatment . . . 338
17.1.4 Prognosis . . . 339
17.2 Obesity . . . 339
17.2.1 Obesity in Survivors of Leukemia . . . 339
17.3 Inferior Outcomes and Obesity . . . 340
17.3.1 Incidence . . . 340
17.3.2 Etiology . . . 341
17.4 Tumor Lysis Syndrome . . . 341
17.4.1 Incidence . . . 341
17.4.2 Etiology . . . 341
17.4.3 Treatment . . . 343
17.4.4 Prognosis . . . 347
17.5 Hypercalcemia . . . 347
17.5.1 Incidence . . . 347
17.5.2 Etiology . . . 347
17.5.3 Treatment . . . 347
17.5.4 Prognosis . . . 348
17.6 Impaired Glucose Tolerance . . . 348
17.6.1 Incidence . . . 348
17.6.2 Etiology . . . 348
17.6.3 Treatment . . . 349
17.6.4 Prognosis . . . 349
References . . . 349

18 Gastrointestinal Tract
Anne Marie Maloney

18.1 Mucositis . . . 354
18.1.1 Incidence . . . 354
18.1.2 Etiology . . . 354
18.1.3 Prevention . . . 357
18.1.4 Treatment . . . 357
18.1.5 Prognosis . . . 358
18.2 Dental Caries . . . 358
18.2.1 Incidence . . . 358
18.2.2 Etiology . . . 358
18.2.3 Prevention and Treatment . . . 359
18.2.4 Prognosis . . . 359
18.3 Nausea and Vomiting . . . 359
18.3.1 Incidence . . . 359
18.3.2 Etiology . . . 359
18.3.3 Prevention . . . 360
18.3.4 Treatment . . . 360
18.3.5 Delayed Nausea and Vomiting . . . 361
18.3.6 Anticipatory Nausea and Vomiting . . . 361
18.3.7 Radiation-Induced Nausea and Vomiting . . . 362
18.3.8 Other Causes of Nausea and Vomiting . . . 363
18.3.9 Nonpharmacological Management . . . 363
18.3.10 Prognosis . . . 364
18.4 Constipation . . . 364
18.4.1 Incidence . . . 364
18.4.2 Etiology . . . 364
18.4.3 Prevention . . . 365
18.4.4 Treatment . . . 365
18.4.5 Prognosis . . . 366

18.5 Diarrhea . . . 366
18.5.1 Incidence . . . 366
18.5.2 Etiology . . . 366
18.5.3 Prevention . . . 368
18.5.4 Treatment . . . 368
18.5.5 Prognosis . . . 369
18.6 Typhylitis . . . 369
18.6.1 Incidence . . . 369
18.6.2 Etiology . . . 370
18.6.3 Prevention . . . 370
18.6.4 Treatment . . . 370
18.6.5 Prognosis . . . 371
18.7 Perirectal Cellulitis . . . 371
18.7.1 Incidence . . . 371
18.7.2 Etiology . . . 371
18.7.3 Prevention . . . 371
18.7.4 Treatment . . . 371
18.7.5 Prognosis . . . 372
18.8 Acute Gastrointestinal Graft Vs. Host Disease . . . 372
18.8.1 Incidence . . . 372
18.8.2 Prevention . . . 372
18.8.3 Treatment . . . 373
18.8.4 Prognosis . . . 374
18.9 Chemical Hepatitis . . . 374
18.9.1 Incidence . . . 374
18.9.2 Etiology . . . 374
18.9.3 Prevention . . . 374
18.9.4 Treatment . . . 374
18.9.5 Prognosis . . . 375
18.10 Pancreatitis . . . 375
18.10.1 Incidence . . . 375
18.10.2 Etiology . . . 375
18.10.3 Prevention . . . 375
18.10.4 Treatment . . . 375
18.10.5 Prognosis . . . 375
References . . . 376

19 Bone Marrow Function
Sandra Doyle

19.1 Introduction . . . 380
19.2 Anemia . . . 380
19.2.1 Incidence and Etiology . . . 380
19.2.2 Treatment . . . 380
19.3 Neutropenia . . . 381
19.3.1 Incidence and Etiology . . . 381
19.3.2 Treatment . . . 382
19.4 Thrombocytopenia . . . 389
19.4.1 Incidence and Etiology . . . 389
19.4.2 Treatment . . . 389
19.5 Transfusion Issues . . . 390
19.5.1 Granulocyte Transfusions . . . 390
19.5.2 Transfusion-Associated Graft vs. Host Disease . . . 391
19.5.3 Cytomegalovirus and Transfusions . . . 392
19.5.4 Platelet Refractoriness . . . 392
19.6 Disseminated Intravascular Coagulation . . . 393
19.6.1 Etiology and Manifestation . . . 393
19.6.2 Treatment . . . 394
19.7 Septic Shock . . . 395
19.7.1 Etiology . . . 395
19.7.2 Treatment . . . 395
19.7.3 Prognosis . . . 396
19.8 Immune Suppression . . . 396
19.8.1 Polymorphonuclear Leukocytes . . . 396
19.8.2 Lymphocytes . . . 397
19.8.3 Spleen and Reticuloendothelial System . 398
19.8.4 Other Factors Contributing to Immunocompromised States . . . 398
References . . . 398

20 Respiratory System
Margaret Parr

20.1 Pneumocystis Pneumonia . . . 401
20.1.1 Incidence . . . 401
20.1.2 Etiology . . . 402
20.1.3 Treatment . . . 402
20.1.4 Prognosis . . . 404
20.2 Pneumonitis . . . 404
20.2.1 Incidence . . . 404
20.2.2 Etiology . . . 404
20.2.3 Prevention . . . 405
20.2.4 Treatment . . . 405
20.2.5 Prognosis . . . 405
20.3 Fibrosis . . . 406
20.3.1 Incidence . . . 406
20.3.2 Etiology . . . 406
20.3.3 Prevention . . . 406
20.3.4 Treatment . . . 406
20.3.5 Prognosis . . . 406
20.4 Compromised Airway . . . 407
20.4.1 Incidence . . . 407
20.4.2 Etiology . . . 407
20.4.3 Prevention . . . 407
20.4.4 Treatment . . . 408
20.4.5 Prognosis . . . 408
References . . . 408

21 Renal System
Fiona Reid

21.1 Nephrectomy . . . 412
21.1.1 Incidence . . . 412
21.1.2 Etiology . . . 412
21.1.3 Treatment . . . 412
21.1.4 Prognosis . . . 416

21.2 Cytotoxic Drug Excretion . . . 417
21.2.1 Pharmacokinetics/Dynamics . . . 417
21.2.2 Metabolism . . . 418
21.2.3 Excretion . . . 418
21.2.4 Drug Interactions . . . 420
21.2.5 Dose Modification . . . 420
21.2.6 Safe Handling of Cytotoxic Excreta . . . 424
21.3 Nephrotoxicity . . . 425
21.3.1 Incidence . . . 425
21.3.2 Etiology . . . 426
21.3.3 Prevention . . . 427
21.3.4 Treatment . . . 430
21.3.5 Prognosis . . . 432
21.4 Hemorrhagic Cystitis . . . 432
21.4.1 Incidence . . . 432
21.4.2 Etiology . . . 433
21.4.3 Prevention . . . 434
21.4.4 Treatment . . . 435
21.4.5 Prognosis . . . 437
References . . . 437

22 Cardiovascular System
Alison Hall

22.1 Cardiac Toxicity/Cardiomyopathy . . . 441
22.1.1 Incidence . . . 441
22.1.2 Etiology . . . 443
22.1.3 Treatment . . . 445
22.1.4 Prevention . . . 445
22.1.5 Prognosis . . . 447
22.2 Veno-Occlusive Disease . . . 447
22.2.1 Hepatic Veno-Occlusive Disease . . . 447
22.2.2 Pulmonary Veno-Occlusive Disease . . . 449
References . . . 450

23 Central Nervous System
Jane Belmore • Deborah Tomlinson

23.1 Spinal Cord Compression . . . 453
23.1.1 Incidence . . . 453
23.1.2 Etiology . . . 453
23.1.3 Treatment . . . 454
23.1.4 Prognosis . . . 454
23.2 Fatigue . . . 454
23.2.1 Incidence . . . 455
23.2.2 Etiology . . . 455
23.2.3 Treatment . . . 456
23.2.4 Prognosis . . . 457
23.3 Cognitive Deficits . . . 458
23.3.1 Incidence . . . 458
23.3.2 Etiology . . . 458
23.3.3 Prevention and Treatment . . . 458
23.3.4 Prognosis . . . 459
23.4 Diabetes Insipidus . . . 459
23.4.1 Incidence . . . 459
23.4.2 Etiology . . . 460
23.4.3 Treatment . . . 460
23.4.4 Prognosis . . . 460
References . . . 460

24 Musculoskeletal System
Deborah Tomlinson • Sue Zupanec

24.1 Bone Tumors . . . 463
24.1.1 Limb Salvage Procedures . . . 463
24.1.2 Amputation . . . 464
24.1.3 Comparison of Limb Salvage and Amputation . . . 469
24.2 Altered Bone Mineral Densityand Increased Fracture Risk . . . 470
24.2.1 Incidence . . . 470
24.2.2 Etiology . . . 471
24.2.3 Prevention and Treatment . . . 471
24.2.4 Prognosis . . . 472
24.3 Osteonecrosis . . . 472
24.3.1 Incidence . . . 473
24.3.2 Etiology . . . 474
24.3.3 Treatment . . . 474
24.3.4 Prognosis . . . 475
References . . . 475

25 Skin: Cutaneous Toxicities
Martina Nathan • Deborah Tomlinson

25.1 Alopecia . . . 477
25.1.1 Etiology . . . 477
25.1.3 Treatment . . . 478
25.1.4 Prognosis . . . 479
25.2 Altered Skin Integrity Associated with Radiation Therapy . . . 479
25.2.1 Incidence . . . 479
25.2.2 Etiology . . . 479
25.2.3 Prevention . . . 479
25.2.4 Treatment . . . 480
25.2.5 Prognosis . . . 481
25.3 Radiation Sensitivity and Recall . . . 481
25.3.1 Incidence . . . 481
25.3.2 Etiology . . . 481
25.3.3 Clinical Features . . . 481
25.3.4 Treatment . . . 481
25.3.5 Prognosis . . . 482
25.4 Ultraviolet Recall Reaction/Photosensitivity . . . 482

25.5 Cutaneous Reactions Associated with High-Dose Cytosine Arabinoside 482
25.5.1 Incidence 482
25.5.2 Etiology 482
25.5.3 Prevention and Treatment 482
25.6 Nail Dystrophies 483
25.7 Graft Vs. Host Disease 483
25.7.1 Incidence and Etiology 483
25.7.2 Prevention 485
25.7.3 Treatment 486
25.7.4 Prognosis 486
References 486

26 Endocrine System
Julie Watson

26.1 Introduction 489
26.2 Hypothalamic–Pituitary Dysfunction 489
26.2.1 Incidence and Etiology 489
26.3 Growth Hormone Deficiency 491
26.3.1 Treatment 492
26.3.2 Prognosis 492
26.4 Hypothalamic–Pituitary–Gonadal Axis 493
26.4.1 Gonadotrophin Deficiency 493
26.4.2 Early or Precocious Puberty 493
26.5 Thyroid Disorders 494
26.5.1 Treatment 494
26.6 Hypothalamic–Pituitary–Adrenal Axis 495
26.6.1 Treatment 495
26.7 Other Pituitary Hormones 495
26.7.1 Fertility 496
26.7.2 Treatment 496
26.7.3 Prognosis 497
References 499

27 Ototoxicity
Colleen Nixon

27.1 Introduction 501
27.2 Prevention and Treatment 505
27.3 Future Perspectives 507
27.4 Prognosis 508
References 508

28 Ocular Complications
Martina Nathan • Deborah Tomlinson

28.1 Ocular Toxicity Associated with High-Dose Cytarabine Arabinoside 511
28.1.1 Incidence and Etiology 511
28.1.2 Prevention 512
28.1.3 Treatment 512
28.1.4 Prognosis 512
28.2 Cataracts 513
28.2.1 Incidence 513
28.2.2 Etiology 513
28.2.3 Prevention 513
28.2.4 Treatment 513
28.2.5 Prognosis 513
References 513

PART V

29 Nutrition and Hydration in Children with Cancer
Cheryl Rodgers • Sara Gonzalez

29.1 Introduction 515
29.2 Nutritional Assessment 516
29.2.1 Hydration Needs 516
29.2.2 Nutrition Needs 516
29.2.3 Nutritional History 517
29.2.4 Physical Examination 518
29.2.5 Anthropometric Measurements 518
29.2.6 Laboratory Evaluation 519
29.3 Principles of Treatment for Dehydration and Malnutrition 519
29.3.1 Rehydration 519
29.3.2 Oral Nutrition Replacement 520
29.3.3 Enteral Nutrition Replacement 520
29.3.4 Total Parenteral Nutrition/Hyperalimentation 521
29.4 Special Considerations 524
29.4.1 Common Hydration Complications 524
29.4.2 Common Complications of Oral/Enteral Nutritional Supplementation 524
29.4.3 Common Complications of Total Parenteral Nutrition/Hyperalimintation . 525
29.4.4 Common Complications of Enteral and Parenteral Nutritional Supplementation . 527
29.4.5 Specific Nutritional Concerns of Long-Term Survivors 527
29.4.6 Specific Nutritional Concerns During Palliative Care 527
References 528

30 Pain in Children with Cancer
Cara Simon

30.1 Introduction 529
30.2 Causes of Pain in Childhood Cancer 529

30.3 Assessment . . . 530
30.4 Cultural Issues . . . 536
30.5 Principles of Treatment . . . 536
30.6 Treatment . . . 537
30.6.1 By the Ladder . . . 537
30.6.2 By the Route . . . 538
30.6.3 By the Clock . . . 538
30.6.4 Opioids . . . 538
30.6.5 Equianalgesia . . . 538
30.6.6 Procedure-Related Pain . . . 540
30.6.7 Patient-Controlled Analgesia (PCA) . . . 540
30.6.8 Adjuvant Medications . . . 542
30.6.9 Nonpharmacologic Treatment . . . 542
References . . . 544

31 Blood Transfusion Therapy
Colleen Nixon

31.1 Introduction . . . 546
31.2 Blood Screening Guidelines . . . 546
31.3 Blood Product Processing . . . 546
31.3.1 Irradiation . . . 547
31.3.2 Washed Red Blood Cells . . . 547
31.4 Transfusion Complications . . . 547
31.4.1 Hemolytic Reactions . . . 547
31.4.2 Febrile Nonhemolytic Transfusion Reactions . . . 548
31.4.3 Allergic Reactions . . . 548
31.4.4 Transfusion Associated Graft vs. Host Disease . . . 549
31.4.5 Circulatory Overload . . . 549
31.4.6 Bacterial Contamination . . . 549
31.4.7 Transfusion-Acquired Infections . . . 550
31.4.8 Iron Overload from Chronic Transfusion . . . 551
31.5 Red Blood Cell Transfusion . . . 551
31.5.1 Packed Red Blood Cells . . . 551
31.5.2 Whole Blood . . . 552
31.5.3 Exchange Transfusion . . . 552
31.6 Platelet Transfusion . . . 552
31.6.1 Indications . . . 552
31.6.2 Procurement . . . 553
31.6.3 Dosing/Transfusion Guidelines . . . 553
31.6.4 Crossmatching . . . 553
31.6.5 Nursing Implications . . . 553
31.7 Granulocyte Transfusion . . . 553
31.7.1 Indications . . . 554
31.7.2 Dosing/Transfusion Guidelines . . . 554
31.7.3 Crosssmatching . . . 554
31.7.4 Nursing Implications . . . 554
31.8 Albumin (5 or 25% solution) and Plasma Protein Fraction (5% solution) . . . 554
31.8.1 Indications . . . 554
31.8.2 Dosing/Transfusion Guidelines . . . 554
31.8.3 Crossmatching . . . 555
31.8.4 Nursing Implications . . . 555
31.9 Fresh Frozen Plasma . . . 555
31.9.1 Indications . . . 555
31.9.2 Dosing/Transfusion Guidelines . . . 555
31.9.3 Crossmatching . . . 555
31.9.4 Nursing Implications . . . 555
31.10 Cryoprecipitate . . . 555
31.10.1 Indications . . . 555
31.10.2 Dosing Guidelines . . . 556
31.10.3 Crossmatching . . . 556
31.10.4 Nursing Implications . . . 556
31.11 Intravenous Immunoglobulin . . . 556
31.11.1 Indications . . . 556
31.11.2 Dosing/Transfusion Guidelines . . . 556
31.11.3 Crossmatching . . . 556
31.11.4 Nursing Implications . . . 556
31.12 Erythropoietin . . . 556
31.13 Indications . . . 557
31.14 Dosing Guidelines . . . 557
31.15 Nursing Implications . . . 557
31.16 Palliative Care Issues for Transfusion Therapy 557
31.16.1 Anemia and Thrombocytopenia . . . 557
References . . . 557

32 Cytokines
Linda D'Andrea

32.1 Principles of Treatment . . . 559
32.2 Future Perspectives . . . 563
References . . . 564

33 Care of the Dying Child and the Family
Angela M. Ethier

33.1 Children's Understanding of Death . . . 565
33.1.1 Infants (0–12 Months) and Toddlers (12–24 Months) . . . 565
33.1.2 Preschool Children (3–5 Years) . . . 566
33.1.3 School-Age Children (6–11 Years) . . . 567
33.1.4 Adolescents (12–19 Years) . . . 567
33.2 Explaining Death to Children . . . 567
33.3 Pediatric Palliative Care . . . 568
33.3.1 Principles . . . 568
33.3.2 Locations of Care . . . 568
33.4 Grief . . . 569
33.4.1 Principles . . . 569
33.4.2 Assessment of Child and Family . . . 569
33.4.3 Interventions . . . 571
33.5 Cultural and Spiritual Care . . . 571

33.5.1 Principles 571
33.5.2 Assessment of Child and Family 571
33.5.3 Interventions 571
33.6 Nearing Death 573
33.6.1 Physical Symptoms Near the End of Life 573
33.6.2 Death-Related Sensory Experiences 574
33.7 Care Following the Child's Death 575
33.7.1 Interventions Immediately Following the Child's Death 575
33.7.2 Bereavement Interventions 575
33.8 Resources 575
33.8.1 Resources for Children 575
33.8.2 Resources for Adults 576
References 576

Subject Index 579

PART I

Leukemia

Sue Zupanec • Deborah Tomlinson

Contents

1.1 Introduction . . . 2
1.2 Acute Lymphoblastic Leukemia . . . 3
1.2.1 Epidemiology . . . 3
1.2.2 Etiology . . . 4
1.2.2.1 Genetic Factors . . . 4
1.2.2.2 Environmental Factors . . . 4
1.2.3 Molecular Genetics . . . 6
1.2.4 Symptoms and Clinical Signs . . . 7
1.2.5 Diagnostics . . . 8
1.2.6 Staging and Classification . . . 9
1.2.6.1 Risk Classification . . . 9
1.2.6.2 Cell Morphology . . . 10
1.2.6.3 Cytochemistry . . . 10
1.2.6.4 Immunophenotyping . . . 10
1.2.6.5 Cytogenetics . . . 11
1.2.7 Treatment . . . 12
1.2.7.1 Induction . . . 13
1.2.7.2 Consolidation . . . 14
1.2.7.3 Reintensification . . . 14
1.2.7.4 CNS-Directed Therapy . . . 15
1.2.7.5 Maintenance/Continuing Treatment . . . 15
1.2.7.6 Allogeneic Stem Cell Transplant . . . 16
1.2.8 Prognosis . . . 16
1.2.9 Follow-Up . . . 16
1.2.10 Future Perspectives . . . 17
1.2.11 Relapsed ALL . . . 17
1.3 Acute Myeloid Leukemia . . . 19
1.3.1 Epidemiology . . . 19
1.3.2 Etiology . . . 19
1.3.2.1 Genetic Factors . . . 19
1.3.2.2 Environmental Factors . . . 20
1.3.3 Molecular Genetics . . . 20
1.3.4 Symptoms and Clinical Signs . . . 20
1.3.5 Diagnostics . . . 21
1.3.6 Staging and Classification . . . 21
1.3.7 Treatment . . . 22
1.3.8 Prognosis . . . 24
1.3.9 Follow-Up . . . 24
1.3.10 Future Perspectives . . . 24
1.4 Chronic Myeloid Leukemia . . . 25
1.4.1 Epidemiology and Etiology . . . 25
1.4.2 Molecular Genetics . . . 25
1.4.3 Symptoms and Clinical Signs . . . 25
1.4.4 Diagnostics . . . 26
1.4.5 Treatment . . . 26
1.4.6 Prognosis . . . 26
1.4.7 Future Perspectives . . . 26
1.5 Juvenile Myelomonocytic Leukemia . . . 26
1.6 Langerhans Cell Histiocytosis . . . 27
1.6.1 Epidemiology and Etiology . . . 27
1.6.2 Diagnostics . . . 28
1.6.3 Symptoms and Clinical Signs . . . 28
1.6.4 Treatment . . . 29
1.6.5 Prognosis . . . 29
References . . . 29

1.1 Introduction

Leukemia is the most common malignancy that affects children, accounting for approximately one-third of cancer diagnoses. It may be defined as a neoplastic disease that affects the blood-forming tissues of the bone marrow, lymph nodes, and spleen.

Normal hematopoiesis occurs in these blood-forming tissues; the development of blood cells is shown in Fig. 1.1. A range of extracellular protein factors regulate the growth and differentiation of pathways of developing cells. This ensures that the mature blood cell types are produced in appropriate proportions. Leukemia is a clonal disease that results from genetic mutations and transformation of a single early progenitor myeloid or lymphoid cell during hematopoiesis. Therefore, the type of leukemia that results is dependent on the cell lineage that is affected by the mutation. Table 1.1 shows the blood cells that can be affected from either lineage. In leukemia, there is an overproduction of immature white blood cells that cannot function effectively. These immature white blood cells are commonly called "blasts," such as the myeloblasts, lymphoblasts, and monoblasts. An

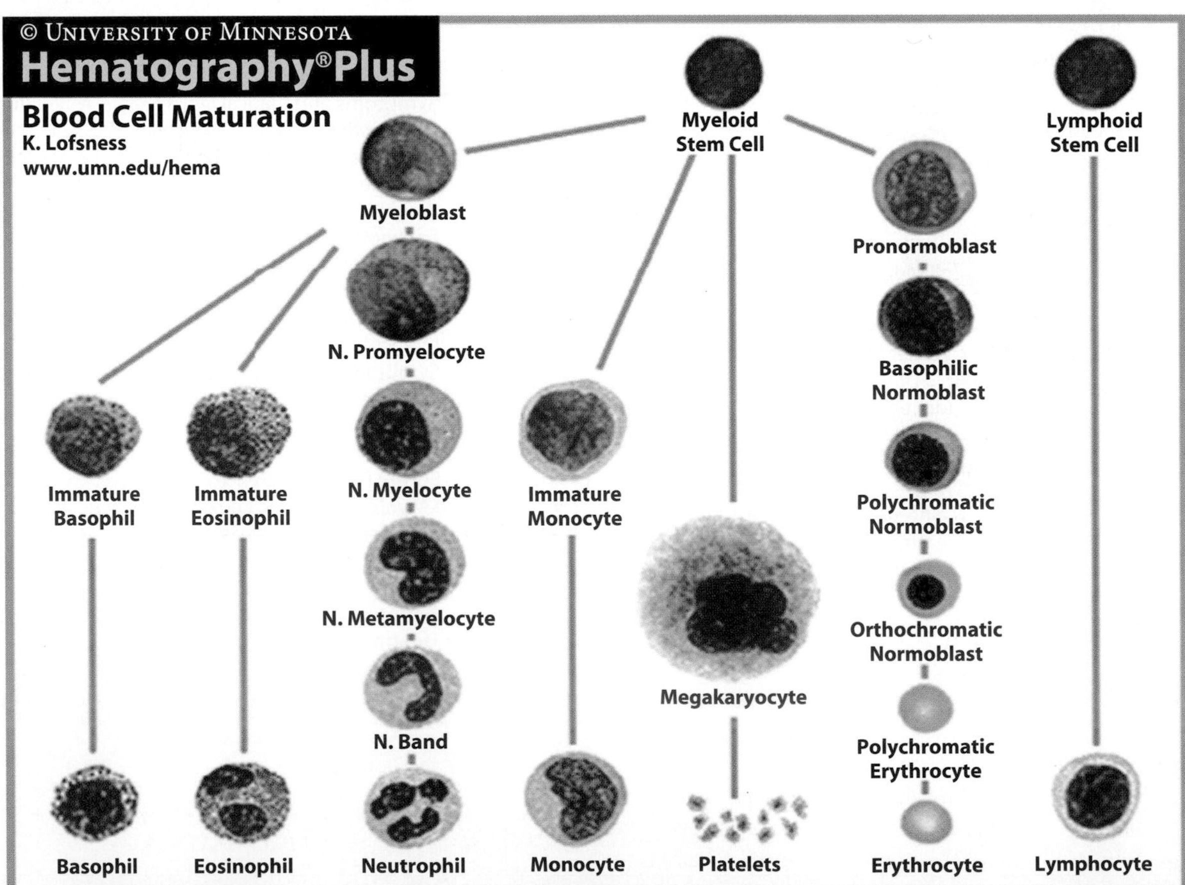

Figure 1.1

Hematopoiesis: The lymphoid stem cell differentiates into T-lymphocytes and B-lymphocytes. Natural Killer (NK) cells are also thought to be derived from the lymphocyte stem cells. Image credit: K. Lofsness, University of Minnesota

Table 1.1. Lineage and function of major types of blood cells

Blood cell	Lineage	Function	Half life
Red blood cells (erythrocytes)	Myeloid	Transport oxygen from lungs to tissue Transport some carbon dioxide from tissues to lungs	About 120 days
Platelets (thrombocytes)	Myeloid	Repair blood vessels and participate in clotting mechanism	7–10 days
White blood cells (leucocytes)		Crucial in immunity	
Monocytes	Myeloid	Can differentiate into macrophages, phagocytosis, antigen presentation, immune regulation	1–3 days in blood 3 months in tissues
Granulocytes			
Neutrophils	Myeloid	Phagocytosis, killing bacteria	6–12 h in blood
Eosinophils	Myeloid	Detoxify products from allergic response, phagocytosis	2–3 days in tissues
Basophils	Myeloid	Involved in allergic response, source of immune inhibitors (e.g., histamine)	Minutes to hours in blood, then in tissue for about 12 days
Lymphocytes	Lymphoid	Role In Immunity	Undetermined cells can move between blood and lymphoid tissues
T-lymphocytes		Attack invaders directly	
B-lymphocytes		Production of antibodies	
Others Null cells, natural killer cells, lymphokine-activated killer cells, and tumour-infiltrating lymphocytes			

abnormal population of immature white blood cells decreases the space available for the production of other healthy blood cells produced by the bone marrow. The blast cells can also enter the blood and may infiltrate the central nervous system (CNS), testicles in males, bones, and other tissues or organs.

The two broad classifications of leukemia are acute and chronic. The most common types of leukemia are:

- Acute lymphoblastic leukemia (ALL), which accounts for 75–80% of childhood leukemia
- Acute myeloid leukemia (AML), also known as acute nonlymphoblastic leukemia (ANLL), which accounts for 20–25% of childhood leukemia

The most common type of chronic leukemia is:

- Chronic myeloid (or myelocytic) leukemia (CML), which accounts for less than 5% of childhood leukemia

1.2 Acute Lymphoblastic Leukemia

1.2.1 Epidemiology

ALL affects slightly more males than females (1.2:1) and peaks between the ages of 2 and 5 years. In infants, higher number of females are observed to be affected.

Globally, the highest incidence of ALL appears to be in Europe and North America, with about 5 cases in 100,000 of 0–14-year-old children. The lowest incidence, of about 0.9 in 100,000, has been observed in Kuwait and Mumbai. There may be a lack of clarity regarding some incidence figures, owing to the lack of true population-based registration of cancer. A recent study has shown that the incidence of leukemia has increased in Europe in the last decades with an average 0.6% annual increase (Kaatsch and Mergenthaler 2008). Generally, higher incidence of ALL is observed in the affluent industrialized nations among white populations. The incidence tends to be lower among the black populations of the same nations.

1.2.2 Etiology

The factors involved in the cause of childhood cancers are still unclear. Many different etiologies have been suggested and investigated, but few are well established. It would be misleading to entirely associate the cause of any childhood malignancy to genetic or environmental factors, but the study of various factors can improve the understanding of events that may lead to leukemia in children.

1.2.2.1 Genetic Factors

Syndromes that have a component of hereditary or genetic predisposition to leukemia have been identified and are listed in Table 1.2. A study by Mellemkjaer et al. (2000) has shown that children of parents with autoimmune disease are slightly more susceptible to leukemia. Family cancer history does not appear to be associated with an increased risk of childhood acute leukemia (Rudant et al. 2007). If one monozygotic twin is diagnosed with leukemia, the other twin will have a 5–25% risk of developing leukemia (Greaves et al. 2003; Kadan-Lottick et al. 2008; Couto et al. 2005).

Table 1.2. Syndromes with a predisposition to leukemia

Genetic bone marrow failure syndromes predisposed to leukemia
Fanconi anemia
Diamond-Blackfan anemia
Shwachman-Diamond syndrome
Dyskeratosis congenita
Kostmann severe congentila neutropenia
Genetic syndromes predisposed to leukemia as one of the illnesses
Chromosomal abnormality
Down's syndrome (trisomy 21)
Chromosome 8 trisomy syndrome
Klinefelter syndrome
DNA repair/tumor suppressor deficiency
Ataxia telangiectasia
Li-Fraumeni syndrome
Neurofibromatosis type 1
Bloom syndrome
Nijmegen/Berlin breakage syndrome

(Table compiled from Mizutani, 1998)

1.2.2.2 Environmental Factors

It has been accepted that ionizing radiation is a causal factor of leukemia. Following the explosion of atomic bombs in Japan, the exposed children acquired an increased risk of developing leukemia. However, those individuals exposed in utero showed no increase in the incidence of leukemia. This finding is in contrast to the suggested results of various studies that showed an increased risk of leukemia and other cancers (by about 40%) among children exposed in utero to diagnostic radiography (Doll and Wakeford 1997). There is no doubt that ionizing radiation is a causal factor in leukemia; however, there are uncertainties regarding various aspects of its effect on leukemogenesis.

Kinlen's theory (1995) states that population mixing, herd immunity, and abnormal response to infection of unusually susceptible children increases the risk of ALL. The "delayed infection" or "hygiene" hypothesis suggests that ALL in children is caused by a lack of exposure to infection in infancy, with an abnormal response to a later common infection incurred after mixing with other children in playgroups or schools. This hypothesis is consistent with Greaves's theory that childhood ALL results from at least two mutations, with the second one more likely to occur in children with a delayed exposure to infection leading to increased immunological stress (Stiller et al. 2008). Therefore, circumstances that alter the pattern of infections in infants may contribute to the etiology of ALL (Stiller et al. 2008).

Table 1.3 highlights the studies that have been undertaken to investigate the various possible factors in the

Table 1.3. Reported environmental links to childhood leukemia and current conclusions

Possible environmental link	Current conclusions
Parental use of tobacco	Studies on parental smoking are controversial. However, several studies support the hypothesis that paternal smoking is associated with an increased risk of ALL (MacArthur et al. 2008; Rudant et al. 2008; Lee et al. 2009; Menegaux et al. 2007; Pang et al. 2003)
Vitamin K prophylaxis in infants	Now disproved; intially inconsistent associations reported. However, confirmed benefits of vitamin K outweigh the hypothetical association with any childhood cancer (American Academy of Pediatrics Committee on Fetus and Newborn 2003; Roman et al. 2002; Ross and Davies 2000; Parker et al. 1998; Passmore et al. 1998)
Living near landfill sites	No excess risk of any cancer reported (Jarup et al. 2002)
Proximity to railways and roads	No association reported between risk of childhood leukemia and railway proximity (Dickinson et al. 2003). Small association with railway density assumed to be the consequence of population mixing and proximity of railways in deprived urban areas. Child cancer initiations may be determined by prenatal or early postnatal exposures to engine exhaust gas (Knox 2006)
In vitro fertilization	No increased risk of childhood cancer reported in studies published (Bergh et al. 1999; Klip et al. 2001). Underlying cause of infertility may be a predisposing factor which may account for some case control studies reporting increased risk of specific cancers (Lightfoot et al. 2005)
Prenatal ultrasound	No association with childhood leukemia found (Naumburg et al. 2000)
Supplementary oxygen	Resuscitation with 100% oxygen immediately postpartum is associated with childhood ALL; further studies warranted (Naumburg et al. 2002a)
Breastfeeding	Contradicting reports of association with a reduced risk of acute leukemia (Bener et al. 2008; Lancashire et al., 2003; UK Childhood Cancer Study Investigators 2001; Shu et al. 1999)
Pet (healthy or sick) ownership	No relationship (Swensen et al. 2001)
Electromagnetic fields (EMF) and power lines	Consensus of available studies does not support hypothesis of an association (Skinner et al. 2002; Schüz et al. 2007)
Natural radionuclides in drinking water, including uranium and arsenic	Results do not indicate increased risk of leukemia (Auvinen et al. 2002; Engel and Lamm 2008)
In utero exposure to metronidazole	No reported increased risk (Thapa et al. 1998)
Allergies or family history of allergies	Reduced risk of ALL; no such pattern seen with AML (Schuz et al., 2003). The reduced risk may be due to an increased infection rate associated with a positive allergy history (Rosenbaum et al. 2005)
Exposure to pesticides	May increase risk (Rudant et al. 2007; Ma et al. 2002)
Perinatal exposure to infection	Some association reported between maternal infection in utero and risk of childhood leukemia (Kwan et al. 2007; Naumburg et al. 2002b)
Population mixing	Increased risk of ALL in children 1–6 years old in high tertile of population mixing (Alexander et al. 1999; Boutou et al. 2002). Further support for the hypothesis of infectious agents involved in etiology of ALL
Parental alcohol consumption	Some studies indicate an increased risk of ALL and increased maternal alcohol consumption (MacArthur et al. 2008; Menegaux et al. 2007)
Parental caffeine consumption	No significant reports of increased risk of childhood ALL and maternal coffee consumption (Menegaux et al. 2007)

etiology of childhood leukemia and other cancers. All the theories surrounding the causes of ALL, or indeed the majority of childhood cancers, are for the most part unexplained, and further studies are necessary to confirm or reject the conclusions of those available.

Because of the public interest that surrounds the majority of these potential risk factors, parents will continue to form theories regarding their children's illnesses (Ruccione et al. 1994). Nurses have a role in eliciting parents' causal explanations so that the content of these concerns can be related to the parents' adjustment and management of their experience of childhood cancer.

1.2.3 Molecular Genetics

Clonal chromosomal abnormalities (originating in a single cell) are detectable in around 90% of childhood ALL cases. The leukemia then evolves by the accrual of mutations within a clone. The abnormalities are responsible for a loss of controlled cell growth, division, and differentiation.

The following is a review on the biology of chromosomes:

- Genes carry instructions to make proteins essential for cell growth, division, and differentiation.
- A deoxyribonucleic acid (DNA) molecule carries the genetic information in coded form.
- DNA is a nucleic acid made of chains of nucleotides.
- Nucleotides have three components – a phosphate group, a pentose sugar, and a base.
- In DNA, the sugar is deoxyribose, and the bases are adenine, guanine, thymine, and cytosine.
- DNA consists of two chains of nucleotides linked across their bases by weak hydrogen bonds. These two complementary strands of nucleotides are linked in a double-helix formation.
- The bases have specific affinities toward each other, and thymine pairs only with adenine, and cytosine pairs only with guanine.
- The base sequence is the key to the control of the cell and is referred to as the genetic code.
- The length of DNA in cells is so great that there is a significant risk of mutations. DNA is packaged into 46 compact manageable chromosomes (23 pairs).
- The complete chromosome complement of a cell is referred to as the karyotype.

Some genes are associated with the transformation of a normal cell to a malignant cell. These are known as oncogenes (or proto-oncogenes) and tumor suppressor genes. Mutations in the DNA of these genes may cause them to produce an abnormal product, or disrupt their control so that they are expressed inappropriately, making products in excessive amounts or at the wrong time. Some oncogenes may cause extra production of growth factors, which are chemicals that stimulate cell growth. Other oncogenes may cause changes in a surface receptor, causing it to send signals as though it were being activated by a growth factor.

The exact number of mutations required to transform a normal cell into a malignant cell is unknown, but research indicates that two or more mutations, or "hits," are involved. The first hit is thought to occur in the womb, which in ALL is likely to be a developmental accident affecting a chromosome. This may then suggest that a second hit after birth is necessary before ALL develops. This theory has arisen mainly from the observed high concordance rates of leukemia in infant monozygotic twins (i.e., if one twin has leukemia, so will the other) and the study of neonatal blood spots or Guthrie cards. In twins, the leukemogenic event is considered to arise in one twin, and the cells from the abnormal clone are presumed to spread to the other via shared placental anastomoses. Polymerase chain reaction (PCR) has been used to identify the same fusion gene sequence in neonatal blood spots similar to that in patients' leukemic cells at diagnosis. In almost all cases of infant leukemia with a fusion of the MLL gene and in many cases of childhood ALL with a fusions of the TEL-AML1 gene, these fusions are detectable at birth. These gene fusions would indicate the first hit or mutation. Table 1.4 shows the classification of types of mutation that can occur. In childhood ALL, reciprocal translocations account for approximately 25% of the chromosomal abnormalities. The translocations involve exchanges of tracks of DNA between chromosomes, resulting in the generation of chimeric or fusion genes. There may also be changes in chromosome number (ploidy), gene deletions, or single nucleotide-base changes in

Table 1.4. Types of mutation to genetic code

Mutation	Description	Presentations
Point mutation	Change in DNA sequence Can occur in base substitution, deletion, or addition May result in wrong amino acid being inserted into protein	Mis-sense mutation, usually a decrease in function
Chromosomal mutation	Alteration in the gross structure of chromosomes Result from cell breakage and reunion of chromosomal material during the cell cycle	Translocation Rearrangement
Genomic mutation	Change in the number of chromosomes in the genome	Amplification Aneuploidy (loss or gain of single chromosome)

genes (the chromosome number is also measurable as the DNA index, in which 46 chromosomes equals a DNA index of 1) .

As discussed earlier, the process by which a normal cell transforms into a leukemic cell is unclear. However, improved molecular analysis techniques have assisted in identifying mechanisms regulating cell growth and differentiation. These include the following:

- PCR
- Fluorescence in situ hybridization (FISH)
- Flow cytometry for immunophenotyping
- Digitized karyotype imaging/multicolor spectral karyotyping
- Microarray profiling of all genes active in a given cell population
- Southern blotting

Molecular analysis has proved indispensable for identifying prognostic factors and therapeutically important genetic subtypes of childhood ALL. The ranges of subtypes are based on gene expression, antigens that delineate the cell type, and chromosomal and molecular abnormalities. There is currently a relatively sophisticated understanding of the genetic basis of ALL, which will be discussed further in the following sections.

1.2.4 Symptoms and Clinical Signs

ALL can be either of T-lymphoblastic lineage or of B-lymphoblastic lineage. Both the subtypes of ALL have similar presenting features. However, T-cell ALL can have some associated symptoms related to the presence of a mediastinal mass. The symptoms and clinical signs of both T-cell and B-cell lineage will be described in the following sections.

ALL usually presents as an acute illness of short onset, but symptoms are occasionally slow and insidious. The symptoms are related to the infiltration of the bone marrow and other affected organs by lymphoblastic cells and the absence of normal blood cells. The presenting features often appear like many childhood illnesses. Parents or children may describe the following:

- Irritability
- Fatigue
- Bone pain, which may present as limping
- Loss of appetite

Initially, symptoms may fluctuate daily, with the child feeling exhausted one day and fine the next day.

Physical findings may include the following:

- Pallor and lethargy
- Pain at the sites of disease infiltration, especially in long bones
- Petechiae
- Bruising or unusual bleeding (including nose bleeds)
- Enlarged liver or spleen, causing the abdomen to protrude
- Enlarged lymph nodes and fever
- Painless testicular swelling

In less than 10% of the cases, the disease is observed to spread to the CNS at diagnosis. This may cause related symptoms of

- Headache
- Poor school performance
- Weakness
- Vomiting
- Blurred vision
- Seizures
- Difficulty maintaining balance

In 60–70% of children with the T-cell type of ALL, there is involvement of the thymus. Enlargement of the thymus caused by an accumulation of white blood cells can give rise to an anterior mediastinal mass that can cause pressure on the trachea, causing coughing, shortness of breath, pain, and dysphagia. In some cases, the pressure may also compress the superior vena cava and cause swelling of the head and arms.

In rare circumstances, acute leukemia may present with extremely high blast cell counts, known as hyperleukocytosis. This state of the disease can cause respiratory failure, intracranial bleeding, and severe metabolic abnormalities – conditions that are the main causes of early mortality. The process that leads to these complications is known as leukostasis. It had been thought that leukostasis was caused by overcrowding of leukemic blasts. However, it is now evident that leukostasis results from adhesive interactions between blasts and the vascular endothelium. Damage to the endothelium is likely, owing to the cytokines that are released. The adhesion molecules displayed by the blasts and their response to the environment are probably more important factors in leukostasis formation than the numbers of cells. Leukopheresis is sometimes used to reduce the leukocyte count in the initial phase when there is hyperleukocytosis. It remains unclear whether this is the most efficient method of treating leukostasis. It is also important to start cytoreductive therapy as soon as possible, and this requires an expedited diagnosis. Further research should indicate the most appropriate use of leukopheresis and the development of practice guidelines for the management of hyperleukocytosis.

1.2.5 Diagnostics

If ALL is suspected following the history and physical examination of the child, then the initial investigations include a complete blood count, serum evaluations of kidney and liver function, electrolyte counts, and a chest X-ray. The blood count may point to a diagnosis of leukemia if there are blast cells present or there is evidence of anemia, thrombocytopenia, or leukopenia. At presentation of leukemia, the white blood cell count (WBC) is often elevated; however, it may also be in the normal range or below normal values. Figure 1.2a shows a normal blood film, and Fig. 1.2b is a blood film from a child with ALL. Blood counts may raise suspicion of leukemia, but the diagnosis is most often confirmed by bone marrow examination. Occasionally, a diagnosis is made on peripheral blood samples, particularly if there is a high WBC and/or the patient is clincally unstable making sedation for diagnostic procedures dangerous. When bone marrow procedure is done, the marrow is mostly aspirated from the iliac bone at the iliac crest. Despite the new technologies available, ALL is still usually diagnosed by an experienced pediatric oncologist and/or pathologist, by examining a Romanowsky-stained bone marrow smear with a high-powered microscope. A higher than 25% blast-cell count in the marrow confirms a diagnosis of leukemia. A portion of the bone marrow aspirate is then analyzed to detect other features of the leukemic cells to help determine what type of leukemia is present. Bone marrow biopsy/trephine may be required for diagnosis if bone marrow aspirate is inconclusive and leukemia is still suspected.

A lumbar puncture (LP) is performed to determine any CNS involvement; a sample of cerebrospinal fluid (CSF) is examined for blast cells. The bone marrow aspirate (BMA) and LP are most often performed together using sedation or anesthetics. Therefore, because of the potential anesthetic difficulties that could develop, a chest X-ray is vital to assist in diagnosing infection or detecting a mediastinal mass. To minimize the risk of bleeding, platelet transfusion may be required prior to an LP. For males suspected of testicular involvement on clinical examination, an ultrasound is indicated. An echocardiogram is often carried out at diagnosis, and is necessary for all patients who are intended to start an induction therapy that included anthracycline chemotherapy.

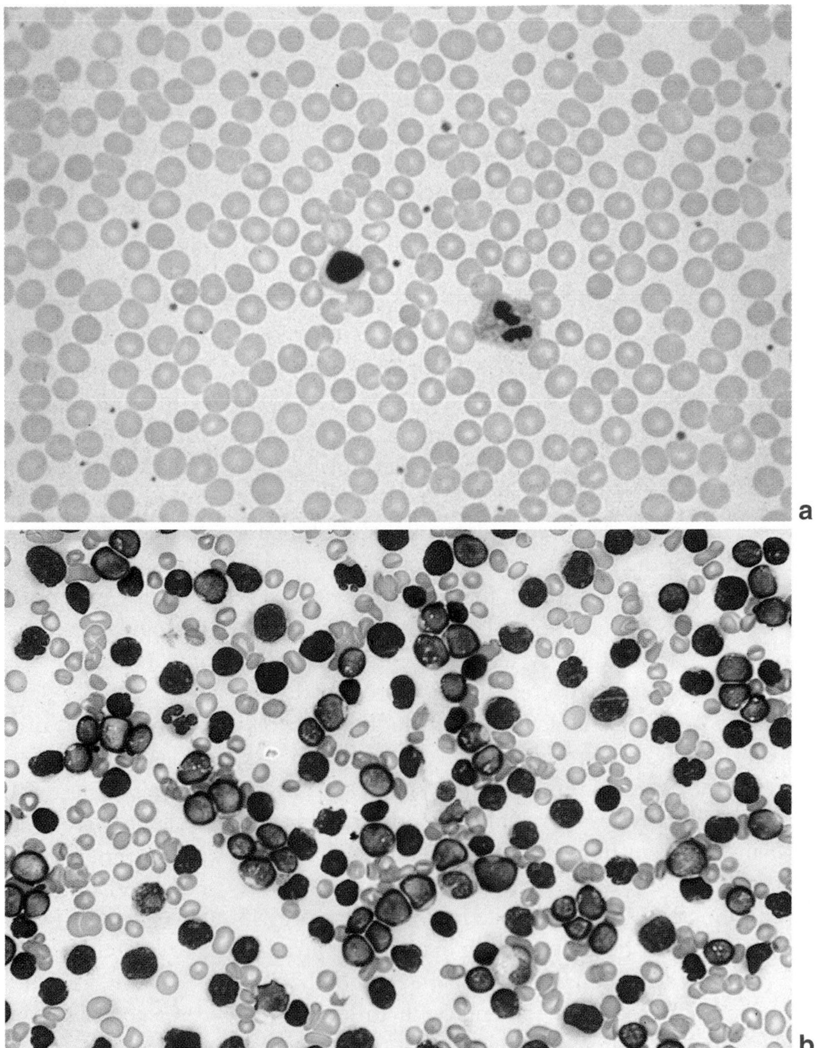

Figure 1.2

(**a**) Normal blood film (×25), (**b**) ALL blood film (×25). Image credit: Dr Angela Thomas, RHSC, Edinburgh

1.2.6 Staging and Classification

1.2.6.1 Risk Classification

Once the diagnosis of ALL has been confirmed, cell morphology, cytogenetics, and immunophenotyping are determined to elicit more defined prognostic factors. Treatment can subsequently focus on "risk-directed" protocols developed through well-designed clinical trials. This strategy uses the child's likelihood of relapse or resistance to treatment, to intensify or reduce the treatment to ensure adequate cell kill within acceptable levels of toxicity. The significance of various reported risk factors has led to some debate. Difficulty also arises when comparing the results among different countries and centers using locally-assigned risk categories. However, over the past few decades, several features have been determined to be more favorable prognostic factors. In 1993, following a previous initiative in Rome, collaborative groups met to establish those features that would indicate "standard risk" of ALL. These are known as the Rome/NCI (National Cancer Institute) criteria:

- WBC <50,000/mm^3
- 1–9 years of age
- non-T/non-B (mature B-cell ALL)

Although risk classification differs by investigator group, most investigators agree on the four identified risk group classifications. These include:

- Standard risk: low (trisomy 4, 10, and TEL-AML1 t(12:21))
- Standard risk (NCI as mentioned earlier)
- High risk (WBC >50,000/mm^3 or age >10 years)
- Very high risk (VHR) (hypodiploid karyotyoe or presence of BCR-ABL/t(9:22) or poor early response to treatment, high minimal residual disease (MRD) level at the end of induction).

Other factors are also used to determine the risk classification, but the number and array of factors used to classify ALL make it difficult to establish any one system. Consequently, there is a lack of precision within most risk classification systems. Varying conclusions have been reported with regard to the prognostic significance of other characteristics, including the presence of Down's syndrome (DS), liver and spleen size, the presence of an anterior mediastinal mass, French–American–British (FAB) subtype, body mass index, CNS involvement, hemoglobin level, and platelet count. Interestingly, traumatic lumbar puncture at diagnosis of childhood ALL may indicate increased risk of CNS relapse and may be an indication to intensify intrathecal (IT) therapy (Gajjar et al. 2000; Rech et al. 2005). However, subgroups of patients with different outcomes can be predicted by blast karyotype, molecular abnormalities, and early response to treatment, with response to treatment proving to be increasingly more important (Schultz et al. 2007). Response to treatment is usually assessed at the end of induction therapy for ALL, and is now determined by measuring the amount of minimal residual disease (MRD). This very sensitve diagnostic test appears to have the greatest strength to predict prognosis when compared with the other biological and clinical features (Pui and Evans 2006). Currently, investigators continue to determine a cutoff value that is indicative of poor prognosis prompting treatment intensification. Presently, an MRD value of 0.01% appears to be highly prognostic, with patients achieving a value less than 0.01% at the end of the induction phase having a predicted excellent treatment outcome. Alternatively, patients who have a greater end of induction MRD value may have a high risk of relapse and will benefit from intensified therapy (Pui and Evans 2006). Patients who have a high MRD value are considered poor early responders (or slow early responders). MRD can be measured using either flow cytometry or PCR techniques.

A VHR classification is assigned to pediatric patients with ALL, who have clinical or biological features associated with a high risk of relapse. Patients with VHR classification are usually recommended for hematopoietic stem cell transplant (HSCT). MLL rearrangement is also considered an VHR feature, but only if there is evidence of a slow early response to treatment and an associated MRD-positive end of induction finding. The MRD value appears to be so strongly prognostic that it is likely to override other biological features of ALL in future therapies.

1.2.6.2 Cell Morphology

Despite other ways of looking at cells, a morphological classification that is still widely applied is the FAB system. This classification is based on the morphology (appearance, structure, and cytochemistry) and number of cells, and it defines three categories (Table 1.5). However, this system is no longer used for prognosis.

1.2.6.3 Cytochemistry

Several biochemical markers have been identified to assist in the classification of leukemia. However, little is added to the morphology of ALL, with the exception of

- Periodic-acid Schiff positivity, seen in around 15% of cases correlating with common ALL
- Acid phosphatase positivity in T-ALL

1.2.6.4 Immunophenotyping

ALL is probably best classified on the basis of immunophenotyping. Antigens on the surface of normal hematopoietic cells express changes as the cells

Table 1.5. French–American–British classification of acute lymphoblastic leukemia

Category	Definition	Features	Percentage of patients
L1	Small cells with scant cytoplasm	Associated with good treatment response	90
L2	Large cells with abundant cytoplasm	Indicates more refractory to therapy if 10–20% L2 cells are present	9
L3	Large cells with prominent nucleoli	Mature B-cell phenotype, frequently presents as lymphoma, poor prognosis	1

mature in the bone marrow. Technology has produced monoclonal antibodies to many of these cluster-of-differentiation (CD) antigen groups. These are each given a classification number prefixed with CD. Some CD antigen groups are related to lymphocyte sublineage (CDs 1–8 mark various stages of T-cell lineage; CDs 19–22, 24, and 79a mark B cells) and some are related to myeloid lineage, whereas others mark more primitive features (CD10 and CD34). CD10 is known as the common ALL antigen (CALLA). Other useful immunologically defined cell characteristics include the following:

- Cytoplasmic immunoglobulins found in pre-B-cell ALL
- Surface immunoglobulins found in mature B-ALL
- Terminal deoxynucleotidyl transferase (TdT) found in immature lymphoid cells

Using these markers enables the classification of ALL into major categories (Table 1.6). ALL cells occasionally express cell antigens usually associated with myeloid lineage. The myeloid antigens may be weakly expressed and are often considered abberant expressions. However, opinion is divided as to whether this is clinically significant.

Table 1.6. Categories of acute lymphoblastic leukemia

Category of ALL	Percentage (approximately)
Common or pre-B	80
T-cell	10
Mature B	7
Null (early B-precursor)	3

1.2.6.5 Cytogenetics

Cytogenetic abnormalities are detectable in most cases of childhood ALL. They can be categorized either by the number of chromosomes (ploidy) or by the structural changes and rearrangements based on the detailed analysis of the karyotype. The assessment of ploidy status is clinically useful in predicting prognosis (Table 1.7).

With regard to structural changes, the identification of translocations and marker chromosomes and the delineation of complex chromosome aberrations are possible with multicolor spectral karyotyping. The most significant chromosome (Ch') translocations identified in childhood ALL include the following:

Table 1.7. Outcome prediction associated with ploidy status of acute lymphoblastic leukemia

Ploidy Status	Number of chromosomes per malignant cell	Percentage of childhood ALL cases	Predictive response to treatment
Hyperdiploidy	>50	25–30	Favorable
Hypodiploidy	<44	5–10	Poor
Near-haploid	<30	<1	Very poor

Important: Fewer than 44 chromosomes is a degree of hypodiploidy that is prognostically relevant

- Ch'12 and Ch'21; that is, t(12:21), resulting in the TEL-AML1 (more recently called ETV6-RUNX1) fusion gene, which has been commonly reported to indicate a good prognosis
- The Philadelphia chromosome, which is translocation t(9:22) and gives rise to the BCR/ABL fusion gene in ALL that indicates a poor prognosis
- t(1:19), giving rise to E2A/PBX1 which is a translocation of pre-B-ALL
- t(4:11), giving rise to MLL/AF4, which is a typical translocation occurring in infant leukemia

Other significant abnormalities include

- Rearrangements of the MLL gene
- Rearrangements of the MYC gene with immunoglobulin genes
- Rearrangements of T-cell receptor genes
- Mutations of p16 (a tumor suppressor gene)
- Mutations of p53 gene (although uncommon in childhood ALL, these mutations are associated with relapse or refractory leukemia)
- Number of chromosomes: hyperdiploidy with trisomy of chromosome 4 and chromosome 10
- Hypodiploidy: less than 45 chromosomes

The effects of these genetic alterations in leukemia help to explain adverse clinical outcomes. For example, the Philadelphia chromosome results in the production of an active kinase enzyme that drives cell proliferation independently of the normal requirements of growth factor, and blocks apoptosis (programmed cell death). Therefore, drug responsiveness pathways may be blocked. Normal p53 protein is required to induce cell death following anoxia or DNA damage from exposure to drugs or irradiation. Mutations in the p53, common in relapse of leukemia, may explain drug resistance in more advanced disease.

Although the risk criteria features must be considered important predictors of outcome, it would appear that they are most beneficial in predicting the risk groups in B-cell lineage, but not consistently in T-cell disease (Eden et al. 2000). Overall, 30–40% of the children with T-lineage ALL relapse within the first 18 months after diagnosis, and approximately 20% of the children with "standard risk" ALL relapse. Some groups of patients require further intensification of therapy. Consequently, more sophisticated approaches to risk classification that incorporate the molecular genetic findings and minimal residual disease measurement have the potential for identifying higher-risk children.

1.2.7 Treatment

The treatment of infant ALL remains a challenge. The current estimated overall survival rate of infant ALL is 50%, and 30–40% for infant ALL with MLL rearrangement (Tomizawa et al. 2007; Pieters et al. 2007). Most investigators treat infants as a unique subgroup on infant ALL protocols, giving multiple drugs at high doses. Investigators are considering the benefit of a hybrid AML/ALL therapy. Intensive systemic and IT treatments seem to provide adequate therapy for the CNS, even in infants with CNS involvement at diagnosis, thus avoiding cranial irradiation. The role of HSCT for infant ALL remains controversial owing to the signficant toxicity and lack of evidence to support improved overall survival, even for infants with high-risk features. At present, HSCT is usually recommended in the event of a first relapse of infant ALL. Future prespectives in infant ALL therapy should include a refined risk stratification, so that therapy in the future can be risk-directed. Presently, there is agreement on high-risk features of infant ALL and these include the following features:

- Age <3 months at the time of diagnosis
- Presence of an MLL rearrangement
- Presenting WBC >300,000 U/L

The remainder of this treatment section will focus on the treatment of ALL for pediatric patients aged over 1 year and less than 18 years at the time of diagnosis. Advances in the treatment of ALL have improved to such a degree that about 80% of childhood ALL is curable. The cytotoxic drugs used have been available for over 20 years, but better understanding of the pharmacology of these drugs has led to more effective protocols being devised that also attempt to avoid and minimize long-term adverse effects. Improvements have also been made in supportive care to reduce morbidity and mortality. The aim of treatment for ALL is to effectively halt the production of abnormal cells and eradicate the disease. The treatment protocols for ALL are being constantly

Table 1.8. Drugs commonly used in the treatment of acute lymphoblastic leukemia

Drugs	Route of administration	Induction/ Reintensification	Consolidation	CNS Prophylaxis	Maintenance
Vincristine	Intravenous	*	*		*
L-asparaginase	Subcutaneous/ intramuscular/ intravenous	*	*		
Prednisone/ Dexamethasone	Oral	*	*		*
					*
Methotrexate	Oral				*
Methotrexate	Intrathecal	*	*	*	*
Methotrexate (with folinic acid rescue)	Intravenous			*	
Daunorubicin	Intravenous	*Possibly	*		
Etoposide or cyclophosphamide	Intravenous	*Possibly for reintensification	*		
Cytarabine	Intravenous		*		
Thioguanine (or mercaptopurine)	Oral		*		
Mercaptopurine	Oral		*Possibly		*

*: drug prescribed

improved in terms of efficacy and long-term toxicity. Protocols for ALL generally include the following features:

1. Induction
2. Consolidation
3. Reintensification
4. CNS-directed therapy
5. Maintenance/continuing treatment

The drugs normally administered during the treatment for ALL are shown in Table 1.8 (Part 3 will detail the cytotoxic drugs further). Treatment for ALL continues for a period of 2–3½ years.

1.2.7.1 Induction

The drugs used initially to induce a remission are vincristine, steroids, and a third drug – L-asparaginase – given over a 4-week period. This three-drug induction usually produces remission in about 95% of children with standard risk classification. A fourth drug is added to pediatric patients who present with initial high-risk features (age >10 years, and WBC >50,000/mm^3).These patients have a four-drug induction that includes the standard three-drug agents along with an anthracycline over a 4–6-week period.Research suggests that early treatment with daunorubicin could achieve a reduced relapse risk if it is not replaced by alternative intensification strategies (Chessells et al. 2002). CNS prophylaxis/treatment is also started during induction with IT chemotherapy. For patients with BCR-ABL-positive ALL, imatinib mesylate (Gleevec), a tyrosine kinase inhibitor, is often added to the induction regimen. It remains unclear if this will improve overall survival, but there is good evidence to suggest that it increases disease-free survival. For patients with T-cell lineage ALL, current trials are investigating the benefit of adding a new agent, 506U78 (nelarabine), in induction, and then again in reinduction and maintenance therapy. 506U78 is an agent that is cytotoxic to T-lymphoblasts. This new agent has some dose-limiting neurological toxicities that include weakness, ataxia, confusion, coma, seizure, and Guillian-Barre syndrome. Investigators will continue to study the optimal dose of this new agent for treating T-cell ALL, and are trying to determine whether intensifying the dose for poor induction responders will improve overall survival.

The steroid of choice is normally prednisone, but research is being carried out to establish the efficacy of dexamethasone. Dexamethasone has more effective CNS penetration and is currently used in some induction regimens but is associated with significant side effects such as increased infections and the development of osteonecrosis.

L-asparaginase can be derived from several sources, including

- Polyethylene-glycol (PEG) L-asparaginase
- *Escherichia coli (E. coli)* L-asparaginase
- *Erwinia* asparaginase (derived from *Erwinia carotovora* or *Erwinia chrysanthemi)*

Each of these L-asparaginase preparations has different pharmacokinetic properties and different toxic tendencies. PEG L-asparaginase has a longer half-life than *E. coli* asparaginase, which in turn has a longer half-life than *Erwinia* asparaginase. When given in equivalent doses, the one with a longer half-life should be more effective, but it is also more toxic. Reports comparing the efficacy of different preparations have debated the clinical significance of the results. Owing to the sources of the preparations, these compounds can all display immunogenicity and cause allergic side effects. However, the presence of antibodies does not necessarily cause an allergic reaction. Other toxicities, including coagulation disorders, liver toxicity, and acute pancreatitis, are related to the inhibition of protein synthesis. Few studies have compared the effect of the various asparaginase preparations on the coagulation proteins. *Erwinia* asparaginase has been reported as having a less pronounced effect on coagulation than *E. coli* asparaginase has. This may be argued to be dose-related rather than preparation-related. Fresh frozen plasma (FFP) was often transfused prior to L-asparaginase, if coagulation screening showed a decrease in any coagulation proteins; however, this is now thought to be of no clinical benefit. Protocols for the treatment of ALL usually specify one particular preparation of L-asparaginase. However, allergic reactions usually require the discontinuation of therapy and subsequent substitution with a different preparation.

When treatment for ALL begins, the lysis of leukemic cells causes an increase in uric acid levels in the blood. Therefore, a uricolytic agent (uric acid depletor) is routinely prescribed. Historically, this agent was allopurinol, but more effective agents such as recombinant urate oxidase (Rasburicase) have been utilized with improved management of tumor lysis syndrome (see Chap. 17).

Because of the risk of *Pneumocystis jiroveci* pneumonia (PCP) in immunocompromised patients, sulfamethoxazole/trimethoprim (SMX/TMP) or cotrimoxazole is given as effective prophylaxis. This is normally administered as an oral preparation (usually 2 or 3 times per week), but may be given intravenously if the patient's condition requires such administration. Occassionally, owing to adverse reactions including prolonged periods of neutropenia, a secondary alternative may be necessary. These alternatives include aerosolized/nebulized pentamidine, oral dapsone, and oral atovaquone. Pentamidine can be given intravenously, but there is controversy regarding its effectiveness when administered IV and there may be greater systemic toxicities with this method of administration.

1.2.7.2 Consolidation

This block of treatment is given following induction, once there is evidence of normal hematopoetic function and remission is confirmed. The length of consolidation therapy ranges from about 4 to 8 weeks. Consolidation therapy has intensive therapy directed to the CNS.

1.2.7.3 Reintensification

Reintensification, which is essentially a repeat of induction chemotherapy, has proven to be an important component of ALL protocols. Common chemotherapeutic agents administered during reintensification include vincristine, steriods, asparginase, and the addition of an anthracycline. In some cases, reintensification may be augmented to include other common chemotherapeutic agents including cyclophosphamide, cytarabine, and methotrexate with mercaptopurine. Owing to the repetition of intensive glucocorticosteroids, the risk of osteonecrosis is escalated particularly for patients over 10 years of age. Owing to this risk, steroid therapy during reintensification is often administered on an alternating week schedule. Reintensification includes CNS-directed therapy.

1.2.7.4 CNS-Directed Therapy

Prophylactic CNS therapy is based on the premise that the CNS provides a sanctuary site for leukemic cells that are undetectable at diagnosis and that can be protected from systemic therapy by the blood–brain barrier. If preventative therapy were not given to children with ALL, over 50% would develop CNS disease. During induction and intensification phases, IT methotrexate is delivered on an intensive schedule. Regular (usually every 12 weeks) lumbar punctures with IT methotrexate are continued throughout maintenance therapy. Additionally, high-dose methotrexate is given intravenously, usually at 2-week intervals between the intensification blocks. High-dose methotrexate infusions with leukovorin rescue were introduced into protocols to replace cranial irradiation because of its associated adverse side effects, and the benefits are still under investigation. Additionally, current ALL trials are comparing the administration of methotrexate on an esclating schedule (Capizzi Methotrexate) every 10 days without leukovorin rescue as outpatient therapy, with the traditional intermediate- or high-dose methotrexate inpatient chemotherapy. Owing to the concern of long-term neurocognitive deficits, endocrinopathy and second malignancies cranial radiotherapy may be reserved for children thought to be especially at high risk of CNS involvement (T-cell with high WBC at diagnosis) or for those with CNS infiltration at diagnosis. The risk of neurocognitive deficits is greater in younger children, particularly children below the age of 3 years. There remains controvery surrounding the optimal dose of cranial radiation. Studies suggest that the prophylaxis dose of cranial radiation is 1,200, and 1,800 cGy for those with overt CNS involvement. Triple IT therapy (including Methotrexate, cytarabine and hydrocortisone) is also under investigation in some protocols.

! Note: It is vital that the IT methotrexate NEVER be confused with the intravenous (IV) vincristine that is normally given on the same day. This would result in fatality.

1.2.7.5 Maintenance/Continuing Treatment

Oral methotrexate administered weekly and oral 6-mercaptopurine administered daily are the mainstay of most continuation regimens. Administering these drugs in the evening appears to give a better clinical outcome. This result may be mainly due to issues surrounding compliance; it may be easier for parents or adolescents to remember medications at this time of day. Studies have indicated the need to give continuation therapy to the limits of tolerance by titrating doses against myelosuppression and reiterating the importance of compliance. This may result in periods of discontinuing therapy during this phase. Therapy is not usually discontinued if there is an episode of elevated liver enzymes that is less than 20 times the upper limit of normal values. Currently, maintenance therapy also includes pulses of IV vincristine and oral steroid pulses at monthly intervals, PCP prophylaxis, and CNS-directed therapy.

Some patients are at risk of increased myleosuppression owing to the administration of mercaptopurine. These patients may have inherited either a heterozygous or homozygous thiopurine purine methyltransferase (TPMT) deficiency. TPMT is an enzyme that catabolyzes mercaptopurine. Therefore, if TPMT is deficient, less mercaptopurine is metabolized to the inactive form and there is higher concentrations of active metabolite, putting patients at risk of hematopoetic toxicity. It is recommended that all patients who require therapy for ALL, which will include mercaptopurine, be tested for TPMT deficiency. Patients who are identified as having a homozygous deficiency (approximately 1/300 patients) of TPMT are recommended to receive a significantly reduced dose of mercaptopurine. Treatment for patients who have a heterozygous deficiency is generally started with the recommended dose with close observation and titration of dose of mercaptopurine to maintain neutrophils within the suggested target range as directed by the protocol.

The progression of each stage of the protocol relies on a degree of return of normal bone marrow function, where the blood component levels are within normal limits. Periods of neutropenia are associated with any ALL treatment protocol during which the child/adolescent becomes immunocompromised. Procedures regarding supportive care are adhered to and are as important as the cytotoxic therapy with regard to ensuring the best outcomes for these children and adolescents.

1.2.7.6 Allogeneic Stem Cell Transplant

Some high-risk leukemias may indicate the need for transplantation from the time of diagnosis, such as BCR-ABL-positive ALL and hypodiploid ALL. Patients who are MRD positive at the end of induction may also be recommended for HSCT. However, as transplantation and chemotherapy are improving, these patients are continually subject to review. Stem cell transplantation has not been shown to improve outcomes for infant ALL in first remission, but is often considered in the event of relapse.

1.2.8 Prognosis

The prognosis of ALL is one of the best among childhood malignancies, with an event-free survival rate (survival free from relapse) of around 80%. Studies have investigated the influence of ethnicity and socioeconomic status on survival. Bhatia et al. (2002) reported an increased risk of treatment failure in Hispanic children treated for ALL (Bhatia et al. 2002). Increasing levels of deprivation were associated with poorer survival from all cancers, including leukemia, but only before other prognostic factors were taken into consideration (McKinney et al. 1999). However, despite continuing improved protocols, the rate of relapse has decreased only slightly over the last decade. The main improvements in survival rates have been because of improved management of relapse, especially for those relapsing off treatment.

The survival rate of 80% is the mean that disguises the rates that range from 60% to 90%. The failure of improved rates of survival has been most notable in high-risk groups. However, the relapse that occurs in standard risk groups must also be explained. The reasons may be pharmacological in cases of noncompliance, or drug resistance. Drug sensitivity testing and greater vigilance may help to identify those at risk and allow for intervention. Other reasons for treatment failure may be due to intrinsically resistant disease or recurrence from residual disease. Testicular relapse of ALL can occur, possibly because this area is a sanctuary site. However, this is a rare event, affecting approximately 1% of boys with ALL, and is normally treated with local radiation therapy and chemotherapy. Approximately 10–13% of pediatric ALL cases have T-lineage phenotype, and approximately 30% of these still relapse during the first 18 months of treatment. More sophisticated approaches to risk classification and measurement of minimal residual disease to capture patients who would benefit from more intense treatment may help to increase overall event-free survival rates.

1.2.9 Follow-Up

Following the completion of therapy for ALL, it is crucial to monitor these children and adolescents for two reasons: relapse of disease and late effects of therapy.

1. Blood counts will be carried out to ensure that signs of relapse can be detected, but with decreasing frequency over a number of years. Follow-up bone marrow evaluations are usually reserved for patients when there is a raised clinical suspicion of disease relapse. Risk of relapse significantly declines after the third year off treatment (Pui et al. 2005).
2. As therapy becomes more successful, late side effects are of increasing concern.

Long-term effects of antileukemic treatment include the following:

- Chronic cardiotoxicity induced by anthracyclines (daunorubicin, doxorubicin), which can manifest as sudden onset of irreversible heart failure. The severity of cardiac dysfunction is related to the cumulative dose of anthracycline. The younger age of the child at the time of anthracycline administration increases the risk of cardiotoxicity (Ruggiero et al. 2008).

- Hypothalamic–pituitary axis and gonadal damage induced by radiation. Growth problems may cause short stature and obesity later in life, and girls may undergo precocious puberty. Growth hormone therapy may be required. It is less clear if chemotherapy alone can impair growth. Testicular radiotherapy renders males sterile, and most will require androgen replacement throughout puberty. Chemotherapy may lead to subfertility, which can improve over time. Ovaries are less sensitive to chemotherapy, but if they are irradiated, estrogen replacement will be necessary. Alkylating agents are also likely to cause gonadal damage.
- Secondary malignancies induced by epipodophyllotoxins (etoposide), radiation, or alkylating agents. Exposure to epipodophyllotoxins has produced an increase in secondary acute leukemia. There has been a marked increase in brain tumors among children who received cranial irradiation before the age of 5 years.
- Osteonecrosis caused by glucocorticoids (prednisolone, dexamethasone). This is most often seen in children over the age of 10 years, with females at greater risk than males (Mattano et al. 2000).
- Altered bone density (osteopenia/osteoporosis) induced by glucocorticoids, which increases susceptibility to fractures.
- Some potential impairment of intellectual development, which is measurable by a fall in IQ of 10–20 points. There may also be subtle neurocognitive late effects that include inattention, hyperactivity, and learning difficulties without significant changes in IQ scores.
- Psychosocial sequelae of the diagnosis of and treatment for leukemia, which are significant. There may be problems regarding relationships, career, insurance, and mortgage application, and emotional issues such as depression, anger, and confusion. Anxiety and post traumatic stress are also potential complications in the post treatment/survivorship phase. Many studies have highlighted the need to include excellent psychosocial care throughout the disease trajectory and beyond.

Approaches to minimize adverse effects without affecting treatment outcome have included the development of new drugs, such as the liposomal formulation of daunorubicin, the use of cardioprotective agents, alternative administration schedules such as continuous infusions/prolonged infusion times (the advantages of which are debatable), and the monitoring of minimal residual disease, which allows for reduction or optimization of drug doses.

1.2.10 Future Perspectives

Remarkable advances have been made by defining the molecular abnormalities involved in leukemogenesis and drug resistance. This has led to the development of promising new therapeutic strategies. Recognition of inherited differences in the metabolism of antileukemic drugs has enabled the selection of optimal drug dosages and scheduling. This could be useful to increase antileukemic effects and to reduce late effects. Future strategies should incorporate more specific risk-directed therapy and greater international collaboration. With subgroups of children with ALL having very favorable features of the disease and a 95% overall survival, the aim of future protocols is likely to focus on how therapy may be decreased to minimize the potential for late effects. The predictive role of MRD will continue to be evaluated. Investigators will need to determine a clinical MRD cut-off value that would define positive or negative early treatment (induction/steroid) response. The development and implementation of monoclonal antibodies in proven ALL protocols for patients with evidence of resistance disease will be important for future trials.

1.2.11 Relapsed ALL

Despite the current excellent survival rate for pediatric ALL, relapsed ALL remains the fourth most common pediatric malignancy and the cause of a significant number of childhood deaths. Although relapse of ALL is more likely in the subgroup of cases of ALL with high-risk features including t(9:22), infants with 11q23 rearrangements, and severe hypodiploidy with chromosomal number less than 44 (Gaynon, 2005), a substantial number of children with relapse were intially diagnosed with standard risk ALL. There are several prognostic features of relapsed ALL which are important for clinical decisions about treatment intensity and specifically, the role of HSCT and selection of suitable transplant donor. These prognostic features include:

- Time of relapse also described as duration of first remission (very early relapse, early relapse, and late relapse)
- Site of relapse (isolated extramedullary relapse (CNS, testicular), isolated bone marrow relapse, combined bone marrow, and extramedullary relapse)
- Immunophenotype (B-lineage vs. T-lineage relapse)

A relapse of T-cell lineage ALL usually occurs early after diagnosis (within the first 18 months post initital diagnosis) and is associated with a very poor overall survival. Patients with relapse of T-cell ALL are generally recommended for HSCT with any available and suitable donor, owing to the significant poor reported survival outcomes.

For relapse of preccursor B-lineage ALL, treatment intensity decisions are based on the site and time of relapse. Investigative groups currently do not use consistent definitions to distinguish between standard and high-risk relapse. The BFM investigative group use a time cut-off of 18 months from initial diagnosis to discern between very early and early relapse. The BFM group defines a relapse occuring beyond 6 months post completion of therapy as a late relapse.

Currently the Children's Oncology Group (COG) uses a time point of 36 months to stratify between a relapse and a high-risk relapse. The COG defines a high-risk relapse as occuring before 36 months from initial diagnosis.

Site of relapse is also prognostic in relapsed ALL. Isolated extrameduallary relapse of pre-B-cell ALL is quite uncommon. However, when an isolated extramedullary relapse occurs and is defined as late, it is often curable without HSCT (Barredo et al. 2006). The prognosis for isolated extrameduallary precursor B-cell ALL is approximately 70%, with further intensified chemotherapy and with radiation to the appropriate site (CNS, testis).

The most common site of ALL relapse is the isolated bone marrow relapse. The timing of the bone marrow relapse followed by the response to salvage chemotherapy are important for clinical decision making. An early bone marrow relapse is generally recommended for HSCT with any suitable donor available. A late relapse is often treated with chemotherapy alone; however, this descision will also depend on the response to treatment. Similar to frontline ALL therapy, an evaluation of remission status by morphology is carried out at the end of the first induction cycle of relapsed therapy.

The definitions of remission are the same as the frontline ALL therapy, with the exception of MRD. Currently, the use of MRD is being evaluated in relapsed ALL clinical trials to determine the specific time point of evaluation that is clinically relevant. The BFM investigative group uses a time point of 5 weeks following the start of relapsed therapy to assess MRD response. At this point, an evaluation of MRD is assessed to determine if further treatment intensity in the form of HSCT is indicated, specifically for the late relapse subgroup. Patients who remain persistantly MRD positive at 5 and 7 weeks post induction therapy for relapsed ALL are generally recommended for HSCT. The MRD-positive post induction therapy for relapsed ALL may represent resistance to disease that has a significantly poor prognosis. The clinical significance of MRD in relapsed ALL remains unclear and clinical trials are ongoing, similar to first-diagnosis ALL treatments.

The goal of relapsed ALL treatment is to induce a remission and then consolidate the remission with either further continuation chemotherapy or HSCT. These treatment goals are similar to those of ALL therapy as previously described. Various relapse induction regimens have been investigated, and it has been reported that a second remission is acheivable in approximately 70% of early relapses and 96% of late relapses of ALL (Harned and Gaynon 2008). The challenge of consolidation and continuation therapy is to maintain the clinical remission, and this is achieved with further chemotherapy and/or HSCT. If HSCT is recommended, it is imnportant to maintain

Table 1.9. New agents in the treatment of ALL and Relapsed ALL

	Mechanism of action	Target subtype of ALL
Monoclonal antibodies		
Rituxamab	Antibody against CD 20	B-lineage ALL
Daclizumab	Antibody IL2 receptor (CD 25)	T-lineage ALL
Epratuzamab	Antibody against CD 22	B-lineage ALL
Alemtuzamab	Antibody against CD 52	B- and T-lineage ALL
Small molecule inhibitors		
Imatinib	Inhibition of BCR-ABL	Philadelphia + ALL
Dasatinib	Inhibition of BCR-ABL	Philadelphia + ALL
Bortezomib	Inhibition of NF-κb	B- and T-lineage ALL
Sirolimus	Inhibition of mTOR	B- and T-lineage ALL
Nucleoside analogues		
Clofarabine	Deoxyadenosine analog	B- and T-lineage ALL
Nelarabine	Deoxyadenosine analog	T-lineage ALL

the remission of leukemia with intensive therapy while the donor search is ongoing. Relapse therapy for ALL is higher in intensity than frontline ALL therapies, and is associated with signficant toxicity.

Treatment of relapsed ALL remains a challenge. Future directions should include the timing and cut-off value of MRD in relapsed ALL. Specifically, issues such as when is an MRD value clinically important and what value indicates a significantly poor prognosis indicating that treatment intensification is necessary should be addressed. New agents will be important in the treatment of relapsed ALL. Clofarabine is one agent that has shown evidence of antileukemic effect in patients with relapsed or refractory ALL (Jeha et al. 2004). Other agents currently being investigated in the treatment of relapsed disease are outlined in Table 1.9.

1.3 Acute Myeloid Leukemia

1.3.1 Epidemiology

AML is most often observed in adults over the age of 40 years, but the annual incidence of childhood AML is approximately 5–7 per million, and is constant from birth to 10 years of age. Incidence peaks slightly in adolescence, and AML is the more common leukemia found in neonates. Both boys and girls appear to be affected equally. It is generally reported that AML is equally distributed among ethnic groups, but a study by McKinney et al. (2003) indicated a significantly higher incidence of AML among South Asians in an urban English city. The FAB classification subtypes are represented equally across racial and ethnic groups; however, the subgroup AML M3 (APML) has a slightly higher incidence in children of Latin or Hispanic decent (Rubnitz et al. 2008). Although the incidence of AML has historically remained stable, a recent increase in the incidence of secondary AML has emerged. The risk of secondary AML is associated with exposure to high cumulative doses of alkylating agents.

Children with Down Syndrome (DS) have a disproportionate and increased risk of AML with an estimated 10–15-fold increase in incidence compared with that of the general childhood population (Hasle et al. 2000). It is estimated that approximately 10% of newborn children with DS will have transient leukemia (TL). This reported incidence may probably be lower than the true value owing to the lack of screening of all newborns with DS. Among these newborns, with DS and TL, approximately 20% may develop AMKL before 5 years of age.

1.3.2 Etiology

1.3.2.1 Genetic Factors

The various conditions that have a predisposition to AML are akin to those of any acute leukemia

(Table 1.2), with the addition of myelodysplastic syndrome (monosomy 7).

1.3.2.2 Environmental Factors

Similarly, the risk factors associated with AML are the same as those for ALL (see Table 1.3). Interestingly, allergy or a family history of allergy (including hay fever, neurodermatitis, asthma, and, to a lesser degree, eczema) has been associated with a decreased risk of ALL, but not of AML (Schuz et al. 2003).

Until recently, a Vietnam-era herbicide, Agent Orange (dioxin), was reported to be a parental exposure link to childhood AML. However, subsequent studies have ruled out any increased risk (Ahmad 2002).

1.3.3 Molecular Genetics

The defect that occurs in AML appears to be an arrest in the differentiation combined with an increase in the proliferation or cell survival. Fusion genes generated by translocations of chromosomes frequently cause these functional effects. These genes can be detected by PCR, and clonal chromosomal abnormalities of dividing bone marrow cells have been identified in more than 70% of children diagnosed with AML. The most common fusion genes detected in AML are:

- AML1/ETO from t(8:21), most often seen in acute myeloblastic leukemia
- MLL/AF10 from t(10:11)
- Inversion of parts of chromosome 16 (creating the fusion gene CBFB-MYH11)
- Trisomy 8
- Monosomy 7
- PML/RARα from t(15:17), the most common fusion gene of acute promyelocytic leukemia (APL)

Fusions involving the MLL gene occur in about 15% of AML cases. These fusions are thought to be fetal in origin, as this fusion is often detected on the Guthrie card or neonatal blood spot of those children who subsequently develop AML. This is possibly the initiating event in childhood AML that requires additional secondary genetic alterations to cause leukemia.

1.3.4 Symptoms and Clinical Signs

AML can have a similar presentation to that of ALL, with symptoms appearing 1–6 weeks before diagnosis. The symptoms of AML result from infiltration of leukemic blasts in the bone marrow and extramedulary sites. The presenting signs and symptoms often include the following:

- Pallor
- Fatigue, weakness
- Petechiae
- Bleeding
- Fever, infection
- Sore throat
- Lymphadenopathy
- Skin lesions
- Gastrointestinal symptoms, including pain, nausea, and vomiting
- Gingival changes (gingival hypertrophy) or infiltrates

Additional signs and symptoms in AML may be caused by chloromas (also called granulocytic sarcomas or myeloblastomas), which are localized collections of leukemic blasts. The presence of a chloroma at diagnosis does not affect overall prognosis. Presentation with bleeding can be due to disseminated intravascular coagulation (DIC) and may be life-threatening in the AML acute promyelocytic leukemia (APL). DIC can occur as a result of the release of procoagulants from abnormal promyelocytic granules (see Chap. 19). Complaints of bone pain are less common in AML, and hepatosplenomegaly is more marked in infants with AML. Testicular involement of AML is rare.

CNS involvement of AML, occurring in 5–15% of cases, can cause symptoms similar to those of CNS involvement in ALL, such as:

- Headache
- Poor school performance
- Weakness
- Vomiting
- Blurred vision
- Seizures
- Difficulty maintaining balance

Hyperleukocytosis can be present at diagnosis of childhood AML and may or may nor require leukopheresis therapy. Similar to ALL, early cytoreductive therapy with chemotherapy is important in patients with hyperleukocytosis.

1.3.5 Diagnostics

If the history and physical examination suggest leukemia, examination of peripheral blood and bone marrow samples is required to confirm the diagnosis. Bone marrow findings include a hypercellular trephine/biopsy sample and an aspirate sample showing more than 20% blast cells. The diagnosis and subtype of AML is determined by morphololgy, immunochemistry, and cytogenetic and molecular evaluation of the blast cells.

The treatment for AML is distinctively different from ALL, making the distinction between these two leukemia types extremely important. Cytochemical staining of bone marrow smears can help to differentiate between AML and ALL. Common stains include Sudan black stain, myeloperoxidase, and non specific esterase. These stains will most often be positive in AML and negative in ALL. Immunophenotyping by flow cytometry provides further information about the originating cell line, further differentiating AML from ALL. Common AML antigens include CD33, CD15, CD14, CD41, CD15, CD11b, and CD36. Additionally, surface cell and cytoplasmic markers will be valuble in distinguishing AML. Monoclonal surface antigen and cytoplasmic immunoglobulin heavy chains are usually absent in AML. Immunophenotyping can also be used to distinguish FAB subtypes of AML. Of these, the HLA-DR antigen is the most useful in identifying the AML M3 (APL) subtype. In AML, the HLA-DR antigen is commonly expressed (75–80%), but rarely expressed in APL.

In AML, it is important to identify subtypes that are treated on unique protocols or require less intensive therapy. The determination of subtype is done by cytogenetic and molecular testing. Specific recurring subtypes of AML associated with a more favorable prognosis are:

- AML with t(8:21)
- AML with inversion 16
- AML with t(15:17) (APL)
- AML in DS (most frequently of the megakaryocytic subtype M7)

Subtypes of AML with chromosomal abnormalities associated with a poor prognosis include:

- Abnormalities with chromosome 3, 5, and 7 (monosomy 7, monosomy 5, and del 5q, inv3 or t(3:3)(q21126))
- AML with FLT 3 mutations

1.3.6 Staging and Classification

There is presently no therapeutically or prognostically meaningful staging system for AML. Risk stratification is less clear in AML compared with ALL. The original FAB classification system categorized AML into major AML subtypes based on morphology and immunophenotyping. The World Health Organization (WHO) classification system for AML is more comprehensive, including clinical, morphologic, cytogenetic, and molecular data.

If the myeloid cell line is involved and a diagnosis of AML is confirmed, the FAB classification system for AML is applied. There are eight different classifications or types of AML (M0–M7), based on the appearance of the diseased cells under the microscope (Table 1.10).

Table 1.10. French–American–British (FAB) classification of acute myeloid leukemia

FAB group	Cell morphology
M0	Myeloid leukemia with minimal differentiation
M1	Myeloblastic leukemia with little differentiation
M2	Myeloblastic leukemia with differentiation
M3	Promyelocytic leukemia with t(15:17) translocation
M4	Myelomonocytic leukemia
M5	Monocytic leukemia: M5a – without differentiation M5b – with differentiation
M6	Erythroblastic leukemia
M7	Megakaryoblastic leukemia

Each subtype refers to the particular myeloid lineage affected and the degree of blast-cell differentiation. This standardization began in 1976, but with improvements in treatment outcome, this approach to classification has limited clinical relevance. Approximately 80% of children less than 2 years of age have either M4 or M5 FAB subtypes. M7 is most common in children under 3 years of age, particularly in those with DS.

Myelodysplastic syndrome (MDS) is a preleukemic syndrome that has a relationship with some types of AML (MDS-related AML or MDR-AML). In children, the majority of AML occurs de novo (see below), and fewer than 15% of childhood AML cases follow MDS. The other main group of AML consists of cases unrelated to MDS, with a suggested name of de novo AML. This led to subclassification of AML based on its relationship with MDS. The WHO attempted to refine the FAB classification by incorporating the AML/MDS relationship. This classification, shown in Table 1.11, has been a cause for debate over the past few years. However, the WHO classification incorporates subcategories of AML with recurring translocations, AML related to MDS, and subsets of treatment-related AML based on their relation to the first two groups. Therefore, this system may assist clinical decisions and be useful in analyzing the biological studies of AML. It may be noted that MDS-AML is more prominent in the elderly, with only 15% of cases observed in children and young adults. The de novo AML group, related to a set of recurring cytogenetic translocations and inversions, has a median age approximating the median age of the population (Head 2002).

1.3.7 Treatment

The most dramatic improvement of outcomes for children with AML has resulted from intensively timed therapy over a brief period of time. Treatment usually includes two phases; an induction phase followed by a consoldiation phase. During both of these phases, CNS-directed therapy in the form of IT chemotherapy is included. A maintenance phase is not required for AML with the exception of APL. The goal of the induction phase is to induce a remission.

Table 1.11. World Health Organization classification of acute myeloid leukemia

Group	Subgroups
Acute myeloid leukemia with recurrent genetic abnormalities	Acute myeloid leukemia with t(8:21) Acute myeloid leukemia with abnormal bone marrow eosinophils inv(16) or t(16:16) Acute promyelocytic leukemia (AML with t(15:17) and variants Acute myeloid leukemia with MLL abnormalities
Acute myeloid leukemia with multilineage dysplasia	Following MDS or MDS/myeloproliferative disorder Without antecedent myelodysplastic syndrome
Acute myeloid leukemia and MDS, therapy related	Alkylating agent-related Topoisomerase type II inhibitor-related Other types
Acute myeloid leukemia not otherwise specified	Acute myeloid leukemia minimally differentiatedAcute myeloid leukemia without maturation Acute myeloid leukemia with maturation Acute myelomonocytic leukemia Acute monoblastic and monocytic leukemia Acute erythroid leukemia Acute megakaryoblastic leukemia Acute basophilic leukemia Acute panmyelosis with myelofibrosis Myeloid sarcoma

Adapted from (Head 2002)

Intensive induction therapy successfully induces remission in 75–90% of children and adolescents with AML. A confirmed remission by the end of the second induction cycle has been found to be independently prognostic with those not achieving remission having evidence of resistant disease and a poor prognosis. Remission in AML is defined by morphologic blast count in the bone marrow. At present, the clinical role of MRD in the treatment of AML has not been clearly determined (Perea et al. 2006). Induction chemotherapy generally consists of two courses of anthracycline and cytarabine in combination with etoposide or thioguanine, intensively timed. Landmark studies have shown that intensive timing of the second induction cycle (delivered approximately 6–10 days following the completion of the first induction cycle), regardless of neutrophil and bone marrow recovery, has shown an improved clinical remission and event-free survival compared with the standard timing (approximately 14 days following completion of first cycle and dependent on bone marrow recovery) (Woods et al. 1996). Owing to this intensive timing, the implemetation and improvement in supportive care guidelines have been crucial. Pediatric patients with AML require blood-product support, aggressive management of infectious complications, and access to a pediatric intensive care unit. Following induction therapy is consolidation, consisting of either continued chemotherpay or allogeneic HSCT. The goal and challenge of consolidation therapy is to prolong and maintain the remission.

Various factors are involved in the decision to recommend HSCT including: cytogenetic features, disease response, and availability of a suitable donor. For the small group of patients with favorable cytogenetics such as t(15:17), t(8:21), or inv(16), intensive continued chemotherapy may be the treatment of choice even if a matched sibling donor is available (Sung et al. 2003). These patients would be transplanted only in the event of a relapse if a second remission is acheived. For children without favorable cytogenetic features of AML, HSCT is recommended if there is an available sibling donor. For pediatric patients who have unfavorable cytogenetic features or who do not achieve a remission status at the completion of the second induction phase, HSCT is recommended regardless of the HSCT donor type available. Therefore, this subgroup of patients would be recommended for an unrelated donor transplant if a family donor is not available. There is no evidence to suggest that autologous transplant is of benefit in pediatric acute leukemia (Part 3 will cover stem cell transplants in detail).

With the current protocols, the overall survival remains poor at approximately 50–60%. Future protocols in development cannot further intensify therapy owing to the current intensive schedule. Therefore, investigators are developing and trialing targeted therapies that will not further add to the current hematopoetic toxicity of therapy. Gemtuzumab ozogamicin (GMTZ) is an example of a current targeted therapy for AML that is in clinical trials. GMTZ is a recombinant anti-CD33 monoclonal antibody linked to the potent cytotoxic agent, calicheamicin.

Two subtypes of AML are treated on unique protocols:

- APL
- AML in young children with DS (age <4 years)

APL (i.e., FAB subtype M3) is treated by chemotherapy protocols that combine all-transretinoic acid (ATRA) with combination chemotherapy (Riberiro 2006). Children and adolescents with APL successully achieve a remission and cure in most children with AML of this type. This outcome is possible due to the translocation of t(15:17) involving a breakpoint that includes the retinoid acid receptor. However, administration of ATRA is associated with the risk of retinoic acid sydrome, known as RAS. RAS occurs approximately 7 days after the start of ATRA therapy (range 1–35 days) and has symptoms of respiratory distress, fever, weight gain, peripheral edema, hypotension, and renal and cardiac insufficiency. A chest X-ray will often show pulmonary infiltrates and pleuropericardal effusions. It is critical to promptly recognize these symptoms so that treatment with steroids, usually dexamethasone can begin. Another common complication of ATRA therapy is pseudotumor cerebri which has presenting symptoms of headache, blurred vision, and papilloedema. The APL subtype is associated with severe coagulopathy at the time of diagnosis. Fatal hemorrhagic complications can occur before or during induction in this subtype. There is a low incidence of CNS disease in children with APL and therefore, an initial diagnostic lumbar puncture is not performed because of the significant risk of bleeding. Pediatric patients with the APL subtype are not recommended for HSCT in first relapse. Most relapse protocols for APL contain arsenic trioxide. Approximately 85% of patients can achieve a second remission with the administration of arsenic trioxide after a first relapse. It must be noted that for patients receiving arsenic trioxide it is important to closely monitor serum electrolyte concentrations and maintain serum potassium and magnesium levels in the normal range. This is due to the potential for arrhythmias (specifically prolonged QT interval) in patients on arsenic trioxide treatment. Current pediatric trials involve the combination of arsenic trioxide with ATRA and chemotherapy as frontline therapy for APL. The goal of introducing arsenic trioxide into the frontline therapies is to hopefully reduce the cumulative dose of anthracyclines.

DS patients less than 4 years of age with AML have a markedly increased responsiveness to therapy. The blast cells of this group of children appear to have a unique biology and are very sensitive to both anthracycline and cytarabine chemotherapy. Owing to this sensitivity, AML protocols have been tailored specifically for this population of children. On tailored protocols, the event-free survival for children with DS less than 4 years of age is approximately 85%. Therefore, in this population HSCT in first remission is not recommended. Children with DS who are diagnosed with AML after the age of 4 years do not maintain this excellent overall survival, and in fact tend to have a prognosis similar to children with AML without DS. The current recommendation for this group is standard AML treatment. Infants with DS are commonly diagnosed with TL or transient myeloproliferative disorder (TMD) during the first few months of life. The blast cells of TL are indistinguishable from the blast cells of AMKL. However, there is spontaneous resolution of TL without intervention with chemotherapy. In rare cases, a short course of low-dose cytarabine is required if the infant has evidence of organ involvement or failure. In approximatley 20% of the cases of TL, the children will develop AML before the age of 3 years (Zwaan et al. 2008). In almost all the cases of TL and AMKL with DS, the leukemic blasts contain *GATA1* mutations.

1.3.8 Prognosis

Despite significant improvements in the outcomes of children with AML, the cure rate is only approximately 50%. About 50% of children are found to have AML relapse, and there remains little information about the best treatment for this group of children.

1.3.9 Follow-Up

Children and adolescents need appropriate and sensitive follow-up. The specific features of follow-up for AML concern the increased incidence of relapse and the increased number of children and adolescents who receive transplant as a standard modality of treatment.

1.3.10 Future Perspectives

The progress in therapy for AML lags behind that for ALL. The estimated overall survival rate for AML of 50–60% is significantly less than the estimated 80% overall survival for childhood ALL. Allogeneic bone marrow transplant appears to remain the best option for most patients who do not present with favorable features of their disease. Only a limited population of children and adolescents with AML present with favorable features of their disease and will not be recommended for transplant in the first remission. Allogeneic transplant from either a matched family donor or an unrelated donor continues to be a significant cause of treatment-related deaths and treatment-related morbidity for children with AML. It will therefore be important to continue to refine the risk classification and assign risk-directed therapy based on the genetics of the leukemia blasts and response to therapy.

Drug resistance is an apparent factor in treatment failure of AML. Investigating causes of drug resistance in AML including the detetion of minimal residual disease continues to be a research and clinical priority. In adult patients with AML, the expression of the multidrug resistance gene (MRD1) defines a poor prognostic group. This is not a similar finding in children with AML .A study by Steinbach et al. (2003) investigated the expression of five of the genes encoding the multidrug resistance-associated proteins (MRP) in children with AML and their response to chemotherapy. Expression of MRP3 was found to be involved in drug resistance, producing a poorer prognosis, and the expression of MRP2 was, to a lesser extent, also associated with poor prognosis. Expression of high levels of both these genes indicated a particularly poor prognosis. This study suggests that these proteins, MRP3 and possibly MRP2, could provide markers for risk-adapted therapy and possible targets for the development of drugs that would overcome multidrug resistance in childhood AML.

AML therapy cannot be further intensified in either dosing or timing of chemotherapy. Alternative approaches to therapy may include risk-directed therapy based on different prognostic criteria, differentiation therapy with all-trans-retinoic acid, immunotherapy with monoclonal antibodies, or tumor vaccines. The effectiveness of targeted therapy, such as Gemtuzamab ozogamicin (GMTZ), and of kinase inhibitors will continue to be an area of clinical research. The activation of FLT 3 mutation portends a poor prognosis in AML, and a targeted small molecule inhibitor has shown promise in adult patients with AML (Brown and Smith 2008). To date, clinical trials of FLT 3 inhibitors in pediatrics are limited and will be an area of future research.

1.4 Chronic Myeloid Leukemia

1.4.1 Epidemiology and Etiology

An increase in the incidence of adult chronic myeloid leukemia (CML) has been observed in three populations:

- The Japanese exposed to radiation released from atomic bombs in Nagasaki and Hiroshima
- Patients with ankylosing spondylitis treated with spine irradiation
- Women with uterine cervical carcinoma who received radiation treatment (Freedman 1994)

Despite this obvious relationship between radiation and CML, only 5–7% of adult cases of CML have documented exposure to excessive radiation, and previous exposure is infrequent in children with CML (Freedman 1994). CML accounts for less than 5% of childhood leukemia diagnoses, making it quite rare. In patients younger than 20 years of age, the incidence is less than 1 in 100,000, with 80% of these cases being over the age of 4 years. In the pediatric age group, CML most commonly occurs in older adolescents.

1.4.2 Molecular Genetics

CML is normally a hematological disease of the elderly, characterized by the BCR/ABL oncogene caused by a translocation between the ABL gene on Ch'9 and the BCR gene on Ch'22. The resulting chromosome 22, with a shortening of the long arm, is known as the Philadelphia (Ph') chromosome. The BCR/ABL gene fusion product is thought to be causative in CML, and has multiple effects on diverse cell functions, such as growth, differentiation, adhesion, and apoptosis.

1.4.3 Symptoms and Clinical Signs

In CML, there are three clinical phases: chronic, accelerated, and blast-crisis. The "chronic phase" of leukemia evolves into a more rapidly progressive phase known as the "accelerated phase" and ultimately "blast crisis." The chronic phase lasts about 3 years, but can range from a few months to 20 years. The accelerated phase generally occurs over a 3–6-month period. The final phase is generally resistant to current treatment and is therefore considered fatal.

The signs and symptoms of CML can vary depending on the phase the disease has reached:

- The *chronic phase* has a nonspecific onset over weeks to months, with complaints of fatigue, anorexia, weight loss, and excessive sweating. Physical presentation includes pallor, bruising, low-grade fever, sternal bone pain, and splenomegaly that is sometimes accompanied by hepatomegaly.
- Signs and symptoms of the *accelerated phase* present over a few months and are similar to those

of the chronic phase, but with more episodes of unexplained fever, lymphadenopathy, bruising, and petechiae caused by thrombocytopenia. The accelerated phase also presents with progressive splenomegaly, and an increasing percentage of peripheral and bone marrow blasts.

- The *blastic phase* presents with symptoms identical to those of acute leukemia.

1.4.4 Diagnostics

CML is characterized by the presence of large numbers of granulocytes in the blood, with mild anemia and thrombocytosis. Furthermore, the numbers of basophils and eosinophils are increased. A characteristic laboratory feature is a marked reduction or absence in the leukocyte alkaline phosphatase (LAP) activity, which results from a decrease in monocytes that normally secrete a factor that induces LAP activity (Freedman 1994).

Cytogenetic analysis of the marrow cells displays the Philadelphia chromosome in over 90% of new patients with CML. Absence of cytogenetic or molecular abnormalities rules out the diagnosis of CML.

1.4.5 Treatment

In children with CML, allogeneic bone marrow transplant has been considered the treatment of choice. This treatment has been providing promising survival rates even in the event of advanced disease and histoincompatibility with donor marrow (Sharathkumar et al. 2002). Another treatment that has produced encouraging results, reported by Millot et al. (2002), uses a combination of interferon and cytarabine for children with Philadelphia-chromosome-positive CML. This may offer an alternative to transplantation in children and adolescents in the chronic phase of CML. Treatment with HSCT is most effective when the transplant is done during the chronic phase of disease. Recently, the introduction of Imatinib mesylate (Gleevec) has significantly changed the treatment of CML (Deininger et al. 2005). Imatinib mesylate can induce a remission both clinically and molecularly when it is administered during the chronic phase of disease. Imatinib mesylate has almost completely replaced interferon in the treatment of CML (O'Brien et al. 2003; Druker et al. 2006). The evidence for imatinib mesylate as the standard of care therapy is strong for adults with CML, but there are limited studies in children. It appears that imatinib mesylate has the same effectiveness in children with CML, although there is no evidence that it is curative, making HSCT the only currently known curative therapy in pediatrics (Champagne et al. 2004). Researchers will continue to evaluate the role of imatinib mesylate in the treatment of CML in children as well as other new agents known as second generation BCR-ABL inhibitors, such as dasatinib and nilotinib.

1.4.6 Prognosis

For children with the adult form of CML, the importance of prognostic factors is difficult to define owing to the low incidence of the disease. Remissions can be induced, but relapse is common and long-term survivors are rare.

1.4.7 Future Perspectives

For children with CML, current efforts should aim to reduce transplant-related deaths. Current trials are attempting to reduce the side effects of myeloblative HSCT by using reduced conditioning regimens. The role of imatinib and other BCR-ABL inhibitors will continue to be investigated both as single agent therapy and in combination with HSCT. Cytogenetic studies to identify further risk factors will assist in the understanding of the biology of this disease.

1.5 Juvenile Myelomonocytic Leukemia

Juvenile myelomonocytic leukemia (JMML) is a rare but distinct form of chilhood leukemia, formerly called juvenile chronic myeloid leukemia (JCML). This subgroup represents less than 1% of cases of childhood leukemia, and has an incidence of 1–2 cases per million annually. Controversy surrounds the classification of this subgroup, and it was also termed as chronic myelomonocytic leukemia (CMML). Most patients are less than 2 years of age, with 95% younger than 4 years (Freedman 1994).

Children frequently present with complaints of malaise, bleeding, or fever, often with localized infection. Less common presentations include pulmonary symptoms (cough, wheezing, tachypnea), abdominal distension and discomfort, weight loss, and occasionally bone pain. On examination, splenomegaly is often observed as a frequent feature, and pallor and hepatomegaly may also be present. Skin manifestations may be seen, with an eczematous rash that is unresponsive to topical treatment. Xanthoma and café-au-lait spots are often associated with JMML. These skins findings are also common in neurofibromatosis, and an interrelationship between neurofibromatosis and JMML has been established (Freedman 1994). JMML is associated with neurofibromatosis type I in 11% of the cases (Niemeyer and Kratz 2008).

The diagnosis of JMML is made on clinical assessment as well as peripheral blood and bone marrow evaluations. Peripheral blood samples show an increasing number of circulating monocytes (monocytosis) in all the cases. The monocyte value must exceed 1×10^9/L to make a diagnosis of JMML. Immature granulocytes, anemia, and thrombocytopenia are also frequently present. The cells in JMML do not contain the Philadelphia chromosome, although other chromosomal abnormalities are present.

Bone marrow findings are not themselves diagnostic, but are consistent with the diagnosis. Bone marrow findings generally will include:

- Bone Marrow hypercellularity with a predominance of granulocytes at all stages of maturation
- Monocytosis, but less pronounced than in the peripheral blood
- Increased blast count but not to the level seen in acute leukemia
- Megakaryoctes are often reduced
- Thrombocytopenia is common

Cytogenetic evaluation will often show a normal karyotype, but in approximately 25% of the cases, monosomy 7 will be present.

Although JMML does not routinely convert to a blast crisis, the disease is considered fatal without treatment by HSCT. There is no current clinical agreement on the antileukemic therapy that is most effective pre-HSCT for patients with JMML. Recent studies have shown that an approximately 50% EFS can be achieved when the child receives HSCT from a matched related donor (Niemeyer and Kratz 2008). Other studies have reported 45% 2-year survival for children with JMML receiving HSCT from an unrelated cord transplant when a matched family donor was unavailable (Madureira et al. 2007). Currently, no data is available on the effectiveness of Haplo stem cell transplant for patients with JMML.

Future directions in the management of JMML will need to include the cooperation of many investigative groups owing to the rarity of this disease. The role and intensity of pre-HSCT treatment will continue to be a focus of research. However, it has been called into question whether high-intensity therapy such as standard AML therapy offers any advantage compared with low-dose therapy with mercaptopurine or no antileukemic therapy prior to transplantation. A better understanding of the biology of the disease will aim at identifying a subgroup of patients with JMML who might be cured without intensive HSCT. Of particular interest will be patients with an RAS mutation, where there is the suggestion of spontaneous remission and hematological improvement (Matsuda et al. 2007).

1.6 Langerhans Cell Histiocytosis

Histiocytosis is not defined as a malignancy, but it is treated with cancer therapies (e.g., chemotherapy, radiotherapy) and pediatric oncology nurses may be involved in the care of a child with Langerhans cell histiocytosis (LCH).

1.6.1 Epidemiology and Etiology

An epidemiology study found that the age-standardized incidence rate of LCH in children aged 0–14 years was 4.1 per million per year with a slight predominance in males (Salotti et al. 2009). However, the Histiocytosis Association of America has reported a higher incidence of 8.9 per million (Histiocytosis Association of America 2009). Incidence rates can also vary significantly by age at diagnosis, with a much higher incidence in children under 1 year of age compared with a significantly lower incidence in the 10–14-year-old group (Alston et al. 2007).

Histiocytes are normal cells in the immune system found in the bone marrow, blood, skin, liver, lungs, lymph glands, and spleen. Histiocytosis identifies a group of disorders that have proliferation of cells of the mononuclear phagocyte (monocytes and macrophages) and dendritic cell systems. In LCH, the histiocytes move into tissues where they are not normally found and cause damage to those tissues. The accumulated cells, with characteristics of epidermal dendritic cells, are called Langerhans cells. The accumulation results in granulomatous, yellow–brown lesions. These lesions are also made up of other cell types such as macrophages, multinucleated giant cells, stromal cells, and natural killer cells. Identification of Langerhans cells requires electron microscopy. All Langerhans cells are differentiated from the bone marrow, but are considered to be derived from lymphoid and myeloid lineages (Grifo 2009).

The cause of LCH is unknown. Suggested hypotheses include the possibility of clonal abnormalities, cytokine or chemokine abnormality causing abnormal expression of Langerhans cells, a combination of oncogenesis and immune dysregulation (Egeler et al. 2004), and lesional Langerhans cells that control the persistence and progression themselves (Annels et al. 2003).

The Histiocyte Society, an international body, was formed in 1987 and has outlined morphology, immunohistiochemistry, and clinical criteria required for LCH.

1.6.2 Diagnostics

A diagnosis of LCH is usually made following a biopsy and microscopic examination of the affected tissue. A complete physical examination will be carries out, to check all of the commonly affected body systems. Other tests may then be necessary to determine the extent of disease, so that a treatment plan can be made. As LCH can be present in many areas of the body, tests can include complete blood count and blood chemistries, radiographs, urine tests, CT scans, and tissue or skin biopsy.

1.6.3 Symptoms and Clinical Signs

The symptoms of LCH are dependent on the body system involved, and are listed in Table 1.12. Single-system (localized) LCH usually disappears on its own without any treatment. This may account for the underestimated incidence rate with some missed cases either diagnosed or undiagnosed. Single-system (predominantly bony involvement) accounts for the largest proportion of cases (Salotti et al. 2009).

Table 1.12. Common symptoms of histiocytosis

System	Symptom
Gastrointestinal	Abdominal pain, vomiting, diarrhea, jaundice, weight loss, esophageal bleeding
Bone	Bone pain, headaches (skull lesions), limp (leg lesions)
CNS (brain)	Diabetes insipidus, mental deterioration, headaches, dizziness, seizures, increased intracranial pressure
CNS (pituitary gland)	Polydipsia, polyuria, dehydration, short stature, delayed puberty
Pulmonary	Feeding problems (infants), chest pain, dyspnea, cough, hemoptysis
Oral	Facial swelling and pain, loss of teeth, swollen and bleeding gingiva, swollen lymph nodes
Skin	Scaly rash
Ear	Inflammed, draining ear canal, rash behind the ears

1.6.4 Treatment

Although treated with chemotherapy, there has been no specific research trial for the use of cytotoxic therapy in LCH. In a small number of children, treatment will be needed and low-dose radiotherapy, surgery, and steroids may be used. Multi-system (disseminated) disease is usually treated with chemotherapy and steroids. The combination and duration of therapy will vary depending on the severity of the illness.

LCH is radiosensitive, but has been restricted in children owing to the late toxicities and potential effects on growth development. It may be considered if there is evidence of disease progression or threat to visceral organs. It may be used for isolated lesions of spine or femur (McClain 2005).

1.6.5 Prognosis

Eighty percent of children who develop LCH will recover from it. A small number of children may develop side effects many years later, because of the treatment they have received. This is more likely to happen when treatments have been intensive. Possible late side effects include reduced growth impairment, infertility, pulmonary and cardiac abnormalities, and second malignancy.

References

American Academy of Pediatrics Committee on Fetus and Newborn (2003) Controversies concerning vitamin K and the newborn. American Academy of Pediatrics Committee on Fetus and Newborn. Pediatrics112(1 Pt 1):191–192

Ahmad K (2002) Agent Orange no longer linked to childhood AML. The Lancet Oncology 3(4):199

Alexander FE, Boyle P, Carli PM, Coebergh JW, Ekbom A, Levi F, McKinney PA, McWhirter W, Michaelis J, Peris-Bonet R, Petridou E, Pompe-Kirn V, Plesko I, Pukkala E, Rahu M, Stiller CA, Storm H, Terracini B, Vatten L, Wray N (1999) Population density and childhood leukaemia: results of the EUROCLUS Study. European Journal of Cancer 35(3):439–444

Alston RD, Tatevossian RG, McNally RJ, Kelsey A, Birch JM, Eden TO (2007) Incidence and survival of childhood Langerhans cell histiocytosis in Northwest England from 1954 to 1998. Pediatric Blood Cancer 48(5):555–560

Annels NE, Da Costa CE, Prins FA, Willemze A, Hogendoorn ERM (2003) Aberrant chemokine receptor expression and chemokine production by Langerhans cells underlies the pathogenesis of Langerhans cell histiocytosis. Journal of Experimental Medicine 197(10):1385–1390

Auvinen A, Kurttio P, Pekkanen J, Pukkala E, Ilus T, Salonen L (2002) Uranium and other natural radionuclides in drinking water and risk of leukemia: a case-cohort study in Finland. Cancer Causes and Control 13(9):825–829

Barredo J, Devidas M, Lauer S, Billett A, Marymount M, Pullen J, Camitta B, Winick N, Carroll W, Ritchey K (2006) Isolated CNS relapse of acute lymphoblastic leukemia treated with intensive systemic chemotherapy and delayed CNS radiation: a pediatric oncology group study. Journal of Clinical Oncology 24(19):3142–3149

Bener A, Hoffmann GF, Afify Z, Rasul K, Tewfik I (2008) Does prolonged breastfeeding reduce the risk for childhood leukemia and lymphomas? Minerva Pediatrica 60(2): 155–161

Bergh T, Ericson A, Hillensjo T, Nygren KG, Wennerholm UB (1999) Deliveries and children born after in-vitro fertilization in Sweden 1982–1995: a retrospective cohort study. Lancet 354(9190):1579–1585

Bhatia S, Sather HN, Heerema NA, Trigg ME, Gaynon PS, Robison LL (2002) Racial and ethnic differences in survival of children with acute lymphoblastic leukemia. Blood 100(6):1957–1964

Boutou O, Guizard AV, Slama R, Pottier D, Spira A (2002) Population mixing and leukaemia in young people around the la Hague nuclear waste reprocessing plant. British Journal of Cancer 87(7):740–745

Brown P, Smith FO (2008) Molecularly targeted therapies for pediatric acute myeloid leukemia: progress to date. Paediatric Drugs 10(2):85–92

Champagne MA, Capdeville R, Krailo MWQ, Peng B, Rosamilia M, Therrien M, Zoellner U, Blaney SM, Bernstein M (2004) Imatinib mesylate (STI571) for the treatment of children with Philadelphia chromosome-positive leukemia: results from a children's oncology group phase 1 study. Blood 104(9): 2655–2660

Chessells JM, Harrison G, Richards SM, Gibson BE, Bailey CC, Hill FG, Hann IM (2002) Failure of a new protocol to improve treatment results in paediatric lymphoblastic leukaemia: lessons from the UK Medical Research Council trials UKALL X and UKALL XI. British Journal of Haematology 118(2):445–455

Couto E, Chen B, Hemminki K (2005) Association of childhood acute lymphoblastic leukemia with cancers in family members. British Journal of Cancer 93(11):1307–1309

Deininger M, Buchdunger E, Druker BJ (2005) The development of imatinib as a therapeutic agent for chronic myeloid leukemia. Blood 105(7):2640–2653

Dickinson HO, Hammal DM, Dummer TJB, Parker L, Bithell JF (2003) Childhood leukaemia and non-Hodgkin's lymphoma in relation to proximity to railways. British Journal of Cancer 88(5):695–698

Doll R, Wakeford R (1997) Risk of childhood cancer from fetal irradiation. The British Journal of Radiology 70:130–139

Druker J, Guilhot F, O'Brien SG, Gathmann I, Kantarjian H, Gattermann N, Deininger MW, Silver RT, Goldman JM, Stone RM, Cervantes F, Hochhaus A, Powell BL, Gabrilove JL, Rousselot P, Reifers J, Cornelissen JJ, Hughes T, Agis H, Fisher T, Verhoef G, Shepherd J, Saglio G, Gratwohl A, Nielsen JL, Radich JP, Simonsson B, Taylor K, Baccarani M, So C, Letvak L, Larson RA (2006) Five year follow-up of patients receiving imatinib for chronic myeloid leukemia. New England Journal of Medicine 355(23):2408–2417

Eden OB, Harrison G, Richards S, Lilleyman JS, Bailey CC, Chessells JM, Hann IM, Hill FG, Gibson BE, on behalf of Medical Research Council Childhood Leukaemia Working Party (2000) Long-term follow-up of the United Kingdom Medical Research Council protocols for childhood acute lymphoblastic leukaemia, 1980–1997. Leukemia 14(12):2307–2320

Egeler RM, Annels NE, Hogendoorn PC (2004) Langherhans cell histiocytosis: a pathological combination of oncogenesis and immune dysregulation. Pediatric Blood Cancer 42(5):401–403

Engel A, Lamm SH (2008) Arsenic exposure and childhood cancer–a systematic review of the literature. Journal of Environmental Health 71(3):12–16

Freedman MH (1994) Chronic myelocytic leukemia in infancy and childhood. In: Pochedly C (ed) Neoplastic diseases of childhood, vol 1. Harwood Academic, Switzerland

Gajjar A, Harrison PL, Sandlund JT, Rivera GK, Ribeiro RC, Rubnitz JE, Razzouk B, Relling MV, Evans WE, Boyett JM, Pui CH (2000) Traumatic lumbar puncture at diagnosis adversely affects outcome in childhood acute lymphoblastic leukemia. Blood 96(10):3381–3384

Gaynon P (2005) Childhood acute lymphoblastic leukemia and relapse. British Journal of Hematology 131:579–587

Greaves MF, Maia AT, Wiemels JL, Ford AM (2003) Leukemia in twins: lessons in natural history. Blood 102(7):2321–2333

Grifo AH (2009) Langerhans Cell Histiocytosis in Children. Journal of Pediatric Oncology 26(1):41–47

Harned TM, Gaynon P (2008) Relapsed acute lymphoblastic leukemia: current status and future opportunities. Current Oncology Reports 10(6):453–458

Hasle H, Clemmensen IH, Mikelsen M (2000) Risks of leukemia and solid tumours in individuals with Down's syndrome. Lancet 355(9199):165–169

Head DR (2002) Proposed changes in the definitions of acute myeloid leukemia and myelodysplastic syndrome: are they helpful? Current Opinion in Oncology 14(1):19–23

Histiocytosis Association of America (2009) LCH in Children. http://www.histio.org/site/c.kiKTL4PQLvF/b.1764433/k.8BCD/LCH_in_Children.htm. Accessed 09 January 2009

Jarup L, Briggs D, de Hoogh C, Morris S, Hurt C, Lewin A, Maitland I, Richardson S, Wakefield J, Elliott P (2002) Cancer risks in population living near landfill sites in Great Britain. British Journal of Cancer 86(11):1732–1736

Jeha S, Gandhi V, Chan KW, McDonald L, Ramirez I, Madden R, Rytting M, Brandt M, Keating M, Plunkett W, Kantarjian H (2004) Clofarabine, a novel nucleoside analog, is active in pediatric patients with advanced leukemia. Blood 103(3):784–789

Kadan-Lottick NS, Dinu I, Wasilewski-Masker K, Kaste S, Meacham LR, Mahajan A, Stovall M, Yasui Y, Robison LL, Sklar CA (2008) Osteonecrosis in adult survivors of childhood cancer: a report from the childhood cancer survivor study. Journal of Clinical Oncology 26(18):3038–3045

Kaatsch P, Mergenthaler A (2008) Incidence, time trends and regional variation of childhood leukaemia in Germany and Europe. Radiation Protection Dosimetry 132(2):107–113

Kinlen LJ (1995) Epidemiological evidence for an infective basis in childhood leukaemia. British Journal of Cancer 71(1):1–5

Klip H, Burger CW, de Kraker J, van Leeuwen FE, OMEGA-project group (2001) Risk of cancer in the offspring of women who underwent ovarian stimulation for IVF. Human Reproduction 16(11):2451–2458

Knox EG (2006) Roads, railways, and childhood cancers. Journal of Epidemiology and Community Health 60(2):136–141

Kwan ML, Metayer C, Crouse V, Buffler PA (2007) Maternal illness and drug/medication use during the period surrounding pregnancy and risk of childhood leukemia among offspring. American Journal of Epidemiology 165(1):27–35

Lancashire RJ, Sorahan T, OSCC (2003) Breastfeeding and childhood cancer risks: OSCC data. British Journal of Cancer 88(7):1035–1037

Lee KM, Ward MH, Han S, Ahn HS, Kang HJ, Choi HS, Shin HY, Koo HH, Seo JJ, Choi JE, Ahn YO, Kang D (2009) Paternal smoking, genetic polymorphisms in CYP1A1 and childhood leukemia risk. Leukemia Research 33(2):250–258

Lightfoot T, Bunch K, Ansell P, Murphy M (2005) Ovulation induction, assisted conception and childhood cancer. European Journal of Cancer 41(5):715–724

Ma X, Buffler PA, Gunier RB, Dahl G, Smith MT, Reinier K, Reynolds P (2002) Critical windows of exposure to household pesticides and risk of childhood leukemia. Environmental Health Perspective 110(9):955–960

MacArthur AC, McBride ML, Spinelli JJ, Tamaro S, Gallagher RP, Theriault G (2008) Risk of childhood leukemia associated with parental smoking and alcohol consumption prior to conception and during pregnancy: the cross-Canada childhood leukemia study. Cancer Causes Control 19(3):283–295

Madureira ABM, Rocha V, Teira P, Champagne M, O'Brien TA, Vora A, Stein J, Olive T, Bonfim CS, Stary J, Bertrand Y, Garnier F, Ionescu I, Niemeyer C, Gluckman E, Locatelli F (2007) Unrelated cord blood transplantation for children with JMML. Bone Marrow Transplantation 39(Suppl 1):10

Matsuda K, Shimada A, Yoshida N, Ogawa A, Watanabe A, Yajima S, Iizuka S, Koike K, Yanai F, Kawasaki K, Yanagimachi M, Kikuchi A, Ohtusuka Y, Hidaka E, Yamauchi K, Tanaka M, Yanagisawa R, Nakazawa Y, Shiohara M, Manabe A, Kojima S, Koike K (2007) Spontaneous improvement of hematologic abnormalities in patients having juvenile myleomonocytic leukemia with RAS mutations. Blood 109:5477–5480

Mattano LA, Harland NS, Trigg ME, Nachman JB (2000) Osteonecrosis as a complication of treating acute lymphoblastic leukemia in children: a report from the Children's Cancer Group. Journal of Clinical Oncology 18(18):3262–3272

McClain KL (2005) Drug therapy for the treatment of langerhans cell histiocytosis. Expert Opinion on Pharmacotherapy 6:2435–2441

McKinney PA, Feltbower RG, Parslow RC, Lewis IJ, Picton S, Kinsey SE, Bailey CC (1999) Survival from childhood cancer in Yorkshire, UK: Effect of ethnicity and socio-economic status. European Journal of Cancer 35(13):1816–1823

McKinney PA, Feltbower RG, Parslow RC, Lewis IJ, Glaser AW, Kinsey SE (2003) Patterns of childhood cancer by ethnic group in Bradford, UK 1974–1997. Eur J Cancer. 39(1):92–7

Mellemkjaer L, Alexander F, Olsen JH (2000) Cancer among children of parents with autoimmune diseases. British Journal of Cancer 82(7):1353–1357

Menegaux F, Ripert M, Hémon D, Clavel J (2007) Maternal alcohol and coffee drinking, parental smoking and childhood leukaemia: a French population-based case-control study. Paediatric and Perinatal Epidemiology 21(4):293–299

Mizutani S (1998) Recent advances in the study of the hereditary and environmental basis of childhood leukemia. Int J Hematol. 68(2):131-43

Millot F, Brice P, Phillipe N, Thyss A, Demeoq F, Wetterwald M, Boccara JM, Vilque J-P, Guyotat D, Guilhot J, Guilhot F (2002) a-Interferon in combination with cytarabine in children with Philadelphia chromosome-positive chronic myeloid leukemia. Journal of Pediatric Hematology/Oncology 24(1):18–22

Naumburg E, Bellocco R, Cnattinigius S, Jonzon A, Ekbom A (2000) Prenatal ultrasound examinations and risk of childhood leukaemia: case-control study. British Medical Journal 320(7230):282–283

Naumburg E, Bellocco R, Cnattinigius S, Jonzon A, Ekbom A (2002a) Supplementary oxygen and risk of childhood lymphatic leukaemia. Acta Paediatrica 91(12):1328–1333

Naumburg E, Bellocco R, Cnattinigius S, Jonzon A, Ekbom A (2002b) Perinatal exposure to infection and risk to childhood leukemia. Medical and Pediatric Oncology 38(6):391–397

Niemeyer C, Kratz C (2008) Paediatric myelodysplastic syndromes and juvenile myelomonocytic leukemia: molecular classification and treatment options. British Journal of Haematology 140:610–624

O'Brien SG, Guilhot F, Larson RA, Gathmann I, Baccarani M, Cervantes F, Cornelissen JJ, Fisher T, Hochaus A, Hughes T, Lechner K, Nielsen JL, Rousselot P, Reiffers J, Saglio G, Shepherd J, Simonsson B, Gratwohl A, Goldman JM, Kantarjian H, Taylor K, Verhoef G, Bolton AE, Capdeville R, Druker BJ (2003) Imatinib compared with interferon and low-dose cytarabine for newly diagnosed chronic-phase myeloid leukemia. New England Journal of Medicine 348(11):994–1004

Pang D, McNally R, Birch JM on behalf of the UK Childhood Cancer Study Investigators (2003) Parental smoking and childhood cancer: results from the United Kingdom Childhood Cancer Study. British Journal of Cancer 88(3):373–381

Parker L, Cole M, Craft AW, Hey EN (1998) Neonatal vitamin K administration and childhood cancer in the north of England: retrospective case-control study. British Medical Journal 316(7126):189–193

Passmore SJ, Draper G, Brownbill P, Kroll M (1998) Case-control studies of relation between childhood cancer and neonatal vitamin K administration. British Medical Journal 316(7126):178–184

Perea G, Lasa A, Aventin A, Domingo A, Villamor N, Queipo P, de Llano M, Llorente A, Junca J, Palacios C, Fernandez C, Gallart M, Font L, Tormo M, Florensa L, Bargay J, Vivancos P, Torres P, Berlanga JJ, Badell I, Brunet S, Sierra J, Nomdedeu JF (2006) Prognostic value of minimal residual disease (MRD) in acute myeloid leukemia (AML) with favorable cytogenetics (t(8:21) and inv 16). Leukemia 20:87–94

Pieters R, Shrappe M, De Lorenzo P, Han I, De Rossi G, Felice M, Hovi L, Leblanc T, Szczepanski T, Ferster A, Janka F, Rubnitz J, Silverman L, Stary J, Campbell M, Li C, Mann G, Suppiah R, Biondi A, Vora A, Valseckli M (2007) A treatment protocol for infants younger than 1 year with acute lymphoblastic leukaemia (Interfant 99): an observational study and a mulitcentre randomized trial. Lancet 370(9583):240–250

Pui CH, Evans WE (2006) Treatment of acute lymphoblastic leukemia. New England Journal of Medicine 354(2): 166–178

Pui CH, Pei D, Sandlund JT, Campana D, Ribeiro R, Razzouk B, Rubnitz J, Howard S, Hijiya N, Jeha S, Cheng C, Downing J, Evans W, Relling M, Hudson M (2005) Risk of adverse events after completion of therapy for childhood lymphoblastic leukemia. Journal of Clinical Oncology 23(31):7936–7941

Rech A, de Carvalho GP, Meneses CF, Hankins J, Howard S, Brunetto AL (2005) The influence of traumatic lumbar puncture and timing of intrathecal therapy on outcome of pediatric acute lymphoblastic leukemia. Pediatric Hematology and Oncology 22(6):483–488

Riberiro R (2006) Update of the management of pediatric acute promyelocytic leukemia. Clinical Advances in Hematology and Oncology 4(4):263–265

Roman E, Fear NT, Ansell P, Bull D, Draper G, McKinney P, Michaelis J, Passmore SJ, von Kries R (2002) Vitamin K and childhood cancer: analysis of individual patient data from six case-control studies. British Journal of Cancer 86(1):63–69

Rosenbaum PF, Buck GM, Brecher ML (2005) Allergy and infectious disease histories and the risk of childhood acute lymphoblastic leukaemia. Paediatric Perinatal Epidemiology 19(2):152–164

Ross JA, Davies SM (2000) Vitamin K prophylaxis and childhood cancer. Medical and Pediatric Oncology 34(6):434–437

Rubnitz J, Gibson B, Smith F (2008) Acute myeloid leukemia. Pediatric Clinics of North America 55:21–51

Ruccione KS, Waskerwitz M, Buckley J, Perin G, Hammond GD (1994) What caused my child's cancer? Parents' responses to an epidemiology study of childhood cancer. Journal of Pediatric Oncology Nursing 11(2):71–84

Rudant J, Menegaux F, Leverger G, Baruchel A, Lambilliotte A, Bertrand Y, Patte C, Pacquement H, Vérité C, Robert A, Michel G, Margueritte G, Gandemer V, Hémon D, Clavel J (2008) Childhood hematopoietic malignancies and parental use of tobacco and alcohol: the ESCALE study (SFCE). Cancer Causes & Control 19(10):1277–1290

Rudant J, Menegaux F, Leverger G, Baruchel A, Nelken B, Bertrand Y, Patte C, Pacquement H, Vérité C, Robert A, Michel G, Margueritte G, Gandemer V, Hémon D, Clavel J (2007) Household exposure to pesticides and risk of childhood hematopoietic malignancies: The ESCALE study (SFCE). Environmental Health Perspectives 115(12):1787–1793

Ruggiero A, Ridola V, Puma N, Molinari F, Coccia P, De Rosa G, Riccardi R (2008) Anthracycline cardiotoxicity in childhood. Pediatric Hematology and Oncology 25(4):261–281

Salotti JA, Nanduri V, Pearce MS, Parker L, Lynn RM, Windebank KP (2009) Incidence and clinical features of langerhans cell histiocytosis in the UK and Ireland. Archives of Disease in Childhood 94(5):376–380

Schultz K, Pullen J, Sather H, Shuster J, Devidas M, Borowitz M, Carroll A, Heerema N, Rubnitz J, Loh M, Raetz E, Winick N, Hunger S, Carroll W, Gaynon P, Camitta B (2007) Risk and response-based classification of childhood B-precursor acute lymphoblastic leukemia: a combined analysis of prognostic markers from the pediatric oncology group (POG) and the childrens cancer group (CCG). Blood 109(3): 926–935

Schüz J, Svendsen AL, Linet MS, McBride ML, Roman E, Feychting M, Kheifets L, Lightfoot T, Mezei G, Simpson J, Ahlbom A (2007) Nighttime exposure to electromagnetic fields and childhood leukemia: an extended pooled analysis. American Journal of Epidemiology 166(3):263–269

Schuz J, Morgan G, Bohler E, Kaatsch P, Michaelis J (2003) Atopic disease and childhood acute lymphoblastic leukemia. International Journal of Cancer 105(2):255–260

Sharathkumar A, Thornley I, Saunders EF, Calderwood S, Freedman MH, Doyle J (2002) Allogenic bone marrow transplantation in children with chronic myelogenous leukemia. Journal of Pediatric Hematology/Oncology 24(3): 215–219

Shu XO, Linet MS, Steinbuch M, Wen WQ, Buckley JD, Neglia JP, Potter JD, Reaman GH, Robison LL (1999) Breast feeding and risk of childhood acute leukemia. Journal of the National Cancer Institute 91(20):1765–1772

Skinner J, Mee TJ, Blackwell RP, Maslanyj MP, Simpson J, Allen SG, Day NE, Cheng KK, Gilman E, Williams D, Cartwright R, Craft A, Birch JM, Eden OB, McKinney PA, Deacon J, Peto J, Beral V, Roman E, Elwood P, Alexander FE, Mott M, Chilvers CE, Muir K, Doll R, Taylor CM, Greaves M, Goodhead D, Fry FA, Adams G, Law G (2002) Exposure to power frequency electric fields and the risk of childhood cancer in the UK. British Journal of Cancer 87(11):1257–1266

Steinbach D, Lengemann J, Voigt A, Hermann J, Zintl F, Sauerbrey A (2003) Response to chemotherapy and expression of the genes encoding the multidrug resistance-associated proteins MRP2, MRP3, MRP4, MRP5, and SMRP in childhood acute myeloid leukemia. Clinical Cancer Research 9(3):1083–1086

Stiller CA, Kroll ME, Boyle PJ, Feng Z (2008) Population mixing, socioeconomic status and incidence of childhood acute lymphoblastic leukaemia in England and Wales: analysis by census ward. British Journal of Cancer 98(5):1006–1011

Sung L, Bucktein R, Doyle JJ, Crump M, Detsky AS (2003) Treatment options for patients with acute myeloid leukemia with a matched sibling donor: a decision analysis. Cancer 97(3):592–600

Swensen AR, Ross JA, Shu XO, Reaman GH, Steinbuch M, Robison LL (2001) Pet ownership and childhood acute leukemia (USA and Canada). Cancer Causes & Control 12(4):301–303

Tomizawa D, Koh K, Sato T, Kinukawa N, Morimoto A, Isoyama K, Kosaka Y, Oda T, Oda M, Hayashi Y, Equali M, Horibe K, Nakahata T, Mizutansi S, Ishii E (2007) Outcome of risk-based therapy for infant acute lymphoblastic leukemia with or without an MLL gene rearrangement, with emphasis on late effects: a final report of two consecutive studies, MLL96 and MLL98, of the Japan Infant Leukemia Group. Leukemia 21(11):2258–2263

Thapa PB, Whitlock JA, Brockman Worrell KG, Gideon P, Mitchel EF Jr, Roberson P, Pais R, Ray WA (1998) Prenatal exposure to metronidazole and risk of childhood cancer: a retrospective cohort study of children younger than 5 years. Cancer 83(7):1461–1468

UK Childhood Cancer Study Investigators (2001) Breastfeeding and childhood cancer. British Journal of Cancer 85(11):1685–1694

Woods WG, Kobrinsky N, Buckley JD, Lee JW, Sanders J, Neudorf S, Gold S, Barnard DR, DeSwarte J, Dusenbery K, Kalousek D, Arthur DC, Lange BJ (1996) Timed-sequential induction therapy improves postremission outcome in acute myeloid leukemia: a report from the Children's Cancer Group. Blood 87(12):4979–4989

Zwaan M, Reinhardt D, Hitzler J, Vyas P (2008) Acute leukemias in children with down syndrome. Pediatric Clinics of North America 55:53–70

Lymphoma

Sue Zupanec

Contents

2.1 **Lymphoma** 33
2.2 **Hodgkin Lymphoma** 33
2.2.1 Epidemiology 34
2.2.2 Etiology 34
2.2.3 Molecular Genetics 34
2.2.4 Symptoms and Clinical Signs 34
2.2.5 Diagnostics 36
2.2.6 Staging and Classification 38
2.2.7 Treatment 39
2.2.8 Prognosis 42
2.2.9 Follow-Up 43
2.2.10 Relapsed/Refractory HL 43
2.2.11 Future Perspectives 44
2.3 **Non-Hodgkin Lymphomas** 44
2.3.1 Epidemiology 44
2.3.2 Etiology 45
2.3.3 Molecular Genetics 45
2.3.4 Symptoms and Clinical Signs 46
2.3.5 Diagnostics 48
2.3.6 Staging and Classification 50
2.3.7 Treatment 50
2.3.8 Prognosis 54
2.3.9 Follow-Up 54
2.3.10 Treatment of Relapsed/Refractory NHL . . 55
2.3.11 Future Perspectives 55
References 56

2.1 Lymphoma

Pediatric lymphomas are the third most common malignancy in North American children, and account for approximately 12% of all childhood malignant diseases (Weitzman and Arceci 2003). Lymphoma in children and adolescents is divided into two major subtypes:

- Hodgkin lymphoma (HL)
- Non-Hodgkin lymphoma (NHL)

HL accounts for 40% of childhood lymphoma diagnoses and NHL accounts for the remaining 60%.

2.2 Hodgkin Lymphoma

HL is a malignant disease of the reticuloendothelial and lymphatic systems. It has a predictable pattern of spread-through contiguous nodes. It does occur, although rarely, in extralymphatic organs. HL can be classified into two distinct disease subtypes:

1. Classical Hodgkin lymphoma (CHL)
2. Nodular lymphocyte predominant Hodgkin lymphoma (NLPHL), which is more uncommon

CHL can be classified based on their sharing of similar neoplastic Reed Sternberg cells (see Sect. 2.1.5). CHL includes the histologic subtypes of nodular sclerosing, mixed cellularity, nodular lymphocytic rich, and lymphocyte depleted HL. Nodular predominant HL has a unique biology distinguishing it from the classic subtype.

2.2.1 Epidemiology

HL accounts for 5–6% of all pediatric malignancies. The overall incidence of HL every year is approximately 6.6 per million children under the age of 15 years, with a peak incidence of 23.1 per million children under 14 years of age (Gurney et al. 1995). HL has a bimodal age distribution that varies with the geographical area. In industrialized countries, the early peak occurs in the young adult with the second peak occuring after the age of 50. In comparison, the first peak in developing coutries occurs prior to adolescence. There appears to be a slight male predominance in the incidence of HL, particularly when HL is diagnosed in the younger childhood age (less than 14 years). This male predominance equals out during the adolescent age group, when the incidence between males and females becomes almost equal. HL is rarely diagnosed before the age of 5. Epidemiology studies of HL have demonstrated clustering of HL cases in families. This may suggest a genetic predispostition or a common exposure to an etiologic agent.

2.2.2 Etiology

In general, HL tends to be diagnosed most frequently in patients with abnormal immune systems. There has been a strong association noted between the development of HL and previous Epstein–Barr virus (EBV) infection, especially with early and prolonged exposure. The virus has been noted in the Reed-Sternberg cells in 50% of HL patients (Hudson and Donaldson 2002). Epidemiological studies have shown that EBV is mostly associated with the mixed cellularity subtype, showing a slight male predominance, and is more frequent in children under the age of 10 (Jarrett 2003). Patients with a history of serologically confirmed mononucleosis have a fourfold increased risk of developing EBV-positive HL, but EBV serologic status alone is not a prognostic factor for HL. HL has been noted with greater frequency in patients with ataxia telangiectasia, or immunodeficiency syndromes such as human immunodeficiency virus (HIV).

2.2.3 Molecular Genetics

Although many cytogenetic abnormalities have been identified in HL, currently, this cytogenetic information does not influence treatment decisions, as is common in other pediatric maligancies.

2.2.4 Symptoms and Clinical Signs

HL usually presents with persistent and painless lymphadenopathy that is characteristically rubbery and firm on clinical examination. In rare cases, the node may be sensitive if it has enlarged quickly. It is common for pediatric patients presenting with HL to have completed several courses of antibiotic therapy prior to their diagnosis of HL, as reactive lymphadenopathy is common in childhood. However, there should be heightened clinical suspicion of a malignant etiology with physical findings of supraclavicular lymphadenopathy. With disease progression of HL, abnormal nodal masses may form, which get anchored to the underlying tissues. Cervical lymphadenopathy is present in approximately 80% of HL. When cervical disease is present, there may be accompanying mediastinal involment in two-thirds of the cases (see Fig. 2.1). Most often patients with intrathoracic HL are asymptomatic, but in some cases, there may be a nonproductive cough, dyspnea, chest pain, or superior vena cava syndrome. It is always important to ensure that a chest X-ray is done to assess the airway patency when there is clinical suspicion of lymphoma, particularly if the diagnostic investigations for the patient requires sedation or general anesthesia. Importantly, for the younger child, it may be difficult to distinguish mediastinal involvment from a normally enlarged thymus. Uncommonly, HL may present with axillary

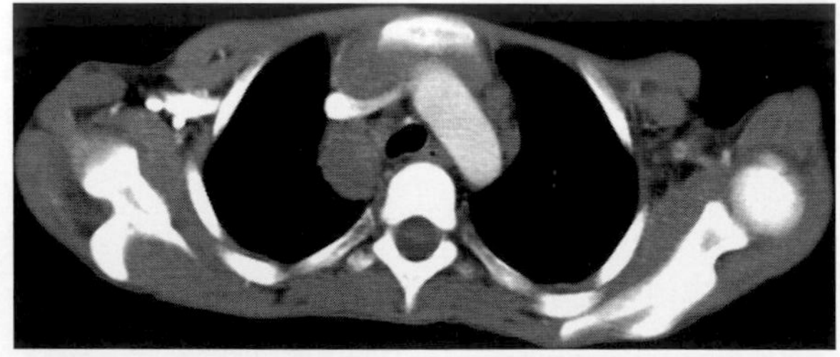

Figure 2.1

HL Stage IVB mediastinal mass by CT scan

or inguinal lymphadenopathy, and very rarely, HL can present with primary subdiaphragmatic disease.

The clinical presentation and specifically the site of nodal involvement of HL is unique to each histologic subtype:

- Nodular sclerosis HL commonly presents with cervical, supraclavicular, and mediastinal nodal involvement. Nodular sclerosing is the most common subtype of HL in adolescents. There is often aggregate or bulky nodal development of this nodular sclerosis subtype that does not always fully regress after completion of therapy (Donaldson 2007).
- Mixed cellularity HL commonly presents as advanced disease with extranodal involvement. The mixed cellularity HL subtype commonly occurs in children under the age of 10 years and has a strong association with the EBV.
- Nodul ar lymphocyte-predominant HL often presents with localized disease in the cervical, axillary, or inguinal regions.
- Nodular lymphocyte-rich HL is more common in males and at younger age.
- Lymphocyte-depleted HL subtype is very rare in pediatrics. However, it may develop in the condition of an aquired immunodeficiency such as HIV or chronic immunosuppression following a solid organ transplant. The lymphocyte-depleted HL subtype commonly has bone and bone marrow involvement.

Systemic symptoms associated with HL are considered to be the result of cytokine production by the Reed–Sternberg cells. Some systemic symptoms that are common at presentation include:

- Fatigue
- Urticaria
- Anorexia
- Mild weight loss
- Pruritis that can often be so severe that it may lead to skin excoriation. Pruritis is more common in females and patients with advanced disease

These nonspecific systemic symptoms, if present, are not prognostic in HL. Other systemic symptoms known as constitutional or B symptoms are present in approximately 30% of pediatric patients, and have been associated with a less favorable prognosis. The determination of B symptoms at presentation will affect the staging and intensity of therapy for patients with HL (see Sect. 2.6). There are three constitutional B symptoms that include:

- Unexplained fever with temperature higher than 38°C for more than 3 days
- Drenching night sweats
- Unexplained weight loss of 10% or more within 6 months preceding diagnosis (Chauvenet et al. 2000)

Splenic enlargement may be observed with abdominal involvement, and splenic disease is present in 30–40% of pediatric patients. Physical examination may reveal an enlarged spleen; however, this does not always indicate splenic involvement. Computed tomography (CT) scanning is helpful to identify splenic lesions (see Fig. 2.2). Hepatic involvement in pediatric HL is rare.

In approximately 2% of pediatric cases, there may be bone involvment of HL. These patients may present with bone pain. In older adolescent patients, there may be severe pain induced at the involved nodes or bones with alcohol ingestion.

Paranchymal lung lesions are also sometimes present and often require biopsy to confirm pathology

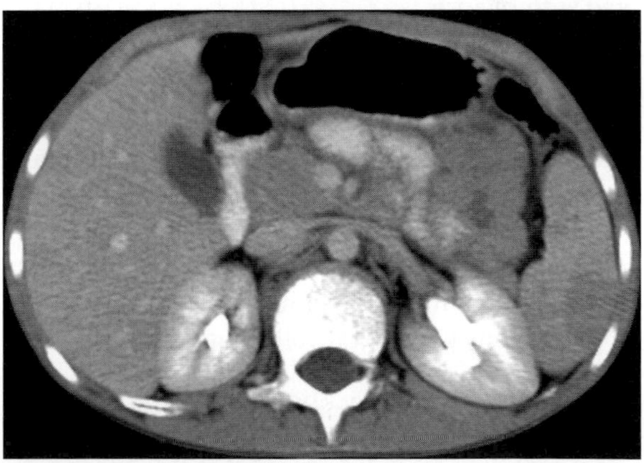

Figure 2.2

Stage IVB splenic lesion and infradiaphragmatic lymphadenopathy on CT scan

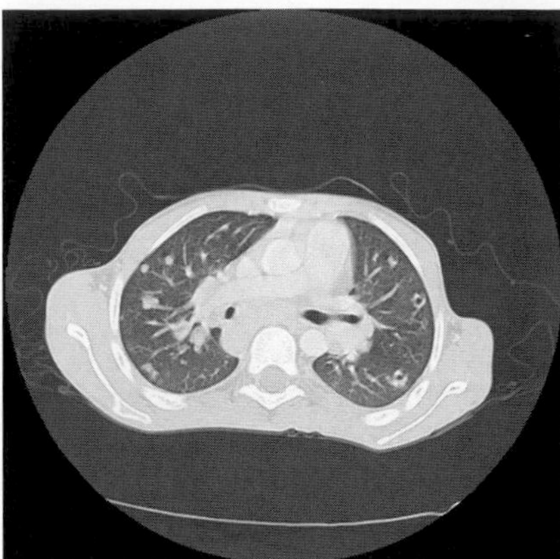

Figure 2.3
HL stage IVB with parenchymal lung metastases

(see Fig. 2.3). Idiopathic thrombocytopenia purpura (ITP) occurs in 1–2% of children with HL, and is often associated with autoimmune hemolytic anemia (Hudson and Donaldson 2002). Thrombocytopenia caused by ITP that is associated with HL can occur at diagnosis, but may also occur on treatment and after completion of treatment. The association of ITP and HL is not prognostic, and ITP that develops after of the completion of therapy for HL has not been associated with relapse.

2.2.5 Diagnostics

The first step in diagnosis is a complete history and physical examination. Physical examination may demonstrate the presence of any significant lymphadenopathy. Table 2.1 summarizes the recommended investigations in the diagnostic work-up of HL. Investigations include the following:

- A chest x-ray quickly provides information about mediastinal involvement and potential complications. A definition of bulky disease can be made from the chest X-ray if the measurement of a mediastinal mass is greater or equal to 33% of the maximum intrathoracic cavity (see Fig. 2.4).

Table 2.1. Diagnostic work-up of HL

Complete blood count with differential count
Erythrocyte sedimentation rate (ESR), C-reactive protein (CRP), serum copper, ferritin
Renal and hepatic function tests
Albumin, lactate dehydrogenase (LDH)
Chest X-ray with measurement of ratio of mediastinal mass to maximum intrathoracic cavity at the dome of the diaphragm
Computed tomography (CT) of neck and chest
Computed tomography (CT) or magnetic resonance imaging (MRI) of abdomen and pelvis
Bone marrow biopsy for all children, expect those in stages IA/IIA
Bone scan recommended for children with bone pain or elevated alkaline phosphatase
Gallium or positron emission tomography (PET) scan

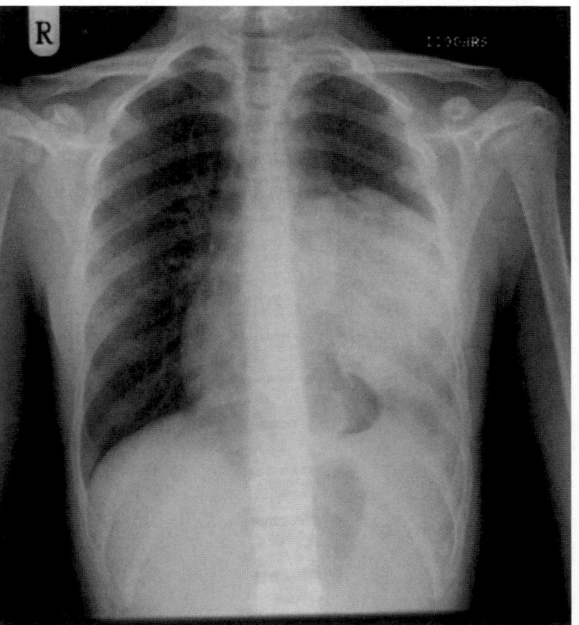

Figure 2.4
Chest X-ray of mediastinal mass HL

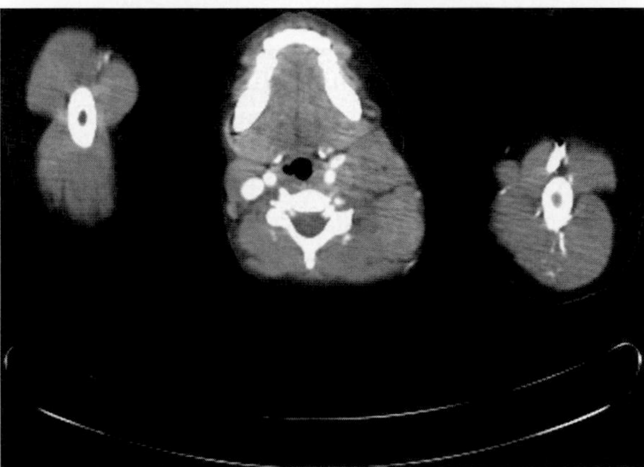

Figure 2.5

HL stage IIA with bulk disease cervical lymphadenopathy on CT imaging

- CT of the neck, chest, abdomen, and pelvis. The CT scan is necessary to evaluate the extent of disease at diagnosis (see Fig 2.5).
- Nuclear imaging such as a gallium scan, and more recently, positron emission tomography (PET) scanning provides additional information on the extent of disease and is subsequently used to assess the response to treatment (see Fig 2.6). PET has largely replaced Gallium scan in the diagnosis and staging of HL. The PET can demonstrate proliferative activity in tumors undergoing anaerobic gycolysis, through the uptake of the radioactive glucose analog, 18-fluoro-2-deoxyglucose (FDG). Often PET is combined with CT and can be easily carried out, with results obtained on the same day. As the PET-CT scan technique requires the patient to remain still, younger children may require sedation.
- Bone scan is not always required, but should be done if clinically warranted; i.e., bone pain, elevated alkaline phosphatase, or evidence of metastatic disease.
- Bilateral bone marrow aspirate and biopsies are necessary to rule out bone marrow involvement; however, this diagnositic test is only recommended for patients with advanced stage of the disease. Specifically patients with stage I–IIA rarely have bone marrow involvement and generally do not require bone marrow biopsy as part of the diagnostic work-up.

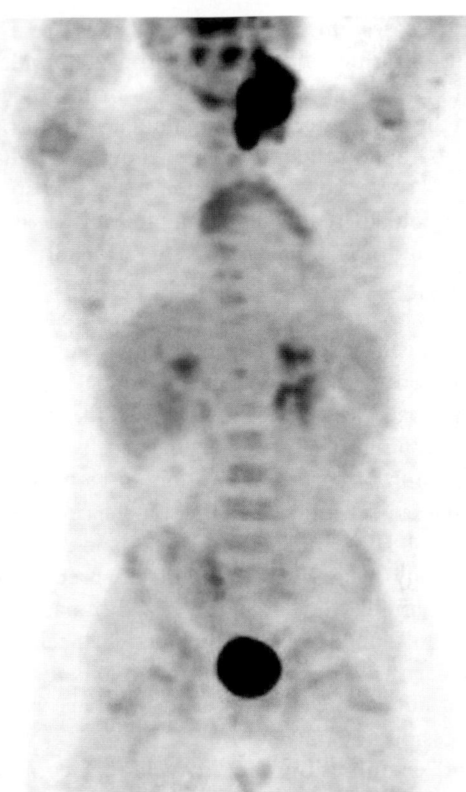

Figure 2.6

Positive PET scan showing uptake in HL

- A biopsy of the affected node is required for diagnosis. An excisional biopsy is preferred over a needle biopsy because it preserves the architecture of the node and because the sample must be large enough to locate the presence of Reed–Sternberg cells. HL is characterized by the presence of Reed–Sternberg cells, which are giant multinucleated cells with abundant cytoplasm, with the nucleo lus having a characteristic "owl's eye" appearance, or large mononuclear cell variants (lymphocytic and histiocytic). In most cases, the Reed Sternberg cells are B-cells that are nonfunctional due to their inability to synthesize immunoglobulin.

In rare cases, the Reed–Sternberg cells are T-cell in origin (Hudson and Donaldson 2002). Malignant cells comprise less than 1% of tumor cells, with the remainder being inflammatory infiltrates. Histopathological studies carried out on Hodgkin tumors consist of hematoxylin, eosin, and special immunohistochemical staining for surface markers, including CD15, CD20, and CD30. Sternberg cells express CD30 and CD15 in 70% of the cases. CD20 is expressed in 5–10% of Reed–Sternberg cells. Reed–Sternberg cells show constitutive activation of the nuclear factor kappa B pathway (NFkappa B) that prevents cell death. Immunophenotyping of Reed–Sternberg cells indicates expression of certain activation antigens, including the IL2 receptor, Ki-1, the transferrin receptor, and HLA-DR (Hudson and Donaldson 2002). The pathology of nodular lymphocyte predominant HL is unique and is characterized by large cells with multilobed nuclei called "popcorn cells." The "popcorn cells" express B-cell antigens including CD20, but are negative for CD15 and have variable expression of CD30.

- Blood examination should include a complete/full blood count (CBC) and a differential count. Cytopenias may be observed with bone marrow diseases. Lymphopenia is more common in patients with advanced-stage diseases, and also in adult patients with HL. Liver and renal function tests should be done to confirm satisfactory hepatic and renal function prior to treatment initiation. Several acute-phase reactants may be elevated at presentation of HL, including erythrocyte sedimentation rate (ESR), serum copper, ferritin, and C-reactive protein (CRP). Of these, the ESR and CRP have been prognostic and are often used during therapy to nonspecifically monitor the response. In addition, an alkaline phosphatase test should be done to screen for bone involvement. Elevations of alkaline phosphatase well beyond the age-controlled limits should prompt investigations for skeletal involvement. Additional chemical parameters that are routinely screened in the diagnostic work-up include hypoabluminemia and elevations of lactate dehydrogenase (LDH).

2.2.6 Staging and Classification

Recently, the classification of HL has been modified from the previous Rye classification by the World Health Organization (WHO) (Stein 2001). This WHO classification system has recognized Hodgkin disease as a lymphoma, and has now stated that HL be used synonymously with Hodgkin disease. In addition, the WHO has classified HL into two distinct classifications:

1. CHL with four subtypes
   - Nodular sclerosing
   - Lymphocyte-rich
   - Mixed cellularity
   - Lymphocyte depletion
2. NLPHL is distinct in its unique biology, histology, and clinical features (Donaldson 2007).

The Ann Arbor Staging Classification System is used to stage the disease (Table 2.2). In the following

Table 2.2. Ann Arbor staging classification for HL (adapted from Pinkerton et al. 1999)

Stage	Characteristics
I	Involvement of a single lymph node region or a single extralymphatic organ or site
II	Involvement of two or more lymph node regions on the same side of the diaphragm or solitary involvement of an extralymphatic organ or site and of one or more lymph node regions on the same side of the diaphragm
III	Involvement of lymph node regions on both sides of the diaphragm, which may be accompanied by localized involvement of extralymphatic organ or site, or by involvement of the spleen, or both
IV	Diffused or disseminated involvement of one or more extralymphatic organs or tissues with or without associated lymph node enlargement

A subfix will be added to the stage number. In HL there is always an A or B included in staging. Sometimes, an additional subfix will be added to the stage in HL. *A* absence of systemic symptoms; *B* presence of systemic symptoms; fever, night sweats and weight loss; *S* splenic involvement; *E* extranodal involvement

Sect. 2.7, the stage of the disease will be described in relationship to the recommended therapy.

It must be noted that along with the stage of the disease, there is a subfix (A,B,E,S) that denotes the presence of diagnostic features.

- The subfix A denotes the absence of unfavorable features.
- The subfix B denotes the presence of B symptoms.
- The subfix E indicates extranodal disease.
- The subfix S indicates splenic involvement.

If there is bulky disease, this information is often added to staging, e.g., stage IIB with bulk disease.

2.2.7 Treatment

The goal of treatment for children and adolescents with HL has become increasingly focused on response-based therapy and on minimizing late effects. Historical treatment regimens for HL resulted in unacceptable musculoskeletal hypoplasia, cardiovascular and pulmonary dysfunction, as well as the development of subsequent cancers (Hudson et al. 2007). Therefore, current treatment protocols aim to maintain an excellent overall survival while reducing the risk of treatment-related morbidity and late effects including second malignancies. Treatment for HL is based on risk where children with favorable disease receive fewer cycles of combination chemotherapy and occasionally, the addition of involved field radiation, compared with children with more advanced and unfavorable clinical presentations.

Chemotherapy is recommended for all children and adolescents with HL with the rare exception. The use of chemotherapy has allowed for the treatment of unrecognized and metastatic sites of disease at presentation and for the reduction of radiation fields and radiation doses known to be harmful in children who continue to grow and develop. The first drug used in the treatment of HL was Nitrogen Mustard, but due to subsequently recognized significant toxicities, specifically a relatively high incidence of secondary malignancies (predominantly acute myeloid leukemia) and sterility/infertility, it is no longer commonly used. Although tumor response can be seen with single-agent chemotherapy, combination chemotherapy for the treatment of HL is the standard recommended therapy. Combination chemotherapy allows for different mechanisms of action and has the ability to overlap chemotherapies to minimize toxicity. For example, current treatment is focused on avoiding the use of alkylators and other drugs with significant long-term sequelae. Most current therapies for children have adopted hybrid cycles of proven regimens; thus, limiting the cumulative doses of anthracyline chemotherapies, etoposide, and bleomycin. Drugs that are predominantly used in the treatment of HL include mechlorethamine (M), vincristine (O), prednisone (P), procarbazine (P), doxorubicin (A), methotrexate (MT) bleomycin (B), vinblastine (V), etoposide (E), dacarbazine (D), and cyclophosphamide (C). See Table 2.3 for a list of chemotherapy regimens currently used to treat pediatric HL.

Radiation therapy also plays a vital role in treating HL. The involved field radiation therapy includes the areas that are clinically involved as well as the surrounding lymph nodes. This involved field approach to radiation is used more commonly now to decrease the radiation field, thereby minimizing the damage to the unaffected tissue and decreasing late effects. Efforts to sheild normal tissue and specifically, the breast, ovaries, testes, lungs, and heart are always considered in the radiation treatment planning. The dose of radiation in pediatric HL generally does not exceed 25 Gy; however, no studies have been carried out to determine the optimal radiation dose for children.

One of the most common and important fields of radiation therapy in HL is mantle radiation. The mantle field encompasses the submandibular, submental, cervical, supraclavicular, infraclavicular, axillary, mediastinal, and pulmonary hilar lymph nodes (Hudson and Donaldson 2002). The mantle field can be expanded to include the cardiac sillouhette and/or lungs; however, the dose of radiation to these organs may be reduced by utilizing a partial transmission block. Owing to the extent of the mantle field, efforts have been taken to sheild the occipital area, mandible, larynx, humeral heads, and spinal cord to avoid both unneccessary treatment and side effects that may be acute and

Table 2.3. Chemotherapy regimens for the treatment of HL (adapted from Hudson et al. 2007)

Name	Drugs	Dosage	Route	Days
MOPP and derivatives				
MOPP	Mechlorethamine	6 mg/m^2	i.v.	1, 8
	Vincristine	1.4 mg/m^2	i.v.	1, 8
	Procarbazine	100 mg/m^2	p.o.	1–15
	Prednisone	40 mg/m^2	p.o.	1–15
COPP	Cyclophosphamide	600 mg/m^2	i.v.	1, 8
	Vincristine	1.4 mg/m^2	i.v.	1, 8
	Procarbazine	100 mg/m^2	p.o.	1–15
	Prednisone	40 mg/m^2	p.o.	1–15
OPPA	Vincristine	1.5 mg/m^2	i.v.	1, 8, 15
	Procarbazine	100 mg/m^2	p.o.	1–15
	Prednisone	60 mg/m^2	p.o.	1–15
	Doxorubicin	40 mg/m^2	i.v.	1, 15
ChlVPP	Chlorambucil	6 mg/m^2	p.o.	1–14
	Vinblastine	6 mg/m^2	p.o.	1, 8
	Procarbazine	100 mg/m^2	p.o.	1–14
	Prednisone	40 mg/m^2	p.o.	1–14
ABVD & derivatives				
ABVD	Doxorubicin	25 mg/m^2	i.v.	1, 15
	Bleomycin	10 U/m^2	i.v.	1, 15
	Vinblastine	6 mg/m^2	i.v.	1, 15
	Dacarbazine	375 mg/m^2	i.v.	1, 15
OEPA	Vincristine	1.5 mg/m^2	i.v.	1, 8, 15
	Etoposide	125 mg/m^2	i.v.	3–6
	Prednisone	60 mg/m^2	p.o.	1–15
	Doxorubicin	40 mg/m^2	i.v.	1, 15
VAMP	Vinblastine	6 mg/m^2	i.v.	1, 15
	Doxorubicin	25 mg/m^2	i.v.	1, 15
	Methotrexate	20 mg/m^2	i.v.	1, 15
	Prednisone	40 mg/m^2	p.o.	1–14
VBVP	Vinblastine	6 mg/m^2	i.v.	1, 8
	Bleomycin	10 U/m^2	i.v.	1
	Etoposide	100 mg/m^2	i.v.	1–5
	Prednisone	40 mg/m^2	p.o.	1–8
DBVE	Doxorubicin	25 mg/m^2	i.v.	1, 15
	Bleomycin	10 U/m^2	i.v.	1, 15
	Vincristine	1.5 mg/m^2	i.v.	1, 15
	Etoposide	(maximum 2 mg)	i.v.	1–5
VEPA	Vinblastine	6 mg/m^2	i.v.	1, 15
	Etoposide	200 mg/m^2	i.v.	1, 15
	Prednisone	40 mg/m^2	p.o.	1–14
	Doxorubicin	25 mg/m^2	i.v.	1, 15

Table 2.3. (Continued)

Name	Drugs	Dosage	Route	Days
Dose-intensive MOPP/ABVD combination derivatives				
COPP/ABV	Cyclophosphamide	600 mg/m^2	i.v.	1
	Vincristine	1.4 mg/m^2	i.v.	1
	Procarbazine	100 mg/m^2	p.o.	1–7
	Prednisone	40 mg/m^2	p.o.	1–14
	Doxorubicin	35 mg/m^2	i.v.	8
	Bleomycin	10 U/m^2	i.v.	8
	Vinblastine	6 mg/m^2	i.v.	8
DBVE-PC	Doxorubicin	25 mg/m^2	i.v.	1,2
	Bleomycin	5/10 U/m^2	i.v.	1/8
	Vincristine	1.4 mg/m^2	i.v.	1,8
	Etoposide	(maximum 2.8 mg)	i.v.	1–3
	Prednisone	125 mg/m^2	p.o.	1–7
	Cyclophosphamide	40 mg/m^2	i.v.	1
		800 mg/m^2		
BEACOPP	Bleomycin	10 U/m^2	i.v.	8
	Etoposide	200 mg/m^2	i.v.	1–3
	Doxorubicin	35 mg/m^2	i.v.	1
	Cyclophosphamide	1,200 mg/m^2	i.v.	1
	Vincristine	2 mg/m^2	i.v.	8
	Procarbazine	(maximum 2 mg)	p.o.	1–7
	Prednisone	100 mg/m^2	p.o.	1–14
		40 mg/m^2		
Stanford V	Mechlorethamine	6 mg/m^2	i.v.	1, 15
	Vinblastine	6 mg/m^2	i.v.	1, 15
	Doxorubicin	25 mg/m^2	i.v.	1
	Etoposide	60 mg/m^2	i.v.	15, 16
	Vincristine	1.4 mg/m^2	i.v.	8, 22
	Bleomycin	(maximum 2 mg)	i.v.	8, 22
	Prednisone	5 U/m^2	p.o.	Every other day
		40 mg/m^2		

long-term. When pelvic radiation is needed, surgical repositioning of the ovaries to a central midline position is sometimes possible, enabling a midline pelvic block to protect the ovaries, minimize toxicity, and preserve fertility. Radiation therapy continues to be an important element of treatment for HL, but due to the long-term risks of hypoplasia, hypothyroidism, cardiopulmonary fibrosis, and breast cancer, investigators are focused on identifying the subsets of patients with HL who can achieve cure without exposure to radiation.

To minimize exposure to chemtherapy and radiation and to maximize event-free survival, a risk-adapted approach for the treatment of HL has been adopted. Risk includes prognostic factors at diagnosis, staging of disease, and response to therapy. Risk designations at diagnosis may vary based on the investigator, but most typically includes low-risk disease, intermediate-risk disease, and high-risk disease categories. In all risk designations, an evaluation of response will factor into treatment decisions at varying timepoints in the therapy.

Low-risk HL is characterized by local nodal involvement (stage I/II) as well as the absence of B symptoms and lymph node bulk disease. It must be noted that the subfix "A" denotes the absense of B symptoms. Low-risk HL is generally stage IA/IIA disease. Many investigators have found that pediatric patients with low-risk HL are good candidates for reduced therapy. Most standard therapies for low-risk HL include 2–4 cycles of chemotherapy, followed by low-dose involved field radiation. The characteristic of the low-risk HL chemotherapy cycles is little or no anthracycline therapy. Pediatric investigators from St. Jude's, Stanford, and Dana Farber have reported excellent outcomes using four cycles of vinblastine, doxorubicin, methotrexate, and prednisone (VAMP) followed by involved field radiation (Donaldson et al. 2002). Other groups including the Pediatric Oncology Group (POG) have used combinations of chemotherapy with reduced anthracyclines substituting etoposide for anthracyclines and alkylators with similar results (Schwartz and Constine 2002). French investigators reported a 5-year EFS of 91.5% for pediatric low-risk HL using VBVP (vinblastine, bleomycin, etoposide, and prednisone), followed by radiation (Landman-Parker et al. 2000). This protocol eliminated both anthracyclines and alkylators. The German–Austrian investigators have demonstrated that gonadal toxicity can be reduced by replacing procarbazine from the OPPA cycle with etoposide, with no effect on disease-free survival (Dorffel et al. 2003). Although there is a concern about secondary acute myeloid leukemia with the substitution of etoposide for anthracycline and alkyling agents, this risk is extremely low and is outweighed by the risk of gonadal and cardiac toxicity in HL survivors. Other pediatric investigators have aimed to eliminate radiation therapy for low-risk pediatric patients with HL. Prospective trials randomizing patients to receive no radiation after chemotherapy cycles based on a good early response to therapy are ongoing.

Intermediate-risk HL is characterized by stage I/II with the presence of unfavorable features at presentation, and sometimes by stage III with the absence of unfavorable features. There is no consensus on the definition of unfavorable features among investigators. However, it is generally agreed that unfavorable features include the presence of B symptoms, lymph node bulk disease, hilar lymph involvment, and extranodal extension to contigous structures (subfix E) (Hudson et al. 2007). High-risk HL is an advanced-stage disease and generally includes stage IIIB and stages IVA and IVB. This group of pediatric patients with high-risk HL receives the most dose intensive chemotherapy followed by involved field low-dose radiation to consolidate the remission. Treatment of both intermediate-risk and high-risk HL most often includes a hybrid combination of COPP and ABVD (see Table 2.3). Treatment for intermediate-risk HL is usually 4–6 cycles of combination chemotherapy over 6 months, often followed by involved field radiation. Similar to the Low-risk HL group, investigators have been trying to eliminate radiation therapy in randomized current trials for the intermediate-risk group. Treamtment for high-risk pediatric HL is 6–8 cycles of chemotherapy followed by involved field radiation. Etoposide has been incorporated into intermediate-risk and high-risk regimens, with the aim of minimizing the exposure to anthracycline and alkylating agents. At this stage, the use of hematopoietic stem cell transplantation (HSCT) is reserved for patients with relapsed or refractory HL, owing to the excellent reported survival with standard treatment approaches.

The standard treatment for nodular lymphocyte predominant HL is chemotherapy along with low-dose involved field radiation, similar to the regimens used to treat CHL. However, owing to the unique natural history of this histologic subtype, there is evidence to support observation following total resection of isolated nodal disease or chemotherapy alone (Hall et al. 2007; Murphy et al. 2003), and this continues to be the focus of current studies.

2.2.8 Prognosis

The overall survival of children and adolescents with HL is 90% (Schwartz 2003). As previously mentionned, adverse prognostic features include the presence of B symptoms, bulky disease, as defined by a mass greater than 6 cm in size for pediatric patients, extranodal extension, elevated ESR, and large mediastinal adenopathy. Smith et al. (2003) described a prognostic factor analysis as reported in two POG studies. They found that advanced-stage disease and the male gender showed an inferior event-free survival. It is difficult to identify prognostic factors across different treatment regimens. The rapidity of response to treatment cycles appears to be prognostic, and is currently being used to stratify therapy between standard or intesified treatment.

2.2.9 Follow-Up

The follow-up for HL must be long-term due to the many potential late effects of treatment. Most relapses occur within the first 3 years after the therapy; however, relapse has been documented as late as 10 years post treatment (Hudson and Donaldson 2002). The recommended schedule for follow-up tests and scans varies among investigators and clinicians. Typically, scans including chest X-ray are taken every 3 months for the first year, and then every 6 months during the second year after therapy. The schedule of CT scans is controversial due to the risk of repeated radiation exposure vs. the benefit of detecting subclinical disease. However, current protocols recommend CT scans of the primary site every 6 months and CT neck, chest, abdomen, and pelvis annually for the first 2 years after therapy.

The late effects of therapy must be monitored carefully. Thyroid dysfunction in the form of nodules, hypothyroidism, and hyperthyroidism occurs more frequently in patients who have been treated with radiation therapy, compared with the general population. The incidence of hypothyroidism is four to five times higher in patients treated with radiation therapy for HL, compared with the general population (Sklar et al. 2000). Thyroid problems usually present within the first 5 years post therapy, but can occur as late as 20 years post therapy. Thyroid-stimulating hormone (TSH) and thyroxine T4 must therefore be monitored routinely, and the schedule is often annual. Echocardiogram and pulmonary function tests must be done routinely to monitor for late cardiomyopathies and pulmonary fibrosis, secondary to anthracycline and bleomycin, respectively (with or without radiation). The risks of secondary tumors at various sites can occur in the two to three decades following treatment (Metayer et al. 2000). Patients treated for HL have the highest incidence of second malignancies of all pediatric cancer survivors. Infertility and primary ovarian failure can also occur following chemotherapy and pelvic irradiation. Aklylating agents used to treat HL also pose an increased risk of goandal dysfuntion and premature menopause (De Bruin et al. 2008). During the follow-up care of pediatric patients treated for HL, counseling must be done regarding lifestyle behaviors, such as smoking, to minimize confounding oncogenic agents/exposure.

2.2.10 Relapsed/Refractory HL

It is estimated that 10–20% of patients with pediatric HL will have a relapse of their disease. Timing of the relapse remains prognostic. However, the most unfavorable is the progession of HL during induction, or a relapse of HL within the first 12 months following completion of therapy. The overall survival for this group has been reported to be less than 30% (Trippet and Chen 2007). Relapses of HL beyond 12 months post therapy have been more responsive to salvage therapies, but still, a poor prognosis has been reported between 30 and 60% (Trippet and Chen 2007). Owing to the poor outlook for relapse and refractory HL, aggressive reinduction chemotherapy followed by autologous HSCT has been used as the standard treatment approach. The role of reinduction chemotherapy for relapsed/refractory HL is to demonstrate disease response and achieve minimal disease status prior to HSCT. A demonstrated disease response to reinduction chemotherapy for relapsed/refractory HL is associated with improved overall survival. Examples of reinduction protocols for relapsed/refractory HL include ICE (ifosphamide, carboplatinum, etoposide), IV (ifosphamide, vinorelbine), Mini Beam (carmutine, melphalan, etoposide, cytarabine), and GEM/VRB (gemcitabine/vinorelbine). The choice for reinduction therapy is based on the reported rate of disease response and also on the ability to mobilize peripheral stem cells for HSCT. Currently, the role of allogeneic HSCT in the treatment of relapsed or refractory HL is a controversial issue.

2.2.11 Future Perspectives

Future trials for HL treatment will continue to focus on tailored risk-adapted disease protocols in an attempt to minimize late effects, while continuing to maintain and exceed current excellent survival data. The quest to eliminate radiation for identified subsets of pediatric patients with HL is ongoing. As more scientific advances are made, immunotherapy, vaccine, and monoclonal antibody therapy may be beneficial in the treatment of HL. An improved understanding of the biology of HL will ultimately lead to the development of more efficacious and less toxic therapies. Identifying subgroups of pediatric HL patients with very unfavorable characteristics, who may benefit from frontline HSCT will also be important for future studies. In addition, identifying if an advantage exists for allogeneic HSCT in patients with refractory or relapsed HL will continue to be investigated.

2.3 Non-Hodgkin Lymphomas

NHLs are a group of malignancies that are derived from lymphocytes and their precursors. They are a heterogenous group of diseases, as malignant clonal proliferation can occur at any stage of lymphocyte differentiation. NHL tumors can be intermediate to high-grade tumors which are clinically aggressive and often present in an advanced stage. NHLs can be classified into three major subtypes:

- Lymphoblastic lymphoma (LL)
- Burkitt lymphoma (BL)
- Large cell lymphoma (LCL)

Subtypes of LCL include diffuse large B-cell lymphoma (DLBCL) and anaplastic large cell lymphoma (ALCL). At present, the technique to distinguish the subtype Burkitt-like lymphoma from BL does not alter the treatment or outcome, and this subtype will be addressed in the following sections as BL. When it is important to distinguish Burkitt-like lymphoma, a special distinction is made. In addition to the common subtypes of NHL in pediatrics, children and adolescents may develop lymphoproliferative disorders in the setting of congenital or aquired immunocompromise. Recent increases in solid organ transplants and HSCTs has resulted in an increase in lymphoproliferative diseases. Post transplant lymphoproliferative disease (PTLD) is usually B-cell lineage proliferations. Non-anaplastic peripheral T-cell lymphoma and gamma/delta lymphomas are rare subtypes in pediatrics, and will not be included in this chapter.

2.3.1 Epidemiology

NHL accounts for approximately 8–10% of all childhood malignancies (Sandlund et al. 1996). NHL is very rare in children less than 2 years of age, suggesting that exposure to environmental agents may be important in the development of pediatric lymphomas (Weitzman and Arceci 2003). The incidence of pediatric NHL varies with sex and race. Males are diagnosed with NHL three times more often than females, and NHL is twice as common in whites compared with blacks. The male predominance is most striking in patients under the age of 15, where three-fourths of NHL cases occur in males (Link and Weinstein 2006). There is an age variation by specific NHL subtype. The most common age at diagnosis for BL is between the age of 5 and 15. The age of diagnosis for LL does not show an age peak/trend and is fairly constant across all age groups. The LCL subtype DLBCL is the most common subtype during adolescence with a peak age of 15–19. There is a geographical variance in incidence, particularly for BL. BL is endemic in equatorial Africa and accounts for approximately 50% of all childhood cancers, affecting 50 children per million. BL in Africa accounts for 80% of all childhood NHL diagnoses (Magrath 2002). In other areas of the world, BL occurs sporadically and is less common, affecting approximately 2 children per million. Overall, the incidence of pediatric NHL appears to be increasing by 3–4% per year, regardless of age, sex, or ethnicity (Sandlund et al. 1996).

Risk for the development of NHL is greater in children with abnormalities of the immune system. Notably, children with congenital or aquired immunodeficiency have an increased risk of developing

NHL. In particular, children with Wiskott–Aldrich syndrome or ataxia-telangectasia have an increased risk of developing NHL, possibly the large cell or Burkitt subtype (Weitzman and Arceci 2003). NHL is the most common malignancy associated with acquired immunodeficiency syndrome (AIDS) in children. Children who have received solid organ transplants and HSCT are also at an increased risk of developing PTLD/NHL due to the associated immunosuppressive therapy (Faye and Vilmer 2005). PTLD is now the third most common form of pediatric NHL in the US (Gross and Shiramizu 2007).

2.3.2 Etiology

The etiology of NHL is unknown. It is suggested and supported by evidence that NHL develops as a result of genetic alterations caused by viral infection. In BL there is a strong association between EBV and the development of malignancy, particularly in endemic (African) cases. The EBV has been found in the DNA of tumor cells in 95% of the cases of endemic BL, compared with only 15% EBV isolated in cases of sporadic BL (Weitzman and Arceci 2003). In PTLD, there is a strong association with EBV demonstrated by the malignant cells containing multiple copies of the EBV genome (Link and Weinstein 2006). The genetic alteration leading to the development of malignancy may also be the result of exposure to previous chemotherapy and/or radiation. Exposure to pesticides as a potential influence on the development of NHL has not been proven.

2.3.3 Molecular Genetics

Cytogenetic abnormalities are commonly found in NHL and assist in the diagnosis of the disease. Rearrangements in immunoglobulin and T-cell receptor genes (TCR) are the most common molecular alterations in pediatric NHL (Weitzman and Arceci 2003). A summary of the major histological categories of NHL with their associated cytogenetic abnormalities is shown in Table 2.4. The following section will provide a brief overview of the common cytogenetic abnormalities by the subtype of pediatric NHL.

In 80% of the cases of BL, there is the translocation of the proto-oncogene, c-myc, on chromosome 8 to the immunoglobulin heavy chain gene locus on chromosome 14 (t(8:14)(q24;q32)) (Weitzman

Table 2.4. Summary of major histological categories, immunophenotypes, common cytogenetic abnormalities, and common sites of disease of NHLs (Magrath 2002; Cairo and Perkins 2000)

Histological category of lymphoma	Immunophenotype	Cytogenetic abnormalities	Common sites of disease
Burkitt's	B-cell (CD19, CD20, CD22, CD79, CD77, CD10)	t(8;14), t(8;2), and t(8;22)	Abdomen, head, neck
Large B-cell	B-cell (CD19, CD20, CD22, CD38, CD79, sometimes CD10) TdT neg	Bcl-6 or bcl-2 t(8;14) in 5–10%	Abdomen, mediastinum
Burkitt's-like	B-cell (MIB-1 positivity)	t(8;14)	Abdomen, head, neck
Lymphoblastic	Pre-T (CD77, CD7, CD5, CD2,CD1, CD3, CD4, CD8, TdT pos) CALLA sometimes observed Pre-B (CALLA, B4, HLA-DR)	T-cell t(11;14) t(7;14), t(8;14), t(10;14) B-cell t(1;19), t(4;11)	Thorax Lymph nodes, bone marrow
Anaplastic large cell	T-cell or null (CD 30) Ki-1+	t(2;5) and variants	Lymph nodes, skin, intrathoracic, soft tissue, CNS
Peripheral T-cell lymphoma	T-cell	Unknown	Variable

and Arceci 2003). In the remaining 20% of the BL cases, c-myc is translated to the κ light-chain gene locus on chromosome 22 (t(2:8)(p11:q24)) or to the λ light-chain locus on chromosome 22 (t(8:22)(q24:q11)). In LL, many different translocations have been identified and usually involve the translocation of TCR on chromosome 14. The most common ones include (t(11:14)(p13;q110), (t(10:14)(q24;q11)) and (t(1:14)(p32–34;q11)). Other common genetic abnormalities for LL include the overexpression of the tal-1 gene found on chromosome 1. Additionally, a common genetic defect in T-cell lymphoma is the inactivation of the multitumor suppression gene (mts1) located on chromosome 9p21 (Weitzman and Arceci 2003). In 30% of the pediatric large B-cell lymphoma, there will be genetic abnormalites of BCL-6 expression. Rearrangements of BCL-6 can lead to overexpression of the gene and proliferation of B-lymphocytes, causing high-grade pediatric B-cell lymphomas. In pediatric ALCL, the majority of cases will demonstrate the translocation (t(2:5)(p23:q35)). This translocation results in the production of the fusion protein, ALK, which may be identified by immunochemistry on fixed tissue. Notably, the primary cutaneous ALCL that is rare in pediatrics will typically be ALK negative.

2.3.4 Symptoms and Clinical Signs

Pediatric NHL is generally an aggressive tumor that grows quickly and spreads rapidly. Most children will therefore present with advanced-stage or metastatic disease. The clinical presentation of NHL is unique to each classification. Table 2.5 outlines the various clinical presentations of NHL.

Endemic or African BL differs in clinical presentation compared with sporadic BL. Endemic BL presents at a peak age of 7 years, with involvement of the jaw/facial bones in approximately 60–70% of the cases (Magrath 2007). Bone marrow involvement is rare in endemic BL, but central nervous system (CNS) involvement is common. A high rate of paraplegia caused by an extradural mass is found at clinical presentation of endemic BL (Magrath 2007). In comparison, sporadic BL presents with abdominal disease in 90% of the cases and has a peak age of 11 years at presentation. The remaining 10% of the cases of sporadic BL arises from B-lymphocytes in Waldeyer's ring. With this presentation, patients may have a history of nasal breathing, change in voice, and frequent draining ear infections. Common symptoms at presentation of sporadic BL with abdominal presentations include abdominal mass, abdominal pain, ascites, nausea, and vomiting. Bowel obstruction may occur as an initial feature of sporadic BL. In females, ovarian involvement of BL is common. Mediastinal involvement of BL is a rare occurrence. BL is a clinically aggressive and rapidly growing tumor with a reported tumor doubling time of 2–3 days. Owing to the rapid growth associated with BL, children will often present with hyperuricemic neuropathy and will subsequently have the highest incidence of tumor lysis syndrome after initiation of chemotherapy.

LL presents with a mediastinal mass and associated pleural and/or pericardial effusions in approximately 50% of pediatric cases (see Figs. 2.7 and 2.8). In addition, these children can present with right ventricular outflow obstruction and/or superior vena cava syndrome. Symptoms can include dyspnea, dysphagia, and swelling of the face, neck, and arms. Lymphadenopathy is common at presentation and is usually cervical, supraclavicular, or axillary in location. In some cases, physical examination may reveal hepatosplenogmegaly. Similar to acute lymphoblastic leukemia (ALL), involvement of the bone marrow and CNS may be present at diagnosis. Patients with positive CNS disease may have no clinical symptoms or may present with facial nerve palsies and/or symptoms of increased intracranial pressure, including headache, visual changes, papilloedema, nausea, and vomiting. CBCs are typically normal or may demonstrate mild cytopenias resulting from the less than 25% of disease infiltration in the bone marrow. Overt testicular involvement is rare at presentation. Patients with LL may also present with bone pain or limp, which may be associated with pathologic fractures or lytic lesions from disease infiltration (Sandlund 2007).

LCLs can present with mediastinal or abdominal involvement and can make the clinical presentation similar to both BL and LL. Bone marrow involvement

Table 2.5. Presentations of NHL

Features	Signs and symptoms	Indication
Meningoencephalitis	Headache Cranial nerve palsies Altered level of consciousness	CNS disease found commonly in BL
Waldeyer's ring involvement	Tonsillar hypertrophy	BL
Jaw lesion	Swelling Pain	Endemic BL
Systemic features	Fever Weight loss Night sweats Anorexia Malaise	Anaplastic LCL
Mediastinal mass	Persistent nonproductive cough Dysphagia Dyspnea Chest pain	Intrathoracic disease, common in T-cell LL
Superior vena cava syndrome	Swelling of the upper extremities Distended neck veins Decreased breath sounds Dyspnea or stridor due to mass pressing on internal structures, pericardial effusion	Intrathoracic lesion Common in T-cell LL
Acute abdomen	Abdominal distension Pain Rebound tenderness Shifting dullness Nausea Vomiting GI bleeding Change in bowel habits Intussusception	Abdominal lymphoma B-cell (Intussusception is not an uncommon presentation for abdominal BL)
Bone pain	Local pain Swelling	Bony disease, can occur in LCLs, LLs, and BLs
Skin involvement	Painful lesions	Particularly anaplastic LCLs
Testicular involvement	Pain Swelling	Localized anaplastic LCL or LL
Pancytopenia	Infection Fatigue Bleeding	Metastatic disease – bone marrow LL or BL Lymphoma common

is less frequent compared with other presentations of NHL, and CNS involvement is rare (Weitzman and Arceci 2003). In the subtype ALCL, the clinical presentation often includes unusual sites such as the bone, skin, and peripheral nodes. ALCL can also present with diffuse pulmonary disease. ALCL often has systemic or "B" symptoms present at the time of initial presentation. B symptoms include fever with a temperature higher than 38 °C for more than 3 days, drenching night sweats, and unexplained weight loss

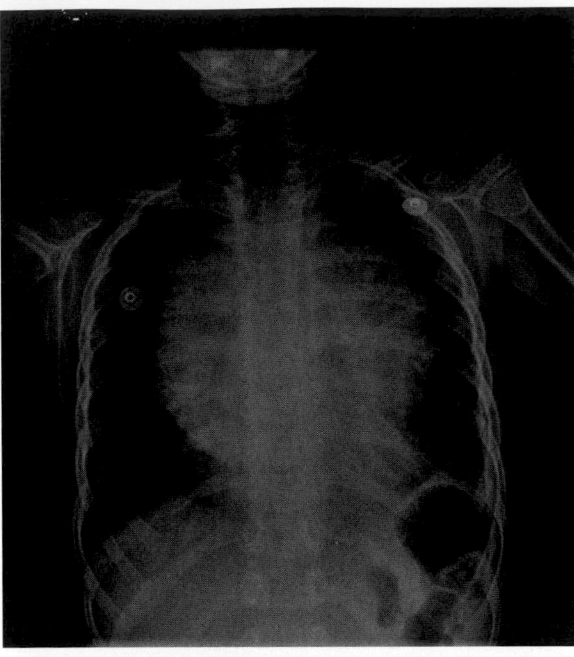

Figure 2.7
Chest X-ray LL with large mediastinal mass

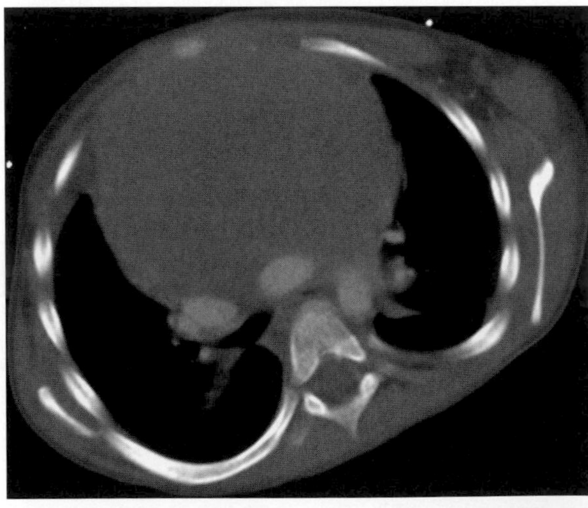

Figure 2.8
LL with large mediastinal mass on CT scan

of more than 10% over 6 months (see Sect. 2.4 in HL) (Chauvenet et al. 2000).

2.3.5 Diagnostics

Owing to the highly aggressive nature of pediatric NHL, it is crucial to make the diagnosis in a timely manner so that appropriate therapy can begin. The first step in the diagnosis is a complete history and physical examination. This may highlight potential sites of disease and determine the priority of diagnostic scans and investigations. Imaging studies are required to assess for potential complications of the tumor at presentation, and also to determine the extent of disease involvement. It is important to both determine and document disease involvement at diagnosis, to assign treatment intensity and allow for the use of subsequent imaging studies to assess for disease response.

Imaging studies vary by institution, but generally will include:

- Chest X-ray
- CT scan of the neck, chest, abdomen, and pelvis
- Abdominal ultrasound
- Echocardiogram (Magrath 2007)

CT of the head or MRI of the brain is indicated for patients with potential CNS disease, as evidenced by their clinical signs and symptoms. Nuclear imaging studies such as gallium, and more recently, PET are used to screen for unrecognized sites or metastatic disease. In addition to determining the extent of the disease, imaging studies also assist the clinical team in determining suitable sites, tissue, or fluid for biopsy, which is required to confirm the diagnosis. In some instances, a fine needle aspiration of the tumor or aspiration of pleural or pericardial fluids can produce enough material to carry out the diagnosis; however, an excisional biopsy is preferred. An excisional biopsy allows for more thorough immunophenotyping, cytogenetic, and molecular genetic testing. Sometimes, significant complications from the presence of a mediastinal mass, such as right ventricular outflow obstruction or superior vena cava syndrome may be present, requiring sedation or general anesthesia to obtain

a biopsy too dangerous. In these cases, corticosteroids have been used for a maximum of 24–36 h to decrease the size of the tumor before a biopsy can be done and the diagnosis can be confirmed. Bone marrow and CSF evaluations should also be done to determine disease involvement. Bone scanning is indicated for patients with clinical symptoms of bone pain and, if positive, should be followed up with X-ray or MRI. Although it is important to identify bone involvement, it currently does not affect disease staging. The required blood examination at diagnosis is often research-protocol driven, but at minimum should include a CBC, serum renal and liver function tests, serum chemistries including uric acid, potassium and calcium, and lactate dehydrogenase (LDH) as a measure of tumor burden. Serologic tests for EBV and HIV are recommended prior to initiating therapy. Although diagnostic studies are similar across disease subtypes of NHL, it is important to pay special attention to physical examination of the soft tissue and skin, as these sites are commonly involved in patients with ALCL. The skin and soft tissue may be isolated ALCL, but all patients with skin or soft tissue involvement should have a complete diagnostic work-up to assess for other potential sites of disease involvement. See Table 2.6 for a list of staging studies suggested for diagnosis of pediatric NHL.

Once the specimen for biopsy has been obtained, the appearance of the cells (morphology) along with immunophenotyping using flow cytometry and chemical staining will help to carry out the diagnosis. Additionally, cytogenetic and molecular testing can confirm the diagnosis by determining the presence of common genetic alterations associated with pediatric NHL. Cytogenetic and molecular alterations in pediatric NHL have been described in a previous section. The following paragraphs briefly outline some of the morphology and immunophenotyping associated with each NHL subtype.

Table 2.6. Staging studies for pediatric NHL

Chest X-ray
CT scan of neck, chest, abdomen, and pelvis
Abdominal ultrasound
PET or Gallium scan
CT head or MRI brain if clinically indicated
Echocardiogram
Bone marrow aspirate/biopsy
CSF collection

BL is the malignant transformation of a relatively mature B-lymphocyte cell. Under the microscope, the BL tumor will demonstrate a diffuse, infiltrative pattern with small- to medium-sized homogenous cells with round to ovoid nuclei, two to five prominent basophilic nucleoli, and basophilic cytoplasm that usually contains lipid vacuoles (Link and Weinstein 2006). Often there are scattered residual normal macrophages interspersed among the malignant cells, giving the classic "starry sky" appearance associated with BL. The nuclei of the malignant cells are often similar or smaller in size compared with histiocytes, and have been categorized as small noncleaved lymphocytes (Weitzman and Arceci 2003). Flow cytometry by immunochemistry demonstrates B-cell markers CD20, CD10 (common ALL antigen), and also IgM surface immunoglobulin. In BL, the terminal deoxynucleotidyl transferase (TdT) is negative. Additionally, expression of the Ki-67 antigen is present in almost all Burkitt malignant cells (Link and Weinstein 2006). The distinction between BL and Burkitt-like lymphoma is difficult to determine by histology, and although it has been shown that Burkitt-like lymphoma is likely to be intermediate between BL and DLBCL, there continues to be no proven benefit clinically from differentiating the Burkitt-like subtype (Weitzman and Arceci 2003).

LL cells are indistinguishable from ALL cells by morphology. Under the microscope, LL demonstrates a diffuse proliferation of medium-sized cells with a high nuclear to cytoplasmic ratio. There will be only scant amounts of basophilic cytoplasm. In approximately 50% of LL cases, the nuclear chromatin will be finely stippled with indistinct nucleoli and some degree of nuclear convolution (Weitzman and Arceci 2003). There is high mitotic activity. The LL cells are strongly positive for TdT and acid phosphatase, observed by cytochemistry.

Immunophenotype studies have identified that LL is 80% T-cell phenotype and only 15–20% precursor B-phenotype. The T LL cells are derived from thymic T-cells, which express the pan-T antigen, CD7 (Weitzman and Arceci 2003). The identification of CD7 is one of the best available tests for identifying T cell LL malignancy. Depending on when the malignant transformation occurs during lymphocyte differentiation, other antigens will also be positive. These may include CD2, CD3, CD45RO, CD4, CD8, and CD10 (Link and Weinstein 2006). While morphologically LL cells are similar to ALL cells, there are subtle differences between the cells which can be observed by immunochemistry. The subtle differences demonstrate that T ALL cells are usually derived from early to intermediate thymocytes, whereas T LL cells are usually derived from intermediate to late stage thymoctye cells. The precursor B LL cells demonstrate the common ALL markers including CD10, CD19, CD22, and HLA-DR (Link and Weinstein 2006).

LCLs include various subtypes including ALCL, DLBCL, and the rare peripheral T-cell lymphoma, observed by Revised European American Lymphoma Classification (REAL) classification. The LCL group of tumors have cells in which the nuclei are larger compared with the nuclei of the surrounding histiocytes (Weitzman and Arceci 2003). LCLs will demonstrate different features by morphology and immunochemistry according to subtype. ALCL that represents approximately 10% of all pediatric NHL, have cells that demonstrate diffuse proliferation characterized by cohesive large cells with abundant basophilic cytoplasm and bizarre pleomorphic cells. Additionally, the ALCL cells have eccentric, horseshoe-shaped nuclei with single or multiple prominent nuclei (Link and Weinstein 2006). The ALCL cells demonstrate positive antigens CD30 (Ki-1) and epithelial membrane antigen (EMA). Commonly, CD25 (IL2-R) is also expressed in ALCL. DLBCLs represent proliferation of large lymphoid cells of B lineage. The nuclei of these cells are two times as large as the nuclei of small lymphocytes. Immunophenotyping of DLBCL demonstrates positive antigens CD19, CD20, CD22, and CD79a, with surface immunoglobulin expression in up to 50% of the cases (Link and Weinstein 2006).

2.3.6 Staging and Classification

Recent classification systems define NHL with regard to morphology, immunophenotype, cytogenetic abnormalities, and clinical presentation. Classifications by REAL and WHO are the most recent systems. Pediatric lymphomas are classified by REAL into three major subtypes: LL, BL, and LCL. LL is morphologically and cytogenetically identical to ALL. The distinction between LL and ALL is made only by the degree of bone marrow involvement. Bone marrow involvement of less than 25% denotes a diagnosis of LL and greater than 25% indicates ALL. According to the REAL classification, 30–40% of North American children with NHL have LL subtype (80% T-cell phenotype and 15–20% B-cell precursor lineage), 40–50% will have BL, and 15–30% will have LCL.

Staging of pediatric NHL is most commonly based on the St. Jude's system (see Table 2.7). This staging system is applicable for all three subtypes of pediatric NHL, and separates patients with localized (stage I/II) and advanced disease (stage III). Stage IV NHL is assigned based on the presence of bone marrow and/or CNS involvement. CNS involvement may include leptomeningeal infiltration or cranial nerve palsy. Accurate staging of pediatric NHL is crucial, as it will determine both intensity and length of therapy. The St. Jude's staging system does not currently apply to endemic BL, where the disease is often isolated to the jaw/face. In endemic BL, stage I is a single facial tumor and stage II is the presence of two or more separate facial masses. Stage III endemic includes involvement of intrathoracic, intra-abdominal, paraspinal, or osseous masses (excluding the jaw). Stage IV endemic BL is assigned when there is involvement of the CNS or BM which is similar to the St. Jude's stage IV assignment.

The National Cancer Institute has provided breakdowns of the incidence in which the various forms of lymphoma can be present (Table 2.8).

2.3.7 Treatment

Treatment for NHL depends on the histologic subtype and stage of the disease. Most protocols now assign patients to risk groups to determine the intensity and length of treatment.

Table 2.7. St Jude staging systems for childhood NHL

Stage I	Single tumor (extranodal) or single anatomic area (nodal) with the exclusion of mediastinum or abdomen
Stage II	Single tumor (extranodal) with regional lymph nodes
	Two or more nodal areas on the same side of diaphragm
	Two single tumors (extranodal) with or without regional lymph node
	A resectable primary GI tumor with or without involvement of mesenteric nodes only
Stage III	Two single tumors (extranodal) above and below the diaphragm
	Two or more nodal areas above and below the diaphragm
	All primary intrathoracic tumors
	All extensive primary intra-abdominal disease
	All paraspinal or epidural tumors
Stage IV	Any of the above with the initial involvement of either the central nervous system and/or the bone marrow (<25%)

Pinkerton et al. 1999

Table 2.8. NHL incidence according to subtype and cell of origin (adapted from Pinkerton et al. 1999)

Cell type	Subgroup	Proportion of NHL (%)
B-Cell	Precursor B neoplasm	
	B lymphoblastic	5
	Peripheral B neoplasm	
	Follicular	0.4
	Diffuse large B-cell	3
	Primary mediastinal	0.4
	Burkitt's	42
	High-grade Burkitt's and Burkitt's-like	4
T-Cell	Precursor T neoplasm	
	T-lymphoblastic	20
	Peripheral T-cell	
	PTL unspecified	1
	Anaplastic large cell	15
	Nonspecific/intermediate	9.2

Surgery is primarily used to obtain tissue for biopsy. Sometimes, however, surgery is required at the time of diagnosis to manage complications of the tumor, particularly, abdominal tumors, such as intussusception or bowel obstrution/perforation. If total resection of a localized abdominal turmor is acheivable at the time of laparotomy, it is advised and should be followed by a short (6 week) course of chemotherapy to achieve excellent overall survival. Surgery for the purpose of debulking should be avoided as it has demonstrated no benefit when compared with chemotherapy (Patte 1997). Any surgical intervention that will delay the initiation of chemotherapy should also be avoided. At present, the role of surgery for assessment of residual tumor is controversial. It is sometimes deemed necessary to perform surgery to determine remission status of patients with questionable residual tumor, who may require further aggressive therapy; however, two-thirds of surgeries to confirm histological disease demonstrate necrotic tissue (Büyükpamukcu 1998).

Radiation therapy has been ommitted from the majority of current treatment protocols for pediatric NHL. Historically, before the advent of effective chemotherapy regimens, radiation as a single modality therapy provided a poor overall survival rate of approximately 20% in patients with localized disease. Presently, owing to the known morbidity associated with radiation therapy and the lack of clinical evidence to support its additional benefit to chemotherapy protocols, the use of radiation is restricted to pediatric NHL cases with proven CNS disease and patients with isolated head and neck primary tumors.

Combination chemotherapy is the standard treatment for pediatric NHL, and the intensity and length of the therapy is based on the subtype and stage of the disease. See Table 2.9 for a review of current NHL treatment summaries. Stage of the disease is most commonly divided between localized (stage I/II) and advanced-stage disease (stage III/IV). Chemotherapy regimens are also based on the immunophenotype of the lymphoma (B-cell vs. T-cell). In general, T-cell lymphomas receive longer and less intense treatments, and B-cell lymphomas are treated for shorter intensive periods, but with higher doses of alkylating agents and antimetabolites. NHLs are sensitive to a variety of chemotherapeutic agents, probably due to the aggressive nature of the disease with its rapid doubling time and high growth fractions. Because of this aggressive nature of the disease, patients with NHL are at a great risk of tumor lysis syndrome. Initial management of NHL is therefore focused on both managing immediate complications of the tumor and the prevention and management of tumor lysis syndrome. Although tumor lysis is reviewed in detail in another chapter of this book (Chap. 17), it is important to highlight the use of more current uricolytic agents that initiate a precipitous drop in uric acid by converting it to

Table 2.9. Treatment summaries for NHL (from Cairo and Perkins 2000; reprinted with permission)

Stage and histology	Chemotherapy regimen	Cooperative group	Length of therapy	Percentage of survival (3–5 years)
Stages I and II (St Jude) or group A (FAB)	COPADA	SFOP	6 weeks	95
B large or SNCCL	COMP	CCG	6 months	85
Lymphoblastic	CHOP COMP BFM-NHL	BFM	8 weeks	90
Stages III and IV or group B and C				
SNCCL	LMB-89	SFOP	6 months	80–90
	Orange	CCG	8 months	70–80
	NCI-89-C-41	NCI	6 months	70–80
	Total-B	POG	4 months	60–70
	BFM-NHL	BFM	4 months	60–80
Lymphoblastic	(AD)COMP	CCG	18–24 months	70
	LSA-L2	CCG/POG	18–24 months	70
	BFM-NHL	BFM	18–24 months	90
Large cell	COMP (D)	CCG	18–24 months	60–70
B-cell	APO (+)	POG	18 months	60–70
	LMB-89	SFOP	4–6 months	90
	ORANGE	CCG	4–6 months	90
	BFM-NHL	BFM	4–6 months	70–80
	NCI-89-C-41	NCI	4–6 months	80–90
Anaplastic	CHOP/MACOOP-B	ST JUDE'S	6 months	75
	BFM-NHL-B	BFM	6 months	80
	HM 89–91	SFOP	6–8 months	60–70

allantoin. The use of urolytic agents such as Rasburicase and Uricozyme has much improved clinical management of pediatric patients with NHL, who have a high risk of tumor lysis (Pui et al. 2001; Coiffier et al. 2008) The following sections will review the current treatment approachs for both localized and advanced-stage disease, and is separated by disease subtype.

The treatment course of low-stage (stage I/II) BL and DLBCL is generally short-course chemotherapy. Recently, the Pediatric Oncology Group (POG) demonstrated excellent survival of greater than 90% with 9 weeks of CHOP (Cyclophosphamide, Doxorubicin, Vincristine, and Prednisone)-based chemotherapy with no added advantage of radiation therapy or maintenance therapy (Link et al. 1997). Similar overall event-free survival was achieved by the investigators of the BFM group (Berlin–Frankfurt–Munich) for localized nonlymphoblastic NHL (Reiter et al. 1995). The SFOP LMB-89 trial demonstrated more than 90% survival rates with two courses of chemotherapy without radiaion therapy for localized nonlymphoblastic lymphoma. These short courses of chemotherapy excluding radiation, although effective for nonlymphoblastic localized NHL, have been proven ineffective for children and adolescents with isolated stage I/II LL. This subgroup of stage I/II LL requires a more aggressive treatment approach. Investigators with the BFM group have demonstrated an event-free survival of more than 90%, utilizing the standard arm of the BFM T-cell protocol (Reiter et al. 2000). This treatment protocol includes a standard induction followed by a consolidation phase of five doses of high-dose (5 g/m^2) methotrexate followed by maintenance therapy for 24 months. These patients achieved excellent survival without a reinduction phase that is common in most T ALL protocols. CNS prophylaxis in the form of intrathecal chemotherapy is reserved for patients with LL subtype and patients with localized head and neck lymphoma, but is no longer required for localized nonlymphoblastic abdominal lymphoma including the BL subtype (Weitzman and Arceci 2003). Cranial radiation is reserved for patients with primary localized head and neck lymphoma. Owing to the current excellent overall survival, future clinical trials in the treatment of low-stage BL and DLBCL should focus on minimizing treatment-related morbidity.

For advanced-stage (stage III/IV) BL and large B-cell lymphoma, the current overall survival exceeds 80%. This has greatly improved in the past two decades, noting that the survival of advanced-stage NHL in the early 1980s was less than 30% (Weitzman and Arceci 2003). This improvement in survival can be partly attributed to the intensification of chemotherapy. Most current and successful protocols use a combination of chemotherapy agents including corticosteroids, high-dose methotrexate, high-dose cytarabine (Ara-C), vincristine, and high-dose cyclophosphamide or ifosphamide with or without anthracycline (Weitzman and Arceci 2003). The cycles of chemotherapy are given over 3–5 days and administered in intensively timed cycles over 3–6 months to prevent regrowth of tumors/malignant cells that are known to have a rapid growth rate. Clinical trials of both BFM and SFOP (Society Francais d'Oncology Pediatrique) groups have demonstrated improved survival of pediatric patients with advanced-stage NHL, by increasing the intensity of chemotherapy such as methotrexate and cytarabine (Patte et al. 1992; Büyükpamukcu 1998). It has been demonstrated in this group of patients that CNS prophylaxis and treatment can be achieved without the use of intrathecal chemotherapy or radiation, owing to the addition of high-dose antimetabolite chemotherapies such as cyclophosphamide/ifosphamide, cytarabine, and methotrexate (Weitzman and Arceci 2003). Similar to other malignancies in childhood, an early response to therapy had been associated with improved survival. It is important to reevaluate primary sites of disease following initial cycles of chemotherapy, to determine disease response. If suspected residual tumor is present after initial cycles, it may be necessary to confirm if the disease persists histologically, as these patients may benefit from further intensified chemotherapy, such as HSCT, to improve their overall survival.

Advances in the treatment of advanced-stage (stage III/IV) T-cell LL result from the realization that LL responds best to chemotherapy protocols designed for the treatment of ALL. Although mediastinal masses are common at presentation of LL, the addition of radiation therapy to the mediastinum has not been proven to be beneficial over systemic chemotherapy (Magrath 2002). An important component of chemotherapy, as proven by several investigative groups, is the administration of high-dose methotrexate in improving overall survival and specifically reducing the incidence of CNS relapse (Patte et al. 1992). Similar to ALL therapies, treatment protocols for LL include an early intensive phase including induction, consolidation, and reinduction, followed by a less-intensive maintenance phase for 1–2 years. Most relapses of pediatric LL occur within 18 months of diagnosis, suggesting that an intensified early-treatment phase may be of more importance than maintenance chemotherapy (Weitzman and Arceci 2003). The addition of cranial radiation is generally recommended only for patients with proven CNS disease at diagnosis. Recently, new agents, such as compound 506U78 (2-amino-6 methoxypurine arabinoside), which is a specific anti T-cell agent, are being tested in combination with proven chemotherapy protocols to assess for improved overall survival. There continues to be concern about neurotoxicity of compound 506U78 and studies are ongoing. Most clinical experts agree that precursor B LL should be treated using the same chemotherapy protocols recommended for T-cell LL.

The treatment of ALCL is dependent on determining primary skin and soft tissue disease from systemic disease. As previously mentioned, this distintion can be made by determining the expression of ALK. Primary skin or soft tissue ALCL is usually ALK negative and systemic ALCL is ALK positive. The current approach for isolated skin ALCL is either surgical removement or local radiation (Link and Weinstein 2006). The current approach for systemic ALCL is combination chemotherapy, and length and intensity varies by stage of disease at presentation. Stage I/II ALCL is treated with three cycles of CHOP chemotherapy (Cyclophosphamide, Adriamyin, Vincristine, and Prednisone) and no radiation therapy (Link and Weinstein 2006). More advanced stages of ALCL, such as stages III/IV, have required more intensive regimens. Most current protocols for advanced-stage ALCL include six cycles of chemotherapy that includes a combination of chemotherapeutic agents, such as methotrexate (moderate to high dose), ifosphamide, cyclophosphamide, cytarabine, etoposide, doxorubicin, and intrathecal chemotherapy.

Oncologists are challenged with decisions regarding the therapy for the treatment of PTLD. This is partly due to the heterogeneity of PTLD. Treatment options include reduced immunosuppression, surgical resection with reduced immunosuppression, anti B-cell antibody (anti CD20 monoclonal antibody, Rituximab), chemotherapy either low-dose or as per NHL protocol if disease persists or progresses, and HSCT (Gross and Shiramizu 2007).

2.3.8 Prognosis

Over the past three decades there has been a dramatic improvement in the overall survival of children and adolescents diagnosed with NHL. The current reported disease-free survival for pediatric NHL, independent of the subtype, is approximately 80% (Gross and Termuhlen 2007). However, the survival can be categorized by stage of the disease at presentation. The survival for pediatric patients with localized NHL (nonlymphoblastic) is reported between 85 and 90% (Link et al. 1997; Weitzman et al. 2002; Cairo et al. 2005). The current reported overall survival for advanced-stage NHL is reported between 80 and 90% (Cairo et al. 2005). For some populations, there are identified poor prognostic features including subtype BL with combined bone marrow and CNS involvement and subtype DLBCL with primary mediastinal disease (Cairo et al. 2005). In addition to the stage as a prognostic feature, the level of tumor burden as defined by LDH has been identified as a prognostic factor. At the time of diagnosis of NHL, an LDH level greater than 400 U/L has been identified as a poor prognostic marker (Shulka and Trippett 2006). The significance of tumor bulk as a prognostic factor in pediatric NHL is currently unclear due to the sussesses achieved by systemic therapies.

2.3.9 Follow-Up

Follow-up for children treated for NHL must include surveillance for both disease recurrence and late effects of treatment. Owing to the great variation of treatment protocols used in pediatric NHL, the risk of late effects is also variable. However, due to the limited use of radiation and the careful consideration of cumulative doses of anthryaclines and alkylating agents, the risks for late effects following NHL therapy is relatively low. The risks for late effects have been reported as similar to those of pediatric ALL therapy, and include neurocognitive deficits, cardiotoxicity, and osteopenia/osteoporosis (Meadows and Friedman 2007). Follow-up screening for cardiotoxicity includes echocardiograms every 2–4 years for patients who received anthracycline therapy. It is important to screen attention to learning and school performance in children who have received high-dose methotrexate, intrathecal chemotherapy, or cranial radiation. For some of these children, neuropsychological testing will identify neurocognitive deficits and recommend specific interventions. There is a low risk of second malignancies in the population of children treated for NHL. Cumulative doses of alkylating agents are generally less than 9 g/m^2 on current NHL protocols, so there is a low risk of infertility and gonadal dysfuntion. Recent guidelines for recommended follow-up for pediatric cancer survivors have been published and are very useful clinical tools in planning follow-up care (Landier et al. 2004).

Surveillance for relapse remains important in post completion of treatment care, as approximately 20% of the patients will unfortunately have a recurrance of disease. It is recommended that scans of the primary tumor be carried out using CT or ultrasound, depending on the tumor's location. Frequency of surveillance scans varies by clinician and is often protocol-driven. Generally, it is suggested that scans of the primary site of the disease be carried out every 3 months for the first year post treatment, and then with decreasing frequency over several years. Gallium or PET scans can be very helpful in the surveillance for NHL recurrence and can be done on a similar schedule to primary tumor imaging. CBCs are necessary, especially in LLs, to look for recurrence of bone marrow disease, which is characterized by blasts in the peripheral smear.

2.3.10 Treatment of Relapsed/Refractory NHL

Despite the excellent overall survival of 80% for pediatric NHL, 10–20% of children will unfortunately have a relapse of their disease. The aim of relapsed/refractory therapy for NHL is to achieve a second clinical remission (CR2). Most relased or "salvage" pediatric NHL protocols utilize intensified combination chemotherapy that includes agents not used in the primary frontline treatment. A CR2 is achieved in approximately 60–70% or relapsed pediatric NHL cases. Once CR2 has been achieved, the remission is consolidated with HSCT, either autologous or allogeneic (Gross and Termuhlen 2007). Even though approximately 60–70% of the relapsed cases will achieve a CR2, the reported overall survival for relapsed NHL in children is only 30–50% (Weitzman and Arceci 2003). This estimated survival is even lower for patients who have disease that does not achieve CR2 with relapsed therapy or who have demonstrated an initial slow response to frontline therapy. The current relapsed protocols for NHL do provide intensified chemotherapy, but additionally, some relapsed protocols may include targeted therapies such as monoclonal antibodies to improve success in achieving CR2. The addition of targeted therapies will continue to be the focus of research for pediatric relapsed NHL.

2.3.11 Future Perspectives

Owing to the excellent overall survival associated with pediatric NHL, one major focus for the future is to develop treatment protocols that aim to minimize toxicity related to therapy without sacrificing cure. Part of minimizing toxicity may result from the use of more targeted therapies such as monoclonal antibodies. Specific to this area is the use of anti CD20 (Rituximab) and anti CD22 antibodies. At present, the use of these monoclonal antibodies is primarily for patients with lymphoproliferative disease, but studies are underway investigating their use in frontline treatment, particularly for B-cell lineage lymphomas. Other examples of targeted therapy includes anti CD30 immunotoxins in the treatment of ALCL. In addition to targeted therapies, it will continue to be a priority to identify those patients with high-risk disease and poor response to standard therapy, who may benefit from earlier intesified treatment or alternative therapies. The development of vaccines to prevent viruses that are associated with the deveopment of lymphoma will probably continue to be an area of research interest (Jacobsen and LaCasce 2006).

References

Büyükpamukcu M (1998) Non-Hodgkins lymphomas. In: Voute PA, Kalifa C, Barrett A (eds) Cancer in children, clinical management, 4th edn. Oxford University Press, New York

Cairo MS, Perkins S (2000) Non-Hodgkin's lymphoma in children. In: Bast RC, Kufe DW, Pollock RE, Weichselbaum RR, Holland JF, Frei E (eds) Cancer medicine, 5th edn. Decker, Hamilton, BC

Cairo MS, Raetz E, Lim M, Davenport V, Perkins S (2005) Childhood and adolescent non-Hodgkin lymphoma: new insights in biology and critical challenges for the future. Pediatric Blood and Cancer 45:753–769

Chauvenet A, Schwarz CL, Weiner MA (2000) Hodgkin's disease in children and adolescents. In: Bast RC, Kufe DW, Pollock RE, Weichselbaum RR, Holland JF, Frei E (eds) Cancer medicine, 5th edn. Decker, Hamilton, BC

Coiffier B, Altman A, Pui C, Younes A, Cairo M (2008) Guidelines for the management of pediatric and adult tumor lysis syndrome: an evidence-based review. Journal of Clinical Oncology 26(16):2767–2778

De Bruin M, Huisbrink J, Hauptmann M, Kuenen M, Ouwens G, van't Veer M, Aleman B, Leeuwen F (2008) Treatment related risk factors for premature menopause following Hodgkin lymphoma. Blood 111(1):101–108

Donaldson SS, Hudson MM, Lamborn KR, Link MP, Kun L, Billett AL, Marcus KC, Hurwitz CA, Young JA, Tarbell NJ, Weinstein HJ (2002) VAMP and low-dose, involved field radiation for children and adolescents with favorable, early-stage Hodgkin's disease: results of a prospective clinical trial. Journal of Clinical Oncology 20(14):3081–3087

Donaldson SS (2007) Introduction and historical background: pediatric Hodgkin lymphoma. In: Weinstein HJ, Hudson MM, Link MP (eds) Pediatric lymphomas, 1st edn. Springer, New York

Dorffel W, Luders H, Ruhl U, Albrecht M, Marcihiak H, Parwaresch R, Potter R, Schellong G, Schwarze E, Wickman L (2003) Preliminary results of the multicenter trial GPOH-HD 95 for the treatment of Hodgkin's disease in children and adolescents: analysis and outlook. Klinische Padiatric 215(3):139–145

Faye A, Vilmer E (2005) Post-transplant lymphoproliferative disorders in children: incidence, prognosis and treatment options. Pediatric Drugs 7(1):55–65

Gurney JG, Severson RK, Davis S, Robinson LL (1995) Incidence of cancer in children in the United States. Cancer 75(8):2186–2195

Gross TG, Termuhlen AM (2007) Pediatric non-Hodgkin's lymphoma. Current Oncology Reports 9:459–465

Gross TG, Shiramizu B (2007) Lymphoproliferative disorders related to immunodeficiencies. In: Weinstein HJ, Hudson MM, Link MP (eds) Pediatric lymphomas, 1st edn. Springer, New York

Hall GW, Katzilakis N, Pinkerton CR, Nicolin G, Ashley S, McCarthy K, Daw S, Hewitt M, Wallace WH, Shankar A (2007) Outcome of children with nodular lymphocyte predominant Hodgkin lymphoma - a Children's Cancer and Leukaemia Group report. British Journal of Haematology 138(6):761–768

Hudson MM, Donaldson SS (2002) Hodgkin's disease. In: Pizzo PA, Poplack DG (eds) Principles and practice of pediatric oncology, 4th edn. Lippincott Williams & Wilkins, Philadelphia

Hudson MM, Schwartz C, Constine L (2007) Treatment of pediatric Hodgkin lymphoma. In: Weinstein HJ, Hudson MM, Link MP (eds) Pediatric lymphomas, 1st edn. Springer, New York

Jarrett RF (2003) Risk factors for Hodgkin's lymphoma by EBV status and significance of detection of EBV genomes in serum of patients with EBV-associated Hodgkin's lymphoma. Leukemia and Lymphoma 44(Suppl 3):S27–S32

Jacobsen E, LaCasce A (2006) Update on the therapy of highly aggressive non-hodgkin's lymphoma. Expert Opinions on Biologic Therapies 6(7):699–708

Landier W, Bhatia S, Eshelman D, Forte K, Sweeney T, Hester A, Darling J, Armstrong F, Blatt J, Constine L (2004) Development of risk-based guidelines for pediatric cancer survivors: the children's oncology group long-term follow-up guidelines from the children's oncology late effects committee and nursing discipline. Journal of Clinical Oncology 22:4979–4990

Landman-Parker J, Pacquement H, Leblanc T, Habrand J, Terrier-Lacombe M, Bertrand Y, Perel Y, Robert A, Coze C, Thuret I, Donadieu J, Schaison G, Leverger G, Lemerle J, Oberlin O (2000) Localized Hodgkin's disease: response-adapted chemotherapy with etoposide, bleomycin, vinblastine, and prednisone before low-dose radiation therapy-results of the French Society of Pediatric Oncology Study MDH90. Journal of Clinical Oncology 18(7):1500–1507

Link M, Weinstein H (2006) Malignant non-Hodgkin lymphomas in children. In: Pizzo PA, Poplack DG (eds) Principals and practice of pediatric oncology, 5th edn. Lippincott Williams & Wilkins, Philadelphia

Link M, Shuster J, Donaldson S et al (1997) Treatment of children and young adults with early stage non-Hodgkin's lymphoma. New England Journal of Medicine 337:1259–1266

Magrath, I (2007) B-Cell Lymphoma/Burkitt Lymphoma. In: Weinstein HJ, Hudson MM, Link MP (eds) Pediatric lymphomas, 1st edn. Springer, New York

Magrath IT (2002) Malignant non-Hodgkin's lymphoma in children. In: Pizzo PA, Poplack DG (eds) Principles and practice of pediatric oncology, 4th edn. Lippincott Williams & Wilkins, Philadelphia

Meadows AT, Friedman DL (2007) Late effects following lymphoma treatment. In: Weinstein HJ, Hudson MM, Link MP (eds) Pediatric lymphomas, 1st edn. Springer, New York

Metayer C, Lynch CF, Clarke EA, Glimelius B, Storm H, Pukkala E, Joensuu T, Van Leeuwen FE, van't Veer MB, Curtis RE, Holowaty EJ, Andersson M, Wiklund T, Gospodarowicz M, Travis LB (2000) Second cancers among long-term survivors of Hodgkin's diagnoses in childhood and adolescence. Journal of Clinical Oncology 18(21):2435–2443

Murphy SB, Morgan ER, Katzenstein HM, Kletzel M (2003) Results of little of no treatment for lymphocyte-predominant Hodgkin disease in children and adolescents. Journal of Pediatric Hematology/Oncology 25:684–687

Patte C (1997) Non-Hodgkin's lymphoma. In: Pinkerton CR, Plowman PN (eds) Paediatric oncology clinical practice and controversies, 2nd edn. Chapman and Hall Medical, London

Patte C, Kalifa C, Flamant F, Hartmann O, Brugières L, Valteau-Couanet D, Bayle C, Caillaud JM, Lemerle J (1992) Results of the LMT81 protocol, a modified LSA2L2 protocol with high dose methotrexate, on 84 children with non-B-cell (lymphoblastic) lymphoma. Medical and Pediatric Oncology, 20(2): 105–113

Pinkerton CR, Michalski AJ, Veys PA (eds) (1999) Clinical challenges in paediatric oncology. ISIS Medical Media, Oxford

Pui C, Mahmound H, Wiley JM, Woods GM, Leverger G, Camitta B, Hastings C, Blaney SM, Relling MV, Reaman GH (2001) Recombinant urate oxidase for the prophylaxis treatment of hyperuricemia in patients with leukemia or lymphoma. Journal of Clinical Oncology 19(3):697–704

Reiter A, Schrappe M, Parwaresch R, Henze G, Muller-Weihrich S, Sauter S, Sykora KW, Ludwig WD, Gadner H, Riehm H (1995) Non-hodgkin's lymphoma of childhood and adolescence: results of a treatment stratified for biological subtype and stage-a report of the BFM group. Journal of Clinical Oncology 13:359–372

Reiter A, Schrappe M, Ludwig W, Tieman M, Parwaresch R, Zimmerman M, Schrig E, Henze G, Schellong G, Gadner H, Riehm H (2000) Intensive ALL type therapy without local radiotherapy provides a 90% event-free survival for children with T cell lymphoblastic lymphoma: a BFM Group report. Blood 95:416–421

Sandlund JT (2007) Precursor B and Precursor T-Cell Lymphoblastic Lymphoma. In: Weinstein HJ, Hudson MM, Link MP (eds) Pediatric lymphomas, 1st edn. Springer, New York

Sandlund JT, Downing JR, Crist WM (1996) Non-Hodgkin's lymphoma in childhood. New England Journal of Medicine 334:1238–1248

Schwartz CL, Constine LS (2002) POG 9425: response based, intensively timed therapy for intermediate/high stage pediatric Hodgkin Disease. Proceedings of American Society of Clinical Oncololgy 21:389

Schwartz CL (2003) The management of Hodgkin's disease in the young child. Current Opinions in Pediatrics 15(1): 10–16

Shulka N, Trippett T (2006) Non-hodgkin's lymphoma in children and adolescents. Current Oncology Reports 8:387–394

Sklar C, Whitton J, Mertens A, Stovall M, Green D, Marina N, Greffe B, Wolden S, Robinson L (2000) Abnormalities of the thyroid in survivors of Hodgkin's disease: data from the childhood cancer survivor study. Journal of Clinical Endocrinology and Metabolism 85(9):3227–3232

Smith RS, Chen Q, Hudson MM, Link MP, Kun L, Weinstein H, Billett A, Marcus KJ, Tarbell NJ, Donaldson SS (2003) Prognostic factors for children with Hodgkin's disease treated with combined-modality therapy. Journal of Clinical Oncology 21(10):2026–2033

Stein H (2001) Hodgkin lymphoma. In: Jaffe ES, Harris NL, Stein H, Vardiman JW (eds) World Health Organization classification of tumors. Tumors of hematopoietic and lymphoid tissues. IARC, Lyon

Trippet TM, Chen A (2007) Treatment of relapsed/refractory Hodgkin lymphoma. In: Weinstein HJ, Hudson MM, Link MP (eds) Pediatric lymphomas, 1st edn. Springer, New York

Weitzman S, Arceci R (2003) Non-Hodgkin's lymphoma of childhood. In: Wiernik P, Goldman J, Dutcher J, Kyle R (eds) Neoplastic diseases of the blood. Cambridge University Press, Cambridge, pp 843–861

Weitzman S, Suryanarayan K, Weinstein H (2002) Pediatric non-hodgkin's lymphoma: clinical and biologic prognostic factors and risk allocation. Current Oncology Reports 4:107–113

3.6.7 Treatment 96
3.6.8 Prognosis 99
3.6.9 Follow-Up 100
3.6.10 Future Directions 100
3.7 Rhabdomyosarcoma 100
3.7.1 Epidemiology 100
3.7.2 Etiology 101
3.7.3 Molecular Genetics 101
3.7.4 Symptoms and Clinical Signs 101
3.7.5 Diagnostics 101
3.7.6 Staging and Classification 103
3.7.7 Treatment 103
3.7.7.1 Local Therapy 104
3.7.7.2 Chemotherapy 105
3.7.8 Prognosis 106
3.7.9 Follow-Up 106
3.7.10 Future Perspectives 106
3.8 Non-Rhabdomyosarcomatous Soft-Tissue Sarcomas 107
3.8.1 Alveolar Soft-Part Sarcoma 108
3.8.2 Desmoid Tumor (Aggressive Fibromatosis) 108
3.8.3 Desmoplastic Small Round Cell Tumor 108
3.8.4 Infantile Fibrosarcoma 109
3.8.5 Infantile Hemangiopericytoma 109
3.8.6 Infantile Myofibromatosis 109
3.8.7 Leiomyosarcoma 109
3.8.8 Liposarcoma 109
3.8.9 Malignant Peripheral Nerve Sheath Tumor 110
3.8.10 Synovial Sarcoma 110
3.9 Germ Cell Tumors 110
3.9.1 Epidemiology 111
3.9.2 Etiology 111
3.9.3 Molecular Genetics 112
3.9.4 Symptoms and Clinical Signs 112
3.9.5 Diagnostics 112
3.9.6 Staging and Classification 113
3.9.7 Treatment 113
3.9.7.1 Surgical Considerations 114
3.9.7.1.1 Ovarian Tumors 114
3.9.7.1.2 Testicular Tumors 114
3.9.7.1.3 Extragonadal Tumors 114
3.9.7.2 Chemotherapy 115
3.9.8 Prognosis 115
3.9.9 Follow-Up 115
3.9.10 Future Perspectives 116
3.10 Rare Tumors 116
3.10.1 Adrenocortical Carcinoma 116
3.10.2 Melanoma 117
3.10.3 Nasopharyngeal Carcinoma 118
3.10.4 Pleuropulmonary Blastoma 118
3.10.5 Thyroid Carcinoma 119
References 119

3.1 Ewing's Sarcoma Family of Tumors

Ewing's sarcoma family of tumors (ESFT) comprises a group of neoplasms that can arise in bone and/or soft tissue, and share similar histologic and molecular features. These tumors include Ewing's sarcoma (ES), extraosseous ES, peripheral primitive neuroectodermal tumor (PPNET), and Askin tumor (chest wall tumor). ES is the more undifferentiated form of the tumor, whereas PPNET is more differentiated. ESFTs are thought to derive from neural crest cells, although the exact cell of origin remains unknown.

3.1.1 Epidemiology

ES is the second most frequently seen primary malignant bone tumor in childhood and represents 3% of all pediatric malignancies (Ludwig 2008). The incidence is approximately 3 per million annually in individuals less than 20 years of age (Esiashvili et al. 2008). ESFT occurs most often in the second decade of life, with the median age of diagnosis being 15 years (Paulussen et al. 2008). ESFT are rare in individuals over the age of 30 and in African and Asian children. There is a male predominance of 1.5:1 for this tumor (Esiashvili et al. 2008).

3.1.2 Etiology

There are no identifiable etiological factors in ES, and there do not appear to be any strong associations with congenital or familial cancer syndromes.

3.1.3 Molecular Genetics

Histologically, ESFT are characterized by small round blue cells with abundant glycogen and absence of cytoplasmic filaments (Zagar et al. 2008). Immunocytochemical staining with CD99 (MIC2) in a membranous pattern is pathognomonic for ES (Lewis et al. 2007). Molecular testing is invaluable in helping to distinguish ESFT from other small round blue cell tumors. Fluorescence in situ hybridization (FISH) and/or reverse-transcriptase polymerase chain reaction (RT-PCR) are used to detect the cytogenetic changes in the tumor. Eighty-five percent of ESFT display a characteristic t(11; 22)(q24; q12) that juxtaposes the EWS with the FLI1 gene (Lewis et al. 2007). There are two fusion types with the t(11; 22). Type-1 fusion involves the union of exons 1–7 of EWS with exons 6–9 of FLI1, and occurs in approximately 60% of the patients. Type-2 fusion involves EWS exons 1–7 joining with exons 5–9 of FLI1. This type of fusion appears to be prognostic, with the type-1 fusion imparting a better prognosis (Ludwig 2008), although this information does not alter the therapy currently. The t(21; 22)(q22; q12) occurs in 10% of cases, and fuses the EWS and the ERG gene (Lewis et al. 2007). The less-frequently observed pairings include EWS–ETV1, ESW–EIAF, and EWS–FEV (Ludwig 2008). There are also more complicated chromosomal rearrangements that are seen in 20% of the patients, and may include trisomy 8, trisomy 12, gain of 1q, deletions of 16q, and mutations of the p53 tumor suppressor gene and the *ink-4A* gene (Ludwig, 2008).

3.1.4 Symptoms and Clinical Signs

Anatomically, the sites of occurrence of ESFT are split into half, with 50% of tumors occurring in the axial skeleton and the other 50% arising in the appendicular skeleton (Paulussen et al. 2008). ESFT may occur in any bone or tissue, including skin, visceral organs, and soft tissues (Caudill and Ardnt 2007). ES occurring in the peripheral skeleton most commonly involve the diaphysis of the bone, unlike osteosarcoma, which more commonly involves the metaphysis. The most common sites of bony disease include (Ludwig 2008):

- Pelvis (26%)
- Femur (20%)
- Tibia/fibula (18%)
- Chest wall (16%)
- Upper extremity (9%)
- Spine (6%)

Children typically present with local symptoms caused by the primary tumor. Bone pain and swelling are often present. A palpable mass is frequently seen in tumors of the peripheral skeleton. It is not uncommon for a child to present after a prolonged history of intermittent pain, especially if the tumor is present in the pelvis, abdomen, or thoracic cavity. In extremity lesions, pain is often initially mistaken for growing pains or traumatic injury, which can delay the diagnosis. Extremity lesions may also present as pathological fractures of the affected bone. Primary ES of the chest wall, also known as Askin tumor, are often large and can present with respiratory symptoms such as cough, dyspnea, and unequal breath sounds. Paraspinal lesions can manifest with neurological impairment including motor weakness progressing to paraplegia. Finally, large pelvic tumors may be accompanied by ureteric obstruction, constipation, and pain.

Approximately 20% of patients present with metastatic disease at diagnosis (Paulussen et al. 2008). Metastases usually follow a hematogenous route, spreading to lungs, bone, and bone marrow. Patients with advanced disease may present with systemic signs such as fever, fatigue, and malaise. Infection, bleeding, and lethargy may reflect pancytopenia, suggesting bone marrow involvement.

3.1.5 Diagnosis

For primary bone tumors, a plain film of the affected area is the first and most revealing diagnostic test. The X-ray appearance of ES is that of a destructive lytic or mixed lytic and sclerotic lesion in the bone that is poorly marginated. The affected bone on imaging may have an onion peel appearance secondary to the perisosteal reaction, which is indicative of the tumor's continued growth despite the bone's efforts to repair itself. Magnetic resonance imaging (MRI) of the primary tumor is required to obtain adequate information about the soft-tissue component of the tumor, marrow extension, edema, lymph nodes, and intimacy to vessels and nerves. MRI is indicated for paraspinal lesions to evaluate the compression of the spinal cord (Fig. 3.1). Computed tomography (CT) of the chest and bone scan are needed to rule out pulmonary and bone metastases (Fig. 3.2). ES and RMS are the only two sarcomas which require bilateral bone marrow biopsies to rule out bone marrow metastatic disease. Whole body fluorodeoxyglucose positron emission tomography (FDG-PET)

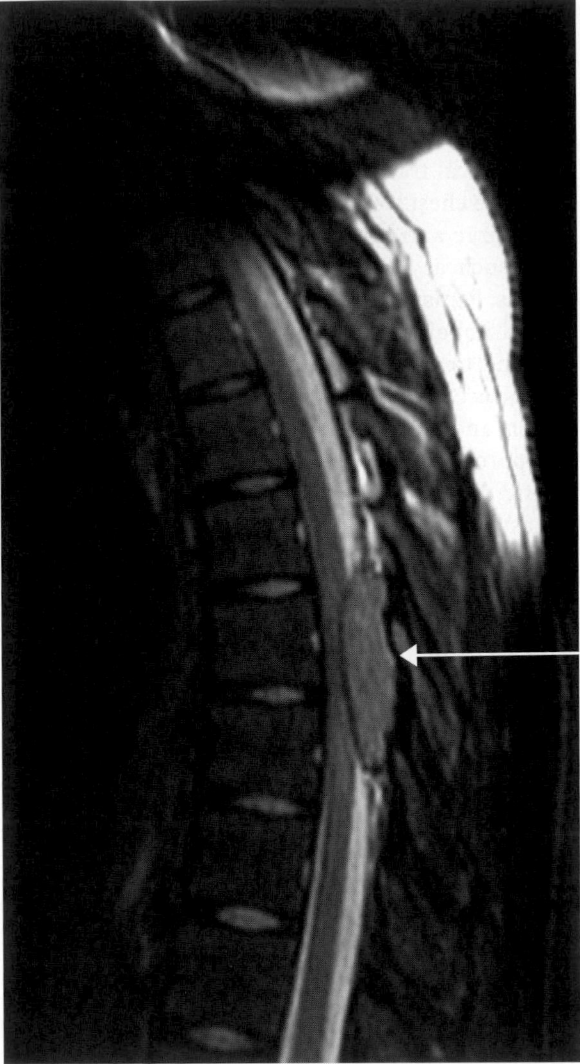

Figure 3.1

Paraspinal Ewing's sarcoma (ES). MRI of the spine shows the ESFT pressing on the spinal cord (*dark area*)

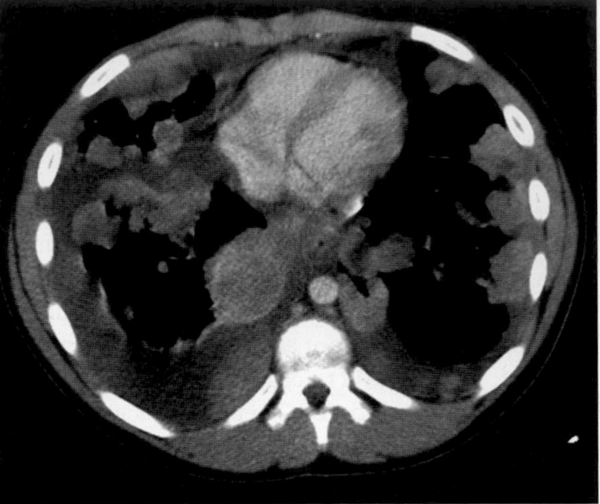

Figure 3.2

Pulmonary metastases. CT demonstrates extensive pulmonary and pleural metastases with pleural effusions in the metastatic ES

is increasingly recommended for staging in patients with ESFT, and may even be superior to bone scan. Positron emission tomography (PET) can also be useful in assessing tumor response to neoadjuvant chemotherapy and in evaluating the possibility of disease recurrence (Meyer et al. 2008). Currently, its limited availability hinders its widespread use, and further studies are required to determine whether changing therapy based on PET–CT results will improve survival.

A biopsy is always indicated to confirm the diagnosis. Tumor histology may be undifferentiated small round blue cells, or show some differentiation in Homer-Wright rosettes. The tumor specimen should be evaluated with routine staining and immunohistochemistry. ESFT almost universally stain positive for CD99, but CD99 positivity is not exclusive to ESFT. Therefore, muscle (myogenin or MyoD1), lymphoid (CD45 or TdT), and neural tissue (neuron-specific enolase) markers should be employed, and must be negative to rule out other small round blue cell tumors (Ludwig 2008). Cytogenetic studies and RT-PCR should be employed to look for the characteristic t(11; 22) or t(22; 21) translocations, discussed earlier.

There are no definitive blood tumor markers for the ESFT; however, an elevated lactate dehydrogenase (LDH) may indicate a large tumor burden or rapid tumor growth. Elevated LDH has also been associated with a less favorable outcome. An elevated white blood cell count or ESR can also be seen at times in advanced disease.

3.1.6 Staging and Classification

There is no specific staging system for ESFT. The tumor is described in terms of the presence or absence of distant metastases.

3.1.7 Treatment

3.1.7.1 Chemotherapy

Chemotherapy, radiation therapy, and surgery all play a role in the treatment of ESFT. Chemotherapy is important for cytoreduction of the primary tumor and for the treatment of micro- and macrometastatic disease. Historically, the standard chemotherapeutic agents used in ESFT included vincristine, actinomycin, doxorubicin, and cyclophosphamide. The addition of ifosfamide and etoposide (IE) to standard chemotherapy in the late 1980s and early 1990s resulted in a significant improvement in the survival of patients with localized disease (Grier et al. 2003). Vincristine, adriamycin, and cyclophosphamide (VADRIAC) alternating with IE now represents the standard backbone of the North American ESFT treatment protocols. Increasing dose intensity through interval compression of chemotherapy cycles, given every 14 days instead of every 21 days, with the support of granulocyte colony stimulating factor, has also improved event-free survival in patients with localized disease without increasing toxicity (Womer et al. 2008).

New drug combinations such as low-dose cyclophosphamide and topotecan have demonstrated activity in recurrent ESFT. A phase II clinical trial by the Pediatric Oncology Group (POG) found that 6 out of 17 patients with heavily pretreated relapsed ESFT responded to this drug combination (Saylors et al. 2001). This study and others have prompted the incorporation of cyclophosphamide and topotecan to standard chemotherapy in phase III trials for upfront therapy in newly diagnosed patients.

3.1.7.2 Surgery

Surgery is the preferred method of establishing local control. It has been very difficult to accurately determine whether radiation alone is as effective as surgery for local therapy, as only large, deep unresectable tumors are ever offered radiotherapy (RT) alone. Therefore, it is difficult to establish whether a poor outcome in radiated tumors is due to the tumor itself or the treatment provided. Despite this, complete surgical resection is always the first choice for local therapy, and is most often utilized for tumors of the extremities. The entire bony or soft tissue lesion needs to be excised using initial imaging studies, to ensure a disease-free margin of at least 1 cm and ideally 2–5 cm around the involved bone. Margins of at least 5 mm are required around fat or muscle planes, and at least 2 mm for fascia planes (Donaldson 2004). Gross or microscopic disease postoperatively requires additional treatment with adjuvant radiation therapy.

3.1.7.3 Radiotherapy

Radiation therapy is often the only viable option for tumors of the central axis, in which radical surgery is not feasible. Doses in the range of 40.4–60 Gy are delivered through intensity modulated radiation therapy (IMRT) in daily fractions (Donaldson 2004). The radiation volume is determined by the extent of tumor at diagnosis, including a 2.0–2.5-cm margin. A boost is then often delivered to the postinduction chemotherapy tumor volume with a 1.5–2.0-cm margin. This approach somewhat minimizes the extent of radiation to healthy tissues, while optimizing the therapy to the tumor itself. In patients who have microscopic residual disease following surgery, the tumor volume requiring radiation includes the site of residual disease or close margin along with a 1.5–2.0-cm margin (Donaldson 2004).

3.1.7.4 Metastatic Disease

The outcomes for patients with metastatic disease are poor, and the best way to treat these patients is still unknown. Sites of residual metastatic disease after completion of chemotherapy are generally treated with surgery and/or radiation therapy. However, the impact of whole lung radiation for pulmonary metastases on survival in ES has not yet been fully delineated (Whelan et al. 2002). Dose intensification regimens for metastatic disease using standard drugs have resulted in increased toxicity, increased secondary malignancies, with no significant improvement in survival (Miser et al. 2007). Standard chemotherapy with VADRIAC alternating followed by high-dose therapy and autologous peripheral blood stem cell support has also been attempted with no significant increase in disease-free survival (Hawkins et al. 2002; Gardner et al. 2008; Kushner and Meyers 2001).

The EURO-EWING 99 trial is attempting to determine the best way to treat ESFT by utilizing a risk-adapted approach. Patients are stratified into three risk groups based on high-risk features that include: patient age, tumor size, site, metastases, and histologic response to chemotherapy. All patients receive induction chemotherapy followed by surgery for local control if feasible. Patients with small tumors or those who are chemoresponsive are randomized to receive consolidation with vincristine, actinomycin-D, and cyclophosphamide (VAC), or vincristine, actinomycin, and ifosfamide (VAI). Patients with high-risk disease based on poor histological response, large size, or presence of lung metastases are randomized to receive VAI chemotherapy (plus whole lung irradiation for patients with lung metastases) vs. myeloablative consolidation with stem cell rescue using busulfan and melphalan (Bu-Mel). Patients with extra-pulmonary metastases are randomized to receive one of the three different conditioning regimens for myeloablative therapy with stem cell rescue (Rodriguez-Galindo et al. 2003) (Fig. 3.3). It is hoped that once this international, multi-center, European–North American study is completed, more definitive answers regarding the optimal treatment of high-risk ESFT will be available.

3.1.8 Prognosis

Prognosis for the ESFT depends on the resectability of the tumor and the presence of metastases at diagnosis. For patients with localized disease, 5-year EFS is approximately 70% (Caudill and Ardnt 2007). If metastases are present at diagnosis, the 2-year disease-free survival rate is less than 30% (Hawkins et al. 2002). Cutaneous, subcutaneous, distal bone, and rib tumors tend to have higher cure rates because of the ease of surgical resection. Tumors of the pelvis

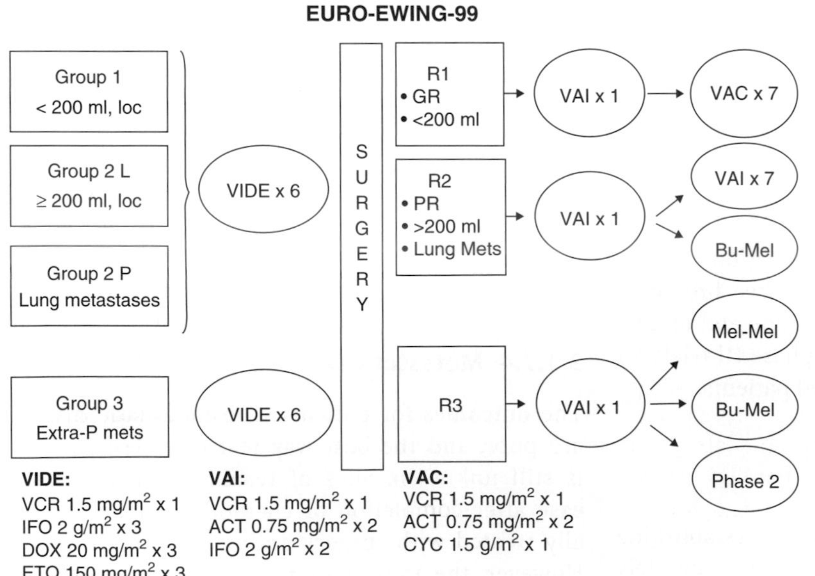

Figure 3.3 EURO-EWING-99 treatment schema. Risk stratification and treatment outline from EURO-EWING-99 study. *loc* localized; *extra-P* extra-pulmonary; *GR* good histological response; *PR* poor histological response; *Mel* melhelan; *Bu* busulfan. Reprinted with Permission Rodriguez-Galindo et al. 2003

are associated with poor outcome, mainly due to their large size and inoperability. Prognosis following relapse is poor, with reported long-term survival of only 13%; however, patients with late recurrence, more than 2 years after initial diagnosis, may be cured (Leavey et al. 2008). Isolated lung metastases and skip metastases in the same bone have better outcomes compared with metastatic disease elsewhere in the body (Ludwig 2008).

The tumor volume, serum LDH, and the amount of tumor necrosis at the time of surgery are of prognostic significance. The subtype of fusion gene is also prognostic, with the type-1 EWS–FLI1 favoring a better outcome than other genetic abnormalities independent of tumor size or location (Ludwig 2008). Patients with localized disease, age less than 15 years, tumor less than 8 cm in size, and extremity sites have shown to be favorable prognostic factors (Ludwig 2008).

3.1.9 Follow-Up

Follow-up requires focus on both recurrent disease and late effects of treatment. Patients are at greatest risk of recurrent disease in the first 3 years following the end of therapy for ESFT, but late recurrences have been reported (Paulussen et al. 2008). Follow-up is recommended every 3 months for the first 2–3 years, then every 6 months until 5 years, and then yearly thereafter (Paulussen et al. 2008). Imaging of the site of the primary tumor, and sites of potential metastatic disease (lungs and bones) should be carried out at regular intervals.

Cardiomyopathy, exercise intolerance, and congestive heart failure (CHF) can occur following anthracycline therapy; therefore, cardiac function should be monitored with echocardiograms. Kidney dysfunction, bladder fibrosis, hemorrhagic cystitis, sexual dysfunction, infertility, and menstrual changes can result from the use of alkylating agents (Lahl et al. 2008). If patients received radiation for local control, they may also have specific late effects related to the body system or site that was treated. It is important that patients are screened for late effects of therapy, so that interventions can be carried out if necessary.

Unfortunately, late effects of therapy also include secondary malignancies and must be considered when following up these patients post therapy. Secondary malignancies at 20 years post therapy are reported to be as high as 9.2%, and for secondary sarcomas, in particular, 6.5% (Kuttesch et al. 1996). The dose of radiation appears to correlate directly with the risk of radiation-induced sarcomas; patients who received less than 48 Gy did not develop secondary sarcomas. Patients are also at an increased risk of developing treatment-related myeloid leukemias and myelodysplastic syndromes (related to the administration of topoisomerase-II inhibitors, alkylating agents); this risk has been reported to be as high as 8% for some of the more intensive protocols (Rodriguez-Galindo et al. 2000).

3.1.10 Future Perspectives

There is a great deal of research looking to improve the outcome of ESFT. Most research efforts have focused on novel therapeutics including antiangiogenic agents targeting blood vessel formation, such as bevacizumab, a monoclonal antibody against vascular endothelial growth factor (VEGF).

Yondelis (Ecteinascidin-743) is a new antitumor agent with a complex transcription-targeted mechanism of action. This has shown promising results in patients in Phase I clinical trials in patients with ESFT, and is currently being studied in a phase II trial (Lau et al. 2005). Recently, there has been much attention given to the insulin-like growth factor (IGF) type-1 receptor pathway in ESFT. There are currently many monoclonal antibodies and some small molecule inhibitors of this pathway that are being investigated in phase I and II trials (Ludwig 2008). The EWS–FLI-1 fusion product may also prove to be a suitable target of molecular therapies, as downstream targets of EWS-fusion transcription factors have been found (Zagar et al. 2008).

3.2 Osteosarcoma

Osteosarcoma is a primary tumor of bone and it is thought to arise from mesenchymal bone-forming cells.

3.2.1 Epidemiology

Osteosarcoma is the most frequently occurring primary bone tumor of children and adolescents. The peak incidence of osteosarcoma is in the second decade of life, a period characterized by rapid linear bone growth. It occurs at an annual rate of approximately 2–3 per million children aged 15–19 years (Bielack et al. 2008), and 5.6 cases per million children less than 15 years (Caudill and Arndt 2007). The incidence is slightly higher in Caucasians and in males (Caudill and Arndt 2007). The incidence of osteosarcoma has increased by 1.4% per year over the last 25 years (Caudill and Arndt 2007).

3.2.2 Etiology

In the majority of cases, the cause of osteosarcoma is unknown. An association between rapid bone growth and the development of osteosarcoma is suggested by the high incidence during the growth spurt in adolescence. Some have postulated that an early growth spurt in addition to tall stature may be important factors in the development of osteosarcoma (Cotterill et al. 2004). While most cases of osteosarcoma are idiopathic, several conditions are associated with an increased incidence of osteosarcoma. Osteosarcoma can be caused by ionizing radiation, and can occur as a secondary malignancy in patients previously treated with radiation therapy for another cancer. This is implicated in 3% of osteosarcomas, and the most common primary malignancies in which this occurs are Ewing's sarcoma (ES), Rhabdomyosarcoma (RMS), Hodgkin's, brain tumors, retinoblastoma (RB), and Wilms' tumor (Koshy et al. 2005). A genetic predisposition exists between hereditary RB and osteosarcoma. The RB gene is a tumor suppressor gene and important in apoptosis. Mutation in one copy of the *RB1* gene is the most frequent genetic change in osteosarcoma, and is observed in 70% of sporadic tumors. Some reports suggest that loss of heterozygosity (LOH) of *RB1* may be associated with an unfavorable outcome in osteosarcoma (Feugeas et al. 1996; Ragland et al. 2002).

Mutations of p53 tumor suppressor gene are also implicated in the development of osteosarcoma (Berman et al. 2008). Acquired p53 mutations are detectable in 25–42% of osteosarcoma cases (Wunder et al. 2005). The p53 mutations are the origin of osteosarcoma development in Li-Fraumeni syndrome, which is characterized by germline mutations of p53 and rendering those affected with an increased risk of developing multiple malignancies, including osteosarcoma (Savage et al. 2007). Other conditions for which there is a higher incidence of osteosarcoma include hereditary multiple exostoses, Rothmund–Thomson syndrome, Paget's disease, Bloom syndrome, fibrous dysplasia, chronic osteomyelitis, multiple osteochondroma, and sites of bone infarcts (Caudill and Arndt 2007).

3.2.3 Molecular Genetics

The diagnosis of osteosarcoma is primarily based on tumor histology. Malignant osteoid is produced by osteosarcoma cells, and its presence confirms the diagnosis (Bielack et al. 2008). Although there is no specific cytogenetic or molecular marker for osteosarcoma, there is a great deal of research in the area of genetics, focusing on improving the understanding of the disease and determining the prognostic factors.

In addition to mutations in p53 and *RB1* described earlier, many other genetic abnormalities continue to be examined to determine their role in the disease. c-Myc is expressed more often in those with osteosarcoma who develop metastatic disease. HER2/neu (human epidermal growth factor receptor 2) is expressed in approximately 40% of patients who develop early pulmonary metastases (Ragland et al. 2002). Cadherin-11 is a molecule that is important in cellular communication. Its level of expression may play a role in metastatic disease and can be a useful marker in predicting survival (Nakajima et al. 2008). MDRI encodes p-glycoprotein, which if over expressed, may indicate an unfavorable outcome, as p-glycoprotein has a propensity to actively pump chemotherapy from tumor cells (Link et al. 2002). Tumor endothelial marker 7 is a protein that is over expressed in osteosarcoma cells, and again, it may represent a gene important in regulating osteosarcoma metastases (Fuchs et al. 2007). Ezrin is a protein that has membrane–cytoskeleton linking functions.

It is important in the cell signaling, growth regulation, and differentiation of cancer cells, and has been shown to regulate the growth and metastatic capacity of cancer. Increased expression of ezrin in osteosarcoma in particular has been shown to correlate with metastases (Park et al. 2006). Survivin is an apoptosis inhibitor gene, for which increased expression has been correlated with poor prognosis in osteosarcoma (Osaka et al. 2007). Important research is being carried out to understand the significance of these findings and whether they may represent future therapeutic targets.

3.2.4 Signs and Symptoms

Osteosarcoma commonly affects the metaphyseal growth plates of the long bones. Although osteosarcoma can occur in any bone, the anatomic sites most commonly affected are the distal femur, the proximal tibia, and the proximal humerus. Osteosarcoma metastasizes most frequently to the lung, followed by bone.

Osteosarcoma typically presents with progressive bone or joint pain, pain at rest, or night pain. Swelling and decreased range of motion in the joint generally follow. The duration of symptoms prior to diagnosis may be as long as 6 months. Symptoms often are reported to start after a sports-related injury that does not heal. Respiratory symptoms at diagnosis may only be present in very advanced pulmonary disease, and are rare. Systemic symptoms of disease, such as fever or weight loss, and lymphadenopathy are also uncommon.

3.2.5 Diagnostics

The workup up of a patient who presents with pain and/or swelling should start with a thorough health history, paying special attention to pain and physical examination. The quality, frequency, timing, duration, and alleviating and exacerbating factors of the pain should be identified. Cancer pain is usually persistent, and does not go away with time. Diagnostic imaging of the affected area and sites of potential metastatic disease, blood tests, and tumor biopsy are required.

The most important investigation in the workup of a suspected bone tumor is a plain X-ray of the area. Plain films of the affected area may reveal a mixed lytic and sclerotic lesion, with indistinct margins, and a sunburst pattern that is characteristic of osteosarcoma (Fig. 3.4). There is sometimes an associated soft-tissue mass that is calcified. Reactive new bone formation can also be seen frequently under the periosteum, forming a "Codman's angle" or "Codman's triangle" (Ragland et al. 2002; Caudill and Arndt 2007). An MRI of the affected area is very important, and will provide further information on tumor boundaries, the soft-tissue component, and the relationship to the joints and neurovascular structures (Fig. 3.5). A CT of the chest is needed to assess for the presence of pulmonary metastases. Pulmonary metastases are present at diagnosis in

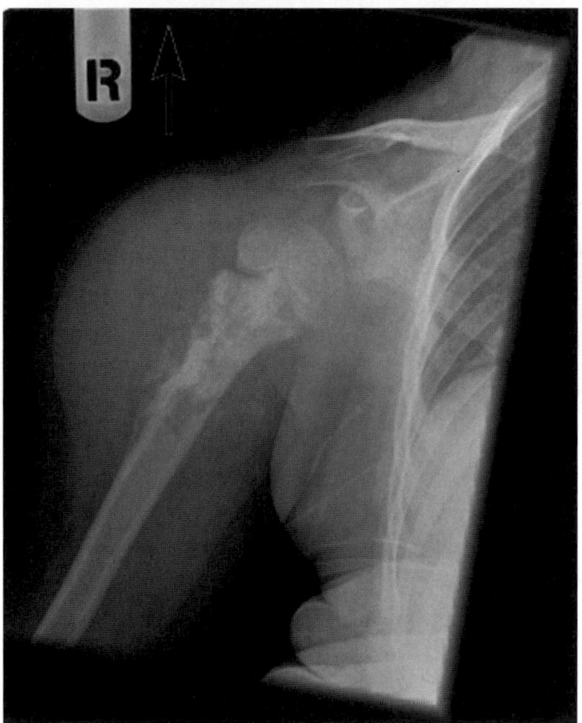

Figure 3.4

Plain film of the patient with osteosarcoma in right humerus. Sunburst periosteal reaction is seen

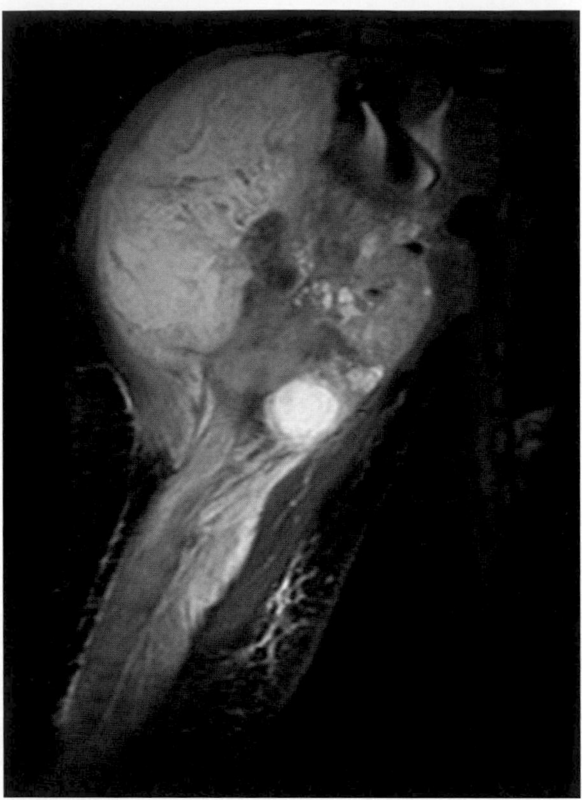

Figure 3.5
MRI of right humerus in the patient with osteosarcoma

15–20% of patients (Kager et al. 2003). A radionucleotide bone scan is also needed to identify areas of skeletal metastases. Bony metastases occur in 10% of patients with osteosarcoma at diagnosis (Link et al. 2002). PET scans are now being more routinely recommended in clinical trials for osteosarcoma (Meyer et al. 2008).

There are no specific blood tumor markers for osteosarcoma. Elevations of alkaline phosphatase and LDH are often seen in osteosarcoma and correlate with adverse outcomes (Bielack et al. 2008). A biopsy is necessary for obtaining definitive diagnosis. Open biopsy is preferred so the surgeon has control over where the biopsy track is placed and to guarantee a sufficient yield of tissue. Histologically, osteosarcoma is characterized by the presence of spindle cells and the production of malignant osteoid (Meyer et al. 2008).

3.2.6 Staging and Classification

There are varied histological patterns of osteosarcoma. Osteoblastic osteosarcoma is the most common type of conventional osteosarcoma, with an incidence of 78%, followed, in descending order of frequency, by chondroblastic, fibroblastic, malignant fibrous histiocytoma-like, giant cell-rich, telangiectatic, low-grade intraosseous, small cell, and juxtacortical types (Caudill and Arndt 2007).

Staging in osteosarcoma is generally straightforward and considers intra and extra compartmental factors (whether tumor extends through cortex to bone), as well as tumor grade and presence of metastases. Table 3.1 shows the Enneking staging system for osteosarcoma. The tumors are divided into low- and high-grade variants depending on the number of mitoses, anaplasia, cellularity, and pleomorphism. The majority of osteosarcomas seen in children are high grade. Stage IIB is the most common presentation of conventional osteosarcoma.

3.2.7 Treatment

The treatment for osteosarcoma consists of surgical resection of the primary tumor and chemotherapy. Historically, osteosarcoma was treated with surgery only. This approach yielded poor outcomes with long-term survival rates less than 20% (Ferrari et al. 2003). This demonstrated that even in the absence of overt metastatic disease, almost all patients have

Table 3.1. Enneking staging system for osteosarcoma

Grade number	Osteosarcoma characteristics
1	Low-grade osteosarcoma
2	High-grade osteosarcoma
3	Osteosarcoma with distant metastases
A	Intracompartmental
B	Extracompartmental

micrometastatic disease at diagnosis, accounting for the high recurrence rate. Currently, with use of neoadjuvant and adjuvant chemotherapy, survival has increased dramatically. High-dose methotrexate, adriamycin, and cisplatin (MAP) are chemotherapy agents that are highly sensitive in osteosarcoma, and represent the backbone of most conventional osteosarcoma treatment protocols. Ifosfamide alone or together with etoposide (IE) have also demonstrated good activity in the disease, although their added benefit to MAP in upfront treatment on newly diagnosed patients is uncertain. Typically, chemotherapy is given for 2–3 months prior to local surgical resection. Following local treatment, an additional 5–6 months of therapy is administered.

Sometimes, despite neoadjuvant chemotherapy, patients do not achieve sufficient tumor necrosis, assessed by pathology review of the resected tumor. Even in patients who do achieve favorable necrosis (>90%), more than 20% of patients still experience relapse. Thus, further clinical trials are needed to improve the outcome of this disease. An international osteosarcoma randomized clinical trial (EURAMOS) is currently being carried out which offers the addition of a biologic agent to standard chemotherapy for patients with favorable necrosis who are considered the "good responders." Good responders are randomized postoperatively to receive standard chemotherapy with MAP vs. MAP plus interferon. The poor responders (<90% necrosis) are being randomized to receive MAP vs. MAPIE (Caudill and Ardnt 2007). The primary question being asked is whether the addition of interferon to patients who have already responded well to MAP chemotherapy will further improve survival. The question being asked with regard to poor responders is whether intensifying chemotherapy by adding IE would improve survival in this high-risk group. Increasing dose intensity of chemotherapy by administering drugs every 2 weeks instead of every 3 weeks does not appear to improve survival in localized osteosarcoma (Ferrari and Palmerini 2007).

A novel agent, muramyl tripeptide phosphatidyl-ethanolamine (MTP–PE) that was studied in a clinical trial by the Children's Oncology Group (COG) in North America, may be useful in osteosarcoma. MTP-PE is a synthetic analog of muramyl dipeptide which is an element of the cell wall in Bacillus Calmette–Guierin (BCG). The drug is delivered selectively to monocytes and macrophages, inducing them to become activated and tumoricidal. The COG study found that patients who received MAP plus ifosfamide and MTP–PE had a statistically significant improvement in OS, compared with those who did not receive MTP–PE (Meyers et al. 2008). It is unclear at this point whether this agent will be studied further.

Surgery for local control consists of three options:

1. Limb salvage: Limb salvage procedures can be done for 90–95% of tumors today (Wittig et al. 2002). They are appropriate when the tumors can be removed effectively with negative margins, that is, the tumor is removed with a rim of healthy tissue around the tumor. To reconstruct the limb and/or joint, an endoprosthesis, allograft, arthrodesis, intercalary allograft, or metallic prosthesis can be used.
2. Amputation: Amputation is usually reserved for tumors that cannot be removed with adequate surgical margins. It is also frequently used in large tumors that do not respond well to chemotherapy and to tumors that have produced skip lesions.
3. Rotationplasty: Rotationplasty is another procedure that is used when there is a large tumor around the knee joint, extensive soft-tissue mass, intraarticular extension of the tumor, or pathologic fractures (Fuchs and Sim 2004). The leg is amputated at the distal femur, and the ankle joint is preserved, rotated 180°, and reattached (Fig. 3.6). This produces an artificial knee joint from which the prosthesis can be effectively secured for a greater range of motion (Fig. 3.7).

It is generally felt that while a limb-sparing procedure offers a more favorable cosmetic outcome, amputation and rotationplasty allow for more aggressive future physical activity (Hopyan et al. 2006), including competitive sport. The initial contemplation of rotationplasty or amputation can be devastating to a patient, and the psychosocial impact of these mutilating surgeries must be taken into consideration when the patient and family are asked to make decisions between these choices (see Chap. 24).

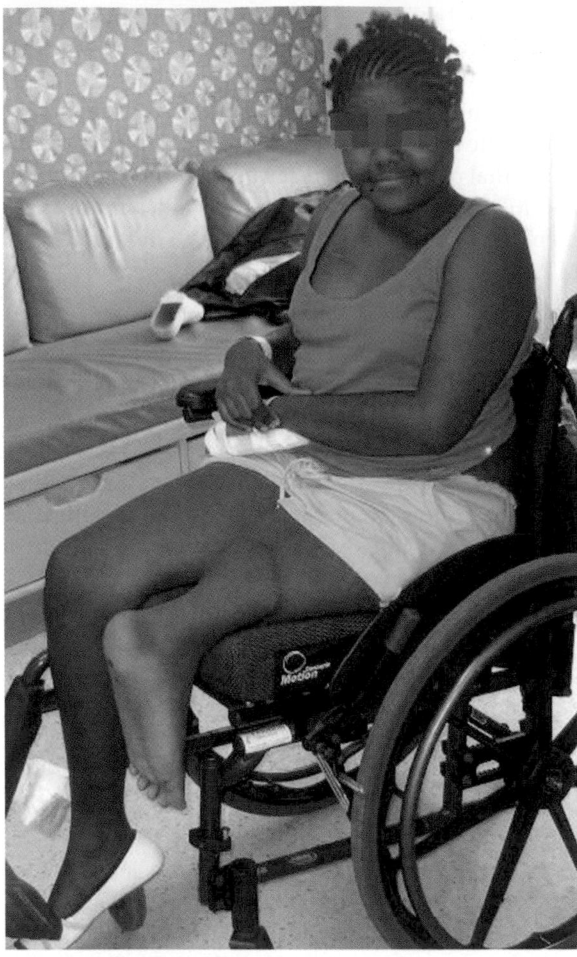

Figure 3.6
Patient with rotationplasty

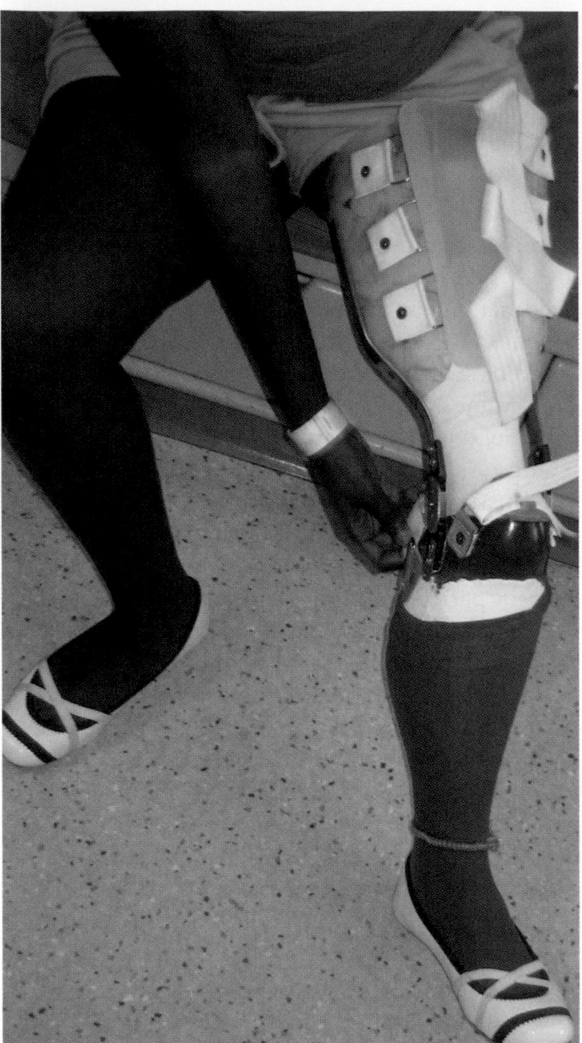

Figure 3.7
Rotationplasty with prosthesis

Radiation therapy does not play a role in the curative treatment of osteosarcoma. Osteosarcoma cells are not sensitive to the doses of radiation that can be safely administered. It is reserved for inoperable axial skeletal tumors and for palliation, especially of painful sites (Bielack et al. 2008).

Metastatic disease at diagnosis predicts a poor outcome. Treatment aims should be the same: chemotherapy and surgical resection of disease. Patients with resectable metastatic disease are also eligible to be treated on the abovementioned randomized trial (EURAMOS), provided all sites of primary and metastatic disease are resectable.

Despite aggressive chemotherapy and surgical resection of nonmetastatic osteosarcoma of the extremities, 30–40% of patients still experience relapse of their disease. The post-relapse survival in this group is poor (<20%) (Bielack et al. 2008). The majority of relapses occur in the lung. Accepted strategies for treatment include surgical resection, sometimes requiring multiple thoracotomies. A retrospective analysis by Ferrari et al. (2003) demonstrated that using ifosfamide may be beneficial in relapsed osteosarcoma, especially in patients with three or more pulmonary nodules. Furthermore, relapsed patients with one or two pulmonary nodules responded better (5-year event-free survival, 24%) than those who had bony metastases or more than two pulmonary nodules. Bony metastases have a poor outcome, and the role of surgical resection for bone metastases remains controversial.

3.2.8 Prognosis

The overall survival (OS) of patients with nonmetastatic disease at diagnosis, with the tumor located in an extremity, is 60–70%, whereas the survival of patients with metastases at diagnosis remains poor, at 15–20% (Bacci et al. 2002). Tumors with greater than 90% necrosis are considered to exhibit a "good response," and long-term survival rates in these patients are higher (75–80%) compared with those with a "poor response" to chemotherapy (<90% necrosis), in whom long-term survival is 45–55% (Bielack et al. 2002; Whelan et al. 2000). Poor prognostic factors in osteosarcoma include age less than 14 years, high serum alkaline phosphatase level at diagnosis, tumor volume greater than 200 mL, inadequate surgical margins, and poor histological response to chemotherapy (Bacci et al. 2006). The site of the tumor plays a role in prognosis, with axial tumors faring worse than skeletal, most likely related to the difficulty in surgical resection of axial tumors.

Several molecular prognostic indicators have been studied, and alterations in the following are associated with inferior survival: increased expression of the gene survivin, increased ezrin expression, LOH at the RB gene locus, over expression of p-glycoprotein, and overexpression of HER 2/erbB-2 (Osaka et al. 2007; Onada et al. 1996; Feugeas et al. 1996; Kim et al. 2007a). The presence of metastatic disease, however, still remains the most significant adverse prognostic indicator.

3.2.9 Follow-Up

Patients need to be followed up for recurrent disease and must be monitored for late effects of the treatment itself. Because of the risk of late recurrences, chest X-rays are recommended every 6 weeks to 3 months for the first 2 years post treatment, followed by every 2–4 months for the third and fourth years post treatment, and then every 6 months until 10 years post therapy (Bielack et al. 2008). Imaging of the primary site should be done every 4 months for 4 years post therapy.

Late effects of chemotherapy include cardiomyopathy related to anthracycline use and hearing impairment and nephrotoxicity secondary to cisplatin chemotherapy. Neurological, hormonal, and psychological late effects should also be considered when assessing patients. Infertility and secondary malignancies may result from the use of high-dose alkylating agents.

3.2.10 Future Perspectives

Novel therapies for osteosarcoma are focusing on biological and alternative agents. Zoledronic acid, a potent bisphosphonate, has shown efficacy against osteosarcoma in preclinical models. It has been found to have antiangiogenic properties (Ferrari and Palmerini 2007). Studies with zoledronic acid and concomitant chemotherapy are currently underway, and its utility in this regard will be observed. The role of mammalian target of rapamycin (mTOR) is also being studied in osteosarcoma. The mTOR inhibitors works by causing growth arrest of the cells in the G1 phase of the cell cycle, and phase II clinical trials showed some encouraging results (Ferrari and Palmerini 2007). Gene therapy using viral vectors have been studied in patients with osteosarcoma and require further investigation, because of several devastating side effects including death and several de novo tumorogenetic events that have occurred in early studies (Dass and Choong 2008). There is also some interest in the antiangiogenic agents that target and impede the tumor's ability to form new blood vessels, thereby inhibiting tumor growth. Thalidomide and celocoxib have been used in this respect, and antecdotal responses have been reported. Granulocyte macrophage colony stimulating factor (GMCSF) is currently being studied to determine its effect on stimulating macrophage activity for lung metastases when administered by inhalation (Postiglione et al. 2003). Finally, the effect of samarium, a bone-seeking radioisotope, is being tested with autologous stem cell transplant for metastatic bony disease (Anderson et al. 2007).

3.3 Liver Tumors

There are a variety of tumors that can develop in the liver, the majority of which (two-thirds) are malignant (Litten and Tomlinson 2008). Malignant tumors include hepatoblastoma (HB), hepatocellular carcinoma (HCC), and less commonly sarcomas, germ cell tumors, and rhabdoid tumors.

3.3.1 Epidemiology

Malignant liver tumors account for just over 1% of pediatric malignancies. HB is an embryonal tumor and is the most common malignant liver tumor of childhood, representing two-thirds of all liver tumors in this population. HB is a disease of infants and young children, with 95% of the cases developing before the age of 4 years; 4% are present at birth (Litten and Tomlinson 2008; Stocker 2001). The mean age at diagnosis is 18 months. There is a male predominance ranging from 1.4:1 to 2.0:1, and Caucasians are affected up to five times more often than African–Americans (Tomlinson and Finegold 2002). There is an increased incidence of HB in the Far East.

HCC accounts for 23% of all childhood liver tumors (Meyers 2007). There is a higher male predominance affected by this tumor, and it most often occurs after the age of 10.

3.3.2 Etiology

There is an association between the development of HB and prematurity. In Japan's registry for pediatric malignancy, the risk for HB is inversely correlated with birth weight (Tomlinson and Finegold 2002). There is also evidence that parental exposure to metals, paints, cigarette smoke, and petroleum may increase the incidence of HB in their offspring (Buckley et al. 1989; Sorahan and Lancashire 2004). There is an association of HB with certain genetic syndromes such as Beckwith–Wiedemann syndrome (BWS), familial adenomatous polyposis (FAP), Li-Fraumeni syndrome, trisomy 18, and glycogen storage disease type I. Syndromes, however, have been reported to be present in less than 20% of liver malignancies (Litten and Tomlinson 2008).

Hepatitis B infection has been shown to be pathogenic in HCC. HCC also develops in the presence of cirrhosis and underlying liver disease. There is some suggestion that parenteral nutrition in infancy is associated with HCC in childhood. The genetic syndromes that are associated with a higher incidence of HCC are glycogen storage disease, hereditary tyrosinemia, neurofibromatosis, ataxia-telangiectasia, Fanconi's anemia, FAP, Alagille syndrome, and other familial cholestatic syndromes (Litten and Tomlinson 2008). Maternal exposure to oral contraceptive pills, fetal alcohol syndrome, and gestational exposures to gonadotropins are environmental factors implicated as possibly leading to HCC (Tomlinson and Finegold 2002).

3.3.3 Molecular Genetics

Several chromosomal abnormalities occur in HB, but very few have been linked to HCC. In HB, the most common chromosomal abnormalities involve trisomy 2, 8, and 20, and a translocation of (1; 4)(q12; q34) (Litten and Tomlinson 2008). LOH at 11p15, which is a known tumor suppressor gene seen in Wilms' tumor, has also been observed in HB. Mutations of the B-catenin/Wnt pathways appear to be involved in the development of HB and require further exploration (Park et al. 2001). Mutations in the tumor suppressor gene (p53) have been reported in HCC and are associated with a shorter survival (Tomlinson and Finegold 2002).

3.3.4 Symptoms and Clinical Signs

The presentations of HB and HCC are often quite similar to those of other abdominal tumors. Symptoms depend on the size of the tumor and can arise from the mass effect of space-occupying lesions. Children most often present with an asymptomatic abdominal mass. On physical examination, a firm, irregular mass may be palpated in the right upper quadrant of the abdomen with extension across the midline or down to the pelvis. Pain, weight loss, anorexia, nausea, vomiting, and constipation may occur in advanced disease. Infants may present with failure to thrive. Severe osteopenia is often seen at diagnosis and is usually detected incidentally on imaging; however, pathologic fractures occur infrequently. An acute abdomen is present in the case of tumor rupture. Precocious puberty may be apparent in children whose tumors secrete beta human chorionic gonadotropin (βHCG). Jaundice and abnormal liver function studies are quite uncommon in HB, but may be presenting features of HCC in the presence of viral hepatitis or cirrhosis. Clinical signs of BWS should be considered, including macroglossia and hemihypertrophy, and a history of hypoglycemia at birth, because of the increased incidence of HB in children with BWS. Patients at risk for developing HB, including those with BWS or FAP, are often placed on a surveillance schedule to observe for the disease, which normally includes ultrasonography of the abdomen and measurements of serum alpha feto-protein (AFP) and βHCG every 3 months until around the age of 7 or 8. Metastases tend to occur in the lung, bone, and brain. Twenty percent of patients present with lung metastases at diagnosis (Meyers 2007).

3.3.5 Diagnostics

The diagnosis of either HB or HCC depends on imaging, blood, physical examination, and ultimately biopsy, to determine tumor histology. X-ray of the abdomen is often one of the first diagnostic tests carried out. A right upper quadrant mass can be seen and calcifications are sometimes present. An ultrasound is useful in identifying a mass with increased echogenicity, which is suggestive of malignancy; Doppler will give information about the tumors vascularity. CT or MRI is needed to assess the extent of the disease, and the presence of local lymph nodes and vascular invasion. Figure 3.8 shows the CT imaging of HB. Tumors often show patchy disease on post-contrast CT, which is differentiated from the normal liver. CT of the chest is necessary to exclude lung metastases. Bone scan can be taken to exclude bony metastases, and MRI of the brain can be taken to rule out intracranial spread; however, these are not standard practice.

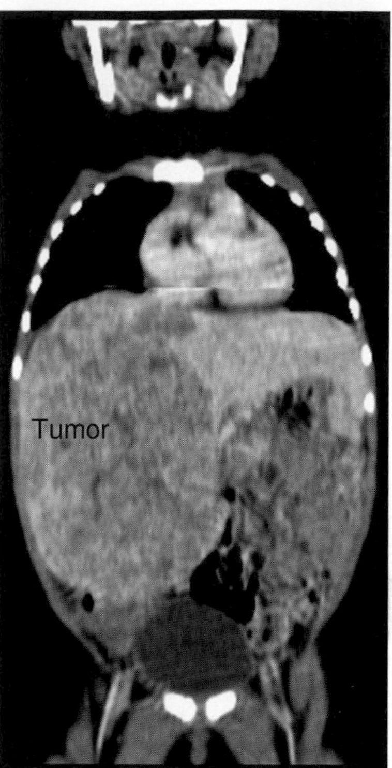

Figure 3.8

CT scan of a patient with Stage III hepatoblastoma. Hepatoblastoma can be seen occupying the right lobe of the liver and extending medially to the left

Serum tumor markers of HB include AFP and βHCG. AFP is a protein that is produced by the fetal liver and is elevated in the blood of infants during the first 8–10 months of life (Corapcioglu et al. 2004). This protein is increased in 90% of HBs, and 60% of HCCs (Meyers 2007; Stocker 2001). In infants being investigated for a liver mass, it may be difficult to distinguish between normal AFP and malignant AFP. It is possible to fractionate the malignant and nonmalignant AFP by immunoelectrophoresis;

however, this lab service in not widely available. The AFP is an important tumor marker in liver tumors and is useful in evaluating response to treatment and recurrent disease. After complete tumor resection, the AFP should return to normal within 6 weeks depending on its initial level; the half-life of AFP is 5–7 days (Lang et al. 1982). βHCG is sometimes elevated in liver tumors and should be evaluated; elevations usually correlate with features of precocious puberty. Similar to AFP, if a tumor secretes βHCG, it should decline following treatment and resection; the half life of βHCG is 24–36 h (Lachman et al. 1986). A complete blood count (CBC) should be carried out, as well as liver and renal function blood tests. Liver enzymes and bilirubin may be elevated in HCC, but is not likely in HB. Seventy percent of children are anemic at diagnosis, and 35% have thrombocytosis (Stocker 2001). Coagulation studies should be carried out prior to any surgical procedure to ensure that liver disease has not interfered with the coagulation pathway.

A biopsy is necessary for definitive diagnosis. HB has five distinct histological subtypes:

- Pure fetal histology (imparts the best prognosis)
- Embryonal
- Mixed epithelial (embryonal and fetal)
- Meseschymal/macrotrabecular
- Undifferentiated small cell (imparts the worst prognosis)

HCC has four main histologic types:

- Trabecular pattern (almost always seen in some part of HCC)
- Compact and pseudoglandular variants
- Scirrhous (rare)
- Fibrolamellar carcinoma is another rare variant of HCC that is not associated with cirrhosis; it shows an increased AFP, and has a male predominance and a more favorable prognosis (Suriawinata and Thung 2002).

3.3.6 Staging and Classification

Staging of liver tumors has been carried out by two different methods by two distinct groups. The North American COG stages HB by the standard postsurgical tumor status. The International Society of Pediatric Oncology (SIOP) uses a pretreatment classification schema called PRETreatment EXTent of disease scoring system (PRETEXT) that helps to determine feasibility of tumor resection based on the number of liver segments involved using preoperative imaging scans (Litten and Tomlinson 2008). Table 3.2 compares and contrasts the two systems.

HCC is staged in a similar manner to HB; however, it is graded differently based on histological differentiation. Stage I HCC resembles normal hepatocytes, Stage II and III cells show moderate differentiation, and Stage IV tumor cells are very poorly differentiated and are often metastatic (Suriawinata and Thung 2002).

Table 3.2. Staging systems for liver tumors (Meyers 2007; Litten and Tomlinson 2008; Malogolowkin et al. 2008)

Stage	Children's Oncology Group staging system (post surgical)	European PRETEXT staging system (presurgical)
I	Tumor completely resected	One quadrant of liver affected
II	Tumor grossly resected with evidence of microscopic residual disease	Two adjoining quadrants of liver affected
III	Unresectable tumor at diagnosis, or positive nodes or intraoperative spill, or incomplete resection	Three adjoining quadrants or two non adjoining quadrants involved
IV	Metastatic disease	Tumor involves all four quadrants or metastases, or ingrowth of the portal vein/vena cava or contiguous extrahepatic disease, or AFP (<↓100)

3.3.7 Treatment

For both HB and HCC, surgical resection is crucial for cure and is the single most important factor predicting survival. The current North American approach advocates tumor resection at diagnosis if surgically feasible; alternatively, the European approach favors preoperative chemotherapy in all patients. Chemotherapy plays an important role in controlling disease and treating micrometastases. Increasingly, liver transplantation is being used for patients with unresectable tumors. The use of radiation with these liver tumors is controversial.

3.3.7.1 Surgery

Surgical resection is the most important part of curative therapy for children with HB. As many as 40–60% of HB tumors are inoperable at diagnosis, and 10–20% have pulmonary metastases (Stocker 2001). Surgery is often not possible at diagnosis if both hepatic lobes are affected, if there is tumor in the porta hepatis, or if bulky lymphadenopathy exists. Presurgical chemotherapy for unresectable lesions renders them resectable 85% of the time (Stocker 2001). Surgical resection may include a lobectomy or trisegmentectomy based on the extent of disease. Lymph nodes and the porta hepatis should be sampled during surgery; the celiac and paraaortic nodes need to be biopsied only if the disease is suspected. In most studies, surgery alone is the only treatment for Stage I tumors with pure fetal histology, which are completely resected at diagnosis. Surgery for patients with HCC is vital, but unfortunately, only 10–20% of these tumors are resectable.

Liver transplantation is now done increasingly in patients with unresectable HB. In the United States, malignancies account for 2% of liver transplants in children. Transplant is often considered, but not limited to instances where tumors are unresectable and have shown chemosensitivity. A recent study showed that children with HB who had unresectable liver tumors at diagnosis and were treated with chemotherapy followed by hepatectomy and liver transplant had post transplant survival rates of 80% (Otte et al. 2005). For patients with HCC, transplant is generally reserved for those without metastatic disease because of the high rate of pulmonary recurrences post transplant (Meyers 2007).

It is somewhat unclear how best to treat pulmonary metastases that persist following chemotherapy. A large multicentre review by Meyers et al. (2007) found that the majority of patients with HB who underwent thoracotomy for persistent pulmonary metastases at some point during initial therapy achieved good long-term survival rates (8/9 patients). They also found that those who underwent thoracotomy for recurrent pulmonary metastases experienced less benefit (4/13) from this aggressive approach. They concluded that thoracotomy should be used more aggressively in patients receiving initial therapy for metastatic disease, and perhaps less in situations of pulmonary relapse (Meyers et al. 2007).

3.3.7.2 Chemotherapy

Survival rates for HB increased significantly in the 1980s after the routine use of platinum-based regimens that remain the backbone of modern treatment protocols (Meyers 2007). Additional chemotherapy agents that have shown utility in the treatment of HB include doxorubicin, ifosfamide, vincristine, and fluorouracil. Irinotecan has showed some activity in phase II trials and recurrent disease. Sequential use of carboplatin, carboplatin–vincristine–fluorouracil (5FU), and high-dose cisplatin–etoposide in a POG phase II study showed response in metastatic HB and in patients with unresectable disease at diagnosis, similar to other regimens, but perhaps with less toxicity (Katzenstein et al. 2002a). Table 3.3 shows current chemotherapy regimens for HB in different parts of the world.

HCC has traditionally been treated with the same chemotherapy agents used in the treatment of HB, but with less success. The results of a POG and Children's Cancer Group (CCG) intergroup study using a prospective trial employing a uniform treatment approach to HCC were published by Katzenstein et al. (2002b). The treatment involved cisplatin, vincristine, and 5FU, or cisplatin and continuous infusion of doxorubicin as determined by randomization. Neither of the regimens was effective in controlling the residual or metastatic disease in children with HCC. Owing

Table 3.3. Current chemotherapy regimens for hepatoblastoma (Meyers 2007; Blouin et al. 2004)

Study group	Study number	Risk	Schema
Children's Oncology Group (COG)	AHEP0731	Pure fetal histology Low Intermediate High	Observation C5V C5V+D C5V+D+VI
International Society Of Pediatric Oncology Liver Tumor Study Group (SIOPEL)	SIOPEL-3 SIOPEL-4	Standard High	Cisplatin PLADO+carbo
German Society For Pediatric Oncology And Hematology (GPOH)	HB-94 HB-99	Standard High	IPA Carbo+VP16
Japanese Study Group For Pediatric Liver Tumor (JPLT)	JPLT-2	Standard High	CITA ITEC+HACE
French Society Of Pediatric Oncology		All risk groups	Carbo+epirubicin

C5V cisplatin + 5FU + vincristine; *D* doxorubicin; *VI* vincristine + irinotecan; *PLADO* cisplatin + doxorubicin; *Carbo* carboplatin; *IPA* ifosfamide + cisplatin + adriamycin; *VP16* etoposide; *CITA* ciplatin + THP-ADR (tetrahydropyranyladriamycin); *ITEC* ifosfamide + THP-ADR + etoposide + carbolatin; *HACE* hepatic artery chemoemboliztion

to the lack of better treatment, most often patients with HCC are treated using the same protocols that are used for treating HB, but with poor results.

3.3.7.3 Radiotherapy

Radiation therapy is sometimes used if there is minimal or gross residual disease, but its utility is controversial and not widely accepted. There are high rates of side effects from tumor irradiation as well.

3.3.8 Prognosis

The most important prognostic factor in HB is complete surgical resection. Pure fetal histology and low mitotic count impart an excellent outcome. Small cell undifferentiated tumors are associated with poor prognosis, and are independent of any other variable. It is also recognized that a low serum AFP at diagnosis (<100 ng/mL) is associated with inferior prognosis, extensive disease, and poor response to therapy (De Ioris et al. 2007).

The long-term survival of children with HB, like other solid tumors, is dependent on the stage of the disease and the treatment regimen used. The European group reported survival rates of 90% for standard risk disease and 50% for high-risk disease as per the International Society of Pediatric Oncology-Liver tumor group II study (Perilongo et al. 2004). The results of the North American INT-0098 trial that randomized patients to receive cisplatin, 5FU, and vincristine (C5V) vs. cisplatin and doxorubicin (CD), demonstrated the following 5-year event-free survival rates of 87 and 95% for Stage I disease, respectively (excludes Pure fetal histology); 100% for Stage II disease; 60 and 68% for Stage III disease, respectively; and 14 and 37% for Stage IV disease, respectively (Malogolowkin et al. 2008). However, it was also found that patients initially treated with C5V had better salvage rates if they recurred, compared with those initially treated with CD.

The survival rates for patients with HCC remain bleak. The therapeutic response to chemotherapy is poor and cure rates are approximately 15% (Meyers 2007).

3.3.9 Follow-Up

Follow-up should be similar for both HB and HCC, and must consist of physical examination, abdominal ultrasound for tumor recurrence, and chest X-ray for evidence of pulmonary metastases. CT scan may be a more sensitive method to monitor for recurrence and metastases post treatment, but this should be decided based on individual patient needs. Surveillance should be done every 3 months for at least the first 2 years, and then with decreasing frequency. Monitoring of the AFP level is essential and is often the first indication that the tumor has recurred.

Monitoring for late effects of the treatment is also necessary. Audiograms should be carried out periodically to assess for hearing loss resulting from cisplatin therapy. Patients should also be monitored for evidence of nephrotoxicity secondary to cisplatin therapy. Echocardiograms should be done following anthracycline therapy, because the potential for cardiac sequelae from treatment exists. If the patient has undergone liver transplantation, secondary lymphoproliferative disorders may occur. Psychological, endocrine, and hormonal issues may need to be addressed as well.

3.3.10 Future Perspectives

New therapies need to be developed to treat patients with high-risk HB. There is hope that targeted therapies may be developed as more is understood about the molecular pathways in HB. Efforts should also be taken to develop standardized surveillance programs for those who carry a genetic predisposition to developing a liver tumor, as early intervention would presumably improve the outcomes for this group of patients.

Undeniably, more effective treatment for HCC needs to be available. Studies have proven that HCC does not respond to chemotherapy as successfully as HB. Novel agents need to be examined for their potential role in treating both these liver tumors. Very recently, Sorafenib, a multikinase inhibitor, has shown activity in advanced HCC in adults, and is now licensed for use in this age group. There are few data available on its effect in pediatric HCC, but it may have promising role in the future (Litten and Tomlinson 2008). Metronomic chemotherapy approaches and antiangiogenic agents are also being investigated (Meyers 2007).

3.4 Neuroblastoma

Neuroblastoma (NBL) is a tumor that arises from neural crest cells that make up the sympathetic or peripheral nervous system. Tumors can grow in the sympathetic ganglia, adrenal medulla, and other sites. NBLs represent a heterogeneous group of tumors that range from a benign ganglioneuroma to a highly malignant NBL. Their behavior is highly variable based on age, stage, histology, and biology.

3.4.1 Epidemiology

NBL is the most common pediatric extracranial malignancy and the most frequently occurring cancer in infancy. Although it accounts for approximately 7% of all childhood malignancies, it accounts for 15% of all pediatric cancer deaths (Maris et al. 2007). It affects boys at a slightly higher rate than girls, and is slightly more predominant in Caucasian children compared with black children. The median age at diagnosis is 18 months, 30% of patients present in the first year of life, and 96% of patients present prior to the age of 10 (Maris and Matthay 1999; Ishola and Chung 2007).

3.4.2 Etiology

The cause of NBL is unknown. According to current evidence, environment does not appear to play a role. Correlation with intrauterine exposure to several agents such as alcohol, medications, and maternal use of hair-coloring products has been proposed, but none of these hypotheses have been confirmed. Although most cases of NBL are sporadic, there seems to be a small group, approximately 1–2%, which is familial. NBL has been identified in other disorders of neural crest cells, such as neurofibromatosis type 1, Hirschsprung's disease, congenital central hypoventilation syndrome, pheochromocytomas, BWS, and DiGeorge syndrome (Maris et al. 2007).

3.4.3 Molecular Genetics

Observations over time have shown that both gains and losses of genetic material are common during NBL evolution. It is known that cytogenetic changes affect survival, differentiation, and apoptosis of NBL cells. Gene amplification, alterations in gene expression, and tumor suppressor gene inactivation are some of the major factors that influence risk determination.

3.4.3.1 Gains in Genetic Material

Ploidy is a general term that is used to describe the overall chromosome number of a cell. A normal diploid cell has a karyotype with 46 chromosomes which is designated as 1. The DNA index is determined by flow cytometry. In infants with favorable NBL, a hyperdiploid (double the number of chromosomes) or near triploid DNA index (ploidy > 1) is observed. When this occurs, there tends to be whole chromosome gains with few structural rearrangements. The majority of advanced NBL tumors have either near diploid or near tetraploid (four times the monoploid number) DNA content. Diploid and tetraploid tumors are characterized by chromosomal rearrangements, including amplification, deletion, and unbalanced translocations. These are associated with a poor prognosis. Ploidy is a significant prognostic factor in children younger than 18 months (George et al. 2005).

The most common genetic abnormality noted in NBL tumors has been observed on the long arm of the chromosome 17. An unbalanced gain at 17q is associated with an adverse prognosis and often occurs in conjunction with deletions of 1p (Tomioka et al. 2003).

MYCN is a proto-oncogene normally expressed in the developing nervous system and selected other tissues. MYCN is found on chromosome 2 band q24, and there are normally two copies in each cell. The gene is considered to be amplified when there are more than ten copies per cell; however, amplification often results in 50–400 copies of the gene per cell. MYCN amplification is associated with advanced disease, rapid progression, and poor prognosis. It occurs in approximately 20% of all NBLs and is a powerful predictor of outcome regardless of stage and age (Maris et al. 2007).

3.4.3.2 Losses of Genetic Material

Loss of genetic information is also an event that happens frequently in the evolution of NBL tumors. If the constitutional DNA of a patient has two alleles at any given locus, but the tumor only has one allele present, then there is a presumptive loss of DNA at that locus. LOH is a term used to describe this loss of genetic information in the tumor. Regions of high-frequency LOH are believed to harbor tumor suppressor genes.

Deletions on the short arm of chromosome 1 (1p36) are often observed in advanced NBL. The deletions vary in their size, and there is a large region on the chromosome that may potentially be affected. Specific areas of deletions probably result in different outcomes. There may be one or more tumor suppressor genes located on the short arm of chromosome 1, and this gene is inactivated in 25–35% of NBL tumors (Maris et al. 2007). Although patients who have deletions of 1p generally also have MYCN amplification and poor survival outcomes, 1p deletion is also an independent prognostic factor especially in young children.

LOH on the long arm of chromosome 11 is seen in 35–45% of NBL tumors and is another negative prognostic marker (Maris et al. 2007). Again, this region is thought to harbor a tumor suppressor gene. Interestingly, 11q deletions are not often seen in patients with MYCN amplification, and therefore, this aberration represents an independent poor prognostic marker.

3.4.3.3 Mutations in Gene Expression

Neurotrophins, including nerve growth factor (NGF), brain-derived neurotrophic factor (BDNF), neurotrophin-3, and neurotrophin-4, are essential for normal neuronal development. They mediate signaling pathways that support cell survival. The signaling of neurotrophins is controlled by the TRK family of tyrosine kinases (Maris and Matthay 1999). Three neurotrophin receptor genes relevant to NBL have been identified: TRK-A, TRK-B, and TRK-C. Aberrant Trk expression and signaling contributes to NBL pathogenesis and clinical prognosis. High TrkA often corresponds to a lack of MYCN amplification, and a favorable outcome. TrkB, however, is expressed in higher-stage tumors that show MYCN amplification and have an unfavorable prognosis. Trk-C is expressed in favorable NBLs that are non-MYCN-amplified. It is preferentially expressed in patients who express TRK-A.

Recently, alterations in the anaplastic lymphoma kinase (ALK) protein have been identified in both inherited and sporadic NBL. ALK abnormalities induce mutations, amplification, and translocations (Chen et al. 2008).

3.4.4 Symptoms and Clinical Signs

NBL tumors can occur anywhere along the peripheral nervous system. The majority of tumors arise in the abdomen (65%), while 32% arise in the adrenal gland (Ninane and Pearson 1997). Other common locations for primary tumors are the thorax, pelvis, and cervical regions. NBL spreads via lymphatic and hematogenous routes, and occasionally by regional lymph node invasion. Common sites for metastases are bone and bone marrow; skin and liver are common in infants. Very rarely, metastases to brain and lung occur. Over 50% of patients present with metastatic disease, and 80% of them may have bone marrow involvement (de Bernardi et al. 2008; Matthay et al. 2005).The clinical signs and symptoms of NBL depend entirely on the tumor location, and adjacent organs, vessels, and nerve involvement. The various presenting signs of NBL and the possible causes are listed in Table 3.4.

There are two paraneoplastic syndromes that children with NBL may present with: opsoclonus-myoclonus ataxia (OMA) and watery diarrhea resulting from secretion of vasoactive intestinal peptide (VIP). OMA syndrome consists of random eye movements, myoclonic jerking movements, and cerebellar ataxia, and occurs in 2–4% of patients with NBL (Maris et al. 2007). The phenomenon is thought to arise because of the production of antineural antibodies that cross-react with the neural cells in the cerebellum or elsewhere in the brain (Bataller et al. 2003). Children presenting with OMA

Table 3.4. Various presentation signs of neuroblastoma and their possible causes (Maris et al. 2007; Ishola and Chung 2007; Brodeur and Maris 2002)

Clinical sign or symptom	Etiology
Abdominal pain, abdominal distension, nausea, vomiting, constipation	Abdominal tumor
"Blueberry muffin" skin lesions	Tumor involving the skin (commonly occurs in infants)
Anorexia, weight loss	Mass effect of midline tumors
Horner's syndrome (ipsilateral ptosis, meiosis, and anhydrosis)	High thoracic and cervical tumors resulting in compromise of descending sympathetic nerve tracks
Respiratory distress	Extensive liver involvement (occurs in infants with Stage IVS disease) or pleural effusions
Proptosis, periorbital ecchymosis "raccoon eyes"	Periorbital tumor involvement
Anemia, thrombocytopenia, frequent infections	Bone marrow involvement
Hypertension	Renal vascular compression
Limp or leg pain	Metastatic bone disease
Decreased motion in legs, muscle weakness, or bowel or bladder disturbances	Spinal or paraspinal disease
Weakness or paraplegia	Compression of spinal cord caused by dumbbell tumors
Watery diarrhea, failure to thrive	Vasoactive intestinal peptide (VIP) secretion (paraneoplastic syndrome)
Ataxia, rapid eye movements, irregular muscle movements	Opsoclonus-myoclonus ataxia (OMA) syndrome (paraneoplastic syndrome)

tend to do quite well from the tumor perspective, and generally present with lower-stage disease; however, long-term neurological and developmental deficits occur in 70–80% of children (Maris et al. 2007). Intractable diarrhea and failure to thrive are a rare presentation caused by tumor secretion of VIP; the symptoms normally disappear with or shortly after tumor resection. VIP-associated NBL often has a favorable prognosis.

3.4.5 Diagnostics

The evaluation of a patient with NBL requires diagnostic imaging, laboratory testing, and pathology. The information obtained from imaging and biopsy results is used to determine the risk stratification based on both clinical stage and biological factors. CT scan is the most common modality used for evaluating tumors of the mediastinum, abdomen, and pelvis; calcifications are often seen within the tumor mass. MRI, however, is superior when investigating the extent of paraspinal/intraspinal tumors. Bone scan is used to determine the presence of skeletal metastases. Metaiodobenzylguanidine (MIBG) scan, using a tracer that concentrates in the secretory granules of NBL cells, is extremely useful in identifying NBL metastases (Fig. 3.9). MIBG imaging is positive in over 90% of NBL tumors (Maris et al. 2007). PET–CT is increasingly being studied in NBL, to determine its use in identifying metastatic disease and tracking treatment response, especially when the tumor is not MIBG avid (Fig. 3.10).

Urinary catecholamine metabolites are produced in the majority (>90%) of NBLs (Kushner et al. 2004). Urinary vanillylmandelic acid (VMA) and homovanillic acid (HVA) are formed from the byproducts of norepinephrine and dopamine breakdown, respectively. They are considered elevated when they are greater than three standard deviations above the upper limit of the normal value (Brodeur and Maris 2002).

NBL tumors produce several substances that can be measured in the blood. Neuron-specific enolase (NSE), GD2 (a cell membrane disialoganglioside), and chromogranin A are produced by NBL tumors, and although not routinely performed at most centers, serum levels of these markers can be measured.

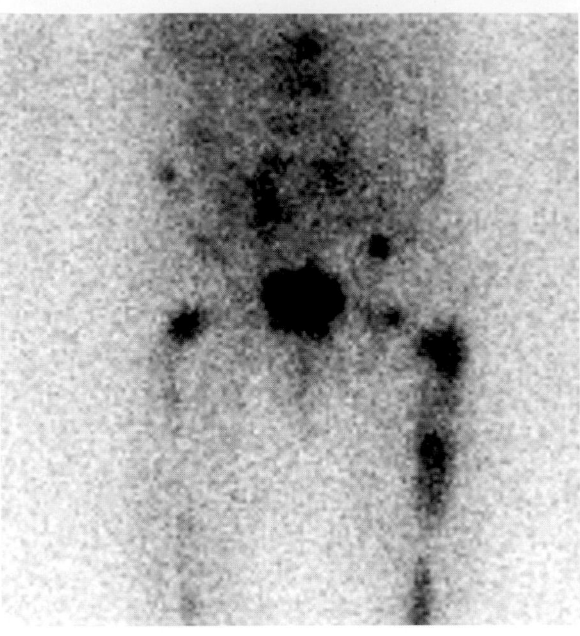

Figure 3.9

MIBG scan in disseminated neuroblastoma (NBL). MIBG avidity is present in the pelvis, femur, and lumbar spine

NSE is a protein associated with neural cells; although nonspecific, OS is worse in patients with elevations of NSE and advanced disease (Matthay and Yamashiro 2000). GD2 can be found on the surface of NBL cells; gangliosides shed from the tumor might be important in accelerating tumor progression (Brodeur and Maris 2002). Similarly, elevations of chromogranin A are associated with unfavorable outcomes. Although nonspecific, serum LDH and ferritin are sometimes elevated in NBL, reflecting rapid cellular turnover; elevations are thought to correlate with unfavorable outcomes (Kushner et al. 2004). A CBC should also be evaluated; any cytopenias that are present may be the result of bone marrow disease.

Tumor biopsy and/or tumor resection are done depending on the stage of the tumor. Tissue samples are sent for molecular and histopathological testing. Stage I and II tumors are usually resected at diagnosis, whereas Stage III and IV tumors are only biopsied. Bilateral bone marrow aspirates and biopsies are also

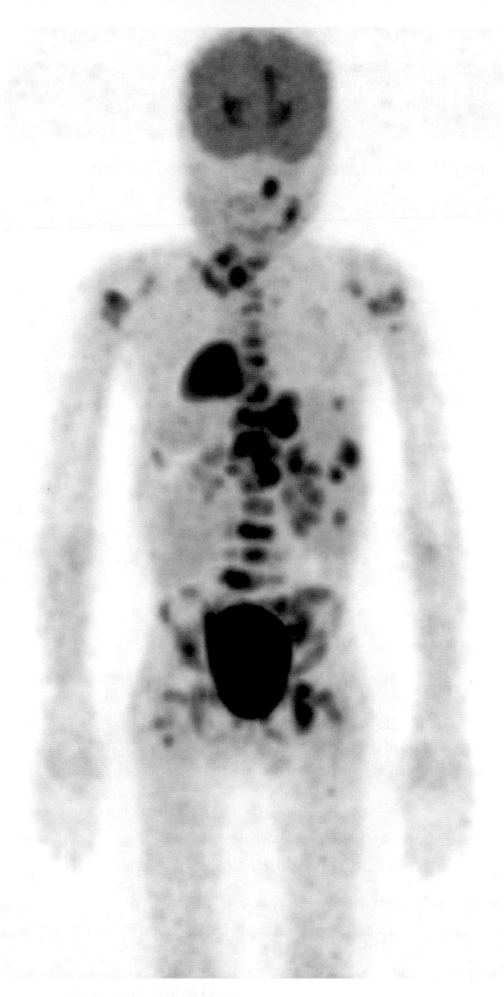

Figure 3.10

PET–CT demonstrating extensive metastatic disease. PET avidity is present in the skull, sinuses, right mandible, left supraclavicular region, right retrocrural region, peripancreatic region, liver, humeral heads, spine, pelvis, and left femur

needed to determine the presence of bone marrow disease. It is generally accepted that if tumor is found in the bone marrow and the child has an elevated VMA/HVA, the diagnosis is NBL and it is not necessary to biopsy the primary tumor. However, valuable information gained via biological markers would not be obtained for risk stratification, which may impact patient care especially in patients younger than 18 months.

Histology is an important determinant in risk stratification for these tumors. NBL is a small blue round cell tumor, and Homer-Wright pseudorosettes are often found within it. It can be distinguished from other small blue round cell tumors because of its distinctive monoclonal antibody staining patterns. NBL stains positively for NSE, neurofilament proteins, and synaptophysin. Shimada et al. (1984) originally developed a pathology staging system for NBL (Shimada et al. 1984); some changes have been made to this earlier system to make it internationally consistent. The histological determination takes into account the mitotic karyorrhectic index (MKI), patient age, the degree of differentiation, and whether the tumor is schwannian stroma poor. Tumors are graded as having favorable histology (FH) or unfavorable histology (UFH) based on the above-mentioned tumor characteristics (see Table 3.5). Figure 3.11 shows the difference in the survival of patients based solely on Shimada histology.

3.4.6 Staging and Classification

NBL is staged according to the international NBL staging system (INSS), which is based on postsurgical interventions for low-grade tumors according to the location and resectability of the tumor (Table 3.6). Extensive involvement of the liver, skin, and/or bone marrow (<10%) in infants reflects Stage IVS disease. The "S" stands for special and this clinicopathological staging is reserved for infants who, along with favorable tumor biology, are considered to have low risk tumours even with advanced disease. Tumors often regress spontaneously with little or no treatment.

Risk classification takes into account clinical features such as stage and age, as well as biological factors, to determine risk stratification. It has been a major focus of cooperative clinical trial groups that study and treat NBL to establish which biological, clinical, and pathological correlates are vital to determine the risk groups, and ultimately to determine the therapy. High-risk tumors naturally include most patients with metastatic disease; however, patients who have Stage II, III, and IVS tumors may also be considered to be at high risk depending on tumor histology and tumor biology.

Table 3.5. International neuroblastoma pathology classification (INPC)

Neuroblastoma histology	Age (years)	International neuroblastoma pathology classification
Favorable	<1.5	Poorly differentiated or differentiating and low or intermediate MKI tumor
	1.5–5.0	Differentiating and low MKI tumor
Unfavorable	<1.5	Undifferentiated tumor, high MKI tumor
	1.5–5.0	Undifferentiated or poorly differentiated tumor, intermediate or high MKI tumor
	>5	All tumors

MKI mitosis-karyorrhexis index (adapted from Shimada et al. 1999)

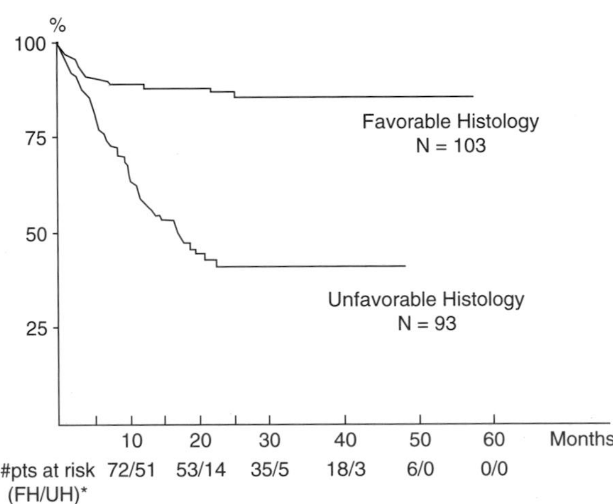

Figure 3.11
Outcome in patients with NBL based on Shimada histology alone Reprinted with permission Shimada et al. 1999

Table 3.6. International neuroblastoma staging system (INSS) (Ishola and Chung 2007)

Stage	Tumor characteristics
I	Localized tumor with gross total resection with or without microscopic residual disease
IIA	Localized tumor with incomplete gross total resection, lymph nodes negative
IIB	Localized tumor with or without gross total resection, with ipsilateral positive nodes
III	Unresectable unilateral tumor which crosses the midline, or unilateral tumor with contralateral regional lymph node involvement
IV	Any primary tumor with dissemination to distant lymph nodes, bone, bone marrow, and/or other organ sites
IVS	Localized primary tumor (I, IIA, IIB), with dissemination limited to skin, liver, and/or bone marrow (<10% involvement) in children less than 12 months

An international effort involving NBL investigators resulted in the development of an International Neuroblastoma Risk Group (INRG) classification system. Data from over 11,000 patients treated in Canada, Europe, Japan, the United States, and Australia were reviewed. The INRG classification schema takes into account INRG stage, age, histologic category, grade of tumor differentiation, MYCN status, presence/absence of 11q aberrations, and tumor cell ploidy (Cohn et al. 2009). This risk classification system will provide the basis for developing future therapies based on stratification, and will provide a common basis for comparing the treatment outcomes internationally.

3.4.7 Treatment

Surgery, chemotherapy, radiation therapy, myeloablative chemotherapy with autologous stem cell rescue (ASCR), differentiation therapy, and more recently, immunotherapy and other biological therapies, are all used in the treatment of NBL depending on the stage of the disease. Treatment intensity depends on risk stratification. Most cooperative groups stratify patients into low-, intermediate-, and high-risk categories; some groups also use an ultra high-risk category. The COG currently uses age, stage, MYCN status, ploidy, and histology to stratify patients (Maris et al. 2007), and have incorporated LOH at 1p and 11q into intermediate-risk protocols. The German NBL studies also use LOH at 1p to stratify patients, in addition to the above-mentioned factors (Oberthuer et al. 2008). Future studies will incorporate the INRG. The approaches to treatment based on risk stratification will be discussed in the following section.

3.4.7.1 Low Risk

Surgical resection and observation is often all that is required for patients with low-risk disease (de Bernardi et al. 2008). This favorable risk group of patients generally includes those with Stage I, II, and sometimes IVS disease, as long as they have favorable biology (no MYCN amplification). NBL has the ability to spontaneously regress or differentiate, and this is the reason for the patients, who have microscopic or residual disease with low-risk characteristics, not requiring adjuvant treatment with radiation or chemotherapy.

There is a group of patients with Stage IVS NBL who may benefit from some minimal therapy; this group comprises infants less than 2 months of age who have rapidly progressing abdominal disease (Nickerson et al. 2000). These patients can often develop respiratory compromise before the natural evolution of Stage IVS, results in spontaneous regression.

Patients who present with OMA–NBL often have low-risk primary tumors, but require therapy for their OMA symptoms. These patients often require treatment with some combination of the following: intravenous gammaglobulin, steroids, adrenocorticotrophic hormone, and chemotherapy (Veneselli et al. 1998; Rudnick et al. 2001). However, the best method to treat OMA remains controversial.

3.4.7.2 Intermediate Risk

Both surgery and neoadjuvant chemotherapy are indicated in the treatment of intermediate-risk NBL. Patients with Stage II, III, IV, and IVS disease may fit into this risk group, depending on the biology. Patients with Stage III disease generally require chemotherapy for cytoreduction prior to surgical resection. The agents that are most often used in intermediate-risk NBL are moderate intensity carboplatin, etoposide, cyclophosphamide, and doxorubicin (Modak et al. 2009). The recent trend in this group of patients is to decrease the amount of systemic chemotherapy used; treatment protocols often tailor the amount of therapy based on the biology and tumor response. The Memorial Sloan Kettering group in New York advocates the use of surgery alone in Stage III patients without MYCN amplification, with good results (Modak et al. 2009).

3.4.7.3 High Risk

Multimodal, intensive therapy is indicated for patients with high-risk NBL. This risk group generally includes patients with Stage IV disease with the exception of young patients (<18 months) with good biology; this group also includes patients with Stage II and III disease with poor biological features (Maris et al. 2007). The treatment plan for these patients with high-risk NBL includes:

- Chemotherapy to decrease the size of both the primary tumor and metastases
- Surgical resection of the tumor
- Myeloablative chemotherapy followed by ASCR
- Radiation therapy to the site of the primary tumor and/or areas of residual disease
- Differentiation therapy with retinoids
- For some immunotherapy and biological therapy

3.4.7.4 Chemotherapy

Induction chemotherapy regimens are intense with the goal of shrinking the size of the primary tumor, ultimately facilitating surgical resection, in addition to immediately controlling metastatic disease. The most common chemotherapy agents that are known to be effective are the following given in some combination: cisplatin, doxorubicin, cyclophosphamide, carboplatin, ifosfamide, and etoposide (George et al. 2006; Ishola and Chung 2007). Cyclophosphamide and topotecan have been used successfully in relapsed disease for several years, and a current phase III study by the COG is incorporating this approach into induction regimens (Maris et al. 2007).

3.4.7.5 Surgery

Surgical resection of the primary tumor is a vital part of the treatment regimen. This is important for local tumor control and it also decreases the number of tumor cells present which can develop drug resistance. The timing of surgery after induction chemotherapy increases the degree of complete excision and decreases surgical complications (Ishola and Chung 2007).

3.4.7.6 Myeloablative Therapy and Autologous Stem Cell Rescue

Consolidation with myeloablative therapy followed by autologous peripheral blood stem cell rescue is now a part of standard high-risk treatment with documented improvements in survival as a result (Matthay et al. 1999). The European bone marrow transplant registry (EBMT) identified from the results of their studies over many years that the most efficacious conditioning regimen for myeloablative therapy are those which included melphalan and busulfan (Ladenstein et al. 2008). Total body irradiation (TBI) is used in some regimens to eradicate micrometastases with similar efficacy compared with chemotherapy conditioning; however, more significant late effects are seen as a result (Ladenstein et al. 2008). More recently, tandem transplants have been studied by various groups; patients receive high-dose therapy followed by stem cell reinfusion, and then receive a second cycle of different high-dose therapy followed by a second stem cell reinfusion. The myeloablative regimens that have been used in this setting use some of the following drugs in a variety of combinations: carboplatin, etoposide, cyclophosphamide, thiotepa, and melphalan in addition to TBI (Grupp et al. 2000; Kletzel et al. 2002). Results of tandem transplants show improved OS rates in multiple published series (George et al. 2006; Ladenstein et al. 2008).

3.4.7.7 Radiotherapy

NBL is a radiosensitive tumor. In cases where the primary tumor cannot be fully resected when there are locally involved lymph nodes, and in cases where microscopic residual disease exists, radiation therapy plays a vital role. It has been shown that radiation to the site of the primary tumor, despite the extent of surgical resection, decreases the local relapse in high-risk tumors (Ishola and Chung 2007). Most of the high-risk protocols that use radiation are carried out after the high-dose therapy. Doses of radiation that are used are in the range of 2,400 cGy (Kletzel et al. 2002). TBI is sometimes used as a conditioning regimen for myeloablation, but shows significant late effects. Doses in the range of 12 Gy have been used in this capacity (Grupp et al. 2000).

MIBG therapy is being used increasingly for high-risk and refractory NBL (Ishola and Chung 2007). MIBG uses higher doses of 131I, compared with those necessary for diagnostic imaging, to deliver targeted RT to NBL tumors. Side effects of MIBG include significant myelosuppression depending on the dose delivered, sometimes necessitating reinfusion of stem cells. More recently, because of this toxicity, the feasibility of delivering MIBG therapy as part of a myeloablative conditioning regimen is being studied, with some preliminary promising outcomes in patients refractory to standard therapy and those with relapsed disease (Ishola and Chung 2007). Finally, radiation is often used and is very effective in controlling bony pain or advanced disease causing distressing symptoms in the palliative setting.

3.4.7.8 Differentiation Therapy

Maintenance therapy for NBL now routinely includes the use of retinoids in most cooperative group trials. Retinoic acid is used to evoke cellular differentiation of NBL cells. In this setting post transplant, it is used to target minimal residual disease. A North American CCG study showed that patients who were randomized to receive 13-*cis*-retinoic acid following either myelablative therapy or consolidation chemotherapy had statistically significant improved 3-year survival rates compared with those who did not receive the retinoid (46 vs. 29% respectively); although myeloablative therapy is also likely to contribute to this superior outcome (Matthay et al. 1999). Most children receive 6 months of therapy according to treatment protocols.

3.4.7.9 Biological Therapies and Immunotherapy

Phase III studies are ongoing to investigate the role of targeted antibody therapy using anti-GD2 antibodies, either alone or together with immunotherapy, in an attempt to target minimal residual disease in the post-transplant or relapsed setting. Ganglioside-GD2 is an antigen that is expressed on the majority of NBL cells, but not on other cells, making it an ideal target for targeted therapy. Anti-GD2 monoclonal antibodies, once administered to the patient, bind with the GD2 antigen, causing cellular death. Immunotherapy comprising interleukin 2 (IL2) and GMCSF is often delivered with antibody therapy in an effort to boost the immune response, thereby working in concert with the antibody (Ozkaynak et al. 2000).

3.4.8 Prognosis

The prognosis in NBL varies widely depending on the child's age and the tumor's stage, location, and biology. Clinical and biological factors that correlate with unfavorable prognosis include: age older than 18 months, advanced stage of the disease (metastases), unfavorable (Shimada) histology, deletions of 1p or 11q, unbalanced gain of 17q, amplification of MYCN, and expression of TrkB (Brodeur 2003). In addition to the tumor markers, serum and urine markers of unfavorable prognosis include LDH greater than 1,500 U/mL, ferritin greater than 42 ng/mL, VMA/HVA ratio of less than 1 (Kushner et al. 2004).

Survival rates are excellent in patients with low-risk, Stage I and II disease treated with surgery only. The SIOP group reported OS and relapse-free survival (RFS) rates of 99 and 94%, respectively, for Stage I disease, and 93 and 83%, respectively, for Stage II disease (de Bernardi et al. 2008). Patients with Stage III or intermediate-risk disease treated with surgery only have demonstrated 10-year OS rates of 85%, and those treated with preoperative chemotherapy followed by surgery had a 10-year OS rate of 97% (Modak et al. 2009). Most groups reported long-term survival rates of less than 40% in patients with high-risk NBL. Infants with Stage IVS, favorable biology, NBL exhibited excellent survival outcomes with little or no therapy, with OS rates of 85–92% (Maris et al. 2007).

3.4.9 Follow-Up

Close observation for recurrent disease is imperative for these children. Most relapse occurs during the first 2 years following the completion of therapy. Follow-up must include imaging, monitoring of urinary catecholamines, blood work, and physical examination. Diagnostic imaging of the primary tumor using CT or ultrasound depending on the location of the tumor is indicated. MIBG scanning is also useful for monitoring for recurrent disease in high-risk patients. Imaging and physical examination should be carried out every 3 months for the first few years after completing therapy, and then with decreasing frequency over several years, or as clinically indicated. Urinary catecholamines should also be measured with the same frequency as radiological imaging. Blood tests such as LDH and ferritin can be monitored easily, and although nonspecific, can be used for screening along with imaging and physical examination. According to the EBMT database, late relapses do occur beyond the fifth year post treatment; however, the chance for long-term survival after 5 years post treatment is 80% (Ladenstein et al. 2008).

Follow-up must also consider treatment-related toxicity and late effects. Ototoxicity is usually significant following cisplatin therapy, and hearing aids are often necessary. Growth and development may be impacted, especially if radiation therapy has been delivered to the spinal area; this should be monitored carefully. Organ toxicity is a potential side effect following chemotherapy, and should be monitored through blood testing where possible. Echocardiograms should be done to screen for cardiomyopathies from anthracycline therapies. If radiation therapy was received, follow-up with a radiation oncologist is imperative. Second malignancies must be considered a risk for long-term survivors of metastatic disease due to the intensive multimodality therapy including radiation that these patients receive. Limited data are available on the late effects of the high-risk cohort because they are a small group to date.

3.4.10 Future Perspectives

Researchers and clinicians continuously attempt to improve risk-stratification criteria for children with NBL, so that treatment intensity may correspond to disease characteristics as new therapies emerge. Gene-expression profiling, targeting abnormal transduction pathways, and the use of biological agents are all areas that are being researched to treat NBL, both in relapsed and primary disease. The following treatments have emerged in recent years and are being investigated for their efficacy in the treatment of NBL:

1. MIBG therapy: This has been used in relapsed NBL, with response rates of 40% (Howard et al. 2005). It is now being studied for refractory disease in upfront therapy. Future trials may combine MIBG therapy with radiosensitizing agents.
2. Retinoids: Fenritinide is a systemic retinoid which does not induce differentiation but apoptosis of NBL cells. This formulation has been developed to provide good exposure while minimizing toxicity. Fenritinide induces responses in tumors that are resistant to 13-*cis*-retinoic acid (Maris et al. 2007).
3. Tyrosine kinase inhibitors: Tyrosine kinase inhibitor therapy is being researched to target TRK A, B, and C expression. CEP-701 is a tyrosine kinase antagonist that has shown to inhibit the growth of NBL cells in vivo, and is being studied in phase I clinical trials (Evans et al. 1999). Drugs that target ALK are also currently being examined in phase I studies (Chen et al. 2008).
4. Antiangiogenic inhibitors: VEGF is a regulator of the blood supply to the tumors. Drugs created to inhibit this growth factor are being studied to determine their role in treating NBL. Imatinib mesylate is one such drug being studied for efficacy in NBL (Ishola and Chung 2007).
5. Cytotoxic agents: Topoisomerase I inhibitors such as topotecan when used in conjunction with cyclophosphamide are known to have good efficacy in relapsed NBL and are currently being studied in upfront disease. Irinotecan and temozolamide are now being investigated for their role in relapsed NBL. ABT-751 is an oral tubulin-binding agent that is also being studied in relapsed and refractory NBL (Maris et al. 2007).

The intension of the current research is to determine agents that are effective against NBL and incorporate these findings into conventional therapy.

3.5 Renal Tumors

Wilms' tumor represents the most commonly occurring malignant tumor arising from the kidney in pediatric patients, representing 85% of all renal tumors (Portugal and Baroda 2008). Renal cell carcinoma (RCC), clear cell sarcoma of the kidney (CCSK), congenital mesoblastic nephroma (CMN), and rhabdoid tumor of the kidney (RTK) are the other less frequently occurring renal neoplasms.

3.5.1 Epidemiology

Wilms' tumor is the fourth most common pediatric malignancy. It occurs at an annual incidence of approximately 8.1 per million individuals (Sonn and Shortliffe 2008). Wilms' tumors can occur bilaterally or unilaterally. Additionally, bilateral tumors occur either synchronously or asynchronously. The incidence is slightly higher in black children, and lower in Asian children when compared with Caucasians, and it occurs slightly more frequently in girls (Dome et al. 2006a). The peak age of diagnosis is between 2 and 3 years.

The other tumors that also arise from the kidney are rare, and they include CCSK, RCC, CMN, and RTK. CCSK, distinct from Wilms' tumor, is the second most commonly occurring renal tumor, and was shown to have an incidence of 4% in a National Wilms' Tumor Study (NWTS) (Beckwith 1998). RCC is a tumor that occurs more frequently in the second decade of life in pediatric patients, but is distinct from both Wilms' tumors and adult RCC (Silberstein et al. 2009). CMN occurs most often in infants with an average age of presentation of 2 months (Pettinato et al. 1989). RTK represents 2% of renal tumors registered with NWTS, and most commonly occurs in children less than 2 years of age (Dome et al. 2006b; Broecker 2000).

3.5.2 Etiology

Wilms' tumors occur sporadically in 95% of these patients. There is, however, a familial form, comprising 1–2% of all Wilms' tumors. These tumors tend to occur bilaterally and earlier, suggesting a germline mutation and loss of a tumor suppressor gene. The familial form is characterized by an autosomal dominant trait with variable penetrance (Grundy et al. 2002). The disease often occurs in the presence of genetic anomalies or as part of a familial predisposition syndrome. Syndromes often associated with Wilms' are the following (Pritchard-Jones and Mitchell 1997):

- Beckwith–Wiedemann syndrome (BWS) (an overgrowth syndrome)
- Denys–Drash (involving genitourinary abnormalities)
- WAGR (Wilms, aniridia, genitourinary anomalies, and mental retardation)

Wilms' tumor has also been described in Bloom syndrome, incontinentia pigmenti, Li Fraumeni, Frasier syndrome, and genetic instability syndromes, but no definite link exists (Grundy et al. 2000; Auber et al. 2009).

3.5.3 Molecular Genetics

Several genes are described in the development of Wilms' tumor. The first Wilms' tumor suppressor gene, WT1, was identified in 1990 and is located on chromosome 11p13 (Grundy et al. 2002). WT1 is important in normal kidney and gonadal development and is also expressed during embryogenesis in the heart, meothelium, and spleen (Auber et al. 2009; May et al. 2007). Its discovery was the result of direct observations of the development of Wilms' tumors in patients with WAGR syndrome. These children with WAGR had heterozygous germline mutations of 11p13, which were found to encode several genes including PAX6 (gene responsible for aniridia) and WT1 (Dome et al. 2006b). Deletions in both the alleles of WT1 are not necessary for the development of Wilms' tumor. A second Wilms' tumor putative gene, WT2, has been identified at chromosome 11p15. The relationship between Wilms' tumor in children with BWS may be the result of this second mutation (Neville and Ritchey 2000). There have been two loci identified in the familial form of Wilms' tumor; at chromosome 17q, labeled FWT1, and chromosome 19q, labeled FWT2. These genes appear to have a role in tumor development. Deletions at chromosome 16q and 1p have been identified as independent adverse prognostic indicators in patients with FH Wilms' tumor. Patients with LOH at these regions have an increased risk of relapse and death (Grundy et al. 2005; Dome et al. 2006a). There has also been an association noted between p53 mutations and anaplastic histology in 65% of cases, which may suggest that mutations underlie the anaplastic phenotype (Dome et al. 2006a).

Patients with CMN often display a characteristic translocation (12; 15)(p13; q25) (Knezevich et al. 1998). RCC have characteristic translocations involving the TFE gene located at breakpoint at Xp11.2 (Dal Cin et al. 1998). No specific molecular changes have been identified in CCSK or RTK.

3.5.4 Symptoms and Clinical Signs

Parents are often the first to notice a painless abdominal mass or abdominal distension in their child. Pain, gross hematuria, fever, and hypertension occur in approximately 25% of children (Grundy et al. 2002). Hypertension is usually attributed to increases in renin activity. Anemia, fever, and rapid abdominal distension can occur if there has been hemorrhage in the tumor, but this occurs rarely. Syndromes such as BWS and WAGR are linked to Wilms' tumor, and hence features associated with these syndromes should be noted (e.g., aniridia, GU anomalies, hemihypertrophy). Rarely, extrarenal Wilms' tumors arise;

they present as a retroperitoneal mass usually adjacent to the kidney. Symptoms of thrombosis should also be considered and any leg swelling and/or prominent veins over abdomen must be noted.

Pulmonary metastases are present in only 15–18% of patients at diagnosis (Nicolin et al. 2008). Liver, bone, and brain are additional potential sites of metastases. Bilateral tumors occur in approximately 7% of patients with Wilms' tumor (Sonn and Shortliffe 2008).

3.5.5 Diagnostics

An abdominal ultrasound is usually the first investigation carried out, which may reveal a mass arising from within the kidney. Doppler ultrasound should also be used to assess the patency of the renal vein and inferior vena cava, as thrombosis can occur. CT of the abdomen should be performed to further assess the extent of the mass, involved lymph nodes, and assess for smaller lesions in the contralateral kidney (Fig. 3.12). The liver should be thoroughly examined as it is a common site for metastases. A CT of the chest is necessary to evaluate for the presence of pulmonary metastases (Fig. 3.13).

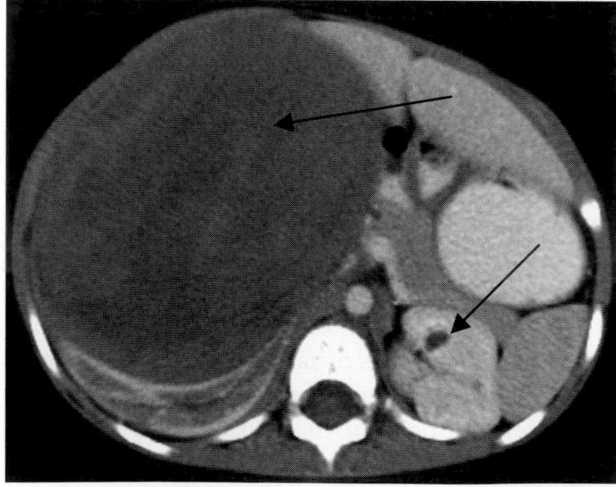

Figure 3.12
CT of abdomen demonstrating bilateral Wilms' tumors

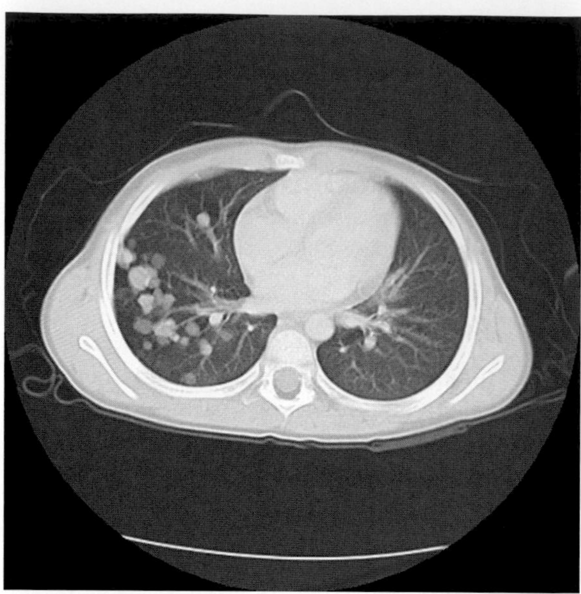

Figure 3.13
CT showing multiple pulmonary metastases

A CT or MRI of the brain should be done after the diagnosis of CSSK or RTK is confirmed, because metastases to the brain can occur. Bone scan and skeletal survey are also indicated in these tumors.

Biopsy vs. tumor resection at diagnosis remains controversial. There are two major Wilms' tumor study groups: the North American National Wilms Tumor Study Group (NWTSG) and International Society of Pediatric Oncology (SIOP) in Europe. The NWTSG recommends resecting the entire tumor and sampling the local lymph nodes at diagnosis. SIOP, however, discourages biopsies and recommends chemotherapy with vincristine and actinomycin, on the basis of radiographic findings, to shrink the tumor to facilitate surgical resection, followed by nephrectomy and staging (Sonn and Shortliffe 2008).

Histologically, Wilms' tumor can comprise blastemal, epithelial, and stromal components. Tumors typically consist of all three components, but one component could predominate. If greater than two-thirds of the tumor composition is of one component, the predominant histological type is assigned to the tumor, as they can behave quite differently (Neville and Ritchey 2000). Monophasic blastemal is a highly invasive type of Wilms' tumor. Cystic or partially differentiated cystic nephromas are less aggressive, and are often cured with surgery alone. Diffuse or focal anaplasia is associated with unfavorable histology (UFH) and is seen is approximately in 5% of tumors (Sonn and Shortliffe 2008). Anaplasia is characterized by large nuclei that are three times the size of the nuclei of other cells, hyperchromasia of enlarged cells, and the presence of bizarre mitotic features. Diffuse anaplasia is characterized by more than one area of anaplasia in tumor sample or in regional nodes or metastases and confers a worse prognosis than focal anaplasia (Neville and Ritchey 2000).

Nephrogenic rests are precursor lesions to Wilms' tumor; they are made up of persistent embryonal nephroblastic tissue with small clusters of blastemal, epithelial, or stromal cells that should no longer be present. They are seen in kidneys of 35% of unilateral Wilms' tumors and in virtually 100% of bilateral Wilms' (Beckwith 1993). The term nephroblastomatosis describes a clinical situation in which there are multiple nephrogenic rests. Although they are not malignant, it is important to know of their presence prior to treating tumors, especially with surgery, because if the contralateral kidney also has these nephrogenic rests, a Wilms' tumor may develop in the future.

CCSK have a distinct histological appearance, but several variant patterns such as classical, epithelioid, myxoid, cystic, sclerosing, palisading, storiform, spindle cell, and anaplastic exist (Ng et al. 2005). CMN has three different histological appearances: cellular, mixed and classic; cellular is the most aggressive variant. RCC in children and adolescents tends to have a papillary architecture (Broecker 2000). RCC of adolescence is very similar in appearance to clear-cell RCC, the adult variant, with copious clear cytoplasm. RTK is thought to be neurogenic in origin. The cells have a prominent acidophilic cytoplasm, resembling rhabdomyoblasts. They are, however, negative for makers of skeletal muscle (Grundy et al. 2000).

There are no specific tumor markers for Wilms' tumor. For the examination of a patient, however, blood should be sent for CBC, liver function tests, creatinine and urea (to assess kidney function), and coagulation screen. It has been noted that acquired Von Willebrand's disease occurs in 8% of Wilms' tumor patients at diagnosis, and treatment with DDAVP may be necessary to correct coagulation prior to surgical intervention (Grundy et al. 2002). Urinalysis should also be carried out to assess for proteinuria and occult blood.

3.5.6 Staging and Classification

There are two staging systems that exist for Wilms' tumor. The NWTSG developed a staging system for Wilms' tumor which is based on imaging and surgical resectability at diagnosis. The SIOP staging system is based on surgical outcomes following neoadjuvant chemotherapy. Table 3.7 highlights the differences between the two systems.

3.5.7 Treatment

The treatment for Wilms' tumors involves surgery and chemotherapy, and sometimes radiation therapy (RT). Less commonly there may be situations when surgery is all that is necessary. Controversy continues regarding the optimal timing of nephrectomy for patients with Wilms' tumor. The SIOP approach recommends nephrectomy following neoadjuvant chemotherapy, whereas the NWTSG advocates for initial nephrectomy followed by adjuvant chemotherapy. It is important to consider, however, that despite the difference in the approach to treatment by the NWTSG and SIOP, outcomes are excellent and comparable between the two groups.

3.5.7.1 Surgery

SIOP asserts that if preoperative chemotherapy is given, the tumor is easier to remove and fewer complications arise, such as intraoperative spill, which has been reported in as many as 20% of patients undergoing primary nephrectomy vs. 5% of patients following preoperative chemotherapy (Graf et al. 2000). Diagnosis is therefore made on clinical and diagnostic imaging only. This approach results in a 5% error in diagnosis (D'Angio 2008). Primary surgery is the approach taken by the NWTSG. This allows for superior staging, including lymph-node sampling. This is important as the involved lymph nodes may be

3.5.7.3 Radiotherapy

RT is routinely used for patients with Stage III disease. This includes patients with intraoperative tumor spill involving the peritoneal surface, positive surgical margins, and regional lymph node involvement. Radiation therapy is delivered most often to the affected flank with doses of 10.8 Gy commonly used; however, whole abdomen radiation is sometimes necessary. Whole lung irradiation is used in patients with pulmonary metastases that do not resolve with induction chemotherapy.

Patients with localized RCC are treated primarily with surgery. The treatment of patients with metastatic disease is difficult. The tumors are not responsive to RT, and there is currently no chemotherapy that is effective. Anecdotal reports of patients responding to cytokine therapy, such as IL-2, have been described (MacArthur et al. 1994). There have, however, been dramatic improvements in the treatment of adults with metastatic RCC in recent years with the advent of novel therapies. Antiangiogenic therapies, with drugs such as bevacizumab in conjunction with interferon, have shown encouraging responses (Escudier et al. 2008). Sunitinib malate, sorafenib, temsirolimus, and everolimus have also shown to improve outcomes in adults in phase III trials by inhibiting VEGF and related pathways (Hutson and Figlin 2008; Cella et al. 2008). Sorafenib is a multikinase inhibitor that is currently licensed for the treatment of metastatic RCC in adults (Wilhelm et al. 2008). Sunitinib is also licensed for the use in metastatic adult RCC. Pediatric phase II clinical trials are currently underway using several of these novel therapies, and it is expected that these agents may also show similar promising results in pediatric RCC.

3.5.8 Prognosis

The OS for patients with localized, FH Wilms' tumor is greater than 90% (Gratias and Dome 2008). The OS of patients with metastatic disease and bilateral disease are both 70% (Pritchard-Jones 2002; Sonn and Shortliffe 2008). Survival rates vary significantly according to stage and histology. Table 3.9 shows the outcomes of the NWTSG trials. Prognostic factors for patients with Wilms' tumors include histology, stage, age, and LOH at 16q and 1p. Fifty to sixty percent of

Table 3.9. Outcomes in patients with Wilms' tumor as per the NWTSG

Stage	Histology	Overall survival (OS) (%)	Event-free survival (EFS) (%)	Relapse-free survival (RFS) (%)	Time interval (years)	NWTSG study
I	FH	98.3	92.4	–	4	V
I	DAH	78.9	68.4	–	4	V
II	FH	–	–	91	–	IV
II	1p and 16q LOH	–	–	75	–	IV
II	DAH	82.6	81.5	–	4	V
III	FH	89	84	–	8	IV
III	DAH	66.7	64.7	–	4	V
IV	FH	80	–	–	4	IV
IV	DAH	33.3	33.3	–	4	V
V	FH	81.7	–	–	4	V
V	UFH	55.2	43.8	–	4	V

FH favorable histology; *DAH* diffuse anaplastic histology; *UFH* unfavorable histology (Sonn and Shortliffe 2008; Dome et al. 2006b; Neville and Ritchey 2000)

patients with relapsed Wilms' tumor can be salvaged (Sonn and Shortliffe 2008).

RTK in the NWTSG III series had an overall 4-year survival rate of 25% and that for CCSK Stages II–IV was 75%. For patients with Stage I RCC, the survival was 90%; however, with Stage IV disease the survival was 0% (Broecker 2000). Outcomes for patients with CMN are excellent. The Cellular variant however, is associated with more aggressive disease including local recurrence and metastases in some patients.

3.5.9 Follow-Up

Follow-up for Wilms' tumor involves regular physical examinations and surveillance scanning, with an abdominal ultrasound and chest X-ray. This is usually done every 3 months for the first 2 years, followed by every 6 months for 2 years, and then with decreasing frequency or as clinically appropriate. In patients with Stage IV disease, imaging with CT scan may be appropriate occasionally in the first 2 years post therapy. Renal function needs to be monitored in the remaining kidney quite carefully, especially if bilateral disease existed and radiation therapy was received.

Follow-up in patients with RCC must occur for many years. The peak time for recurrence occurs within the first 5 years, and 93% of patients who recur do so within this time period. However, recurrences as late as 30 years have been noted (Chin et al. 2006).

Late effects of radiation therapy and specific chemotherapeutic agents should be assessed. Renal failure is a devastating effect that can occur more commonly in patients with bilateral disease who have undergone bilateral nephrectomies. Patients who received anthracycline therapy should be monitored for cardiomyopathy or CHF. The cumulative incidence of CHF at 20 years following therapy for patients who received doxorubicin as part of their initial therapy was between 1.2 and 4.4% (Green et al. 2001, Breslow et al. 2004). Cardiac sequelae might be exacerbated in those patients who also received lung radiation. Altered pulmonary function may also occur in those who have received whole lung irradiation. Patients who have been treated with VP16 need to be screened for secondary myeloid leukemias. The risk of secondary malignancies within the radiation field has been documented to be as high as 12.2% in patients by the age of 50 (Cozzi et al. 2004). Ovarian failure is a possible late effect resulting from alkylating agents.

3.5.10 Future Perspectives

The outcomes in children with Wilms' tumor are relatively favorable. Future efforts should continue to focus on tailoring therapy by decreasing chemotherapy and radiation therapy whenever possible to minimize treatment-related toxicity, based on risk stratification. It is necessary to identify prognostic markers, whether biologic or genetic, in this regard. Topotecan has shown efficacy in the treatment of relapsed Wilms' tumor and may play a role in upfront therapy in the future (Metzger et al. 2007). Stem cell transplantation has shown promising results in relapsed disease and may be useful in a cohort of patients with adverse prognostic features and relapsed disease (Dallorso et al. 2008).

New therapies distinct from the protocols for Wilms' tumor need to be developed for RCC and RTK. The success using therapies targeting VEGF in adults will likely lead to new and efficacious therapies for pediatric patients with metastatic RCC. Studies using novel agents such as sorafenib and sunitinib are underway.

3.6 Retinoblastoma

RB is a rare cancer in the retina. It develops almost exclusively in infants and young children. It represents an important tumor; as much has been learned about tumoriogenesis from RB1 - the first cancer gene to be discovered.

3.6.1 Epidemiology

RB represents 4% of all pediatric malignancies (Abramson 2005). It occurs at an incidence of approximately 1 in 18,000 children less than 5 years of age (Chintagumpala et al. 2007). In some developing countries in Central America, RB is one of the most common pediatric malignancies. Almost all children are diagnosed before the age of 6, the age at which retinal differentiation is complete. Sixty percent of patients have unilateral disease and no predisposing germline mutation (nonheritable RB). Forty percent of patients present with either bilateral or multifocal disease, indicating a germline mutation (heritable RB). The majority of germline mutations are sporadic or de novo, with only approximately 20% of patients having a family history (familial RB) (Balmer et al. 2006; Knudson 2001). Metastatic disease occurs in only approximately 5% of patients in developed countries such as Europe or North America, in contrast to some developing countries where more than 50% of patients have extra ocular disease at diagnosis (Rodriguez-Galindo et al. 2007).

3.6.2 Etiology

The heritable form of RB, presenting as either bilateral or multifocal disease, is associated with errors in transcription, translocations, or deletions of genetic information on chromosome 13q14, which is now referred to as *RB1*. Bilateral RB can occur in utero, and up until the age of approximately 4 years, with the average age of presentation being 7 months, in contrast to unilateral RB, which tends to develop slightly later with an average age of diagnosis of 24 months (Balmer et al. 2006). Bilateral RB can occur asynchronously in infants; therefore, conservative management should be used in infants who present with disease in one eye only, as there is a potential for tumors to develop in the second eye.

Knudson (1971) developed his "two-hit" theory of cancer development after observing the evolution of RB, noting that bilateral RB occurred at a younger age compared with unilateral RB. He subsequently hypothesized that there must be two events that occur before RB tumors develop. In unilateral RB, the two somatic events are considered to occur in the single retinal cell. In bilateral RB, the first mutation is inherited and therefore the *RB1* mutation may be present in every cell of the patient's body (germline), and the second event affects the somatic retinal cells, resulting in tumor development (Gallie et al. 2007; Knudson 2001). Germline mutations are most often de novo mutations that occur at conception or less frequently can be inherited from an affected parent. Errors in transcription occur more often in the paternal allele, suggesting that germline mutations occur more often in spermatogenesis than oogenesis. RB is transmitted as an autosomal dominant trait, with high penetrance (90%) (Balmer et al. 2006). There is a 45% chance that an affected parent may pass on the disease to his or her child. Healthy parents who have a child with bilateral RB also have a 7% chance of having a second child with RB because of germline mosaicism, with each pregnancy (Abramson and Schefler 2004; Chintagumpala et al. 2007). The heritable form of the disease, characterized by the *RB1* germline mutation, predisposes children to the additional risk of developing sporadic secondary malignancies and a much higher risk of developing radiation-induced secondary malignancies.

There is an association between RB and other congenital abnormalities involving the long arm of chromosome 13. When there are large deletions of 13q–, not only can RB develop, but a host of other manifestations including severe developmental delay, congenital anomalies, and dysmorphic features (Brichard et al. 2008). This manifestation of symptoms has been called 13q– syndrome.

3.6.3 Molecular Genetics

Molecular analysis has become increasingly sensitive in detecting chromosomal aberrations. The *RB1* gene is located at chromosome 13q14. The *RB1* gene is a tumor suppressor gene and is important in apoptosis. It is a key regulator of the cell cycle and therefore, governs the proliferation of tumor cells. In RB, deregulation of cell proliferation occurs as a result of the inactivation or absence of RB1 protein, and the constraint that is normally exerted over the cell cycle is lost (Rodriguez-Galindo and Pappo 2003). Advanced mutational analysis can locate the exact RB gene mutation in approximately 90% of patients, which is important for genetic counseling (Rodriguez-Galindo et al. 2007).

3.6.4 Signs and Symptoms

The most common signs of RB are:

1. Leukocoria (cat's eye reflex): This is caused by the tumor, which is white and occludes the normal red retina reflex and is a late sign of the disease (Fig. 3.14).
2. Strabismus: The tumor's placement over the macula causes loss of central vision and causes the affected eye to drift or become crossed.

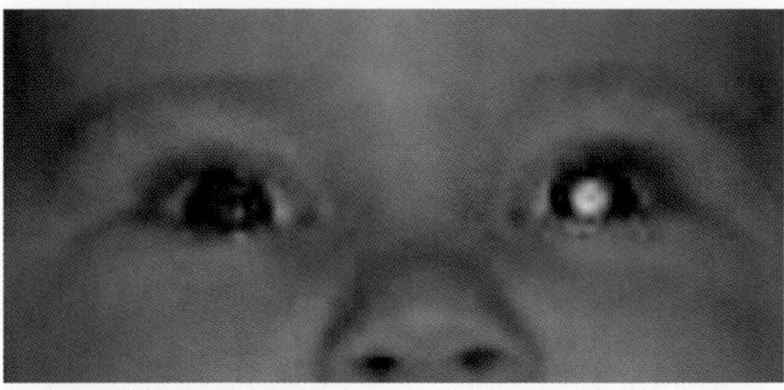

Figure 3.14

Leukocoria as seen on flash photography. The *red* retinal is obscured by the chalky appearing RB tumor, appearing in the left eye

3. Glaucoma: Caused by increased intraocular pressure due to the tumor, and is a sign of advanced disease.
4. Decreased vision in one eye: This is caused by the tumor covering the macula or from retinal detachment.

Some other less common presenting signs of RB include heterochromia (different colored iris), orbital cellulitis, and hyphema (blood in the anterior chamber (Chintagumpala et al. 2007; Balmer et al. 2006)).

Metastatic dissemination of RB occurs by several ways. Tumor can spread posteriorly through the optic nerve directly to the brain and the cerebrospinal fluid. Patients with intracranial disease may present with signs of increased intracranial pressure such as headaches, vomiting, and altered consciousness. RB can also spread through the choroid and vascular layer and disseminate through the blood to bone and bone marrow. These children may present with pain or a mass if bone metastases are present; or with lethargy, fever, anemia, and thrombocytopenia if the bone marrow is involved. Direct extension can also occur through sclera into the orbit, and is quite obvious presenting with proptosis or a mass. In the developed world, less than 5% of the patients present with extraocular disease, in stark contrast to the 50% observed in some developing countries (Rodriguez-Galindo et al. 2007).

RB can also present as a trilateral disease. In addition to the ocular tumors, an intracranial neuroblastic tumor develops in the pineal gland, suprasellar site, or parasellar site. This is relative, with an incidence of 0.5% in unilateral RB, 5–13% in sporadic bilateral RB, and as high as 15% in familial RB (Popovic et al. 2007). Trilateral RB can even be seen years after successfully treated ocular disease and is a major cause of mortality in these children in the first 5 years after diagnosis of bilateral RB. Typically, these patients present with signs of increased intracranial pressure.

3.6.5 Diagnostics

The diagnostic workup for RB begins with a thorough history, paying particular attention to the duration of the symptoms and changes in the eye's appearance. Special attention should be given to any familial history of RB. Physical examination should assess the visual acuity (cranial nerve II), extraocular movements (cranial nerves III, IV, and VI), strabismus, and leukocoria. Direct and indirect fundoscopic examination should be done under anesthesia. The pupils should be well dilated to allow for complete visualization of the fundus. Ultrasound is a common test that is performed on eyes affected by RB and shows the tumor in reference to anatomical structures. Fundoscopic pictures are also taken during the examination under anesthesia (Fig. 3.15). Fluoresceine angiography can be useful in accurately visualizing all the tumors' blood supply.

CT of the brain and orbits is needed to detect distal spread of the tumor and to identify areas of calcification, although there is a trend to avoid radiation in patients with a germline mutation who are predisposed to develop second malignancies. MRI of the brain has been shown to be an excellent method for visualizing tumor extension into the optic nerve and orbital area. CT and MRI are also needed to rule out intracranial tumors. A bone marrow aspirate is often done to detect metastatic disease, if there is an apparent risk for hematogenous spread such as choroidal involvement or when there is an abnormal blood count (Chintagumpala et al. 2007). A lumbar puncture is needed to determine if there is metastatic extension to the cerebrospinal fluid; this is necessary when there is a concern of optic-nerve involvement.

The diagnosis of RB is made by ophthalmoscopic, radiologic, and ultrasonographic appearance of the tumor; pathological confirmation is unnecessary. RB

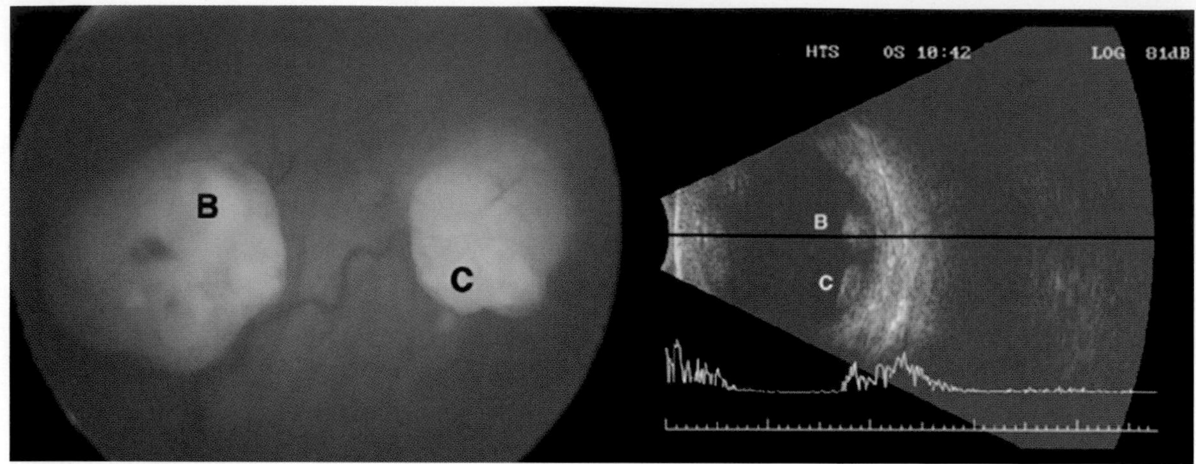

Figure 3.15

Retcam and corresponding ultrasound of RB tumor in the left eye. B and C represent RB tumors prior to treatment; their corresponding position can also be seen in the ultrasound image. Photo captured by Cynthia VandenHoven, The Department of Ophthalmology and Vision Sciences, Hospital for Sick Children

is a small blue round cell tumor consisting of densely packed cells. Calcifications are pathognomonic for RB. It is mitotically active; when the eye is enucleated, Flexner-Winterstein rosettes are present, which are highly characteristic of RB.

3.6.6 Staging and Classification

There are several common growth patterns of RB tumors. In an endophytic pattern, the tumor arises from the retina and grows into the vitreal cavity. These tumors usually fill the cavity and float in the vitreous and are known as vitreal seeds. Exophytic tumors grow from the retina into the subretinal space and cause serious detachments of the retina. From the retina, they can proceed to invade the choroid or the blood supply. A mixed presentation of endophytic and exophytic patterns is the most common occurrence (Balmer et al. 2006).

Historically, RB was staged according to the Reese–Ellsworth (RE) classification system that groups tumors based on the likelihood of losing an eye after external beam RT. In recent years, a new staging system has been developed which takes into account the recent change in the treatment, which has shifted away from the external beam RT in favor of chemotherapy and focal therapies. Murphree et al. (2005) developed a staging system that predicts the prognosis of ocular salvage with chemotherapy. This new system has been called the International Intraocular Retinoblastoma Classification (IIRC) system. Eyes are grouped from A to E, with group A eyes having the best prognosis of salvage following chemotherapy and focal therapies, and group E eyes having the worst prognosis (Gombos and Chevez-Barrios 2007; Gallie et al. 2007) (Fig. 3.16).

3.6.7 Treatment

The goals of treatment for RB are to preserve useful vision without compromising the patient's survival. The major treatment modalities for RB include surgical enucleation, radiation, and chemotherapy, in addition to focal cryotherapy and photocoagulation therapy. The treatment of RB requires a multidisciplinary approach including ophthalmologists, oncologists, radiation oncologists, as well as nurses, social workers, prosthesis makers, and sometimes occupational therapists.

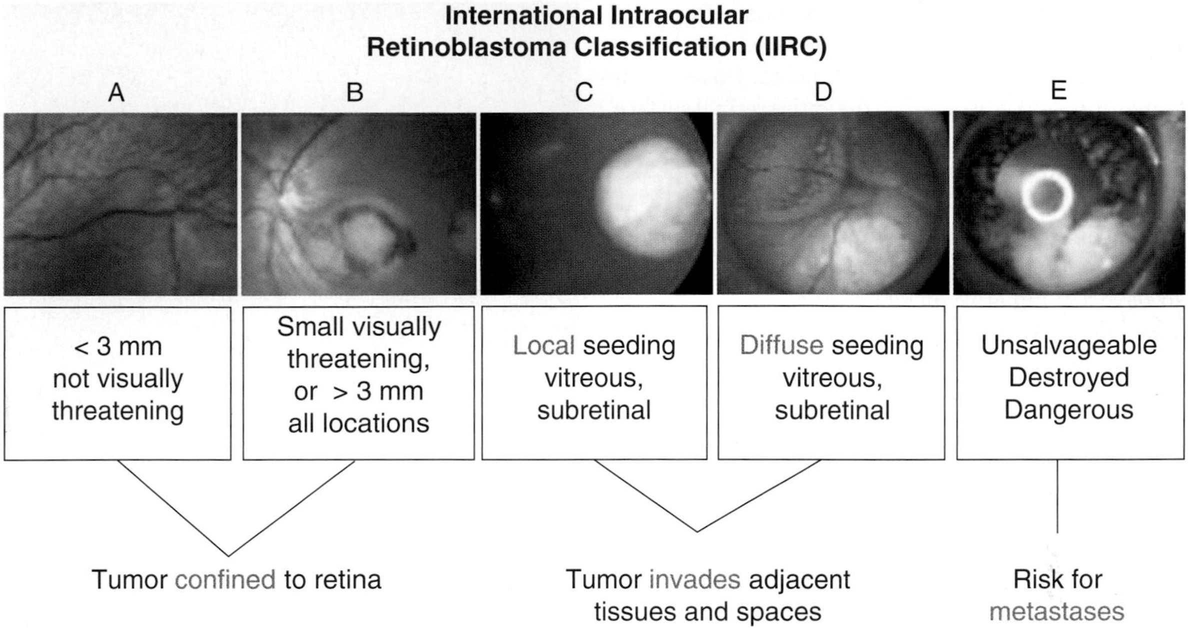

International Intraocular Retinoblastoma Classification (IIRC)

A
< 3 mm
not visually
threatening

B
Small visually
threatening,
or > 3 mm
all locations

C
Local seeding
vitreous,
subretinal

D
Diffuse seeding
vitreous,
subretinal

E
Unsalvageable
Destroyed
Dangerous

Tumor confined to retina

Tumor invades adjacent tissues and spaces

Risk for metastases

Figure 3.16

International intraocular retinoblastoma classification (IIRC) Reprinted with permission Gallie et al. 2007

Enucleation is often the treatment indicated for unilateral RB, as these patients tend to present with advanced disease (Fig. 3.17). Other indications for enucleation in patients who have bilateral disease include: advanced disease in one eye that does not respond to therapy, active tumor in an eye with no vision, glaucoma, anterior tumor invasion, tumor that invades the optic nerve, choroid, sclera, and tumor extending beyond the orbit, and when direct tumor visualization is obstructed by hemorrhage, coroneal opacity, or cataract (Chintagumpala et al. 2007). When the eye is enucleated, an orbital implant is surgically placed and the rectus muscles are attached to allow for some movement of the eventual prosthesis.

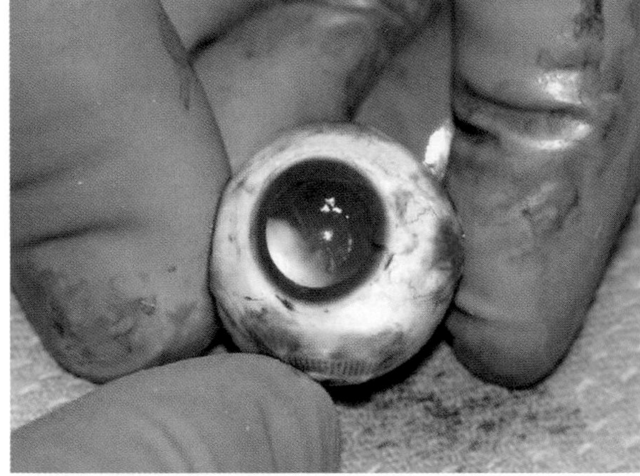

Figure 3.17

Enucleated eye-tumor is visible through the dilated sclera. Photo captured by Cynthia VandenHoven, The Department of Ophthalmology and Vision Sciences, Hospital for Sick Children

External beam radiation therapy (EBRT) was historically the primary therapy used to salvage eyes in patients with intraocular RB, as it was quite effective because RB is a radiosensitive tumor. EBRT is used sparingly today because of the increased associated risks of developing a secondary malignancy in the radiation field. Currently, EBRT is most often used when firstline treatment modalities such as chemotherapy and focal therapies have failed. Doses in the range of 40–45 Gy are used on the entire retinal surface. Its disadvantages include facial hypoplasia, cataract development, retinopathy, and increased risk of secondary tumors in the radiation field (Rodriguez-Galindo et al. 2007). Children who carry the germline RB mutation and receive radiation therapy are reported to have a cumulative incidence of second malignancies of 35–36%; moreover, patients who receive radiation in the first year of life are at an additional risk again of developing a secondary malignancy compared with those who receive radiation therapy after 1 year of age (Chintagumpala et al. 2007; Kleinerman et al. 2005). More recently, stereotactic radiation has been used to target some intraocular tumors, removing the need to radiate the entire orbit. The incidence of cataracts is lessened with this approach.

Plaque RT is another form of radiation therapy. With this form of radiation treatment, cobalt or iodine plaques are surgically implanted at the scleral base of the tumor. The plaque remains in place for 2–4 days and then is surgically removed. Doses in the range of 30–45 Gy are delivered to the tumor, with less scatter to the healthy tissues, compared with EBRT. This treatment is used on medium-sized tumors situated away from the optic nerve and macula (Rodriguez-Galindo et al. 2007). Plaque RT is most often used as a secondary treatment after another form has failed.

Focal therapies are used alone or as adjuvant treatment with chemotherapy. Cryotherapy can be effectively used to manage small anterior tumors. A cryoprobe is placed transclerally in the region of the tumor and it penetrates the retina. The tumors are frozen and subsequently allowed to thaw multiple times in a session, resulting in coagulation of the tumors' blood supply (Rodriguez-Galindo et al. 2007). It is usually performed at monthly intervals. Photocoagulation therapy is used for small posterior tumors. Laser burns are made around the tumor which effectively cut the blood supply to the tumor, ultimately causing cell death (see Fig. 3.18 for a RB tumor post treatment).

Chemotherapy was originally used in the treatment of intraocular RB, with initial good responses followed by tumor recurrence; it was therefore abandoned for many years. In the early 1990s, in an effort to avoid the long-term risks associated with radiation, its use re-emerged, and it has been shown to play a vital role in reducing the size of RB tumors so that they can be further managed with focal therapies such as laser and cryotherapy. This use has been termed cytoreduction or chemoreduction therapy. Although the exact number of treatments has not yet been determined, most groups use 4–6 cycles of agents such as carboplatin, etoposide, and vincristine (CEV) (Kim et al. 2007a). Cycles are administered every 3–4 weeks, while focal therapies are often administered during examination under anesthesia prior to each cycle. The treatment is tailored somewhat based on individual patient responses. Chan et al. (2005) also studied the use of cyclosporin A, in conjunction with these standard chemotherapy agents to prevent p-glycoprotein multidrug resistance (MDR). In vitro, p-glycoprotein has been shown to actively pump chemotherapy agents out of tumors; however, high concentrations of cyclosporin have shown to reverse this process. A current phase III multi-center

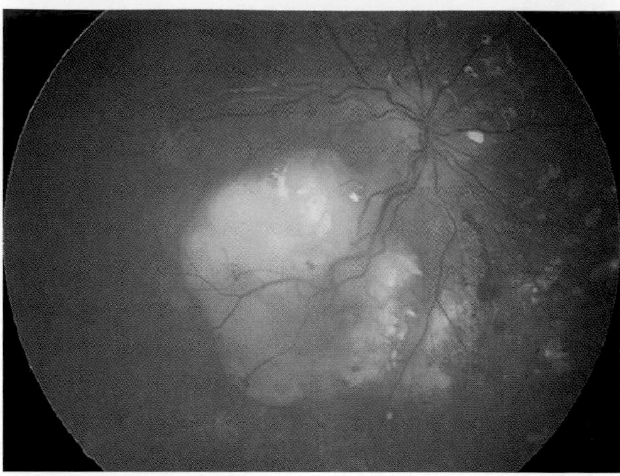

Figure 3.18

Retcam photo of OD following chemotherapy. This photo shows calcification following treatment with chemotherapy and focal therapies. Photo captured by Cynthia VandenHoven, The Department of Ophthalmology and Vision Sciences, Hospital for Sick Children

trial is ongoing to evaluate the efficacy of high-dose cyclosporin in conjunction with the chemotherapy agents, vincristine, carboplatin, and etoposide; preliminary results have shown good efficacy in conjunction with focal therapies (Chan et al. 2005).

Adjuvant chemotherapy is often indicated in patients who have undergone enucleation but whose pathology reveals high-risk features, or if there is overt orbital disease. High-risk features that may necessitate chemotherapy include: massive choroidal involvement, invasion of the ciliary body/iris or anterior changer, scleral disease, and retrolaminar optic nerve invasion (Rodriguez-Galindo et al. 2007).

Chemotherapy can also be delivered by subtenon or subconjunctival injection that delivers therapy locally. This type of local chemotherapy has the advantage of causing less systemic toxicity, and appears to be locally effective on vitreous lesions. Carboplatin, to date, is the agent that has been typically used in this regard (Rodriguez-Galindo et al. 2007).

Chemotherapy has always played a role in the treatment of extraocular RB and in patients with metastatic disease. Generally, the same drugs that are used in intraocular RB are used for metastatic disease – CEV. Other agents that have also shown responses are: cisplatin, cyclophosfamide, doxorubicin, and ifosfamide (Rodriguez-Galindo et al. 2007). In patients with metastatic disease, high-dose chemotherapy followed by stem cell rescue is often used, but is most effective when complete local control of metastatic disease has been obtained. Intrathecal administration of cytarabine and topotecan has also been successfully used to clear metastatic disease in the cerebrospinal fluid, in antecdotal reports.

In recent years, larger cooperative group and multicenter trials have been developed to address outstanding questions regarding the management of RB. These larger trials are likely to yield important information in a timely manner. The following are the trials carried out by the COG, United Kingdom Children's Cancer Study Group, and the Toronto Group (Gombos and Chevez-Barrios 2007; Gallie et al. 2007):

1. COG-ARET0332: A group phase III study of unilateral RB with and without high-risk features and the role of adjuvant chemotherapy. This study hopes to identify the high-risk pathological features that require adjuvant chemotherapy, and these patients will receive uniform treatment.
2. COG-ARET0231: A phase III limited-institution single-arm study for patients with groups C and D eyes, using systemic and subtenon chemotherapy. The goal is to intensify local therapy by administering periocular carboplatin in conjunction with systemic therapy (six cycles of CEV).
3. COG-ARET0331: A phase III limited-institution study using systemic neoadjuvant chemotherapy for group B intraocular RB. This study uses two drug therapy (carboplatin and vincristine) for six cycles in low-risk eyes in conjunction with focal therapies, to determine if reduced therapy is possible in favorable prognosis eyes.
4. UKCCCSG-RB-2005-11: This is a study on patients with unilateral RB who have undergone enucleation. Patients who have high-risk features, but no tumor at the cut end of the optic nerve will receive four cycles of CEV, and those with high-risk features and tumor at the cut end of the nerve will receive six cycles of CEV with intrathecal cytarabine if needed, followed by orbital radiation.
5. Toronto multi-center Trial: This phase II study addresses treatment of groups B, C, and D eyes with CEV chemotherapy, in addition to a 3-h infusion of high-dose cyclosporin. Six cycles are given to patients with groups C and D eyes, and three for group B eyes, to determine the proportion of eyes that remains relapse-free while avoiding enucleation and EBRT.

3.6.8 Prognosis

Documented 5-year survival rates in the US and Europe are reported to be between 87 and 99% in patients who present with intraocluar disease (Kim et al. 2007b). However, these results are not true for patients who live in the underdeveloped countries who often present with more advanced disease. For patients with locoregional and orbital involvement, the cure rate is 60–85% with systemic chemotherapy and radiation. For patients with CNS disease, despite the use of chemotherapy, radiation, intrathecal chemotherapy, and myeloablative chemotherapy with stem cell rescue, the results are dismal with only antecdotal survivors. Long-term survival is far superior in patients with extracranial metastatic disease when high-dose therapy is used; some report cure rates as high as 75% (Abramson 2005; Pandya et al. 2002).

3.6.9 Follow-Up

Close ongoing follow-up of children with RB is needed well after tumor control has been established. Children with hereditary disease are at risk of developing new tumors until retinal differentiation is complete, around the age of 7. Following the treatment of RB, fundoscopic examinations are imperative to detect recurrent or new disease quickly. Eye examinations are generally done under anesthesia while the child is receiving active therapy and routinely thereafter, until a child is able to cooperate for an awake eye examination, has no active disease, and requires no treatment. Once a child is only being monitored and is able to cooperate, eye examinations can be moved to the outpatient setting.

A child treated with chemotherapy and/or radiation therapy must be followed up for late effects of their treatment. Patients may have visual deficits resulting from their primary tumor and/or treatment, and may benefit from the use of visual-assisted devices. Carboplatin can cause hearing disturbances, and therefore audiograms must be a regular part of the follow-up regimen. It is vital to minimize the amount of sensory deficits, especially if patients also have visual defects. With the use of chemotherapy, a few descriptions of secondary leukemias developing in patient treated with etoposide are emerging (Kim et al. 2007b; Zage et al. 2008).

Children who harbor a germline mutation are at a life-long risk of acquiring another malignancy in their lifetime. This risk is magnified in patients who receive radiation therapy as part of their treatment, especially before the age of 1; however, it exists in all patients with a germline mutation. The secondary malignancies that have been described in RB patients include: osteosarcoma, soft-tissue sarcomas, pineoblastoma, melanoma, brain tumors, Hodgkin's disease, and epithelial cancers such as lung and breast cancer (Abramson and Schefler 2004). Families must be taught to be conscientious in reporting any changes in their children's health. Education regarding prevention of secondary cancers should focus on: avoiding radiation, both diagnostic such as CT scans and RT unless absolutely indicated, especially in patient less than 1 year of age; avoiding sun (UV) exposure; avoiding cigarette smoking; and avoiding the use of growth hormone (Abramson 2005).

3.6.10 Future Directions

Topotecan is a relatively new agent that is being studied to determine if it has a role in the treatment of RB. Preclinical studies suggest that it is active and clinical studies are underway using systemic, subconjunctival, and intraventricular/intrathecal topotecan in both intraocular and metastatic RB (Gallie et al. 2007; Rodriguez-Galindo et al. 2007). Research is also being carried out to inhibit the MDMX-p53 pathway. Nulin-3 is a small molecule that targets this pathway, leading to apoptosis both in in vitro and in vivo studies. Suicide gene therapy delivered by periocular injection has been studied in phase I trials to determine its ability to treat vitreal tumors (Rodriguez-Galindo et al. 2007).

3.7 Rhabdomyosarcoma

Rhabdomyosarcoma (RMS) develops from a primitive mesenchymal cell committed to muscle differentiation, and although they can occur anywhere in the body, they have a predeliction for certain sites in the body which are unique to this tumor.

3.7.1 Epidemiology

RMS is the most common soft-tissue sarcoma that occurs in children. It affects approximately 4.3 per million children and adolescents less than 20 years of age (Paulino and Okcu 2008). It is the third most common extracranial solid neoplasm of childhood and represents 5–8% of pediatric cancers (Lewis et al. 2007). Males have a very slightly higher incidence. Two-thirds of children present with RMS before the age of 6. Younger children tend to present with the embryonal subtype of RMS, whereas the alveolar subtype occurs throughout childhood.

3.7.2 Etiology

The cause of RMS is unknown. However, an association has been observed with other genetic syndromes including Rubinstein–Taybi syndrome, Costello syndrome, Noonan syndrome, and Gorlin basal cell nevus syndrome, but most notably, in neurofibromatosis (NF1), Li-Fraumeni syndrome, and BWS (Paulino and Okcu 2008). A higher incidence of RMS has also been noted in patients with congenital anomalies of the gastrointestinal, genitourinary, and central nervous system (CNS). Some studies have shown that parental use of marijuana and cocaine during the year prior to the child's birth leads to a two- to fivefold increased risk of developing RMS (Paulino and Okcu 2008).

3.7.3 Molecular Genetics

Morphologically, RMS is a small blue round cell tumor composed of characteristic rhabdomyoblasts. RMS can be differentiated from tumors with similar morphology based on electron microscopy, immunocytochemistry, and cytogenetic analysis. RMS has three distinct pathological subtypes: embryonal, alveolar, and pleomorphic with embryonal having the most favorable outcome. Sixty percent of RMS are of the embryonal subtype, of which 5% are the botryoid variant (found in hollow organs, such as vagina or bladder) or spindle cell variant (often seen in the paratesticular area). Of the remaining 40, 20% are the alveolar subtype, and 20% are undifferentiated (Pappo et al. 1997). The pleomorphic subtype occurs very rarely in children, is more common in older adults (>45 years), and is characterized by the presence of anaplastic cells in large sheets (Paulino and Okcu 2008).

Alveolar RMS has a characteristic t(2;13) seen in approximately 55% of patients, which fuses the PAX3 gene on chromosome 2q35 with the FKHR gene on chromosome 13q14. A second translocation, t(1;13), occurs in 22% of patients, whereby PAX7 on chromosome 1p36 and the FKHR gene are fused (Lewis et al. 2007). PAX3 and PAX7 are important in muscle development during embryogenesis. Patients with metastatic disease and PAX7–FKHR fusion gene have a different pattern of metastases, and may have a more favorable course than patients with the PAX3–FKHR (Pappo et al. 1997). The presence of even a few foci of alveolar histology warrants a diagnosis of alveolar subtype, rather than embyronal subtype, and warrants treatment intensification. Approximately 20% of patients with alveolar histology will not have a recognized translocation, and diagnosis is based on immunohistological studies and morphology.

The embryonal subtypes have not revealed any translocations but characteristically have shown LOH at the 11p15 locus (Pappo et al. 1997).

3.7.4 Symptoms and Clinical Signs

RMS can occur anywhere in the body, and is not limited to those places where skeletal muscle exists. The prevalence of the tumors according to primary tumor and the correlating clinical symptoms are listed in Table 3.10. In general, patients tend to present with signs of the mass compressing on nearby structures. Patients rarely have systemic illness, and do not tend to have fever or weight loss, except in the occasional patients with metastatic disease. Approximately, in 15% of the patients, RMS occurs as a metastatic disease. RMS spreads via hematogenous and lymphatic routes. The most common sites for metastases are lung, bone marrow, lymph nodes, and bone (Oberlin et al. 2008).

3.7.5 Diagnostics

The necessary diagnostic tests in the investigation of a patient thought to have RMS include:

- MRI and/or CT of the primary site and draining lymph nodes
- CT of the chest to look for pulmonary metastases
- Bone Scan
- Tumor biopsy
- Bilateral bone marrow aspirates and biopsies
- Lumbar puncture with cytology in patients with a parameningeal primary
- Blood tests (CBC, LDH)

For patients with parameningeal primaries, CT and MRI are both indicated, as CT imaging is superior

Table 3.10. Rhabdomyosarcoma (RMS): Prevalence, histology, age, and clinical symptoms according to primary site

Site	Incidence (%)	Most common histology	Median age at presentation (years)	Clinical signs and symptoms
Orbit	10	Embryonal	6.8	Exophthalmos, palpebral swelling, diplopia, decreased visual acuity, ptosis
Parameningeal sites (nasopharynx, nasal cavity, paranasal sinus, middle ear-mastoid region, infratemporal fossa, pterygopalatine fossa)	15	Embryonal	5	Nasal obstruction, congestion, bloody discharge, diplopia, decreased vision, headache, papilledema Involvement of abducens (VI), oculomotor (III), trochlear (IV), facial (VII), or acoustic (VIII) cranial nerves
Other head and neck (scalp, cheek, external ear, parotid, larynx, oral cavity, and oropharynx)	10	Alveolar/embryonal	5	Swelling, mass, pain, facial nerve palsy, trismus, obstructive symptoms
Bladder	10	Embryonal	4.5	Urinary tract obstruction, hematuria, dysuria, polyuria, abdominal mass
Prostate			5.1	Regional lymph-node involvement Tenesmus (inability to empty bowel at defecation)
Paratesticular	7	Embryonal	6	Painless scrotal mass Regional lymph-node involvement
Vagina and vulva	3.5	Embryonal/boytroid	5.2	Bleeding, protrusion of grape-like cluster from vagina
Uterine and cervix			15	May have urinary or bowel obstruction Vulvular inflammation, labial nodule Bleeding, pelvic mass, pedunculated polyp
Extremity	20	Alveolar/embryonal	Teenage	Mass, swelling, limp Regional lymph-node involvement
Trunk (chest wall, paraspinal, abdominal wall)	6	Alveolar	12.5	Mass, swelling, weakness, bowel and bladder disturbance, pain
Retroperitoneum	5–6	Embryonal	6	Late symptoms because of expansion of abdominal cavity
Biliary tree	0.8	Embryonal	3.4	Jaundice, abdominal swelling, extrahepatic biliary obstruction, fever, loss of appetite

(Paulino and Okcu 2008: Pappo et al. 2006; Raney et al. 2008)

at evaluating bony erosion and MRI is important for evaluating intracranial extension. A biopsy is necessary and can be done either via a core or open biopsy. The specimen should be sent for cytogenetics with FISH (or reverse transcriptase-polymerase chain reaction (RT-PCR), when FISH is not available) to look for translocations discussed earlier. Light microscopy reveals rhabdomyoblasts or cross-striations, which are both seen in the skeletal muscle. On immunohistochemistry, RMS cells stain positive for desmin, vimentin, myoglobin, actin, and myogenin (Pappo et al. 1997).

There are no specific serum tumor markers for RMS. Rarely, cytopenias may be present, possibly indicating bone marrow involvement.

3.7.6 Staging and Classification

Staging normally follows two distinct systems. The tumor node metastases (TNM) system takes into account size, local invasiveness, and presence of nodes and metastases, and for RMS, site is also taken into account, allowing clinicians to stratify patients by stage (Table 3.11) (Andrassy 2002). The Intergroup Rhabdomyosarcoma Study Group (IRSG) system stratifies patients based on post-surgical pre-chemotherapy or RT residual tumor volume (Table 3.12). Both TNM stage and IRSG are then used to determine the exact therapeutic strategy. Survival also correlates with clinical group and stage.

3.7.7 Treatment

The IRSG is a cooperative group that have been conducting studies in RMS patients over the past 4 decades, with the aim of exploring the biology of RMS and improving treatment outcomes by conducting coordinated clinical trials. IRS-I, IRS-II, IRS-III, and IRS-IV were carried out sequentially from 1972 until 1997, and have led to important discoveries about the role of surgery, radiation, and chemotherapy in the treatment of RMS (Raney et al. 2008). Table 3.13 presents the most common treatment for RMS based on the site of primary disease.

Similar to other solid tumors in children, treatment for RMS includes systemic therapy to prevent the development of metastases and local therapy. RMS, especially of the embryonal subtype, is extraordinarily radiosensitive, and thus, both

Table 3.12. Intergroup Rhabdomyosarcoma Study Group (IRSG) postsurgical grouping classification

Clinical group	Extent of disease and surgical result
I	Localized disease, completely resected, no microscopic residual
II	Gross total resection with microscopic residual diseaseRegional disease with involved nodes, completely resected with or without microscopic residual
III	Incomplete resection or biopsy with gross residual
IV	Distant metastatic disease

Table 3.11. TNM pretreatment staging classification for RMS

Stage	Sites	T Invasiveness	T Size	N	M
I	Orbit, head and neck (excluding parameningeal),[c] genitourinary[d]	T1 or T2	a[a] or b[b]	N0 or N1 or NX	M0
II	Bladder/prostate, extremity, cranial parameningeal, other[d]	T1 or T2	a[a]	N0 or NX	M0
III	Bladder/prostate extremity, cranial parameningeal, other[e]	T1 or T2	a[a] b[b]	N1 N0 or N1 or NX	M0 M0
IV	All	T1 or T2	a[a] or b[b]	N0 or N1	M1

T tumor; *T1* confined to anatomic site of origin; *T2* extension; *N0* not clinically involved; *N1* clinically involved; *NX* clinical status unknown; *M0* no distant metastases; *M1* distant metastasis present

[a] ≤5 cm in diameter

[b] >5 cm in diameter

[c] Excluding parameningeal

[d] Non-bladder/non-prostate, includes trunk, retroperitoneum, etc.

Table 3.13. Common treatment approaches for specific sites as per the IRS studies

Site	Most commonly used local control modality	Chemotherapy
Orbit	Orbital radiation (chemotherapy alone used in some SIOP trials)	VA ± cyclophosphamide
Parameningeal	Radiation	VAC
Other head and neck	Surgery and/or radiation	VA ± cyclophosphamide
Bladder/prostrate	Radiation partial cystectomy (pelvic exenterative procedures avoided)	VAC ± doxorubicin
Paratesticular	Surgery: radical inguinal orchidectomy and resection of involved scrotal tissue + consideration for retroperitoneal lymph-node dissection	VA ± cyclophosphamide
Gynecologic	Surgery (hysterectomy) and/or radiation	VAC
Extremity	Surgery with lymph-node dissection or sentinel lymph-node mapping	VAC ± topotecan VADRAC +cislatin VAI or VIE
Retroperitoneum	Surgery (debulking) + radiation	VAC
Biliary tree	Radiation ± surgery	VAC

(Paulino and Okcu 2008; Pappo et al. 2006)
VAC vincristine, dactinomycin, cyclophosphamide; *VA* vincristine, dactinomycin; *VADRAC* vincristine, doxorubicin, dactinomycin, cyclophosphamide; *VAI* vincristine, dactinomycin, ifosfamide; *VIE* vincristine, ifosfamide, etoposide

surgery and/or radiation therapy are used effectively in RMS. The type of local therapy offered in RMS depends on the location of the tumor. Treatment for RMS is stratified based on the risk group (described earlier) and histology into low-, intermediate-, and high-risk protocols, with varying treatment intensity.

3.7.7.1 Local Therapy

The IRSG advocates for upfront surgical resection to establish local control, whenever possible, to render treatment to patients in group I. However, as RMS is a radiosensitive tumor, deforming or mutilating surgery is not warranted, and patients with tumor of the orbit, for example, receive radiation alone as their form of local therapy. The algorithm dictating which patients require adjuvant RT is complex, and depends on the amount of residual tumor after initial resection, histology, and site of primary disease.

The timing of RT is variable depending on the protocol used. In patients with parameningeal RMS, fewer local failures were noted if RT was delivered earlier (2 weeks from diagnosis) (Bisogno et al. 2008). Radiation is very useful in patients who require urgent tumor reduction secondary to involvement of vital structures such as cranial nerves or spinal cord. In RMS, radiation dose ranges from 30 to 55.8 Gy with 1.5-cm margins. Intensity-modulated RT (IMRT) is an advanced technique that results in improvement of dose distribution to the tumor and offers decrease dose exposure to the tissues outside the target volume. The result is that healthy tissue is spared compared with the standard three-dimensional planning. IMRT has resulted in improved local control compared with the traditional radiation therapy (Wolden et al. 2005). Figure 3.19 shows an example of radiation planning using IMRT. Hyperfractionated RT (given twice daily) vs. daily fractions was studied by the IRSG; however, there was no significant difference in the outcome (Raney et al. 2008; Crist et al. 2001). Thus, RT in daily fractions remains the standard of care. European studies have attempted to avoid radiation altogether in orbital RMS, with promising survival and salvage rates (Stevens et al. 2005).

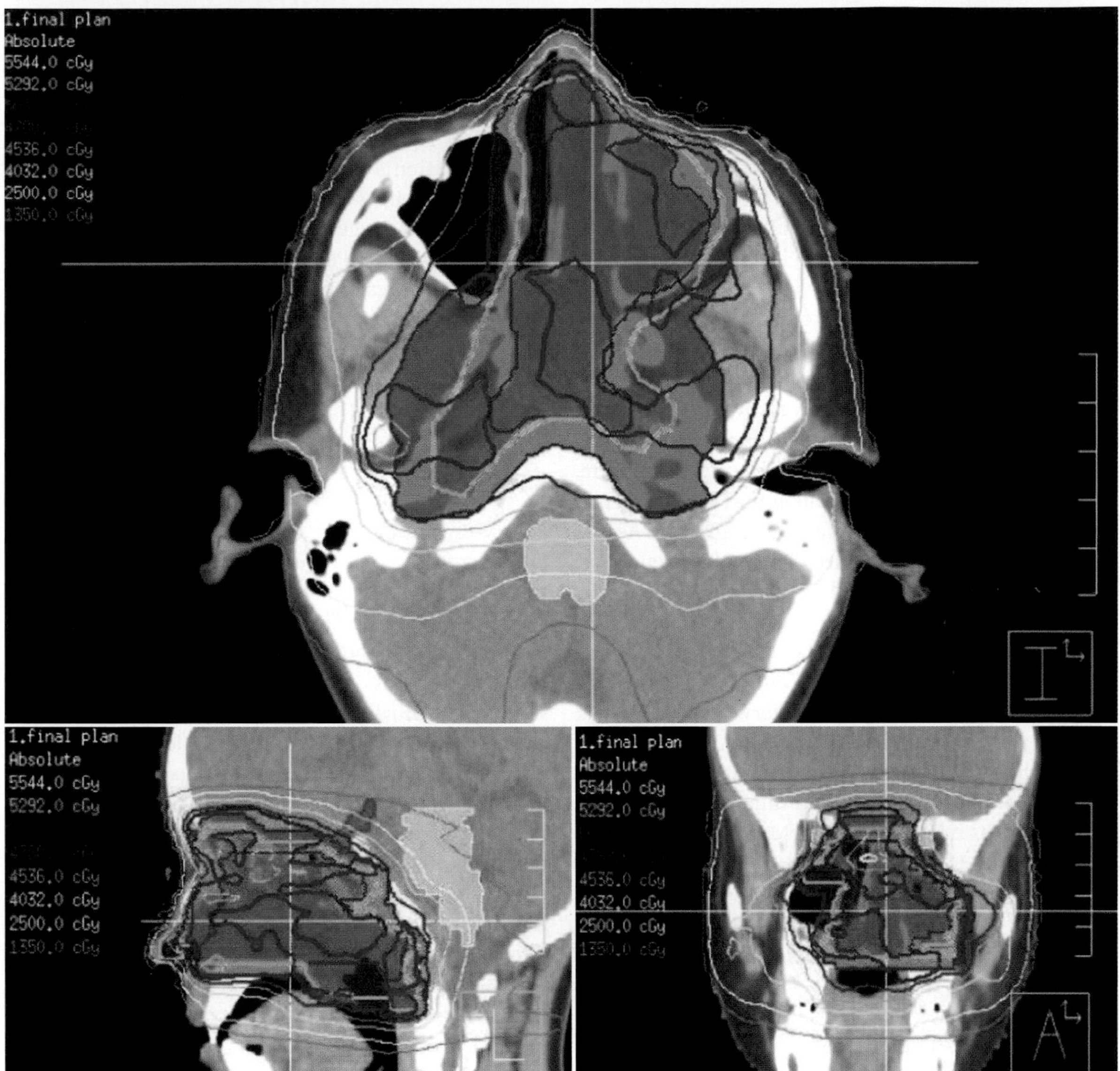

Figure 3.19

Nasopharyngeal RMS: Planning for RT. This CT scan shows the planning doses of IMRT RT conforming to the tumors bed in addition to larger margins

3.7.7.2 Chemotherapy

The chemotherapy agents most commonly used in the treatment of RMS include: vincristine, actinomycin, and cyclophosphamide (VAC), and represent the backbone of most treatment protocols. For patients with favorable site and histology, the IRSG is attempting to reduce the amount of alkylating agent (cyclophosphamide) and yet maintain excellent survival. For example, current treatment protocols for clinical group I tumors, or favorable sites such as orbit and paratesticular, require only vincristine and actinomycin. In contrast, the addition of alkylating agent is still crucial in patients with tumors of unfavorable site, stage, or histology (Stevens et al. 2005; Pappo et al. 2006). Irinotecan has been shown to be a very effective drug in RMS (Wexler et al. 2002), and for clinical group II and III tumors, irinotecan is now being incorporated into the VAC backbone for patients with newly diagnosed disease.

The combination of IE, known to be effective in other sarcomas, including ES, was investigated by the IRSG. The IRSG compared VAI (vincristine, actinomycin, and ifosfamide), VIE (vincristine, ifosfamide, and etoposide), and VAC, and found no difference in the outcome among these three regimens. As the administration of IE requires longer hospital stays, VAC remains the standard of care for RMS (Crist et al. 2001; Stevens et al. 2005). For patients with metastatic disease (group IV disease), VAC still remains a part of therapy; however, IE and doxorubicin are now being explored, due to the very poor prognosis in this group of patients (Pappo et al. 2006). Chemotherapy has traditionally been given for longer duration in RMS than in other solid tumors, approaching 12–24 months in IRSG studies (McDowell 2003).

3.7.8 Prognosis

Prognosis in RMS is directly related to the grouping of the tumor. In the last IRSG (IV) study, the 3-year event-free survival (EFS) was 83, 86, 73, and 25% for groups 1, 2, 3, and 4, respectively (Paulino and Okcu 2008). Prognosis is also dependent on tumor location. OS for various sites is as follows: paratesticular, 90%; bladder/prostate, 85%; orbital, 90%; and extremity, 66% (Andrassy 2002). For groups I, II, and III RMS, SIOP reported an OS and EFS of 71 and 57%, respectively (Stevens et al. 2005). Current data from the IRSG and European cooperative groups cite the OS and EFS for patients with metastatic disease to be 34 and 27%, respectively (Oberlin et al. 2008).

In addition to stage and group described earlier, several prognostic factors have been identified in patients with RMS. Indicators that are well recognized are those that go into staging and grouping the patients: tumor location, size, invasiveness, regional nodal involvement, and metastases. However, histology and age are also important. Age is a very important prognostic indicator, with patients between 1 and 9 years of age having the best outcome (OS = 83%), compared with infants less than 1 year of age (OS = 55%) or patients older than 9 years (OS = 68%) (Paulino and Okcu 2008). Histology is also a significant prognostic factor. Patients with embryonal histology experience superior outcomes (OS = 83%), compared with OS of 66% in patients with alveolar histology, and 55% in patients with undifferentiated sarcomas (Paulino and Okcu 2008).

3.7.9 Follow-Up

Follow-up for children completing therapy for RMS must screen for local recurrence and late effects of treatment. The generally accepted current standard of care includes physical examination, chest CT to look for lung metastases, and CT or MRI of the primary, every 3 months for the first year post therapy. During the second and third year, screening may be offered with decreasing frequency, as deemed clinically appropriate. Follow-up must incorporate late effects of all treatments including, site-specific radiation, surgery, as well as chemotherapy. Patients who have undergone RT as part of their treatment have the highest risk of late effects. In patients with head and neck or parameningeal primaries, late effects of radiation commonly include xerostomia, dental abnormalities, endocrine dysfunction, visual and auditory disturbance, and growth retardation of treated tissues. Bowel obstruction, musculoskeletal growth delay, and gonadal dysfunction can occur in patients with pelvic radiation. Extremity radiation increases the risk of fractures, growth alterations, fibrosis, and decreased range of motion in joints (Paulino and Okcu 2008). Children who have received radiation have the potential for developing secondary tumors later in life and require ongoing follow-up (Andrassy 2002).

3.7.10 Future Perspectives

Patients with metastatic alveolar RMS continue to respond poorly to standard treatment protocols, and new targeted therapy needs to be developed. Molecular gene fusions such as the PAX3–FKHR oncogene may be a therapeutic target in the future (Sorensen et al. 2002). RMS has been shown to express vascular endothelial growth factor (VEGF), and when this pathway is blocked, RMS proliferation is delayed (Oberlin et al. 2008). Antiangiogenic therapies, therefore, may play a role in future RMS therapy. Dysregulation of other pathways including the mammalian target of rapamycin pathway (mTOR), epidermal growth factor receptor (EGFR), and erbB-2 have been observed in RMS, and continue to be targets for future drug development (Oberlin et al. 2008; Pappo et al. 2006). Recognizing that chemotherapy and RT in RMS work by inducing apoptosis (programmed cell death), research is being done to overcome defects in apoptosis, which may contribute to treatment failure. Molecularly targeted therapies are being considered to restore apoptosis sensitivity in RMS (Fulda 2008).

3.8 Non-Rhabdomyosarcomatous Soft-Tissue Sarcomas

Non-rhabdomyosarcomatous soft-tissue sarcomas (NRSTS) are a heterogeneous group of tumors that arise from mesenchymal tissues, such as muscle, bone, fat, nerve, and connective tissues. Collectively, they account for approximately 7.4% of cancers occurring in childhood and adolescence (Okcu et al. 2006). They occur slightly more often in males compared to females and in blacks compared to Caucasians. There is an association between several cancer predisposition syndromes and/or environmental exposures and the development of NRSTS. These syndromes include Li-Fraumeni syndrome, germline *RB1* gene mutations, neurofibromatosis-1, in addition to exposure to ionizing radiation (Spunt et al. 2006). NRSTS may occur anywhere in the body, but in children, they most often arise in the extremities and trunk, and present as a painless mass. Metastatic disease is present at diagnosis in 15% of patients, with the lung being the most common distant site by far. Metastases to other sites include bone, liver, mesentery, and regional lymph nodes, although they occur less commonly (Spunt et al. 1999).

In pediatrics, NRSTS are staged according to the IRSG surgicopathologic staging system (Table 3.12). The IRSG system is limited; however, it neither takes into account the unique and heterogeneous features of each tumor type, nor the prognostic features such as tumor size and grade. Grading is based on histological subtype, amount of necrosis, number of mitoses, the degree of cellularity, and nuclear features. A score is given from 1 to 3, with 3 representing high grade, aggressive tumors (Miser et al. 2002). Prognostic factors for risk of local and distant recurrence and decreased survival are outlined in Table 3.14.

The treatment approach for NRSTS is similar regardless of the tumor type. Primary treatment consists of wide surgical excision of the tumor. A surgical margin of 1 cm is considered adequate if free of all microscopic diseases (Loeb et al. 2008). RT is sometimes required, especially in the presence of inadequate

Table 3.14. Prognostic factors in the NRSTS (Okcu et al. 2006)

	Factors associated with increased risk of local relapse	Factors associated with increased risk of distant metastases	Factors associated with decreased survival
Microscopicallypositive margins	X		X
Tumor >5 cm	X	X	X
High histologic grade		X	X
Intra-abdominal primary tumor	X		X
No radiotherapy	X		
Invasive tumor		X	

surgical margins including microscopic or macroscopic residual disease. RT can be administered preoperatively or postoperatively depending on the situation, with distinct advantages for each. Preoperative RT can potentially offer reduction in tumor size, decrease the risk of intraoperative contamination, and is delivered to a nonhypoxic tumor bed. Postoperative radiation allows for immediate surgery, avoids the risk of delay related to radiation-induced wound healing prior to surgery, and allows for exact interpretation of tumor size and extent (Okcu et al. 2006). In contrast to other childhood sarcomas such as RMS or ES, RT alone (in the absence of good surgical resection) in NRSTS is ineffective for local control, with recurrence rates of 70–75% (Spunt et al. 2006). The lack of chemosensitivity of NRSTS makes this group of tumors very different from all other pediatric solid tumors. Nonetheless, chemotherapy can be used in patients with tumors that are high-grade, unresectable, incompletely excised, and/or metastatic. In some situations, such as synovial sarcoma (SS), chemotherapy is offered even in resectable, localized disease, to decrease the chance of development of metastases. Ifosfamide and doxorubicin are the most effective agents (Loeb et al. 2008; Spunt et al. 2006) in NRSTS. Metastatic NRSTS do poorly and require new therapies.

Local control rates with surgery plus RT approach are 95% in patients with localized extremity tumors (Loeb et al. 2008). Although the OS of children with completely resected tumors is excellent, patients with inadequate local control are at risk for recurrence and death. It is important to recognize those tumors with a high potential for local and distant recurrence so that appropriate adjuvant treatment is utilized during the initial treatment.

Specific NRSTS in children will be briefly discussed, with typical features unique to each tumor summarized.

3.8.1 Alveolar Soft-Part Sarcoma

This tumor is a very rare tumor and is found most often in late adolescence, with a higher incidence in females. It represents less than 1% of all soft-tissue sarcomas in adults and children (Miser et al. 2002). Alveolar soft-part sarcoma (ASPS) most commonly arises in the deep soft tissue of the thigh and buttocks (Coffin et al. 1997). The head and neck regions are also a common site in children. ASPS metastasizes to lung, bone, and CNS. This disease has an indolent course, and relapses can occur very late (Folpe and Deyrup 2006). Imaging generally shows a large intramuscular mass with prominent vascularity. Chromosomal abnormalities have been identified at der(17) t(x; 17)(p11.2q25) (Spunt et al. 2006). Prognosis is best for head and neck tumors, but poor in general.

3.8.2 Desmoid Tumor (Aggressive Fibromatosis)

These rare tumors arise in the connective tissue and represent locally aggressive but benign lesions. They can arise in any age group, with a female predilection in adults (Ballo et al. 1999). Patients with FAP are at risk for abdominal desmoid tumors (Clark et al. 2008). Tumors commonly arise in the extremities, head and neck, shoulder, and chest wall. Some tumors display a trisomy on chromosome 8 (Okcu et al. 2006). Surgery is the primary treatment, although recurrence rates can be high (79%) even with presumed total excision (Okcu et al. 2006). Adjuvant RT can diminish the risk of recurrence. Drugs such as methotrexate along with vinblastine and tamoxifen have been effective in both relapsed and unresectable tumors, although they tend to work slowly over time. Newer therapies such as interferon and imatinib mesylate are being studied (Stengel et al. 2008).

3.8.3 Desmoplastic Small Round Cell Tumor

The tumor is seen most often in adolescents and adults with a significant male predominance and is a highly aggressive sarcoma. These tumors characteristically present in the abdominal/retroperitoneal region. Desmoplastic small round cell tumor (DSRCT) is characterized by the presence of t(11; 22)(p13; q12), although the specific breakpoint is different than that of ES (Okcu et al. 2006). Definitive surgery is often difficult owing to the abdominal/retroperitoneal location of these tumors. Treatment is therefore complex with some centers using high-dose chemotherapy in addition to aggressive surgery and radiation with varying responses (Kushner et al. 1996).

3.8.4 Infantile Fibrosarcoma

This spindle cell tumor affects young infants and children. Congenital or infantile fibrosarcoma are generally found in the distal extremities and the head and neck regions; these tumors grow rapidly but rarely metastasize. These tumors are characterized by a t(12; 15)(p13; q25) (Spunt et al. 2006). Occasionally, infantile fibrosarcoma tumors have been observed to undergo spontaneous regression, and may not require adjuvant therapy in the face of postoperative microscopic margins. VAC chemotherapy can be used in instances where upfront surgical resection is not possible, to reduce tumor bulk and facilitate definitive surgery. The overall 5-year survival with infantile fibrosarcoma is 84–93% (Miser et al. 2002).

3.8.5 Infantile Hemangiopericytoma

This neoplasm represents approximately 3% of all soft-tissue sarcomas in children (Miser et al. 2002). This is a vascular tumor that often displays the cytogenetic abnormalities of t(12; 19)(q13; q13.3) and t(13; 22)(q22; q11)(Okcu et al. 2006). It often presents as a solitary lesion in the oral cavity, chest wall, and head and neck of infants in the first year of life; it is usually associated with an excellent outcome with complete resection and is considered to be relatively benign in this age group (Spunt et al. 2006). In older children and adults, the tumor is found more often in the lower extremities and retroperitoneum, and is usually more aggressive and associated with metastatic disease and poor outcome (Miser et al. 2002). This tumor can metastasize to lung and bone.

3.8.6 Infantile Myofibromatosis

Myofibromas and myobribromatosis are tumors of the soft tissue, characterized by malignant proliferation. They often occur in infancy. Nonspecific chromosomal-8 abnormalities have been observed in these tumors. Tumors arise equally in the trunk, extremities, and head and neck. They can also appear as bluish/purplish macules. These tumors have been known to spontaneously regress. Survival is more than 90% with surgery or conservative management alone (Okcu et al. 2006).

3.8.7 Leiomyosarcoma

This malignant smooth-muscle tumor accounts for less than 2% of NRSTS in children. Radiation therapy may predispose a child to leiomyosarcoma. The development of leiomyosarcoma in children has been associated with states of immunocompromise, such as organ transplantation, immunosuppression, and human immunodeficiency virus (HIV). Epstein–Barr Virus (EBV) has been linked to leiomyosarcoma in children with HIV. A t(12; 14) translocation has been observed in this tumor (Okcu et al. 2006). Leiomysarcomas can arise in any vascular structure or soft tissue. Surgical resections of these tumors alone normally have favorable outcomes.

3.8.8 Liposarcoma

Liposarcoma, similar to leiomyosarcoma, is a tumor normally affecting older adults, but rarely can occur in children and adolescents, with a slight male predominance. The deep soft tissues of the lower extremities account for about half of the pediatric cases, and the second most common site of occurrence is the trunk (retroperitoneum). Metastases are not common but can occur in the lung, liver, lymph nodes, and brain, with a higher predilection to extrapulmonary sites compared with other soft-tissue sarcoma. Liposarcomas can be of myxoid, round cell, well differentiated, or pleomorphic subtypes (Coffin et al. 1997). The myxoid variant, which is the most commonly seen variant in pediatrics, carries the most favorable prognosis, and has a characteristic t(12;16)(q13;p11) (Swanson and Dehner 1991; Loeb et al. 2008). Liposarcomas are locally invasive and treatment is surgery alone if resectable. Liposarcomas, especially of the myxoid subtype, can sometimes respond to chemotherapy, but the exact role for chemotherapy to prevent metastatic disease has not been fully defined. Radiation may be important in large tumors, especially where there is a risk of close margins. Outcomes are dependent on adequate surgical margins, size, and subtype of tumor.

3.8.9 Malignant Peripheral Nerve Sheath Tumor

Malignant peripheral nerve sheath tumors (MPNSTs) arise from the peripheral nerve sheaths, as their name suggests, and they are also referred to as neurofibrosarcomas. They are among the most common of the soft-tissue sarcomas occurring during childhood, representing 10% of all NRSTS (Okcu et al. 2006). They most commonly occur in the second decade of life, with females being affected slightly more often. There is a well established association between neurofibromatosis I and the development of this tumor, and they can develop in pre-existing neurofibromas. Mutations of p53 and alteration of chromosome 7p, 9p, 17q, and 22q have been noted in these tumors, but are not useful diagnostically (Spunt et al. 2006). The most common anatomic sites of presentation of MPNSTs are the extremities and trunk, with the sciatic nerve being the most common site (Fig. 3.20). Metastases are present at diagnosis in 15% of the cases (Okcu et al. 2006). MPNSTs also occur in sites prior to RT. Unresectable or metastatic MPNST are rarely curable, and chemotherapy is often not useful, and only produce responses in 25% of patients (Okcu et al. 2006).

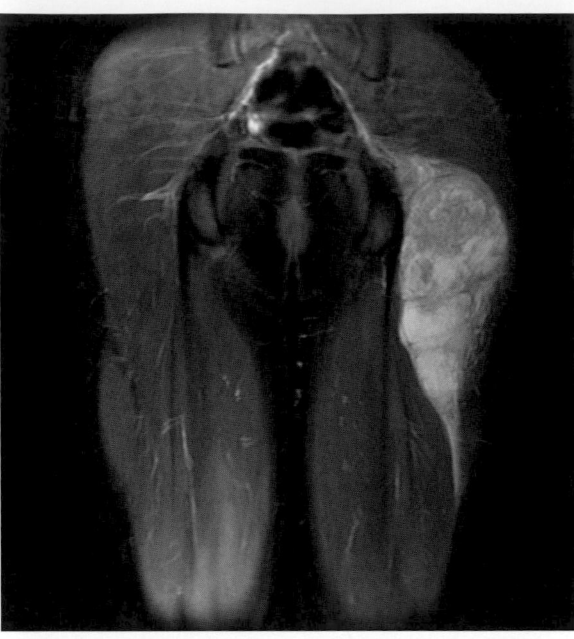

Figure 3.20
MRI showing MRNST arising from the left sciatic nerve

3.8.10 Synovial Sarcoma

Synovial sarcoma (SS) is the most commonly occurring NRSTS in older children and young adults (Miser et al. 2002). There is a very slight male predominance in the development of SS. It has three histological subgroups: biphasic, which is the most common and represents 60% of cases, monophasic-epithelial, and monophasic-fibrous. SS carries a characteristic genetic alteration t(X;18) which is found in over 90% of patients (Spunt et al. 2006; Loeb et al. 2008). SS normally occurs in close proximity to a joint, tendon, or bursa. The lung is the most common site for metastases, but lymph nodes can also be involved. Metastatic disease is present at diagnosis in 10% of patients (Okcu et al. 2006). Diagnostic imaging usually shows a mass with calcification. SS is one of the more chemosensitive NRSTS. Surgery is the primary treatment; however, chemotherapy is usually offered, especially when tumors are large in size, to decrease the risk of metastatic disease. Similar to other NRSTS, RT may be indicated depending on the size and resectability of the disease. Outcomes in patients with small localized and regional disease is excellent (88 and 75%, respectively); however, patients showing metastases have inferior outcomes at 5 years (<20%) (Okcu et al. 2003).

3.9 Germ Cell Tumors

GCTs are a heterogeneous group of neoplasms that arise from primordial germ cells (Palmer et al. 2008). Germ cells develop during the fourth week of embryonic life, where they begin to migrate from their place of origin to the gonadal ridge. Ovarian or testicular differentiation then occurs depending on the sex of the individual. The differences in the presentation and malignant potential of GCT depend on the location and stage of development of the germ cell when the malignant transformation occurs. GCTs range from benign teratomas to aggressive malignancies. Extragonadal GCTs result from germ cells migrating aberrantly during fetal development. Figure 3.21 shows the schema for the differentiation pathway for GCTs. Intracranial GCT will be discussed in the CNS tumors chapter.

3.9.1 Epidemiology

The majority of GCTs are benign, with only 20% being malignant (Horton et al. 2007). Malignant GCT comprises 3% of all childhood neoplasms and occurs at an annual incidence of approximately 2.4 per million children (Terenziani et al. 2007; Gobel et al. 2000; Lo Curto et al. 2003). There is a bimodal peak in the ages of occurrence, with the first peak occurring in children less than 5 years and the second in adolescents aged 15–19 years. Females are affected more often with benign GCT, and males are more often affected by malignant GCT.

3.9.2 Etiology

GCTs are thought to occur from sporadic genetic mutations. There are two conditions that are known to predispose a patient to developing GCT: cryptorchidism (undescended testes) and gonadal dysgenesis. The incidence of GCT is as high as 30% in patients with gonadal dysgenesis and there is a three to ninefold increased risk in patients with cryptorchidism (Horton et al. 2007). There is also an association between mediastinal GCT and Kleinfelters syndrome (Cushing et al. 2006). Although several environmental factors such as maternal chemical/solvent exposure, cigarette smoking, pesticide exposure, and alcohol consumption have been hypothesized to correlate with an increased incidence of GCT, there have been no definitive studies to support this. One COG study did find an increased risk for GCT associated with maternal urinary tract infection during gestation (Horton et al. 2007).

Figure 3.21

Schema for differentiation pathway for the germ cell tumor (GCT)

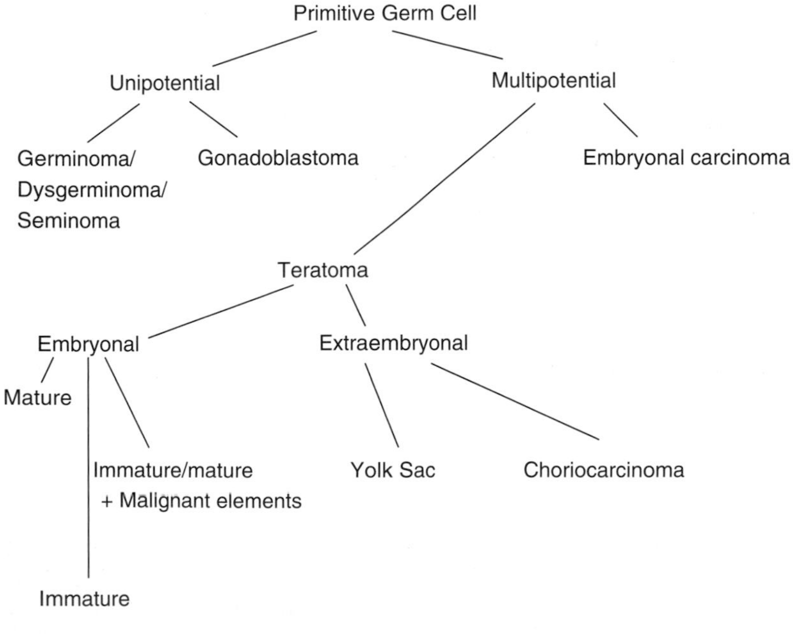

3.9.3 Molecular Genetics

Several characteristic genetic abnormalities predominate in GCT. These can be divided into four groups, each with its distinct molecular characteristics: tumors of the adolescent testes, tumors of infancy, extragonadal tumors of adolescents, and tumors of the adolescent ovary (see Table 3.15).

3.9.4 Symptoms and Clinical Signs

Clinical symptoms of the disease depend on the location of the tumor. Tumors arise either in gonadal or extragonadal midline sites. GCTs occur in the gonads (ovary and testis) in 50% of the and in extragonadal locations in the other 50% cases, with the sacrococcygeal region and brain being the most common extragonadal sites followed by the retroperitoneal, pelvic, and neck regions (Rodriguez-Galindo and Pappo 2003). GCTs metastasize via both hematogenous and lymphatic spread. The common sites of metastasis are lung and liver.

Testicular tumors usually present as a mass or swelling in the scrotum and are usually not painful. A hydrocele may also be present. Ovarian tumors usually present with symptoms such as pain, tenderness, and abdominal swelling. Occasionally ovarian torsion may be present. The duration of symptoms in ovarian yolk sac tumors are often short (2–4 weeks), indicative of a rapidly increasing mass which may cause ascites (Dallenbach et al. 2006). Mediastinal disease may cause symptoms of respiratory distress. Sacrococcygeal tumors can present with symptoms of urinary retention and constipation or as a visible gluteal mass.

3.9.5 Diagnostics

An ultrasound is usually done initially to investigate abdominal and pelvic tumors, and is helpful in differentiating solid from cystic masses (Palenzuela et al. 2008). CT of the chest, abdomen, and pelvis is recommended to assess the extent of primary disease and the presence of metastases, especially in the setting of elevated serum tumor markers (Fig. 3.22). A bone scan may be indicated if bone pain is a presenting feature; however, GCTs rarely metastasize to bone.

There are serum tumor markers for some of the GCT. Onco-feto proteins, such as alpha feto-protein (AFP) and βHCG are used for screening. Elevations in AFP are seen in endodermal sinus tumor (EST), also called yolk sac tumor, and embryonal carcinoma; and increases in βHCG are seen in choriocarcinoma. Serum onco-feto proteins should decline

Table 3.15. Common genetic alterations associated with germ cell tumors (GCTs) (Cushing et al. 2006)

GCT Tumor Group	Ploidy	Chromosomal Alterations
Tumors of the adolescent testes	Aneuploid	Isochromosome 12p [i(12p)] loss of 13 gain of 8, 21,1q
Tumors of infancy		
Teratomas	Diploid	Normal karyotype
Yolk Sac tumor	Diploid or tetraploid	Abnormalities at 1, 3, 6, and 20; loss 6q, 1p; gain 20q, 1q
Extragonadal tumors of adolescents		
Mediastinum	Diploid or tetraploid	Some have i(12p)
Tumors of the adolescent ovary		
Mature teratoma	Diploid	95% karyotypically normal (5% show gains or losses of an entire chromosome)
Immature teratoma	Aneuploid	No consistent changes
Malignant ovarian GCT		i(12p) gains of 21 and 1q

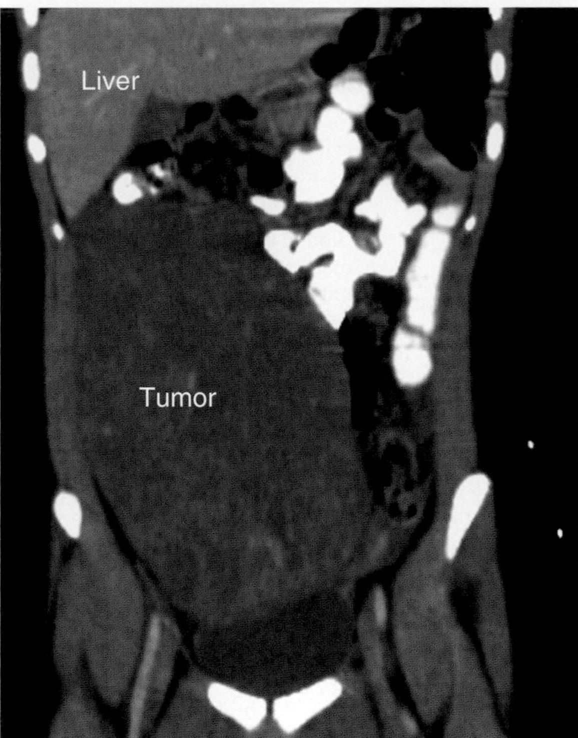

Figure 3.22

CT scan of a large right ovarian GCT. Large right abdominal/pelvic mass can be seen arising from the right ovary

within a half-life following the removal of a tumor, which, for AFP is 5–7 days, and for βHCG is 24–36 h (Lang et al. 1982; Lachman et al. 1986). Failure of the tumor marker levels to decrease may indicate persistent disease. Nonspecific markers such as LDH are often examined, and elevated levels are thought to correlate with growth of solid tumors. Placental alkaline phosphatase is the isoenzyme of alkaline phosphatase and is used as a screening test at some centers; increases are seen in seminomas and some EST. Increases in calcium-125 can also be seen in EST (Dallenbach et al. 2006).

A biopsy, or preferably a tumor resection, is necessary for both pathological diagnosis and treatment of GCT.

3.9.6 Staging and Classification

Germ cells develop from a primordial germ cell. There are many different morphological subtypes, which reflect the pathway of differentiation to which the cell was dedicated prior to malignant transformation. GCT can be either malignant or benign. Benign GCTs are called teratomas, and can be either mature or immature. Teratomas often comprise all three embryologic layers. Well-differentiated cell types such as skin, hair, and teeth are found in mature teratomas, whereas immature teratomas contain immature remnants of embryonal tissue (Horton et al. 2007). Immature teratomas sometimes recur and therefore may have some malignant potential (Lo Curto et al. 2007). Malignant GCT include: ovarian dysgerminomas, testicular seminomas, extragonadal germinomas, ESTs or yolk sac tumors, choriocarcinomas, and embryonal carcinoma (Palmer et al. 2008). It is not uncommon for tumors to contain mixed cells. Characteristics that are associated with the different histological subtypes of GCT are summarized in Table 3.16.

Separate staging systems exist for ovarian and testicular tumors. However, staging of both is similar to that for other solid tumors (Horton et al. 2007; Cushing et al. 2006):

- Stage I indicates localized disease confined to primary site, completely resected
- Stage II implies some degree of microscopic residual disease or nodal involvement (<2 cm)
- Stage III is characterized by gross residual disease or lymph-node involvement (>2 cm)
- Stage IV denotes distant metastases

3.9.7 Treatment

The primary treatment of both malignant and benign GCT is surgical resection. Mutilating surgery should be avoided because GCTs are chemosensitive, and at times, neoadjuvant chemotherapy is indicated to facilitate surgical resection. Adjuvant chemotherapy is used for patients with intermediate- and high-risk tumors. Table 3.17 highlights the risk stratification for malignant GCT. Radiation is sometimes used for residual disease post chemotherapy, as in the case of bulky mediastinal disease post chemotherapy.

Table 3.16. GCTs: Subtypes, Disease Sites, and Specific Characteristics (Cushing et al. 2002, 2006)

Malignant category	Subtype	Common sites of disease	Specific characteristics
Benign GCT	Mature teratomas	Ovary/testis Sacrococcygeal area Mediastinum	Mature elements of all three germ cell layers Neuroglial implants may occur (do not affect prognosis)
GCT of intermediate behavior	Immature teratomas	Ovary/testis	Graded based on degree of maturation/neuroepithelium present (0–2 show benign behavior) ±AFP
Malignant GCT	Germinoma	Ovary (dysgerminoma) Testes (seminoma)	Chemosensitive Radiosensitive
	Endodermal sinus tumor (yolk sac tumor)	Sacrococcygeal Testis/ovary	AFP Chemosensitive
	Embryonal carcinoma	Testis/ovary Mediastinum	AFP ± bHCG
	Choriocarcinoma	Mediastinum Ovary/testis	bHCG
	Mixed	Ovary/testis	AFP and bHCG may be present

Table 3.17. Risk stratification for GCTs (Horton et al. 2007)

	Low risk	Intermediate risk	High risk
Testicular GCT	Stage I	Stage II–IV	
Ovarian GCT	Stage I	Stage II–IV	
Extragonadal GCT		Stage I and II	Stage III and IV

3.9.7.1 Surgical Considerations

3.9.7.1.1 Ovarian Tumors

The recommended surgical intervention includes unilateral salpingo-ooporectomy including biopsies of the omentum, peritoneum, and peritoneal washings for cytology (Dallenbach et al. 2006). The contralateral ovary is always inspected and biopsied if concerning lesions exist. Lymph-node sampling is done for any enlarged, firm, or suspicious retroperitoneal lymph nodes. Omentectomy is generally not felt to be indicated unless it is grossly affected by the tumor (Horton et al. 2007). Often surgery can be done by laparotomy, but occasionally, tumors are too large and require a transabdominal approach.

3.9.7.1.2 Testicular Tumors

An inguinal approach to orchioectomy is the preferred surgical method for tumor resection. Retripperitoneal lymph node sampling is generally indicated for nodes greater than 2 cm in size (Horton et al. 2007).

3.9.7.1.3 Extragonadal Tumors

Surgical management of saccrococcygeal GCT includes total resection often including the coccyx. Mediastinal GCTs are often located in the anterior mediastinum and are not amenable to upfront surgical resection. Operative approaches, when possible include median sternotomy or lateral thoracotomy.

Retroperitoneal GCTs are often large by the time they are detected. Complete surgical resection is necessary, but neoadjuvant chemotherapy is almost always indicated to facilitate surgery (Horton et al. 2007).

3.9.7.2 Chemotherapy

Over the past two decades, the introduction of platinum-based (cisplatin or carboplatin) chemotherapeutic regimens has resulted in major improvements in survival in patients with malignant GCT, and these are now considered to be the standard of care. Other chemotherapeutic agents that are used to treat malignant GCT include actinomycin, vinblastine, bleomycin, doxorubicin, and etoposide. Chemotherapy regimens used in both North America and Europe are similar, comprising: cisplatin, etoposide, and bleomycin (PEB) or carboplatin, etoposide, bleomycin (JEB). The COG previously used four cycles of PEB, administered over 5 days, every 3 weeks for patients with Stage II, III, and IV disease, with excellent outcomes (Cushing et al. 2004). Current COG protocols are studying whether delivering PEB over 3 vs. 5 days, and reducing the number of cycles from four to three will result in optimal outcomes, while decreasing toxicity (Horton et al. 2007). This is being studied based on the results of studies done by both European and American Cooperative Groups, which showed similar outcomes with reduced dose and length of treatment (Saxman et al. 1998; de Wit et al., 2001).

Low-risk patients are generally treated with surgical resection alone with no adjuvant therapy, but these patients require close follow-up. Those with intermediate-risk disease receive surgery and adjuvant treatment with PEB or JEB for three to four cycles, depending on the treating center. High-risk patients require more intensive therapy, often with six cycles of PEB in addition to surgery. Intergroup studies (POG and CCG) in the United States studied the use of high-dose cisplatin in conjunction with standard-dose bleomycin and etoposide, compared with standard-dose cisplatin in high-risk GCTs. EFS, but not OS, was improved, but the cisplatin-associated toxicity (ototoxicity and nephrotoxicity) was severe, precluding its use (Cushing et al. 2004). High-dose therapy with stem cell rescue is also being studied for the upfront therapy in high-risk GCTs with promising results (Kumano et al. 2007).

3.9.8 Prognosis

The 5-year OS of those with mature and immature teratoma is 100% (Cushing et al. 2002). The OS for patients with testicular GCT treated with surgery and platin-based protocols is 100% for Stage I–III disease, and 90% for Stage IV disease (Horton et al. 2007). The OS for patients with Stage I ovarian GCT is 95%, Stages II–III is 94%, and Stage IV is 93% (Horton et al. 2007; Cushing et al. 2004). Patients with extragonadal disease have a somewhat poorer prognosis depending on the location of the tumor. With the use of adjuvant chemotherapy, the CCG and the POG have reported OS rates of 90% in stages of sacrococcygeal GCT, 88% in retroperitoneal GCT, and 71% in mediastinal GCT (Horton et al. 2007).

3.9.9 Follow-Up

Close surveillance, clinical as well as regular tumor marker (AFP, βHCG) assessment, should occur following the surgical resection of teratomas for up to 5 years because disease recurrence is possible. Malignant GCTs should have regular follow-up with either CT or ultrasound imaging of abdominal and pelvic primary sites indicated every 3 months for the first year, followed by a decreasing frequency of scans over the next several years. Chest X-rays are recommended at regular intervals for metastatic surveillance. Tumor marker bloodwork is also indicated, if positive at diagnosis.

Follow-up must also consider late effects of treatment. Cisplatin therapy is associated with a risk of significant hearing loss, and follow-up audiograms are imperative. Nephrotoxicity can also be a problem during and following cisplatin therapy, and renal function studies should be monitored after the completion of therapy. Hypomagnesemia and hypocalcemia are among the more common renal sequelae. Pulmonary fibrosis may result from bleomycin therapy, and pulmonary function studies should be done regularly during follow-up. Survivors should avoid exposure to high-oxygen concentrations or pressure, and must avoid cigarette smoking. Secondary malignancies including myeloid leukemias have been noted after treatment with chemotherapy, especially etoposide.

3.9.10 Future Perspectives

The excellent survival outcomes in malignant GCT with existing agents have prompted the re-evaluation of the amount of therapy that these patients receive, because toxicity from chemotherapy remains a real problem. The formal development of agreed-upon risk groups is needed to stratify the treatment further. The role of carboplatin, ifosfamide, and topotecan may also be used to determine their utility in relapsed GCT. Effective treatment for high-risk patients remains controversial, and the role of high-dose chemotherapy with stem cell rescue is being examined.

3.10 Rare Tumors

There are numerous tumors that occur very infrequently in children and adolescents. Most of these rarely occurring neoplasms are seen more often in the adult population. Several of the more commonly occurring rare tumors will be summarized here.

3.10.1 Adrenocortical Carcinoma

Adrenocortical carcinoma (ACC) is a very rare and aggressive tumor. It occurs more often in females and peaks in the first and fourth decades of life. The incidence of this tumor is very high in Brazil, 10–15 times of that observed in the United States, where only approximately 14 new patients are diagnosed annually according to the Surveillance Epidemiology End Results (SEER) database (Michalkiewicz et al. 2004; Zancanella et al. 2006). ACC is associated with syndromes such as Li-Fraumeni and BWS (van Ditzhuijsen et al. 2007). De novo or inherited germline mutations of the p53 tumor suppressor gene are found in over 70% of children with ACC, though these are much less common in adults (Birch et al. 2001). Interestingly, a unique germline p53 mutation occurs in almost all children with ACC in the Curitiba province of Brazil, where the incidence is exceedingly high. This mutation has been reported only once outside Brazil (DiGiammarino et al. 2002).

Cushing syndrome, characterized by upper body obesity, rounded face, excessive hair growth, and an increase of fat around the neck ("buffalo hump"), reflects an excess of hormonal activity and is a presenting sign of ACC in 60% of patients (van Ditzhuijsen et al. 2007). Evidence of the development of secondary sex characteristics, or virilization, occurs as a presenting sign in 95% of the patients younger than 5 years (Koch et al. 2002). It is not uncommon for patients to present with both virilization and Cushing's features. Clinical signs in patients whose tumors are not hormonally active include those of the mass itself: abdominal pain, fullness, and gastrointestinal symptoms such as nausea. Some patients present with fever, anorexia, and weight loss.

Elevations in dehydroepiandrosterone sulfate (DHEAS) and testosterone in women and 17-β-oestradiol in men are indications of ACC (van Ditzhuijsen et al. 2007). In 40% of children whose tumors do not secrete active hormones, their inactive steroid precursors such as pregnenolone, 11-deoxycortisone, and 17-hydroxypregnenolone can still be found in blood and urine (Koch et al. 2002). ACC can present as a localized disease, but may spread regionally to the adjacent lymph nodes or the retroperitoneum in 20% of cases. Distant metastases to lung and bone can also occur.

Diagnostic work up should include CT scan or MRI of the abdomen. Calcifications can be seen in some ACCs. Chest imaging with CT or X-ray is necessary to identify pulmonary metastases. FDG-PET imaging is being increasingly used to detect regional spread as well as distant metastases. Staging is based on tumor size and degree of spread. Generally, Stage I are completely resected tumors (volume < 200 cm^3), and hormone levels can be normalized after surgery; Stage II are those with a tumor volume greater than or equal to200 cm^3; Stage III are those with residual disease or inoperable tumors; and Stage IV have distant metastases (Sandrini et al. 1997; Michalkiewicz et al. 2004). Biopsy or preferably resection is needed to determine the pathology.

Curative treatment depends on early wide total excision of the tumor while it is still encapsulated. Repeated surgeries are warranted if isolated recurrences occur. For patients without surgically curable disease, mitotane therapy is often initiated, which is meant to cause tumor necrosis and disease regression. It also has the ability to inhibit steroid synthesis, which reduces unpleasant endocrine manifestations in the majority of patients (Zancanella et al. 2006). Chemotherapy agents such as fluorouracil, etoposide, doxorubicin, and cisplatin are also sometimes used with or without mitotane. These approaches, although they may increase the length of survival, are not usually curative. The prognosis for patients with ACC is poor with OS rates correlating with the stage of the disease: Stage I >90%; Stage II 58%; Stage III 24%; and Stage IV <10% (Vassilopoulou-Sellin and Schultz 2001).

3.10.2 Melanoma

Melanoma accounts for 1–3% of childhood neoplasms; it represents the second most common carcinoma found in children (Chao et al. 2005). Conditions that are associated with melanoma in children include congenital melanomas, giant congenital melanocytic nevi, xeroderma pigmentosum, immunosuppression, neurocutaneous melanosis, and mole phenotype (atypical moles) (Pratt and Pappo 2002). Melanoma can develop into a congenitally acquired nevi, or arise as a new lesion. Risk factors for developing melanoma include female sex, white race, and increased environmental ultraviolet radiation exposure, as reported by the SEER database (Strouse et al. 2005).

Presenting signs may include a mole that has changed in size or color, accompanied by bleeding, ulceration, or itching, with a palpable subcutaneous mass or lymphadenopathy (Pappo 2003). Common sites are the trunk, head, and neck (Fig. 3.23). Metastases generally occur via regional lymph node spread prior to lung, bone, and brain. Disease is typically categorized as being localized, having nodal spread, or distant metastases. The American Joint Committee on Cancer (AJCC) staging system of melanoma takes into account tumor thickness, ulceration, nodal disease, and metastases (Balch et al. 2001). Children with thick melanoma of more than 4 mm and those with lymphadenopathy should undergo imaging with CT of the chest and abdomen to evaluate for metastatic disease. MRI of the brain is only indicated for symptomatic patients. More recently, positron emission tomography (PET) scanning has shown to be useful in identifying melanoma metastases.

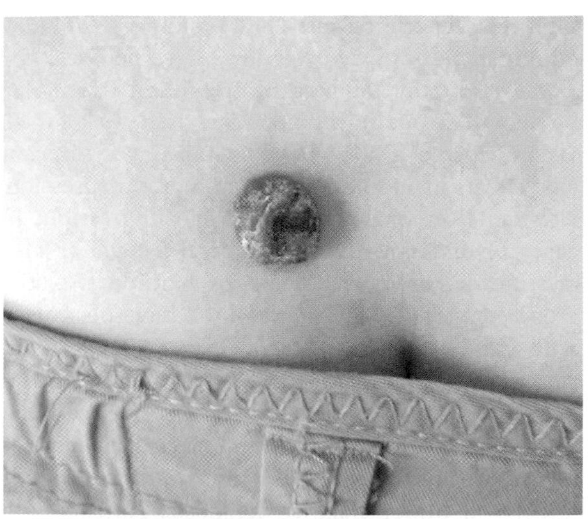

Figure 3.23
Melanoma of the lower back in a 9-year-old girl

Wide excision, with adequate margins of the lesion is necessary for cure. For lesions less than 1 mm in thickness, a resection with a 1-cm margin is adequate. Lesions that are greater than 1 mm in thickness require a 2-cm margin (Downard et al. 2007). Intraoperative lymphatic mapping with sentinel node biopsy has been shown to be highly sensitive at identifying nodal disease and is usually done for lesions greater than 1 mm in thickness. Lymph-node resection is routinely done if microscopic disease is present in the sentinal node.

Alpha-interferon therapy has been used routinely in adult patients with "high risk" resected melanoma with evidence of improving RFS and OS (Pappo 2003). It works via immunomodulatory mechanisms. A similar approach has been used in pediatric patients whereby patients are treated with high-dose interferon alfa-2b, 20 million IU/m2/day administered intravenously for 5 days per week for 4 weeks initially, followed by 10 million IU/m2/day by subcutaneous injection 3 days per week for 48 weeks (Chao et al. 2005). This therapy has significant side effects including flu-like symptoms, depression, elevated liver enzymes, and myelosuppression. In cases of disseminated disease, agents such as vincristine, dactinomycin, cyclophosphamide, cisplatin, etoposide, DTIC, and interleukin-2 have been used with varying rates of success (Pappo 2003). Radiation does not play a role in the treatment of melanoma with the exception of patients with head and neck disease who are at risk of cervical metastases or in those with brain metastases. Prognosis depends largely on tumor stage at diagnosis. Patients with localized Stage I disease have survival rates of 95%, whereas those with thick melanomas (>4 mm) have survival rates ranging from 25 to 70% depending on the treatment (Balch et al. 2001).

3.10.3 Nasopharyngeal Carcinoma

Nasopharyngeal carcinoma (NPC), or lymphoepithelioma, accounts for only 1% of pediatric malignancies (Mertens et al. 2005). This tumor occurs in the epithelium of the nasopharynx, generally affecting males more often than females. There is a strong association of EBV infection with the development of NPC, especially in pediatric patients (Zheng et al. 2007). Increased amounts of EBV latent membrane protein correlate with tumor progression and distant metastatic disease (Lee et al. 2007). This tumor has three distinct subtypes and children are usually affected by the undifferentiated type. It arises in the fossa of Rosenmuller and can spread via direct extension through the oropharynx to the base of the skull and result in cranial nerve palsies (Pratt and Pappo 2002). The only clinical sign of this disease may be cervical lymphadenopathy, indicating regional metastases. Many patients present with advanced locoregional disease, and the most common sites of distant metastases are the lung and bone.

The tumor is staged as per the TNM classification system. CT and MRI of the head and neck are necessary to assess the extent of disease. CTs of the chest and bone scan are indicated to look for distant metastases. Surgery is often not possible for NPC because of its anatomical location. RT is the primary treatment modality and doses in excess of 60 Gy appear to be necessary for disease control (Haimi et al. 2005). Adjuvant chemotherapy is often used in children, and the tumor shows response to agents such as fluorouracil, cisplatin, vincristine, doxorubicin, carboplatin, methotrexate, and bleomycin. Treatment regimens vary significantly depending on the treatment center and location. Multiple researchers have noted survival rates to be 75% for T1 and T2 tumors, but only 37% for T3 and T4 tumors (Pratt and Pappo 2002). The late effects of radiation such as xerostomia, muscle atrophy, fibrosis of the neck, and hypothyroidism can be significant in this population.

3.10.4 Pleuropulmonary Blastoma

Pleuropulmonary blastoma (PPB) is a rare tumor that arises in the lung or pleura. It generally occurs in young children, with the median age at diagnosis being 34 months (Pappo and Furman 2006). PPBs have a tendency to occur in families where there is a strong cancer history. There are three types of PPB: type I is entirely cystic; type II has both solid and cystic components; type III is purely solid. PPB can evolve from a cystic mass to a solid tumor and therefore, from type I to III. The presentation of PPB is variable and can range from cough, a chest infection, and pain to pneumothorax and respiratory distress. CT imaging of the thorax is needed to diagnose PPB. PPB can often be confused with benign congenital cysts. Type I PPB confers a more favorable prognosis, whereas type II and III are characterized by more aggressive disease and metastases. This tumor can spread to brain and bone and therefore, a bone scan and MRI or CT of the brain are indicated in the work up of type II and III disease.

PPB requires adjuvant treatment with chemotherapy and surgical resection. Chemotherapy agents that have been useful in the treatment of PPB are vincristine, dactinomycin, cyclophosphamide, doxorubicin, ifosfamide, and cisplatin (Fosdal 2008). Radiation is sometimes used in unresectable type II an III disease. The International Pleuropulmonary

Blastoma Registry (http://www.ppbregistry.org) is a great resource for patients and health professionals regarding the management of PPB. While patients with type I disease tend to have survival rates approaching 90% when treated with chemotherapy and radiation, the prognosis is poor for patients with type II and III disease with OS rates of only about 50% (International PPB registry 2008).

3.10.5 Thyroid Carcinoma

Thyroid carcinoma represents approximately 1% of malignant tumors in patients less than 15 years (Koch et al. 2006). It generally occurs more often in females, with a peak in incidence between the ages of 7 and 12 years. It is well established that neck irradiation is a causative factor in the development of thyroid carcinoma. It may occur as a secondary malignancy following the treatment of other pediatric malignancies such as Hodgkin's disease and CNS tumors (Gow et al. 2003). Thyroid carcinomas can also occur sporadically and they are sometimes associated with other conditions such as Hashimotos thyroiditis or familial cancer syndromes such as multiple endocrine neoplasia (MEN) IIA and IIB. Cervical adenopathy, thyroid nodules, and goiter are often the presenting clinical signs. In contrast to adults, children tend to present with more advanced disease. Locoregional spread occurs in the lower cervical and upper mediastinal nodes in approximately half of the pediatric patients with 20% having pulmonary metastases (Koch et al. 2006). Despite this, the prognosis is good.

There are several different subtypes of thyroid carcinoma: papillary, follicular, medullary, and anaplastic. Seventy percent of the patients present with the papillary subtype that does not tend to produce an excess of hormones (Koch et al. 2006). Follicular tumors can either have increases in T_3 and sometimes T_4. Increases in calcitonin can be seen in the medullary subtype. Imaging of the primary is generally done with ultrasound and thyroid scintiscan, and chest X-ray or a CT of the chest is performed to rule out lung metastases. A biopsy is needed to confirm malignancy and histology. Complete surgical resection (thyroidectomy) and lymph-node dissection, if nodes are noted pre or intraoperatively, is the treatment of choice for thyroid carcinoma. Radioiodine (131I) therapy is used postoperatively to ablate any residual functioning thyroid and/or metastatic disease. Thyroid hormone needs to be supplemented in these patients.

Recurrence rates in children with thyroid carcinoma are quite high, but the salvage rate with mutimodality therapy remains good (Grisby et al. 2002). Hence, patients need to be followed closely and require ongoing long-term follow-up with physical examination, chest X-ray, and annual measurements of thyroglobulin. The OS in thyroid carcinoma approaches 90%, and metastatic disease does not confer a worse prognosis with the use of radioiodine therapy (Koch et al. 2006).

These tumors that have been briefly described are relatively rare in pediatrics. With the exception of PPB, they have histopathologic similarities to adult tumors. Unlike most pediatric tumors, therapy is highly dependent on successful resection, compared with the pediatric tumors where chemotherapy plays a vital role, regardless of the extent of the resection in most instances.

References

Abramson DH (2005) Retinoblastoma in the 20th century: past success and future challenges the Weisenfeld lecture. Investigative Opthalmology & Visual Science 46(8):2684–2691

Abramson DH, Schefler AC (2004) Update on retinoblastoma. Retina 24(6):828–848

Anderson P, Nuñez R (2007) Samarium lexidronam (153Sm-EDTMP): skeletal radiation for osteoblastic bone metastases and osteosarcoma. Expert Review of Anticancer Therapy 7(11):1517–1527

Andrassy RJ (2002) Advances in the surgical management of sarcomas in children. American Journal of Surgery 184(6):484–491

Auber F, Jeanpierre C, Denamur E et al (2009) Management of Wilms tumors in Drash and Frasier syndromes. Pediatric Blood & Cancer 52(1):55–59

Bacci G, Ferrari S, Longhi A, Forni C, Zavatta M, Versare M, Smith K (2002) High-grade osteosarcoma of the extremity: differences between localized and metastatic tumors at presentation. Journal of Pediatric Hematology/Oncology 24(1):27–30

Bacci G, Longhi A, Verari M, Mercuri M, Briccoli A, Picci P (2006) Prognostic factors for osteosarcoma of the extremity treated with neoadjuvant chemotherapy: 15-year experience in 789 patients treated at a single institution. Cancer 106(5):1154–1161

Balch CM, Buzaid AC, Soong SJ et al (2001) Final version of the American joint committee on cancer staging system for cutaneous melanoma. Journal of Clinical Oncology 16(16):3635–3648

Ballo MT, Zagars GK, Pollack A et al (1999) Desmoid tumor: prognostic factors and outcome after surgery, radiation therapy, or combined surgery and radiation therapy. Journal of Clinical Oncology 17:158–167

Balmer A, Zografos L, Munier F (2006) Diagnosis and current management of retinoblastoma. Oncogene 25(38):5341–5349

Bataller L, Rosenfeld MR, Graus F, Vilchez JJ, Nai-Kong V, Cheung NV, Dalmau J (2003) Autoantigen diversity in the opsoclonus-myoclonus syndrome. Annals of Neurology 53:347–353

Beckwith JB (1993) Precursor lesions of Wilms' tumor: clinical and biological implications. Medical and Pediatric Oncology 21:158–168

Beckwith JB (1998) Nephrogenic rests and the pathogenesis of Wilms' tumor: developmental and clinical considerations. American Journal of Medical Genetics 79:268–273

Berman SD, Calo E, Landman AS, Danielian PS, Miller ES, West JC, Fonhoue BD, Caron A, Bronson R, Bouxsein ML, Mukherjee S, Lees JA (2008) Metastatic osteosarcoma induced by inactivation of Rb and p53 in the osteoblast lineage. Proceedings of the National Academy of Sciences of the United States of America 105(33):11851–11856

Bielack SS, Kempf-Bielack B, Delling G et al (2002) Prognostic factors in high-grade osteosarcoma of the extremities or trunk: an analysis of 1,702 patients treated on neoadjuvant cooperative osteosarcoma study group protocols. Journal of Clinical Oncology 20:776–790

Bielack S, Carrie D, Jost L (2008) Osteosarcoma: ESMO clinical recommendations for diagnosis, treatment and follow-up. Annals of Oncology 19(Suppl 2):ii94–ii96

Birch JM, Alston RD, McNally RJ et al (2001) Relative frequency and morphology of cancers in carriers of germline TP53 mutations. Oncogene 20(34):4621–2628

Bisogno G, de Rossi C, Gamboa Y et al (2008) Improved survival for children with parameningeal rhabdomyosarcoma: results from the AIEOP soft tissue sarcoma committee. Pediatric Blood & Cancer 50:1154–1158

Blouin P, Brugieres L, Tabone MD et al (2004) Carboplatin-epirubicin regimen for the treatment of hepatoblastoma. Pediatric Blood & Cancer 42:149–154

Breslow NE, Ou SS, Beckwith JB, Haase GM, Kalapurakal JA, Ritchey ML, Shamberger RC, Thomas PR, D'Angio GJ, Green DM (2004) Doxorubicin for favorable histology, stage II–III Wilms tumor: results from the National Wilms Tumor Studies. Cancer 101(5):1072–1080

Brichard B, Chantrain C, Gala JL, Sibille C, Vermylen C, De Potter P (2008) Retinoblastoma and deletion of the long arm of chromosome 13: an underestimated diagnosis? Pediatric Blood & Cancer 50(3):694–696

Brodeur GM (2003) Neuroblastoma: biological Insights into a clinical enigma. Nature reviews. Cancer 3:203–216

Brodeur GM, Maris JM (2002) Neuroblastoma. In: Pizzo PA, Poplack DG (eds) Principles and practice of pediatric oncology, 4th edn. Lippincott Williams & Wilkins, Philadelphia

Broecker B (2000) Non-Wilms' renal tumors in children. Urologic Clinics of North America 27(3):463–469

Buckley JD, Sather H, Tuccione K et al (1989) A case-control study of risk factors for hepatoblastoma. A report from the Children's Cancer Study Group. Cancer 61:1169–1176

Caudill JSC, Arndt CAS (2007) Diagnosis and management of bone malignancy in adolescence. Adolescent Medicine 18:62–78

Cella D, Li JZ, Cappellerie C et al (2008) Quality of life in patients with metastatic renal cell carcinoma treated with sunitinib or interferon alfa: results from a phase III randomized trial. Journal of Clinical Oncology 26(22):3763–3769

Chan HSL, Gallie BL, Munier FL, Popovic MB (2005) Chemotherapy for retinoblastoma. Opthalmology Clinics of North America 18(1):55–63

Chao MM, Schwartz JL, Wechsler DS et al (2005) High-risk surgically resected pediatric melanoma and adjuvant interferon therapy. Pediatric Blood & Cancer 44:441–448

Chen Y, Takita J, Choi YL, Kato M, Ohira M, Sanada M, Wang L, Soda M, Kikuchi A, Igarashi T, Nakagawara A, Hayashi Y, Mano H, Ogawa S (2008) Oncogenic mutations of ALK kinase in neuroblastoma. Nature 455(7215):971–974

Chin AR, Lam JS, Figlin RA, Belldegrun AS (2006) Surveillance strategies for renal cell carcinoma patients following nephrectomy. Reviews in Urology 8(1):1–7

Chintagumpala M, Chevez-Barrios P, Paysse EA, Plon SE, Hurwitz R (2007) Retinoblastoma: review of current management. The Oncologist 12(10):1237–1246

Clark SK, Neale KF, Landgrebe JC et al (2008) Desmoid tumours complicating familial adenomatous polyposis. British Journal of Surgery 86:1185–1189

Coffin CM, Dehner LP, O'Shea PA (1997) Pediatric soft tissue tumors a clinical pathological and therapeutic approach. Williams & Wilkins, Baltimore

Cohn SL, Pearson AD, London WB, Monclair T, Ambros PF, Brodeur GM, Faldum A, Hero B, Iehara T, Machin D, Mosseri V, Simon T, Garaventa A, Castel V, Matthay KK, INRG Task Force (2009) The International Neuroblastoma Risk Group (INRG) classification system: an INRG task force report. Journal of Clinical Oncology 27(2):289–297

Corapcioglu F, Turker G, Aydogan A et al (2004) Serum alpha fetoprotein levels in healthy full-term neonates and infants. Marmara Medical Journal 17(1):1–7

Cotterill SJ, Wright CM, Pearce MS, Craft AW (2004) UKCCSG/MRC Bone Tumor Working Group: stature of young people with malignant bone tumors. Pediatric Blood & Cancer 42:59–63

Cozzi F, Schiavetti A, Morini F, Cozzi DA (2004) Re: partial nephrectomy for unilateral Wilms' tumor: results of the study SIOP 93-01/GPOH. Journal of Urology 171(6 Pt 1):2383

Crist WM, Anderson JR, Meza JL et al (2001) Intergroup rhabdomyosarcoma study-IV: results for patients with nonmetastatic disease. Journal of Clinical Oncology 19(12):3091–3102

Cushing B, Perlman EJ, Marina NM, Castleberry RP (2002) Germ cell tumors. In: Pizzo PA, Poplack DG (eds) Principles and practice of pediatric oncology, 4th edn. Lippincott Williams & Wilkins, Philadelphia

Cushing B, Giller R, Cullen JW et al (2004) Randomized comparison of combination chemotherapy with etoposide, bleomycin, and either high-dose or standard-dose cisplatin in children and adolescents with high-risk malignant germ cell tumors: a pediatric intergroup study – Pediatric Oncology Group 9049 and Children's Cancer Group 8882. Journal of Clinical Oncology 22(13):2691–2700

Cushing B, Perlman EJ, Marina NM, Castleberry RP (2006) Germ Cell Tumors. In: Pizzo PA, Poplack DG (eds) Principles and practice of pediatric oncology, 5th edn. Lippincott Williams & Wilkins, Philadelphia

D'Angio GJ (2008) Pre-or postoperative therapy for Wilms' tumor? Journal of Clinical Oncology 26(25):4055–4057

Dal Cin P, Stas M, Sciot R et al (1998) Translocation (X;1) reveals metastasis 31 years after renal cell carcinoma. Cancer Genetics and Cytogenetics 101:58–61

Dallenbach P, Bonnefoi H, Pelte MF, Vlastos G (2006) Yolk sac tumours of the ovary: an update. European Journal of Surgical Oncology 32:1063–1075

Dallorso S, Dini G, Faraci M, Spreafico F (2008) SCT for Wilms' tumor. Bone Marrow Transplantation 41:S128–S130

Dass CR, Choong PFM (2008) Gene therapy for osteosarcoma: steps towards clinical studies. Journal of Pharmacy and Pharmacology 60:405–413

de Bernardi B, Mosseri V, Rubie H et al (2008) Treatment of localized resectable neuroblastoma. Results of the LNESGI study by the SIOP Europe neuroblastoma group. British Journal of Cancer 99:1027–1033

de Ioris M, Brugieres L, Zimmermann A et al (2007) Hepatoblastoma with a low serum alpha-fetoprotein level at diagnosis: the SIOPEL group experience. European Journal of Cancer 44(4):545–550

de Wit R, Roberts JT, Wilkinson PM, de Mulder PHM, Mead GM, Fosså SD, Cook P, de Prijck L, Stenning S, Collette L (2001) Equivalence of three or four cycles of bleomycin, etoposide and bleomycin chemotherapy and of a 3- or 5-day schedule in good prognosis germ cell cancer: a randomized study of the European organization for research and treatment of cancer genitourinary tract cancer cooperative group and the medical research council. Journal of Clinical Oncology 19(6):1629–1640

DiGiammarino EL, Lee AS, Cadwell C, Zhang W, Bothner B, Ribeiro RC, Zambetti G, Kriwacki RW (2002) A novel mechanism of tumorigenesis involving pH-dependent destabilization of a mutant p53 tetramer. Nature Structural Biology 9(1):12–16

Dome JS, Cotton CA, Perlman EJ et al (2006a) Treatment of anaplastic histology Wilms; Tumor: results from the fifth National Wilms' tumor study. Journal of Clinical Oncology 24(15):2352–2358

Dome JS, Perlman EJ, Ritchey ML et al (2006b) Renal Tumors. In: Pizzo PA, Poplack DG (eds) Principles and practice of pediatric oncology, 5th edn. Lippincott Williams & Wilkins, Philadelphia

Donaldson SS (2004) Ewing sarcoma: radiation dose and target. Pediatric Blood & Cancer 42:471–476

Downard CD, Rapkin LB, Gow KW (2007) Melanoma in children and adolescents. Surgical Oncology 16:215–220

Escudier B, Cosaert J, Pisa P (2008) Bevacizumab: direct anti-VEGF therapy in renal cell carcinoma. Expert Review of Anticancer Therapy 8(10):1545–1557

Esiashvili N, Goodman M, Marcus RB (2008) Changes in incidence and survival of Ewing sarcoma patients over the past 3 decades. Surveillance epidemiology and end results data. Journal of Pediatric Hematology and Oncology 30(6):425–430

Evans AE, Kesselbach KD, Yamashiro DJ et al (1999) Antitumor activity of CEP-751 (KT-6587) on human neuroblastoma and medulloblastoma xenografts. Clinical Cancer Research 5:3594–3602

Ferrari S, Palmerini E (2007) Adjuvant and neoadjuvant combination chemotherapy for osteogenic sarcoma. Current Opinion in Oncology 19:341–346

Ferrari S, Briccoli A, Mercuri M, Bertoni F, Picci P, Tienghi A, Brach Del Prever A, Fagioli F, Comandone A, Bacci G (2003) Postrelapse survival in osteosarcoma of the extremities: prognostic factors for long-term survival. Journal of Clinical Oncology 21(4):710–715

Feugeas O, Buriec N, Babin-Boilletot A et al (1996) Loss of heterozygosity of RB gene is a poor prognostic factor in the patients with osteosarcoma. Journal of Clinical Oncology 13:467–472

Folpe AL, Deyrup AT (2006) Alveolar soft-part sarcoma: a review and update. Journal of Clinical Pathology 59:1127–1132

Fosdal MB (2008) Pleuropulmonary blastoma. Journal of Pediatric Oncology Nursing 25(5):295–302

Fuchs B, Sim FH (2004) Rotationplasty about the knee: surgical technique and anatomical considerations. Clinical Anatomy 17:245–353

Fuchs B, Mahlum E, Halder C, Maran A, Yaszemski M, Bode B, Bolander M, Sarkar G (2007) High expression of tumor endothelial marker 7 is associated with metastasis and poor survival of patients with osteogenic sarcoma. Gene 399(2):137–143

Fulda S (2008) Targeting apoptosis resistance in rhabdomyosarcoma. Current Cancer Drug Targets 8(6):536–544

Gallie BL, Zhao J, Vandezande K, White A, Chan HSL (2007) Global issues and opportunities for optimized retinoblastoma care. Pediatric Blood & Cancer 49:1083–1090

Gardner SL, Carreras J, Boudreau C, Camitta BM, Adams RH, Chen AR, Davies SM, Edwards JR, Grovas AC, Hale GA, Lazarus HM, Arora M, Stiff PJ, Eapen M (2008) Myeloablative therapy with autologous stem cell rescue for patients with Ewing sarcoma. Bone Marrow Transplantation 41(10):867–872

George RE, London WB, Cohn SL, Maris JM, Kretschmar C, Diller L, Brodeur GM, Castleberry RP, Look AT (2005) Hyperdiploidy plus nonamplified MYCN confers a favorable prognosis in children 12 to 18 months old with disseminated neuroblastoma: a Pediatric Oncology Group study. Journal of Clinical Oncology 23(27):6466–6473

George RE, Le S, Medeiros-Nancarrrow C et al (2006) High risk neuroblastoma treated with tandem autologous peripheral-blood stem cell-supported transplantation: long-term survival update. Journal of Clinical Oncology 24(18):2891–2896

Gobel U, Schneider DT, Calaminus G et al (2000) Germ cell tumors in childhood and adolescence. Annals of Oncology 11:263–271

Gombos DS, Chevez-Barrios P (2007) Current treatment and management of retinoblastoma. Current Oncology Reports 9(6):453–458

Gow KW, Lensing S, Hill DA et al (2003) Thyroid carcinoma presenting in childhood or after treatment of childhood malignancies: an institutional experience and review of the literature. Journal of Pediatric Surgery 38(11):1574–1580

Graf N, Tournade MF, de Kraker J (2000) The role of preoperative chemotherapy in the management of Wilms' tumor. The SIOP studies. International Society of Pediatric Oncology. Urologic Clinics of North America 27:443–454

Gratias EJ, Dome JS (2008) Current and emerging chemotherapy treatment strategies for Wilms tumor in North America. Paediatric Drugs 10(2):115–124

Green DM, Grigoriev YA, Nan B, Takashima JR, Norkool PA, D'Angio GJ, Breslow NE (2001) Congestive heart failure after treatment for Wilms' tumor: a report from the National Wilms' Tumor Study group. Journal of Clinical Oncology 19(7):1926–1934

Grier HE, Krailo MD, Tarbell NJ et al (2003) Addition of ifosfamide and etoposide to standard chemotherapy for Ewing's sarcoma and primitive neuroectodermal tumor of bone. The New England Journal of Medicine 348(8):694–701

Grisby PW, Gal-or A, Michalski JM, Doherty GM (2002) Childhood and adolescent thyroid carcinoma. Cancer 95(4): 724–729

Grundy PE, Green DM, Breslow NE, Ritchey ML, Thomas PRM (2000) Renal tumors of childhood. In: Bast RC, Kufe DW, Pollock RE, Weichselbaum RR, Holland JF, Frei E (eds) Cancer medicine, 5th edn. B.C. Decker, Hamilton

Grundy PE, Green DM, Breslow NE, Ritchey ML, Perlman EJ, Macklis RM (2002) Renal tumors. In: Pizzo PA, Poplack DG (eds) Principles and practice of pediatric oncology, 4th edn. Lippincott Williams & Wilkins, Philadelphia

Grundy PE, Breslow NE, Li S et al (2005) Loss of heterozygosity for chromosomes 1p and 16q is an adverse prognostic factor in favorable-histology Wilms' tumor: a report from the National Wilms' Tumor Study Group. Journal of Clinical Oncology 23(29):7312–7321

Grupp SA, Stern JW, Bunin N et al (2000) Tandem high dose therapy in rapid sequence for children with high-risk neuroblastoma. Journal of Clinical Oncology 18(13):2567–2575

Haimi M, Arush MWB, Bar-Sela G et al (2005) Nasopharyngeal carcinoma in the pediatric age group. The northern Israel (Rambam) medical center experience, 1989–2004. Journal of Pediatric Hematology and Oncology 27(10)):510–516

Hawkins DS, Feigenhauer J, Park J et al (2002) Peripheral blood stem cell support reduces the toxicity of intensive chemotherapy for children and adolescents with metastatic sarcomas. Cancer 95(6):1354–1365

Hopyan S, Tan JW, Graham HK, Torode IP (2006) Function and upright time following limb salvage, amputation, and rotationplasty for pediatric sarcoma of bone. Journal of Pediatric Orthopedics 26(3):406–408

Horton Z, Schlatter M, Schultz S (2007) Pediatric germ cell tumors. Surgical Oncology 16:205–213

Howard JP, Maris JM, Kersun LS et al (2005) Tumor response and toxicity with multiple infusions of high dose ^{131}I-MIBG for refractory neuroblastoma. Pediatric Blood & Cancer 44:232–239

Hutson TE, Figlin RA (2008) Experimental therapy for advanced renal cell carcinoma. Expert Opinion on Investigational Drugs 17(11):1693–1702

International Pleuropulmonary Blastoma Registry. http://www.ppbregistry.org Retrieved 29 Dec 2008

Ishola TA, Chung DH (2007) Neuroblastoma. Surgical Oncology 16:149–156

Kager L, Zoubek A, Potschger U, Kastner U, Flege S, Kempf-Bielack B, Branscheid D, Kotz R, Salzer-Kuntschik M, Winkelmann W, Jundt G, Kabisch H, Teichardt P, Jurgens H, Gadner H, Bielack SS (2003) Primary metastatic osteosarcoma: presentation and outcome of patients treated on neoadjuvant cooperative osteosarcoma study group protocols. Journal of Clinical Oncology 21(10):2011–2018

Katzenstein HM, Krailo MD, Malogolowkin MH, Ortega JA, Liu-Mares W, Douglass EC, Feusner JH, Reynolds M, Quinn JJ, Newman K, Finegold MJ, Haas JE, Sensel MG, Castleberry RP, Bowman LC (2002a) Hepatocellular carcinoma in children and adolescents: results from the pediatric oncology group and the children's cancer group intergroup study. Journal of Clinical Oncology 20(12):2789–2797

Katzenstein HM, London WB, Douglass EC, Reynolds M, Plaschkes J, Finegold MJ, Bowman LC (2002b) Treatment of unresectable and metastatic hepatoblastoma: a pediatric oncology group phase II study. Journal of Clinical Oncology 20(16):3438–3444

Kim JW, Abramson DH, Dunkel IJ (2007a) Current management strategies for intraocular retinoblastoma. Drugs 67(15):2173–2185

Kim MS, Song WS, Cho WH et al (2007b) Ezrin expression predicts survival in stage IIB osteosarcomas. Clinical Orthopaedics and Related Research 459:229–236

Kleinerman RA, Tucker MA, Tarone RE et al (2005) Risk of new cancers after radiotherapy in long term survivors of retinoblastoma: an extended follow-up. Journal of Clinical Oncology 23(10):2272–2279

Kletzel M, Kazenstein HM, Haut PR et al (2002) Treatment of high-risk neuroblastoma with triple-tandem high-dose therapy and stem cell rescue: results of the Chicago Pilot II study. Journal of Clinical Oncology 20(9):2284–2292

Knezevich SR, McFadden DE, Lim JF et al (1998) A novel ETV6-NTRK3 gene fusion in congenital fibrosarcoma. Nature Genetics 18:184–187

Knudson AGJ (1971) Mutation and cancer: statistical study of retinoblastoma. Proceedings of the National Academy of Sciences of the United States of America 68(4):820–823

Knudson AG (2001) Two genetic hits (more or less) to cancer. Nature Reviews. Cancer 1(2):157–162

Koch CA, Pacak K, Chrousos GP (2002) Endocrine tumors. In: Pizzo PA, Poplack DG (eds) Principles and practice of pediatric oncology, 4th edn. Lippincott Williams & Wilkins, Philadelphia

Koch CA, Pacak K, Chrousos GP (2006) Endocrine tumors. In: Pizzo PA, Poplack DG (eds) Principles and practice of pediatric oncology, 5th edn. Lippincott Williams & Wilkins, Philadelphia

Koshy M, Ac P, Mai WY, Teh BS (2005) Radiation-induced osteosarcomas in the pediatric population. International Journal of Radiation Oncology, Biology, Physics 63(4):1169–1174

Kumano M, Miyake H, Hara I et al (2007) First-line high-dose chemotherapy combined with peripheral blood stem cell transplantation for patients with advanced extragonadal germ cell tumors. International Journal of Urology 14(4):336–338

Kushner BH, Meyers PA (2001) How effective is dose-intensive/myeloablative therapy against Ewing's sarcoma/primitive neuroectodermal tumor metastatic to bone or bone marrow? The Memorial Sloan-Kettering experience and a literature review. Journal of Clinical Oncology 19(3):870–880

Kushner BH, LaQuaglia MP, Wollner N et al (1996) Desmoplastic small round-cell tumor: prolonged progression-free survival with aggressive multimodality therapy. Journal of Clinical Oncology 14:1526–1531

Kushner BH, LaQuaglia MP, Kramer K, Cheung NV (2004) Radically different treatment recommendations for newly diagnosed neuroblastoma: pitfalls in assessment of risk. Journal of Pediatric Hematology and Oncology 26(1):35–39

Kuttesch JF Jr, Wexler LH, Marcus RB, Fairclough D, Weaver-McClure L, White M, Mao L, Delaney TF, Pratt CB, Horowitz ME, Kun LE (1996) Second malignancies after Ewing`s sarcoma: radiation dose-dependency of secondary sarcomas. Journal of Clinical Oncology 14(10):2818–2825

Lachman MF, Kim K, Koo B (1986) Mediastinal teratoma associated with Klinefelter's syndrome. Archives of Pathology and Laboratory Medicine 110:1067

Ladenstein R, Potschger U, Hartman O et al (2008) 28 years of high-dose therapy and SCT for Neuroblastoma in Europe: lessons from more than 4000 procedures. Bone Marrow Transplantation 41:S118–S127

Lahl M, Fisher VL, Laschinger K (2008) Ewing`s sarcoma family of tumors: an overview from diagnosis to survivorship. Clinical Journal of Oncology Nursing 12(1):89–97

Lang PH, Vogelzang NG, Goldman A et al (1982) Marker half-life analysis as a prognostic tool in testicular cancer. Journal of Urology 128:708

Lau L, Supko JG, Blaney S et al (2005) A phase I and pharmacokinetic study of ecteinascidin-743 (Yondelis) in children with refractory solid tumors. A Children's Oncology Group Study. Clinical Cancer Research 11(2 Pt 1):672–677

Leavey PJ, Mascarenhas L, Marina N et al (2008) Prognostic factors for patients with Ewing sarcoma (EWS) at first recurrence following multi-modality therapy: a report from the Children`s Oncology Group. Pediatric Blood & Cancer 51:334–338

Lee DC, Chua DT, Wei WI, Sham JS, Lau AS (2007) Induction of a matrix metalloproteinases by Epstein–Barr virus latent membrane protein 1 isolated from nasopharyngeal carcinoma. Biomedicine and Pharmacotherapy 61(9):520–526

Lewis TB, Coffin CM, Bernard PS (2007) Differentiating Ewing`s sarcoma from other round blue cell tumors using a RT-PCR translocation panel on formalin-fixed paraffin-embedded tissues. Modern Pathology 20:397–404

Link MP, Gebhardt MC, Meyers PA (2002) Osteosarcoma. In: Pizzo PA, Poplack DG (eds) Principles and practice of pediatric oncology, 4th edn. Lippincott Williams & Wilkins, Philadelphia

Litten JB, Tomlinson GE (2008) Liver tumors in children. The Oncologist 13:812–820

Lo Curto M, Lumina F, Alaggio R et al (2003) Malignant germ cell tumors in childhood: results of the first Italian cooperative study "TCG91". Medical and Pediatric Oncology 41:417–425

Lo Curto M, D'Angelo P, Cecchetto G et al (2007) Mature and immature teratomas: results of the first paediatric Italian study. Pediatric Surgery International 23:315–322

Loeb DM, Thornton K, Shokek O (2008) Pediatric soft tissue sarcomas. Surgical Clinics of North America 88:615–627

Ludwig JA (2008) Ewing sarcoma: historical perspectives, current state of the art and opportunities for targeted therapy in the future. Current Opinion in Oncology 20(4):412–418

MacArthur CA, Issacs H, Miller JH et al (1994) Pediatric renal cell carcinoma: a complete response to recombinant interleukin-2 in a child with metastatic disease at diagnosis. Medical and Pediatric Oncology 23:365–371

Malogolowkin MH, Katzenstein HM, Krailo M et al (2008) Redefining the role of doxorubicin for the treatment of children with hepatoblastoma. Journal of Clinical Oncology 26(14):2379–2383

Maris JM, Matthay KK (1999) Molecular biology of neuroblastoma. Journal of Clinical Oncology 17(7):2264–2279

Maris JM, Hogarty MD, Bagatell R, Cohn SL (2007) Neuroblastoma. Lancet 369:2106–2120

Matthay KK, Yamashiro DJ (2000) Neuroblastoma. In: Bast RC, Kufe DW, Pollock RE, Weichselbaum RR, Holland JF, Frei E (eds) Cancer medicine, 5th edn. B.C. Decker, Hamilton

Matthay KK, Villablance JG, Seeger RC et al (1999) Treatment of high-risk neuroblastoma with intensive chemotherapy, radiotherapy, autologous bone marrow transplantation, and 13-cis-retinoic acid. The New England Journal of Medicine 341(16):1165–1173

Matthay KK, Versteeg R, Reynolds CP (2005) High risk neuroblastoma: beyond intensification to novel therapy. American Society of Clinical Oncology Education session 787–795.

May RJ, Dao T, Pinilla-Ibarz J et al (2007) Peptide epitopes from the Wilms' tumor 1 oncoprotein stimulate CD4+ and CD8+ T cells that recognize and kill human malignant mesothelioma tumor cells. Clinical Cancer Research 13(15):4547–4555

McDowell HP (2003) Update on childhood rhabdomyosarcoma. Archives of Disease in Childhood 88(4):354–357

Mertens R, Granzen B, Lassay L et al (2005) Treatment of nasopharyngeal carcinoma in children and adolescents. Definitive results of a multicentre study (NPC-91-GPOH). Cancer 104(5):1083–1089

Metzger ML, Stewart CF, Freeman BB et al (2007) Topotecan is active against Wilms' tumor: results of a multi-institutional phase II study. Journal of Clinical Oncology 25(21):3130–3136

Meyer JS, Nadel HR, Marina N (2008) Imaging guidelines for children with Ewing sarcoma and osteosarcoma: a report from the Children`s Oncology Group Bone Tumor Committee. Pediatric Blood & Cancer 51:163–170

Meyers RL (2007) Tumors of the liver in children. Surgical Oncology 16:195–203

Meyers RL, Katzenstein HM, Krailo M, McGahren ED III, Malogolowkin MH (2007) Surgical resection of pulmonary metastatic lesions in children with hepatoblastoma. Journal of Pediatric Surgery 42(12):2050–2056

Meyers PA, Schwartz CL, Krailo MD et al (2008) Osteosarcoma: the addition of muramyl tripeptide to chemotherapy improves overall survival – a report from the Children's Oncology Group. Journal of Clinical Oncology 26(4):633–638

Michalkiewicz E, Sandrini R, Figueiredo B et al (2004) Clinical and outcome characteristics of children with adrenocortical tumors: a report from the international pediatric adrenocortical tumor registry. Journal of Clinical Oncology 22(5):838–845

Miser JS, Pappo AS, Triche TJ, Merchant TE, Rao BN (2002) Other Soft Tissue Sarcomas of Childhood. In: Pizzo PA, Poplack DG (eds) Principles and practice of pediatric oncology, 4th edn. Lippincott Williams & Wilkins, Philadelphia

Miser JS, Goldsby RE, Chen Z, Krailo MD, Tarbell NJ, Link MP, Fryer CJ, Pritchard DJ, Gebhardt MC, Dickman PS, Perlman EJ, Meyers PA, Donaldson SS, Moore SG, Rausen AR, Vietti TJ, Grier HE (2007) Treatment of metastatic Ewing sarcoma/primitive neuroectodermal tumor of bone: evaluation of increasing the dose intensity of chemotherapy–a report from the Children`s Oncology Group. Pediatric Blood & Cancer 49(7):894–900

Modak S, Kushner BH, LaQuaglia MP, Kramer K, Cheung NV (2009) Management and outcome of stage 3 neuroblastoma. European Journal of Cancer 45:90–98

Murphree AL (2005) Intraocular retinoblastoma: the case for a new group classification. Opthalmology Clinics of North America 18:41–53

Nakajima G, Patino-Garcia BS et al (2008) CDH11 expression is associated with survival in patients with osteosarcoma. Cancer Genomics & Proteomics 5:37–42

Neville HL, Ritchey ML (2000) Wilms' tumor: overview of national Wilms' tumor study group results. Urologic Clinics of North America 27(3):435–442

Ng A, Jenkinson H, Morland B, Grundy R (2005) Clear cell sarcoma: a dilemma on pathological staging and clinical management. Pediatric Hematology and Oncology 22:257–261

Nickerson HJ, Matthay KK, Seeger BC et al (2000) Favorable biology and outcome of stage IV-S neuroblastoma with supportive care or minimal therapy: a children's cancer group study. Journal of Clinical Oncology 18(3):477–486

Nicolin G, Taylor R, Baugh C et al (2008) Outcome after pulmonary radiotherapy in Wilms' tumour patients with pulmonary metastases at diagnosis: a UK Children's Cancer Study Group, Wilms' Tumour Working Group Study. International Journal of Radiation Oncology, Biology, Physics 70(1):175–180

Ninane J, Pearson ADJ (1997) Neuroblastoma. In: Pinkerton CR, Plowman PN (eds) Paediatric oncology clinical practice and controversies, 2nd edn. Chapman & Hall, London

Oberlin O, Rey A, Lyden E et al (2008) Prognostic factors in metastatic rhabdomyosarcomas: results of a pooled analysis from United States and European cooperative groups. Journal of Clinical Oncology 26(14):2384–2389

Oberthuer A, Kaderali L, Kahlert Y et al (2008) Subclassification and individual survival time prediction from gene expression data of neuroblastoma patients by using CASPAR. Clinical Cancer Research 14(20):6590–6601

Okcu MF, Munsell M, Treuner J et al (2003) Synovial sarcoma of childhood and adolescence: a multicenter, multivariate analysis of outcome. Journal of Clinical Oncology 21: 1602–1611

Okcu MF, Hicks J, Merchant TE, Andrassy RJ, Pappo AS, Horowitz ME (2006) Nonrhabdomyosarcomatous soft tissue sarcomas. In: Pizzo PA, Poplack DG (eds) Principles and practice of pediatric oncology, 5th edn. Lippincott Williams & Wilkins, Philadelphia

Onada M, Matsuda S, Higaki S et al (1996) ErbB-2 expression is correlated with poor prognosis for patients with osteosarcoma. Cancer 77:71–78

Osaka E, Suzuki T, Osaka S, Yoshida Y, Sugita H, Asami S, Tabata K, Sugitani M, Nemoto N, Ryu J (2007) Survivin expression levels as independent predictors of survival for osteosarcoma patients. Journal of Orthopaedic Research 25(1):116–121

Otte JB, deVille de Goyet J, Teding R (2005) Liver transplantation for hepatoblastoma: indications and contraindication in the modern era. Pediatric Transplantation 9:557–656

Ozkaynak MF, Sondel PM, Krailo MD et al (2000) Phase I study of chimeric human/murine anti-ganglioside GD2 monoclonal antibody (ch14.18) with granulocyte-macrophage colony-stimulating factor in children with neuroblastoma immediately after hematopoietic stem-cell transplantation: a children's cancer group study. Journal of Clinical Oncology 18(24):4077–4085

Palenzuela G, Martin E, Meunier A et al (2008) Comprehensive staging allows for excellent outcome in patients with localized malignant germ cell tumor of the ovary. Annals of Surgery 248(5):836–841

Palmer RD, Barbosa-Morais NL, Gooding EL et al (2008) Pediatric malignant germ cell tumors show characteristic transcriptome profiles. Cancer Research 68(11):4239–4247

Pandya J, Valverde k, Heon E, Blaser S, Gallie BL, Chan HSL (2002) Predilection of retinoblastoma metastases for the mandible. Medical and Pediatric Oncology 38(4):271–273

Pappo AS (2003) Melanoma in children and adolescents. European Journal of Cancer 39:2651–2661

Pappo AS, Furman WL (2006) Management of infrequent cancers of childhood. In: Pizzo PA, Poplack DG (eds) Principles and practice of pediatric oncology, 5th edn. Lippincott Williams & Wilkins, Philadelphia

Pappo AS, Shapiro DN, Crist WM (1997) Rhabdomyosarcoma biology and treatment. Pediatric Clinics of North America 44(4):953–972

Pappo A, Barr FG, Wolden SL (2006) Pediatric rhabdomyosarcoma: biology and results of the North American Intergroup Trials. In: Pappo A (ed) Pediatric bone and soft tissue sarcomas. Springer, Germany

Park WS, RR OH, Park JY et al (2001) Nuclear localization of bea-catenin is an important prognostic factor in hepatoblastoma. Journal of Pathology 193:483–490

Park J, Jung WW, Bacchini P et al (2006) Ezrin in osteosarcoma: comparison between conventional high-grade and central low-grade osteosarcoma. Pathology, Research and Practice 202:509–515

Paulino AC, Okcu MF (2008) Rhabdomyosarcoma. Current Problems in Cancer 32:7–34

Paulussen M, Bielack S, Jurgens H, Jost L (2008) Ewing`s sarcoma of the bone: ESMO clinical recommendations for diagnosis, treatment and follow-up. Annals of Oncology 19(Suppl 2):ii97–ii98

Perilongo G, Shaffor E, Maibach R et al (2004) Risk adapted treatment for childhood hepatoblastoma: final report of the second study of the internal society of pediatric oncology, SIOPEL 2. European Journal of Cancer 40:411–421

Pettinato G, Manivel JC, Wicks MR et al (1989) Classical and cellular (atypical) congenital mesoblastic nephroma. A clinicopathologic, ultrastructural, immunohistochemical, and flow cytometric study. Human Pathology 20:682–690

Pinkerton CR (1997) Malignant germ cell tumours. In: Pinkerton CR, Plowman PN (eds), Paediatric oncology clinical practice and controversies 2nd edn. Chapman and Hall, London

Popovic MB, Diezi M, Henri K et al (2007) Trilateral retinoblastoma with suprasellar tumor and associated pineal cyst. Journal of Pediatric Hematology and Oncology 29(1): 53–56

Portugal R, Barroca H (2008) Clear cell sarcoma, cellular mesoblastic nephroma and metanephric adenoma: cytological features and differential diagnosis with Wilms tumor. Cytopathology 19:80–87

Postiglione L, Di Domenico G, Giordano-Lanza G, Ladogana P, Turano M, Castaldo C, Di Meglio F, Cocozza S, Montagnani S (2003) Effect of human granulocyte macrophage-colony stimulating factor on differentiation and apoptosis of the human osteosarcoma cell line SaOS-2. European Journal of Histochemistry 47(4):309–316

Pratt CB, Pappo AS (2002) Management of infrequent cancers of childhood. In: Pizzo PA, Poplack DG (eds) *Principles and practice of pediatric* oncology, 4th edn. Lippincott Williams & Wilkins, Philadelphia

Pritchard-Jones K (2002) Controversies and advances in the management of Wilms' tumour. Archives of Disease in Childhood 87(3):241–244

Pritchard-Jones K, Mitchell CD (1997) The genetic basis of children's cancers. In: Pinkerton CR, Plowman PN (eds) *Paediatric oncology clinical practice and* controversies, 2nd edn. Chapman & Hall, London

Ragland BD, Bell WC, Lopez RR, Siegal GP (2002) Cytogenetics and molecular biology of osteosarcoma. Laboratory Investigation 82(4):365–373

Raney B, Anderson J, Breneman J et al (2008) Results in patients with cranial parameningeal sarcoma and metastases (Stage 4) treated on intergroup rhabdomyosarcoms study group (IRSG) protocols II-IV, 1978–1997: report from the Children`s Oncology Group. Pediatric Blood & Cancer 51(1):17–22

Rodriguez-Galindo C, Pappo AS (2003) Less-frequently encountered tumors of childhood. In: Bast RC, Kufe DW, Pollock RE, Weichselbaum RR, Holland JF, Frei E (eds) Cancer medicine, 6th edn. B.C. Decker, Hamilton

Rodriguez-Galindo C, Poquette CA, Marina NM, Head DR, Cain A, Meyer WH, Santana VM, Pappo AS (2000) Hematologic abnormalities and acute myeloid leukemia in children and adolescents administered intensified chemotherapy for the Ewing sarcoma family of tumors. Journal of Pediatric Hematology and Oncology 22(4):321–329

Rodriguez-Galindo C, Spunt SL, Pappo AS (2003) Treatment of Ewing sarcoma family of tumors: current status and outlook for the future. Medical and Pediatric Oncology 40(5):276–287

Rodriguez-Galindo C, Chantada GL, Haik BG, Wilson MW (2007) Treatment of retinoblastoma: current status and future perspectives. Current Treatment Options in Neurology 9(4):294–307

Rudnick E, Khakoo Y, Antunes NL et al (2001) Opsoclonus-myoclonus-ataxia syndrome in neuroblastoma: clinical outcome and antineuronal antibodies-a report from the Children's Cancer Group. Medical and Pediatric Oncology 36:612–622

Sandrini R, Ribeiro RC, DeLacerda L (1997) Childhood adrenocortical tumors. The Journal of Clinical Endocrinology and Metabolism 82(7):2027–2031

Savage SA, Burdett L, Trosisi R, Douglass C, Hoover RN, Chanock SJ, National Osteosarcoma Study Group (2007) Germline genetic variation of TP53 in osteosarcoma. Pediatric Blood & Cancer 49(1):28–33

Saxman SB, Finch D, Gonin R, Einhorn LH (1998) Long-term follow-up of a phase III study of three versus four cycles of bleomycin, etoposide, and cisplatin in favorable-prognosis germ-cell tumors: the Indian University experience. Journal of Clinical Oncology 16(2):702–106

Saylors RL, Stine KC, Sullivan J et al (2001) Cyclophosphamide plus topotecan in children with recurrent or refractory solid tumors: a Pediatric Oncology Group Phase II study. Journal of Clinical Oncology 19(15):3463–3469

Shimada H, Chatten J, Newton WA Jr et al (1984) Histopathologic prognostic factors in neuroblastic tumors: definition of subtypes of ganglioneuroblastoma and an age-linked classification of neuroblastoma. Journal of the National Cancer Institute 73:405–413

Shimada H, Ambros IM, Dehner LP et al (1999) The neuroblastoma pathology classification (the Shimada system). Cancer 86(2):364–372

Silberstein J, Grabowski J, Saltzstein SL, Kane CJ (2009) Renal cell carcinoma in the pediatric population: results from the California cancer registry. Pediatric Blood & Cancer 52(2):237–241

Sonn G, Shortliffe LMD (2008) Management of Wilms tumor: current standard of care. Nature Clinical Practice. Urology 5(10):551–560

Sorahan T, Lancashire RJ (2004) Parental cigarette smoking and childhood risks of hepatoblastoma: OSCC data. British Journal of Cancer 90:1016–1018

Sorensen PHB, Lynch JC, Qualman SJ, Tirabosco R, Lim JF, Maurer HM, Bridge JA, Crist WM, Triche TJ, Barr FG (2002) PAX3-FKHR and PAX7-FKHR gene fusions are prognostic indicators in alveolar rhabdomyosarcoma: a report from the children's oncology group. Journal of Clinical Oncology 20(11):2672–2679

Spunt SL, Poquette CA, Hurt YS, Cain AM, Rao BN, Merchant TE, Jenkins JJ, Santana VM, Pratt CB, Pappo AS (1999) Prognostic factors for children and adolescents with surgically resected nonrhabdomyosarcoma soft tissue sarcoma: an analysis of 121 patients treated at St Jude children's research hospital. Journal of Clinical Oncology 17(12):3697–3705

Spunt SL, Wolden SL, Schofield DE, Skapek SX (2006) Non-Rhabdomyosarcoma Soft Tissue Sarcomas. In: Pappo A (ed) Pediatric bone and soft tissue sarcoma. Springer, Germany

Stengel G, Metze D, Dorflinger B, Luger TA, Bohm M (2008) Treatment of extra-abdominal aggressive fibromatosis with pegylated interferon. Journal of the American Academy of Dermatology 59(2 Suppl 1):S7–S9

Stevens MGG, Rey A, Bouvet N et al (2005) Treatment of nonmetastatic rhabdomyosarcoma in childhood and adolescence: third study of the International Society of Paediatric Oncology–SIOP Malignant Mesenchymal Tumor 89. Journal of Clinical Oncology 23(12):2618–2628

Stocker JT (2001) Liver tumors: hepatic tumors in children. Clinics in Liver Disease 5(1):259–281

Strouse JJ, Fears TR, Tucker MA, Wayne AS (2005) Pediatric melanoma: risk factor and survival analysis of the surveillance, epidemiology and end results database. Journal of Clinical Oncology 23(21):4735–4741

Suriawinata AA, Thung SN (2002) Malignant liver tumors. Clinics in Liver Disease 6(2):527–554

Swanson PE, Dehner LP (1991) Pathology of soft tissue sarcomas in children and adolescents. In: Maurer HM, Ruymann FB, Pochedly C (eds) Rhabdomyosarcoma and related tumors in children and adolescents. CRC Press, Florida

Terenziani M, Spreafico F, Collini P, Meazza C, Massimino M, Piva L (2007) Endodermal sinus tumor of the vagina. Pediatric Blood & Cancer 48:577–578

Tomioka N, Kobayashi H, Kageyama H, Ohira M, Nakamura Y, Sasaki F, Todo S, Nakagawara A, Kaneko Y (2003) Chromosomes that show partial loss or gain in near-diploid tumors coincide with chromosomes that show whole loss or gain in near-triploid tumors: evidence suggesting the involvement of the same genes in the tumorigenesis of high- and low-ri. Genes, Chromosomes & Cancer 36:139–150

Tomlinson GE, Finegold MJ (2002) Tumors of the liver. In: Pizzo PA, Poplack DG (eds) Principles and practice of pediatric oncology, 4th edn. Lippincott Williams & Wilkins, Philadelphia

van Ditzhuijsen CIM, Can de Weijer R, Haak HR, on behalf of the Dutch Adrenal Network (2007) Adrenocortical carcinoma. Netherlands Journal of Medicine 65(2):55–59

Vassilopoulou-Sellin R, Shultz PN (2001) Adrenocortical carcinoma. Clinical outcome at the end of the 20th century. Cancer 92:1113–1121

Veneselli E, Conte M, Biancheri R, Acquaviva A, De Bernardi B (1998) Effect of steroid and high-dose immunoglobulin therapy on opsoclonus-myoclonus syndrome occurring in neuroblastoma. Medical and Pediatric Oncology 30:15–17

Wexler LH, Crist WM, Helman LJ (2002) Rhabdomyosarcoma and the undifferentiated sarcomas. In: Pizzo PA, Poplack DG (eds), Principles and practice of pediatric oncology, 4th edn. Lippincott Williams & Wilkins, Philadelphia

Whelan J, Weeden S, Uscinska B et al (2000) Localised extremity osteosarcoma: mature survival data from two European Osteosarcoma Intergroup randomized clinical trials. Proceedings of the American Society of Clinical Oncology 19:1281a

Whelan JS, Burcombe RJ, Janinis J, Baldelli AM, Cassoni AM (2002) A systematic review of the role of pulmonary irradiation in the management of primary bone tumors. Annals of Oncology 13:23–30

Wilhelm SM, Adnane L, Newell P et al (2008) Preclinical overview of sorafenib, a multikinase inhibitor that targets both Raf and VEGF and PDGF receptor tyrosine kinase signaling. Molecular Cancer Therapeutics 7(10):3129–3140

Wittig JC, Bickel J, Priebat D, Jelined J, Kellar-Graney K, Shmookler B (2002) Osteosarcoma: a multidisciplinary approach to diagnosis and treatment. American Family Physician 65(6):1123–1132

Wolden SL, Wexler MD, Kraus DH, Laquaglia MP, Lis E, Meyers PA (2005) Intensity-modulated head and neck rhabdomyosarcoma. International Journal of Radiation Oncology, Biology, Physics 61(5):1432–1438

Womer RB, West, DC, Krailo M, Dickman PS, Pawel B; for the Children's Oncology Group AEWS0031 Committee (2008) Randomized comparison of every-two-week v. every-three-week chemotherapy in Ewing sarcoma family tumors (ESFT). Journal of Clinical Oncology 26(155):10504. (2008 ASCO Annual Meetings proceedings (Post Meeting Edition))

Wunder JS, Gokgoz N, Parkes R et al (2005) TP53 mutations and outcome in osteosarcoma: a prospective, multicenter study. Journal of Clinical Oncology 23(7):1483–1490

Zagar TM, Triche TJ, Kinsella TJ (2008) Extraosseous Ewing`s sarcoma: 25 years later. Journal of Clinical Oncology 26(26):4230–4232

Zage PE, Reitman AJ, Seshadri R et al (2008) Outcomes of a two-drug chemotherapy regimen for intraocular retinoblastoma. Pediatric Blood & Cancer 50(3):567–572

Zancanella P, Pianovski MAD, Oliveira BH et al (2006) Mitotane associated with cisplatin, etoposide, and doxorubicin in advanced childhood adrenocortical carcinoma. Mitotane monitoring and tumor regression. Journal of Pediatric Hematology and Oncology 28(8):513–524

Zheng H, Li L, Hu D, Deng Z, Cao Y (2007) Role of Epstein–Barr virus encoded latent membrane protein 1 in the carcinogenesis of nasopharyngeal carcinoma. Cellular & Molecular Immunology 4(3):185–197

Central Nervous System Tumors

Nancy E. Kline • Joan O'Hanlon-Curry

Contents

4.1 Causes/Epidemiology . . . 129
4.2 Distribution/Classification . . . 129
4.3 Staging . . . 130
4.4 Molecular Genetics of Brain Tumors . . . 130
4.5 Diagnosis . . . 130
4.6 Specialist Referral . . . 130
4.7 Hydrocephalus . . . 130
4.8 Treatment . . . 131
4.8.1 Surgery . . . 131
4.8.2 Radiotherapy . . . 131
4.8.2.1 Conventional Radiotherapy . . . 131
4.8.3 Chemotherapy . . . 132
4.9 Prognosis . . . 132
4.10 Specific Tumors . . . 132
4.10.1 PNETs/Medulloblastomas . . . 132
4.10.2 Astrocytomas/Glial Tumors . . . 133
4.10.3 Malignant Gliomas . . . 134
4.10.4 Other High-Grade Gliomas . . . 134
4.11 Follow-Up . . . 138
4.11.1 The Late Effects and Rehabilitation of Survivors . . . 138
4.11.2 Palliative Care . . . 139
4.11.3 Future Perspectives/New Innovations . . . 139
References . . . 140

4.1 Causes/Epidemiology

The cause of childhood brain tumors remains largely unknown, although there is correlation with a family history of cancer, and there may be hereditary factors as well. Children with neurofibromatosis have an increased risk of developing optic gliomas and those with tuberous sclerosis have an increased risk of astrocytoma or other benign brain tumors.

Environmental factors such as electric and magnetic fields, radio frequency radiation, chemicals, and cellular telephones have been suggested as causative factors in the development of brain tumors. There remains, however, no evidence to support these claims. Ionizing radiation is a known cause of brain tumors, with secondary local malignancies (e.g., meningiomas) being a small but significant side effect of cranial radiotherapy (Umansky et al. 2008).

4.2 Distribution/Classification

Approximately 60% of childhood brain tumors are infratentorial and include medulloblastoma, cerebellar astrocytoma (WHO grades I–IV), brain stem glioma, and ependymoma. Supratentorial tumors include low-grade astrocytomas, primitive neuroectodermal tumors (PNETs), germ cell tumors, hypothalamic and optic nerve gliomas, and craniopharyngiomas.

The most common central nervous tumors are low-grade gliomas, with cerebellar astrocytomas being the largest of this group. In terms of malignant brain tumors, medulloblastomas occur most frequently.

Classification of pediatric brain tumors may be misleading as low-grade tumors may have devastating effects due to their location. Therefore, using the terms benign and malignant does not always correlate with the outcome.

4.3 Staging

Currently, there is no universal staging system in regard to brain tumors. The only tumor group that does utilize a staging process is medulloblastoma. The Chang operative system is used (Laurent et al. 1985; Verlooy et al. 2006). For other tumors, histological grade, age, site of disease, and areas of dissemination are the main prognostic factors.

4.4 Molecular Genetics of Brain Tumors

The molecular genetics of childhood brain tumors are poorly understood, not only in terms of the pathophysiology but also in terms of the characterization of tumor-specific molecular abnormalities that predict biologically favorable or unfavorable disease.

4.5 Diagnosis

Diagnosing a brain tumor may be difficult. Diagnosis is often complicated by a vague history of symptoms that the parents, general practitioner, or local pediatrician may have attributed to common childhood illnesses. Children who have a long insidious history of symptoms are more likely to have a lower-grade tumor. Those who present with a short history and obvious symptoms are much more likely to have biologically aggressive disease. The site, severity of disease, and the child's age and development will have an impact on presenting symptoms. For example, those children with posterior fossa disease often have signs of increased intracranial pressure (ICP):

- Headaches
- Early morning vomiting
- Blurred vision
- Ataxia
- Poor concentration
- Changes in vital signs (late sign)

Children with supratentorial tumors, however, are more likely to present with hemiparesis, hemisensory loss, and/or seizures. Fundoscopic examination often reveals increased ICP and MRI of the brain confirms the diagnosis. In children with infratentorial tumors, MRI of the spine and cerebrospinal (CSF) sampling are necessary to determine the presence of spinal leptomeningeal disease or metastasis. If the presence of an intracranial germ cell tumor is suspected, serum and CSF levels of alpha-fetoprotein (AFP) and human chorionic gonadotropin (HCG) will be measured as well. This possibility should be considered in all suprasellar and pineal region tumors. If the tumor is not surgically resectable, a stereotactic biopsy may be used to confirm the diagnosis.

4.6 Specialist Referral

While other childhood tumors have routinely been referred to specialist pediatric oncology centers since the 1970s, many children with brain tumors continued to receive treatment outside of specialist units. This practice resulted in less than 40% being treated within clinical trials until after 1997 (UKCCSG/SBNS 1997), when a joint report recommended the centralization of care for children with brain and spinal disease. In the US, children with brain tumors are typically treated at NCI-designated cancer centers or on a cooperative group protocol.

4.7 Hydrocephalus

A significant number of children with brain tumors will develop associated hydrocephalus. Noncommunicating hydrocephalus is most commonly observed in children with brain tumors and is a result of mass effect. This may present as a surgical emergency around the time of diagnosis, requiring immediate management. The most likely symptoms are headache, vomiting on arising in the morning, nausea, and ataxia. Debulking or removal of the tumor may be sufficient to relieve the obstruction and allow normal flow of CSF. Other surgical options are external ventricular drainage, ventriculoperitoneal (VP) shunting, and ventriculostomy. Medical management may include corticosteroids to decrease tumor-associated edema, or acetazolamide (Diamox®) to decrease CSF production.

Children with VP shunts are at risk for potential complications. Shunt malformation, infection, and, although rare, tumor dissemination may occur, and the nurse should consider any sign of increased intercranial pressure (e.g., vomiting, lethargy, ataxia, cranial nerve deficits) as a possible shunt malfunction.

4.8 Treatment

The best method for diagnosing, treating, and managing childhood CNS tumors is through a broad-based multidisciplinary team. Such a team includes the collaboration of pediatric neurosurgeons, oncologists, endocrinologists, nurses, psychologists, radiotherapists, social workers, child life specialists, and physical and occupational therapists. Coordinating these services should be a dedicated neuro-oncology nurse specialist or nurse practitioner.

Treatment options typically involve surgical resection, radiotherapy, and/or chemotherapy, but will be individualized based on histology, degree of resection, and location (inlcuding metastatic sites).

4.8.1 Surgery

Primary surgery remains the mainstay of management for pediatric brain tumors. Depending on the site and extent of the tumor, surgical options range from biopsy alone to complete removal. With most malignant tumors, complete resection is an important surgical goal. There is, however, a balance to be struck between complete excision and the risk of surgical morbidity. For some tumor types, complete surgical excision seems to be of particular prognostic importance (i.e., ependymoma medulloblastoma). Debulking alone, however, may relieve local compression and improve the child's symptoms while histology is sought and other treatment modalities are explored (Ueoka et al. 2009). In other germ cell tumors, chemotherapy now has a primary role, and the indications for surgery are more circumspect (Nicholson et al. 2003).

4.8.2 Radiotherapy

A significant number of children with brain tumors will require radiotherapy, which aims to deliver optimal doses of radiation to tumor cells while sparing surrounding normal tissue.

4.8.2.1 Conventional Radiotherapy

Despite precise planning and delivery of treatment, significant long-term squeal may lead to significant impairment of quality of life. These squeals are particularly profound following whole brain treatment and irradiation of preschool-age children. Internationally, neuro-oncologists recognize the detrimental effects of radiotherapy on the developing brain and have advocated delaying radiation treatment in infants and young children whenever possible. A recent study of long-term survivors of childhood cancer in Canada found that those who received cranial radiation, regardless of age, were at increased risk of poor educational outcomes (Lorenzi et al. 2009).

An added complication for young children is their inability to remain motionless during the delivery of radiotherapy, necessitating the use of daily anesthesia to ensure dose accuracy (Chap. 10). The prolonged use of anesthesia is not optimal but at times unavoidable. When possible, utilizing child-life specialists to assist with radiation treatments to avoid anesthesia should be explored. Dose reductions and modified fractionations, to limit the toxicity of craniospinal irradiation, are features of recent investigation.

Techniques that have been used to increase the therapeutic index (the tumor to normal tissue dose) include:

- Stereotactic radiotherapy
- Brachytherapy
- Radiosurgery

4.8.3 Chemotherapy

Despite the belief that chemotherapy drugs do not cross the blood–brain barrier, there have been multiple studies suggesting there is efficacy in utilizing chemotherapy for a variety of brain tumors. Chemotherapy is now considered a valuable treatment modality as part of the prospective treatment package facilitating cure in children with nonmetastatic medulloblastoma (Taylor et al. 2002; Abd-El-Aal 2006). For example, chemotherapy is advantageous in treating those children less than 5 years of age for whom radiation therapy would cause many side effects. Multi-agent regimens can delay the need for radiotherapy and its associated late effects. Likewise, stabilization of an incompletely resected tumor can be achieved by the use of chemotherapy.

In addition to management with conventional chemotherapy regimens, children with brain tumors, high-grade gliomas, and medulloblastomas are now being treated with high-dose chemotherapy with stem cell rescue. Intensifying treatment is thought to improve the permeability of the blood–brain barrier, and its role continues to be debated as clinical trials continue.

4.9 Prognosis

Survival data may be misleading. Percentage figures quoted to families can be misleading because they are often based on the evaluation of treatment strategies that lag behind current practice.

4.10 Specific Tumors

4.10.1 PNETs/Medulloblastomas

Undifferentiated neuroectodermal tumors of the cerebellum have historically been referred to as medulloblastomas, while tumors of identical histology in the pineal region are diagnosed as pineoblastomas, and cerebral tumors are referred to as PNETs. Microscopically, both medulloblastomas and PNETs consist of small round cells with disproportionately large hyperchromatic nuclei. These cells are often clustered into rosettes.

Medulloblastoma

Epidemiology
- Twenty-five percent of pediatric brain tumors
- Most common between 3 and 7 years and in males
- Arises from primitive neuroepithelial cells

Etiology
- Commonly arises in cerebellar vermis
- Invades fourth ventricle with associated hydrocephalus
- Can disseminate via the CSF

Symptoms
- Headache
- Morning vomiting
- Cranial nerve deficits
- Ataxia

Diagnostics
- Craniospinal imaging
- CSF analysis for free-floating tumor cells
- Bone scan and bone marrow aspiration to detect metastatic spread

Treatment
- Primary surgery: gross total excision optimal
- Craniospinal radiotherapy + boost to the primary tumor site (optimal dose and mode of administration under investigation) ± chemotherapy
- Children under 5: chemotherapy
- National treatment strategies predominantly seeking to reduce irradiation

Prognosis
- Nonmetastatic disease: 70–80% overall survival
- Metastatic disease: trials with craniospinal radiotherapy, high-dose chemotherapy, and stem cell rescue are currently being evaluated

Supratentorial PNETs

These are the supratentorial counterpart of medulloblastoma, having the same histological appearance
- Occur mainly <5 years of age
- The majority arise in the cerebral hemispheres/pineal region

Supratentorial PNETs (continued)

- Treatment considerations are similar to medulloblastoma, with survival being lower

Prognosis

Age-related:

- Less than 3 years: Very poor
- Three years: Site-dependent

4.10.2 Astrocytomas/Glial Tumors

The majority of these tumors are supratentorial and slow-growing and are referred to as low-grade astrocytomas, pilocytic astrocytomas, oligodendrogliomas, mixed gliomas, or gangliogliomas. Less common are malignant gliomas of the supratentorium (i.e., anaplastic astrocytomas and glioblastoma multiforme).

The Kernohan grading system is used to grade glial tumors and uses a grade I to grade IV scale, with I being favorable histology and grade IV being disease associated with a fatal outcome. Anaplastic astrocytomas are histologically recognizable by more frequent mitosis, cellular pleomorphism, and general cellularity of the tumor. Glioblastoma multiforme is diagnosed when areas of necrosis and highly undifferentiated cells are present.

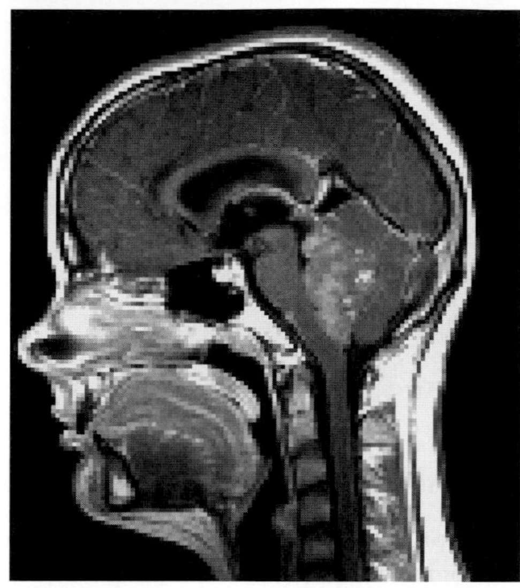

Age at diagnosis	15 years
Diagnosis	Medulloblastoma
Presenting symptoms	3-4 week of double vision and dizziness Early morning vomiting Decreased consciousness

Figure 4.1

Cranial MRI of medulloblastoma

Cerebellar Astrocytoma

Epidemiology

- Commonly occurs in the first decade of life
- More common in boys

Symptoms

- Midline cerebellar signs

Diagnosis

- History
- Neurological examination
- MRI commonly shows cystic tumor with mural node

Treatment

- Complete surgical removal of the tumor is treatment of choice

Cerebellar Astrocytoma (continued)

- Interval MRI scans to monitor for signs of progression
- Radiotherapy

Prognosis

Over 90% of children with a fully resected pilocytic astrocytoma will survive with only surgical intervention. Those with partially resected diffuse disease who have had radiotherapy have only a 50–60% chance of survival.

Poor prognostic features include

- Diffuse histology
- Incomplete resection
- Brain stem involvement

Supratentorial Astrocytoma

Epidemiology
- Twice as common in boys

Treatment
- Complete surgical removal is optimal
- Radiotherapy is indicated for all than the lowest-grade, completely resected tumors

Prognosis
- Varies widely

4.10.3 Malignant Gliomas

Classified primarily by anatomic location and second by histologic phenotype. For those diagnosed within the supratentorium, treatment consists of optimal surgical excision/radiotherapy and chemotherapy. Despite aggressive treatment strategies, survival in this group of patients remains poor.

Brain Stem Glioma

Epidemiology
- Gender incidence equal
- Common presenting age: 5–10 years

4.10.4 Other High-Grade Gliomas

The clinical behavior of supratentorial and cerebellar gliomas is more difficult to predict on the basis of radiological and clinical characteristics, with prognosis being more related to histologic phenotype and grade. After resection, radiotherapy is the treatment of choice. Long-term survival remains poor, with 40% overall survival for grade III and 10% for grade IV (Ueoka 2009).

Brain Stem Glioma (continued)

Etiology
- Arise in the medulla, pons, midbrain, and cerebral peduncles
- Diffuse pontine gliomas are rapidly infiltrative in nature
- Most commonly found in the pons, with equal distribution of histological varieties
- Low-grade tumors constitute <10% of brain stem tumors

Symptoms
- High-grade disease: short history
  - Multiple cranial nerve palsies
  - Ataxia
  - Hemiparesis
- Low-grade disease: long history
  - Minimal or a focal cranial nerve deficit
  - Raised ICP

Diagnostics
Location, radiological appearance (Fig. 4.2), and clinical features are usually diagnostic

Treatment
- Treat hydrocephalus
- High-grade disease: steroids to alleviate neurological symptoms in short pulses
- Radiotherapy is palliative, producing a mean survival of 8–10 months. Chemotherapy and hyperfractionated radiotherapy have failed to make an impact on outcome
- Low-grade disease: surgical debulking
  - Observation
  - Radiotherapy and/or chemotherapy may be indicated

Prognosis
- High-grade disease: median survival 8–10 months

Intracranial Ependymoma

Epidemiology
- Paraventricular lesions usually occur in the first decade of life
- Fifty percent occurring <5 years of age
- Spinal ependymomas present slightly later

Etiology
- Predominantly arise from ependymal tissue within the ventricular system, most commonly the fourth ventricle
- Can disseminate (more frequently with infratentorial and high-grade disease)
- Hydrocephalus common at presentation

Divided into the following categories:
- Subependymoma (WHO grade I)
- Ependymoma (WHO grade II); variants include cellular, papillary, epithelial, clear cell, and mixed
- Malignant/anaplastic ependymoma (WHO grade III)

Symptoms
Depend on site and extent of disease
- Neck pain
- Increased ICP
- Cranial nerve deficits
- Ataxia

Diagnostics
- MRI (whole brain and spine) to establish extent of disease
- CSF cytology when possible

Treatment
- Surgery
- Treat hydrocephalus
- Adjuvant treatment is age-related: *>5 years of age*
- No residual disease or disseminated disease: radiotherapy to the tumor bed
- Residual disease, no disseminated disease: re-resection

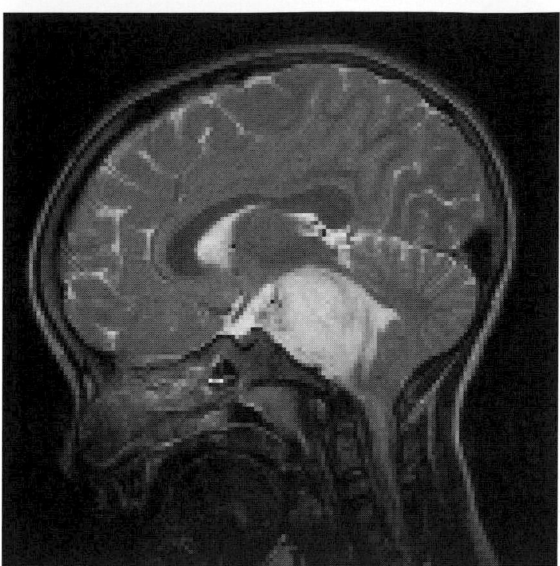

Age	5 years
Diagnosis	Diffuse pontine glioma
Presenting Symptoms	3 week history of gradual onset of left sided weakness, headache, diffculty swallowing

Figure 4.2
Diffuse pontine glioma

Intracranial Ependymoma (continued)

  - Radiotherapy (no spinal)
  - Trials are ongoing to determine role of chemotherapy
- CNS disseminated disease: radiotherapy to entire CNS
  - Trials underway looking at role of chemotherapy *<5 years of age*
- Chemotherapy
- Second-look surgery

Intracranial Ependymoma (continued)

Prognosis

- Overall survival: 40–60% at 5 years
- Good prognostic factors: minimal residual disease post surgery
- Poor prognostic factors: young age
- Subtotal resection

Craniopharyngiomas

Epidemiology

- Eight percent of all childhood brain tumors
- Most commonly seen <18 years
- Mean age at diagnosis 8 years

Etiology

- Arise from neural ectoderm and epithelial elements in Rathke's pouch
- Can be located anywhere in the primitive craniopharyngeal duct
- Ninety percent suprasellar, 10% intrasellar
- Benign and slow-growing

Symptoms

Presenting symptoms relate to pressure on adjacent structures:

- Visual fields and acuity defects
- Endocrine dysfunction
- Hydrocephalus is possible

Diagnosis

- History
- MRI scan

Treatment

- Presurgical neuroendocrine and ophthalmic work-up are essential
- Treatment of hydrocephalus
- Complete resection optimal

Prognosis

Although classified as benign, they can result in considerable morbidity

Craniopharyngiomas (continued)

Associated problems

- Endocrine dysfunction
- Diabetes insipidus
- Hypothyroidism
- Growth and sex hormone deficits
- Excessive weight gain
- Visual disturbances
- Neuropsychological dysfunction
- Psychosocial problems

Intracranial Germ Cell Tumors

Germ cell tumors arising intracranially are histologically indistinguishable from the gonadal varieties.

Intracranial germ cell tumors can be divided into two main groups:

- Germinomas: 60% of total number of germ cell tumors
- Nongerminomatous germ cell tumors (NGGCTs; also referred to as secreting germ cell tumors)

Both groups have the potential for CSF dissemination.

Epidemiology

- For all intracranial germ cell tumors there is a male prevalence
- Intracranial germinomas primarily present in the second decade of life
- NGGCTs tend to occur earlier

Etiology

- Germinomas occur predominantly in the suprasellar region
- NGGCTs occur mainly as pineal tumors

Symptoms

Pineal tumors

- Raised ICP is commonly seen
- Headache
- Vomiting

Intracranial Germ Cell Tumors (continued)

Suprasellar tumors
- Visual disturbances (fields/acuity)
- Diabetes insipidus
- Hypopituitarism
- Headache
- Vomiting

Diagnostics
- Germinoma: MRI and biopsy
- NGGCT: MRI (radiological features are characteristic)
- Serum and CSF levels for AFP and HCG

Treatment

Germinomas
- Surgery has a limited role
- Chemotherapy followed by local radiotherapy

NGGCTs
- Chemotherapy has improved rates of cure; nevertheless, local radiotherapy is still considered necessary to achieve cure
- Surgery for difficult residual disease

Prognosis
- Germinomas: 90–100%
- NGGCTs: 60–70%

Visual Pathway Gliomas

Epidemiology
- Seventy-five percent of isolated optic nerve gliomas occur <10 years
- Peak incidence: 2–6 years
- Occurs in 20% of patients with neurofibromatosis (NF1)

Etiology
- Can present anywhere along optic tracts
- May extend to the pituitary fossa, causing hypopituitarism, or to the hypothalamus, resulting in precocious puberty

Visual Pathway Gliomas (continued)

- Hydrocephalus may be present
- Natural history is unpredictable

Symptoms

Symptoms relate to tumor pressure on the optic nerve and adjacent structures and infiltration:
- Decreased visual acuity or fields
- Squint
- Nystagmus
- Precocious puberty

Diagnostics
- MRI
- Neurological examination
- Frequent neuro-ophthalmological testing (see below)

Treatment
- Treat hydrocephalus
- Observation if disease and symptoms are stable (spontaneous regression has been reported)
- Treatment should be considered to stabilize vision
- Surgery has limited role
- Less then 8 years of age + NF1: chemotherapy
- Greater then years of age: radiotherapy
- The lack of randomised trials makes it difficult to know whether chemotherapy and radiotherapy make a difference

Prognosis
- Isolated optic nerve tumors have a better prognosis than those that extend along the visual pathway or involve the chiasm
- Children with neurofibromatosis, particularly those who are asymptomatic at diagnosis, have improved prognosis

Neuro-Ophthalmological Testing

Visual assessment is frequently used to determine the need for treatment, with deterioration in visual fields or visual acuity indicating the need for intervention. This can be a particular problem in infants and young children,

Neuro-Ophthalmological Testing (continued)

as it can be difficult to obtain accurate results, particularly regarding visual fields. Experience has shown that even in school-age children, results can fluctuate, and it may be unclear whether this fluctuation relates to disease progression or to variable patient compliance.

Germinoma

Comprise 60% of the total number of germ cell tumors

Epidemiology
- Intracranial germinomas primarily present in the second decade of life

Etiology
- Occur predominantly in the suprasellar region

Symptoms
- Visual disturbances (fields/acuity)
- Diabetes insipidus
- Hypopituitarism
- Headache
- Vomiting

Diagnostics
- MRI
- Biopsy

Treatment
- Surgery has a limited role
- Chemotherapy
- Radiation

Prognosis
- Ninety to hundred percent

Nonsecreting germ cell tumors (NSGCTs)

Epidemiology
- NGGCTs tend to occur earlier

Etiology
- NGGCTs occur mainly as pineal tumors

Symptoms
- Raised ICP is commonly seen
- Headache
- Vomiting

Diagnostics
- MRI (radiological features are characteristic)
- Serum and CSF levels for AFP and HCG

Germinoma (continued)

Treatment
- Sensitive to a range of chemotherapy agents
- Chemotherapy has improved rates of cure
- Local radiotherapy is, however, still necessary to achieve cure
- Surgery for difficult residual disease

Prognosis
- Sixty to seventy percent

Spinal Tumors

Primary spinal tumors are rare in children, so spinal tumors that develop are usually "drop metastasis" from a brain tumor. Low-grade astrocytomas are usually intramedullary, requiring extensive surgical removal. Radiotherapy and chemotherapy may be required. High-grade astrocytomas of the spine require radiotherapy and, like similar disease in other sites, surgery has little role. Prognosis for spinal ependymoma (Fig. 4.3) is optimal with total surgical excision. Radiotherapy is routine, with residual disease necessitating chemotherapy.

4.11 Follow-Up

Children treated for a brain tumor will require lifelong follow-up care provided by healthcare providers who are familiar with long-term effects of cancer treatment. Interval MRI scanning and neurological examinations will be important indicators of progress in the early months and years following treatment. Late effects of treatment, such as cognitive deficits and endocrine dysfunction, may only become apparent in subsequent years.

4.11.1 The Late Effects and Rehabilitation of Survivors

It is clear that children who have been treated for brain tumors may have significant long-term problems relating both to the tumor itself and to treatment

(Lorenzi et al. 2009). Side effects are both physical and psychological and include growth problems and weight gain relating to endocrine dysfunction, lack of energy, poor body image, low self-esteem, and decreased overall fitness (Bonato et al. 2008). Adolescent survivors in particular describe feelings of isolation from their peer group and may lack confidence socially. Problems translate into functional difficulties, such as poor attendance at school, attention deficit, and eating disorders. Adolescent survivors of brain tumor treatment can benefit psychosocially from a rehabilitation program targeting their unique needs (Fitzmaurice and Beardsmore 2003).

4.11.2 Palliative Care

Children with brain tumors have specific needs at end-of-life. Symptom mamagement for children with brain tumors may include pain, steroid dependency, spinal involvement, seizure control, reduced mobility, and speech, language, and swallowing difficulties. Involvement of palliative care nurse specialists or hospice providers are important for the care of these patients.

4.11.3 Future Perspectives/New Innovations

New innovations include the following:

- Boron neutron capture therapy, which is an experimental form of radiotherapy that injects a chemical compound containing boron into the bloodstream, which then concentrates in the brain tumor tissue. Radiotherapy with neutrons is then directed at the cancer, and when the neutrons come into contact with the boron, high-energy radiotherapy is released with low penetrance that spares normal tissue.
- Growth factor inhibitors to prevent the effects of the growth factors that allow a cancer to grow.
- Angiogenesis inhibitors to prevent the formation of new blood vessels that nourish the cancers.
- Immunotherapy to stimulate the body's own immune system to fight the cancer.
- Advanced MR techniques such as MR spectroscopy, diffusion MR, and dynamic contrast-enhanced MR to give noninvasive information on tumor function, i.e., metabolism, relation to white matter, and blood flow.

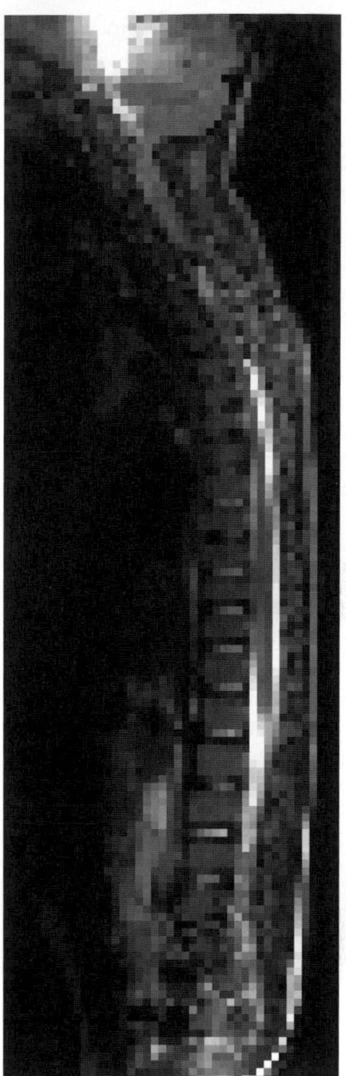

Age	6 years
Diagnosis	Spinal ependymona
Presenting Symptoms	2 month history of intermittent back pain

Figure 4.3
Spinal ependymoma

- Conformal radiotherapy that uses three-dimensional planning. The volume of radiation therapy is irregular and "conforms" to the tumor. Shaped fields of treatment are used, which minimize the amount of normal tissue within the radiotherapy field. This in turn results in a decrease in acute and late morbidity.

References

Abd-El-Aal HH (2006) Pre-irradiation chemotherapy in high risk medulloblastoma. Journal of the Egyptian National Cancer Institute 18(4):357

Bonato C, Severino RF, Elnecave RH (2008) Reduced thyroid volume and hypothyroidism in survivors of childhood cancer treated with radiotherapy. The Journal of Pediatric Endocrinology 21(10):943

Fitzmaurice N, Beardsmore S (2003) The rehabilitation of adolescent survivors of brain tumor treatment. Cancer Nursing Practice 2((5):26–30

Lorenzi M, McMillan AJ, Siegel LS, Zumbo BD, Glickman V, Spinelli JJ et al (2009) Educational outcomes among survivors of childhood cancer in British Columbia, Canada: report of the Childhood/Adolescent/Young adult cancer survivors (CAYACS) program. Cancer 115(10):2234–2245

Nicholson JC, Punt J, Hale J, Saran F, Calaminus G; Germ Cell Tumor Working Groups of the United Kingdom Children's Cancer Study Group (UKCCSG) and International Society of Paediatric Oncology (SIOP) (2003) Neurosurgical management of paediatric germ cell tumors of the central nervous system–a multi-disciplinary team approach for the new millennium. Journal of Clinical Oncology 21(8):1581–1591

Taylor RE, Bailey CC, Robinson K, Weston CL, Ellison D, Ironside J, Lucraft H, Gilbertson R, Tait DM, Walker DA, Pizer BL, Imeson J, Lashford LS; International Society of Paediatric Oncology; United Kingdom Children's Cancer Study Group (2002) Results of a randomized study of preradiation chemotherapy versus radiotherapy alone for nonmetastatic medulloblastoma: The International Society of Paediatric Oncology/United Kingdom Children's Cancer study group PNET-3 study. British Journal of Neurosurgery 16(2):93–95

Ueoka DI, Nogueira J, Campos JC, Filho PM, Ferman S, Lima MA (2009) Brainstem gliomas–retrospective analysis of 86 patients. Journal of Neurological Sciences 281:20–23

UKCCSG/SBNS United Kingdom Children's Cancer Study Group and Society of British Neurological Surgeons (1997) Guidance for services for children and young people with brain and spinal tumors. Report of working party of UKCCSG and the Society of British Neurological Surgeons

Umansky F, Shoshan Y, Rosenthal G, Fraifeld S, Spektor S (2008) Radiation-induced meningioma. Neurosurgical Focus 24(5):E7

Verlooy J, Mosseri V, Bracard S, Tubiana AL, Kalifa C, Pichon F et al (2006) Treatment of high risk medulloblastomas in children above the age of 3 years: A SFOP study. European Journal of Cancer 42(17):3004

PART II

Anemias

Rosalind Bryant

Contents

5.1 Anemia . . . 142
5.2 Iron-Deficiency Anemia . . . 146
5.2.1 Epidemiology . . . 146
5.2.2 Etiology . . . 146
5.2.3 Molecular Genetics . . . 146
5.2.4 Symptoms/Clinical Signs . . . 146
5.2.5 Diagnostic Testing . . . 147
5.2.6 Treatment . . . 148
5.2.7 Transfusion . . . 148
5.2.8 Erythropoietin (Epogen) . . . 148
5.2.9 Prognosis . . . 149
5.3 Sickle Cell Disease . . . 149
5.3.1 Epidemiology . . . 149
5.3.2 Etiology . . . 149
5.3.3 Molecular Genetics . . . 149
5.3.4 Symptoms/Clinical Signs . . . 149
5.3.5 Diagnostic Testing . . . 150
5.3.6 Complications of SCD . . . 151
5.3.6.1 Vaso-Occlusive Crisis/Episode . . . 151
5.3.6.1.1 Diagnostic Test/Differential Count . . . 152
5.3.6.1.2 Treatment . . . 152
5.3.6.2 Acute Sequestration Crisis . . . 152
5.3.6.3 Aplastic Crisis . . . 152
5.3.6.4 Infection . . . 153
5.3.6.5 Acute Chest Syndrome . . . 154
5.3.6.6 Acute Abdominal Pain . . . 155
5.3.6.7 Acute Central Nervous System Event . . . 155
5.3.6.8 Preparation for Surgery . . . 157
5.3.6.9 Hydroxyurea Therapy . . . 157
5.3.7 Prognosis . . . 158
5.3.8 Future Perspectives . . . 158
5.4 Thalassemia . . . 158
5.4.1 Alpha (α)-Thalassemia . . . 158
5.4.1.1 Epidemiology . . . 158
5.4.1.2 Etiology . . . 158
5.4.1.3 Molecular Genetics . . . 158
5.4.2 Beta Thalassemia (Cooley Anemia) . . . 159
5.4.2.1 Epidemiology . . . 159
5.4.2.2 Etiology . . . 159
5.4.2.3 Molecular Genetics . . . 159
5.4.3 Diagnostic Testing . . . 160
5.4.4 Treatment . . . 160
5.4.5 Treatment of Hemosiderosis (Iron Overload) . . . 160
5.4.6 Chelation Therapy . . . 161
5.4.6.1 Initiation of Chelation Therapy . . . 161
5.4.6.2 Chelation Regimens . . . 161
5.4.6.3 Complications of Chelation Medications . . . 161
5.4.7 Clinical Advances (Hemosiderosis) . . . 161
5.4.8 Prognosis . . . 161
5.4.9 Follow-Up . . . 162
5.4.10 Future Perspectives . . . 162
5.5. Hemolytic Anemia . . . 162
5.5.1 Hereditary Spherocytosis . . . 162
5.5.1.1 Epidemiology . . . 162
5.5.1.2 Etiology . . . 162
5.5.1.3 Molecular Genetics . . . 162
5.5.1.4 Symptoms/Clinical Signs . . . 162
5.5.1.5 Diagnostic Testing . . . 163
5.5.1.6 Treatment . . . 163
5.5.1.7 Prognosis . . . 163
5.5.1.8 Follow-Up . . . 163
5.5.1.9 Future Perspectives . . . 163
5.5.2 Autoimmune Hemolytic Anemia . . . 164
5.5.2.1 Epidemiology . . . 164
5.5.2.2 Etiology . . . 164
5.5.2.3 Molecular Genetics . . . 164
5.5.2.4 Symptoms/Clinical Signs . . . 164
5.5.2.5 Diagnostic Testing . . . 164
5.5.2.6 Treatment . . . 164
5.5.2.7 Prognosis . . . 165
5.5.2.8 Future Perspectives . . . 165
5.5.3 Glucose-6-Phosphate Dehydrogenase Deficiency . . . 165
5.5.3.1 Epidemiology . . . 165
5.5.3.2 Etiology . . . 165

5.5.3.3 Molecular Genetics 165
5.5.3.4 Symptoms/Clinical Signs . . . 166
5.5.3.5 Diagnostic Testing 166
5.5.3.6 Treatment. 166
5.5.3.7 Prognosis 167
5.6 Bone Marrow Failure Syndromes 167
5.6.1 Aplastic Anemia. 167
5.6.1.1 Acquired Aplastic Anemia . . 167
5.6.1.1.1 Epidemiology 167
5.6.1.1.2 Etiology 167
5.6.1.1.3 Molecular Genetics 167
5.6.1.1.4 Symptoms/Clinical Signs 167
5.6.1.1.5 Diagnostic Testing 167
5.6.1.1.6 Treatment 168
5.6.1.1.7 Supportive Treatment 169
5.6.1.1.8 Prognosis 169
5.6.1.2 Inherited Aplastic Anemia . . 169
5.6.1.2.1 Epidemiology 169
5.6.1.2.2 Etiology 169
5.6.1.2.3 Molecular Genetics 169
5.6.1.2.4 Symptoms/Clinical Signs 169
5.6.1.2.5 Diagnostic Testing 169
5.6.1.2.6 Treatment 170
5.6.1.2.7 Prognosis 170
References 170

5.1 Anemia

Anemia is defined as a reduction in the red cell mass due to decreased production, increased loss/decreased survival, or increased destruction of red blood cells (RBCs). As most of the oxygen is transported by the RBCs to the body tissues, a reduction in the red cell mass causes reduced oxygen supply to the body cells. Consequently, anemia is a sign of an underlying pathological process, which is usually discovered during a routine health maintenance visit. The investigation of anemia to determine the underlying diagnosis includes a combination of medical history, family history, physical examination, and the initial laboratory assessment, including the evaluation of the full/complete blood count (FBC/CBC), RBC indices/morphology, reticulocyte count, and the peripheral smear (Table 5.1; Figs. 5.1, 5.2 slide 1). More extensive tests may be needed to verify the diagnosis, such as an iron panel, osmotic fragility, hemoglobin (Hgb) electrophoresis, or a

Table 5.1. Normal RBC values in children (adapted from Pesce 2007, p 2944)

Age	Hemoglobin (g/dL)		MCV (fl)	
	Mean	–2 SD	Mean	–2 SD
Birth (cord blood)	16.5	13.5	108	98
1–3 days (capillary)	18.5	14.5	108	95
1 week	17.5	13.5	107	88
2 weeks	16.5	12.5	105	86
1 month	14.0	10.0	104	85
2 months	11.5	9.0	96	77
3–6 months	11.5	9.5	91	74
0.5–2 years	12.0	10.5	78	70
2–6 years	12.5	11.5	81	75
6–12 years	13.5	11.5	86	77
12–18 years, female	14.0	12.0	90	78
12–18 years, male	14.5	13.0	88	78
18–49 years, female	14.0	12.0	90	80
18–49 years, male	15.5	13.5	90	80

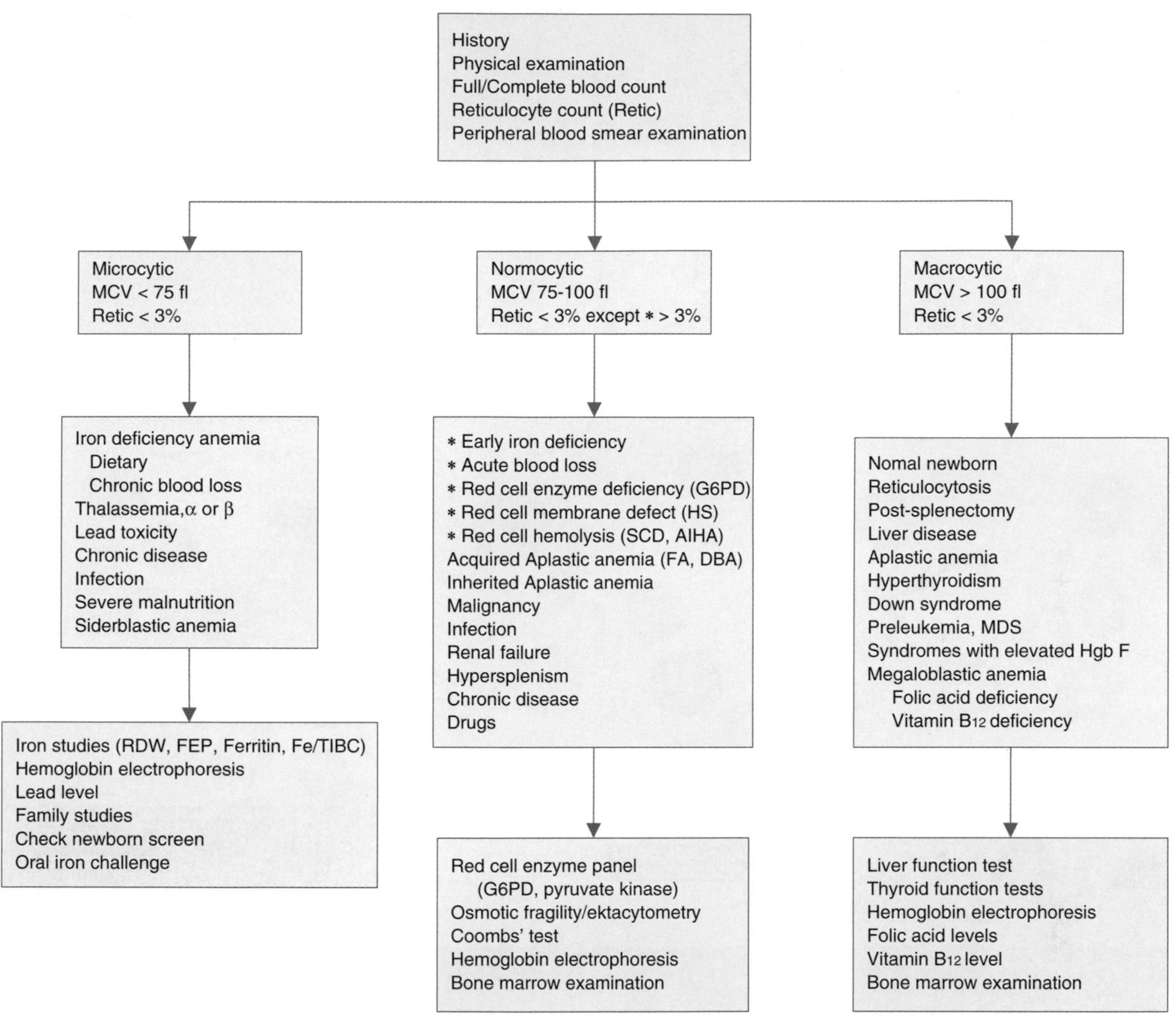

Figure 5.1

The diagnostic approach to the child with anemia

bone marrow examination (Fig. 5.1). It is important to establish whether anemia is related to one cell line (e.g., RBCs, white blood cells [WBCs], or platelets) or multiple cell lines (e.g., RBCs, WBCs, and platelets). If multiple cell lines are affected, this may indicate bone marrow production problem (i.e., leukemia, aplastic anemia, or metastatic disease). If a single cell line is affected, then this usually indicates a peripheral destruction problem such as autoimmune disorders (e.g., immune thrombocytopenic purpura or autoimmune hemolytic anemia).

Anemia is classified into two main categories, which constitute the morphological and etiological (physiological or functional) basis for anemia. The mean corpuscular volume (MCV) and reticulocyte count are the most useful tools for the morphological category. The morphological category classifies the RBC morphology or size into normocytic (normal-size RBC),

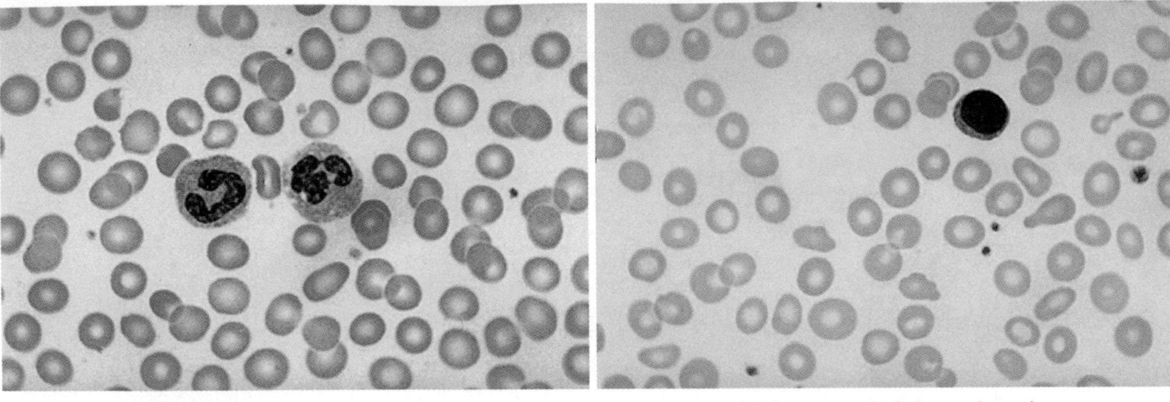

Slide 1: Normal Red Blood Cell

Slide 2: Iron Deficiency Anemia

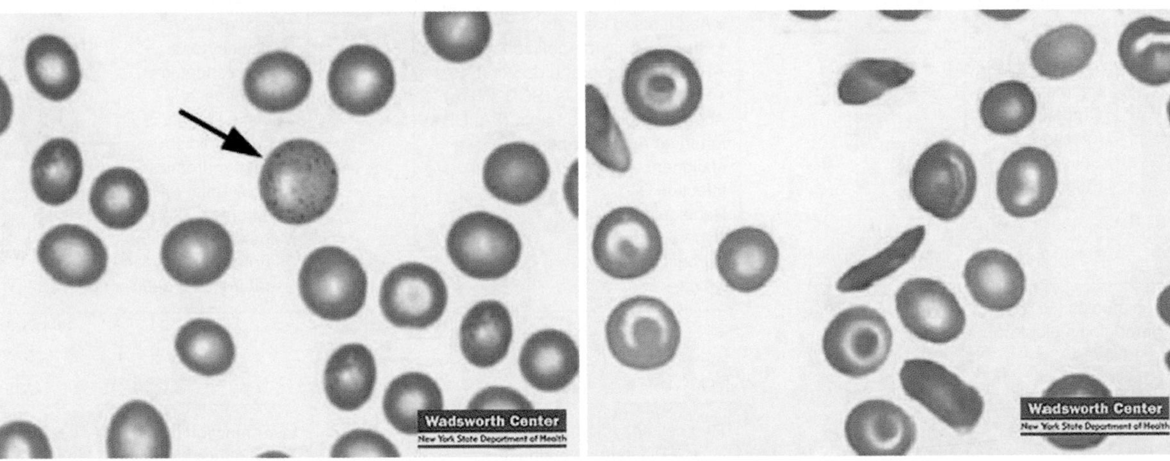

Slide 3: Lead Poisoning

Slide 4: Sickle Cell Anemia

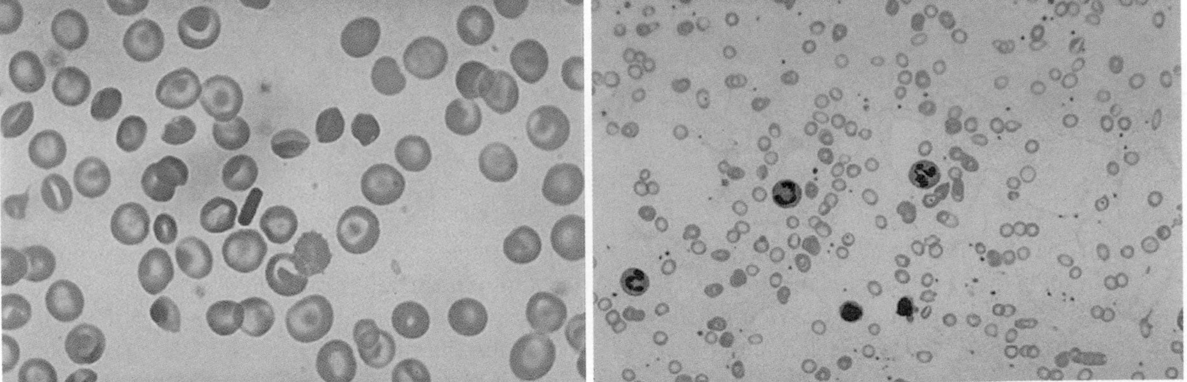

Slide 5: Hemoglobin SC

Slide 6: Thalassemia

Figure 5.2

The diagnostic RBC smears. Courtesy and copyright © of the Clinical Chemistry and Hematology Laboratory, Wadsworth Center, NY State Department of Health (http://www.wadsworth.org/chemheme)

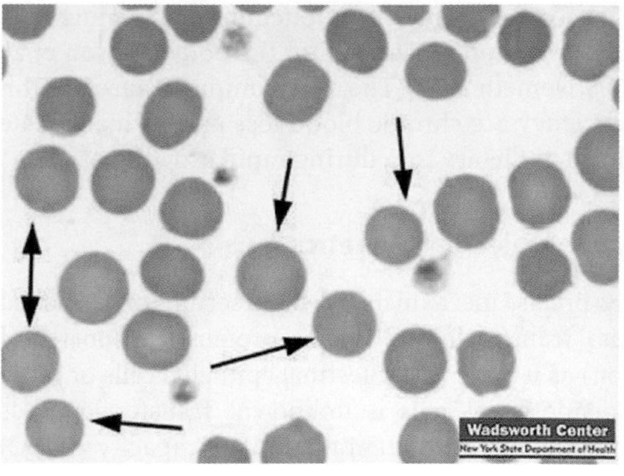

Slide 7: Hereditary Spherocytosis

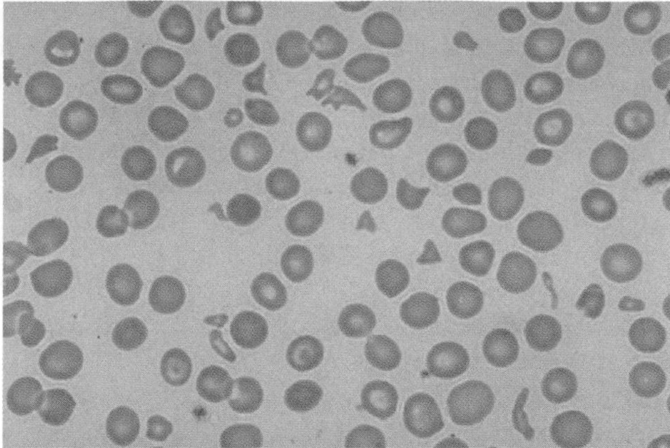

Slide 8: Autoimmune Hemolytic

Figure 5.2
(Continued)

microcytic (smaller than normal RBC), and macrocytic (larger than normal-size RBC) anemias correlated with the reticulocyte count (Fig. 5.1).

These categories are not mutually exclusive for a given type of anemia because anemia may present as normocytic and then revert to macrocytic or develop a combination of RBC sizes. Reticulocytes are immature RBCs released from the bone marrow into the circulating blood which indicate either an adequate or inadequate production of RBCs. The etiological category is divided according to (1) decreased or ineffective production of RBCs, (2) destruction of RBCs, or (3) loss of RBCs. Generally, in the etiological category, there is one basis for anemia, but some anemias may have more than one basis.

Iron-deficiency anemia (IDA) may have more than one basis and more than one morphological presentation (Fig. 5.1). The usual etiological category for IDA is decreased production of RBCs; however, this anemia may also develop because of an increased loss of RBCs. Iron deficiency is usually morphologically classified as microcytic anemia with reticulocytopenia (decreased number of immature RBCs), yet early iron deficiency is classified as normocytic anemia with a slight reticulocytosis (increased number of immature RBCs) (Fig. 5.1).

Sickle cell hemoglobinopathies represent a group of genetic diseases that are all related to the presence of Hgb S. The most common type of sickle cell disease (SCD) is homozygous Hgb SS, which is morphologically classified as normocytic anemia when oxygenated, and as macrocytic anemia in the presence of reticulocytosis. Hgb SS is defined as a protein substitution on the β-globin gene that causes destruction of RBCs.

Thalassemia is a type of anemia that lacks alpha or beta production and is therefore etiologically classified as ineffective RBC production. Morphologically, thalassemic RBCs are classified as microcytic anemia with reticulocytopenia.

Hemolytic anemias are divided into intracorpuscular defects (e.g., glucose-6-phosphate dehydrogenase deficiency [G-6PD], hereditary spherocytosis) and extracorpuscular defects (e.g., autoimmune hemolytic anemia) that cause RBC destruction. Hemolytic anemia is morphologically classified as normocytic, but if it has more than 20% reticulocytes, it is classified as macrocytic.

Lastly, aplastic anemia (AA), which is a bone marrow failure syndrome, is divided into inherited (e.g., Fanconi's anemia [FA], Diamond-Blackfan anemia) or acquired anemia (e.g., moderate or severe), characterized by reduced or absent production of RBCs, WBCs, and platelets. Morphologically, it is classified as normocytic, but most often it is considered as macrocytic anemia with reticulocytopenia. The macrocytosis develops because of stress erythropoiesis, which produces erythrocytes with fetal characteristics that tend to be more pronounced in the inherited types of AA (Bessler et al. 2009).

5.2 Iron-Deficiency Anemia

IDA is defined as a reduction in the red cell mass due to decreased production and/or loss of RBCs (Fig. 5.1). Infants usually have adequate iron stores at birth, unless they were born prematurely or maternal iron stores were inadequate. The iron stores of full-term infants gradually deplete in about 4 months unless replenished with iron-fortified formula or breast milk supplemented with iron.

5.2.1 Epidemiology

IDA, as the most common form of nutritional deficiency, is a major public health problem affecting 30% of the global population with the majority living primarily in developing countries (Glader 2007). In developing countries, IDA is attributed to nutritional deficiency that tends to worsen by chronic blood loss associated with parasitic infections such as hockworm infestation (Glader 2007). Although the prevalence of IDA has declined during infancy in the United States, it is highest among young children between the ages of 12 months and 3 years, and in women of childbearing age (particularly adolescent girls and pregnant women). The increased susceptibility to IDA within these age groups is primarily due to their increased demand for iron with a decreased iron intake.

5.2.2 Etiology

Iron is present in all body cells. Iron balance is maintained between dietary intake (approximately 10% elemental iron is absorbed in the duodenum and jejunum) and iron loss (from sloughing of the skin and mucosal cells). As there is no organ that regulates iron excretion, the majority of dietary iron that is absorbed from the duodenum and jejunum is conserved and reused within the body (Edison et al. 2008, Nemeth 2008). The most common causes of iron deficiency are chronic blood loss and/or inadequate intake of dietary iron during rapid growth periods.

5.2.3 Molecular Genetics

The precise mechanism by which serum iron is loaded onto transferrin (the major protein transporter of iron) as it leaves the intestinal epithelial cells or reticuloendothelial cells is unknown. Transferrin binds with the iron (total iron binding capacity = TIBC) and releases the iron into the cell. Once inside the cell, the iron conjugates with free erythrocyte portoporphyrins (FEP or EP) to form heme, and binds with the globin protein to form Hgb. The Hgb attracts the oxygen and carries it to the body cells for metabolism. The remaining iron is stored as ferritin (soluble protein) or hemosiderin (an insoluble protein complex). Both of these complexes are found in the liver, bone marrow, spleen, and skeletal muscles. Reticuloendothelial cells acquire iron primarily by phagocytosis and breakdown of aging red cells. The iron is then extracted from the heme and returned to the circulation to bind to transferrin and to repeat the cycle.

5.2.4 Symptoms/Clinical Signs

Iron deficiency produces microcytic, hypochromic anemia that impairs tissue oxygen transport to the body cells and may cause weakness, fatigue, palpitations, lightheadedness, pallor, lethargy, tachycardia, and tachypnea that may be detected on physical examination, and while obtaining a thorough history. Pica, a craving for unusual substances such as starch, clay, toilet paper, and paint chips, may be detected during the history and is frequently associated with IDA. Adolescents and children less than 36 months are at the highest risk for developing IDA. Severe IDA is associated with impairment of growth and intellectual development, and may cause decreased motor activity and social interaction. The lack of iron causes damage to the epithelial cells, which has been associated with gastrointestinal blood loss and/or increased absorption of heavy metals including lead (Andrews et al. 2009). Thus, iron deficiency may enhance lead absorption and inadvertently cause lead toxicity in children who ingest lead-containing substances such as soil and lead paint chips. Lead is toxic to the bone marrow and affects erythropoiesis by interfering with the heme synthetic pathway in all cells (Glader 2007, Richardson 2007).

5.2.5 Diagnostic Testing

A blood smear may reveal microcytic, hypochromic (decreased iron content) RBCs with poikilocytosis (varying red cell shapes), anisocytosis (different red cell sizes), and target cells (which resemble a bull's eye target; Fig. 5.2 slide 2). The lead poisoning smear differs from iron deficiency by the presence of coarse basophilic stippling (coarse granules studding the cytoplasm; Fig. 5.2 slide 3) with microcytic hypochromic RBCs. In contrast, a chronic disease anemia smear consists primarily of normocytic and normochromic RBCs with approximately 20% of microcytic cells.

The iron status of the body can be assessed using several laboratory tests. During mild iron deficiency (Hgb >10 g/dL) when the stores are depleted, Hgb may not decrease. Elevated FEP has been used as a screening test for early iron deficiency. The FEP is also elevated in lead poisoning, but usually to a greater level than in iron deficiency. Moderate iron deficiency occurs with a decreased Hgb of 6–10 g/dL and decreased MCV, compared with the age-matched results. Severe iron deficiency is associated with decreased Hgb (<6 g/dL) and decreased MCV compared with age-matched results (Table 5.1).

The test most commonly used regardless of whether iron deficiency is mild, moderate, or severe is the Hgb/hematocrit (Hct) concentration. Although Hgb concentration and Hct cannot be used to determine the cause of anemia, if Hgb concentration or Hct increases after a course of therapeutic iron supplementation, the diagnosis of IDA can be made even with mild iron deficiency (Segel et al. 2002). A newly evaluated screening tool known as reticulocyte hemoglobin content (CHr) can also detect iron deficiency with or without anemia and efficiently predict iron-treatment response (Brugnara et al. 2006, Kim et al. 2008, Mateos et al. 2008). CHr is an iron-containing protein within the reticulocyte that can be measured using the flow cytometer (Brugnara et al. 2006). Other laboratory tests (including decreased reticulocytes, increased RBC distribution width [RDW], decreased serum iron, decreased transferrin saturation, elevated total iron binding capacity [TIBC], positive guaiac, and Hgb electrophoresis) can be used to differentiate IDA from anemia of other causes. Serum ferritin concentration is an early indicator of iron-store depletion, yet is also an acute-phase reactant to chronic infection, inflammation, or diseases, which may obscure the results. The MCV and reticulocyte count (retic count) are the most useful tools for the classification of anemias (Fig. 5.1). A decreased MCV, retic count, and RBC with increased RDW may indicate IDA, whereas a decreased MCV, retic count, and increased or normal RBC with normal RDW may indicate thalassemia minor (Demir et al. 2002). To accurately differentiate between IDA and thalassemia minor, a total iron status and hemoglobin A_2 should be attained (Beyan et al. 2007).

There are nutritional anemias that affect normal red cell production that should be differentiated from iron deficiency (Fig. 5.1). As a common worldwide anemia associated with malnutrition, megaloblastic anemia (B_{12} and folate deficiency) may coexist with IDA. Vitamin B_{12} deficiency may develop in the child on a strict vegetarian diet or in the totally breastfed infant by a strict vegetarian mother. A child is usually treated with cobalamin injections 100 µg/24 h for 10–15 days, and then changed to a maintenance dose of at least 60 µg/month (Lee et al. 2008).In children with inherited defects of cobalamin metabolism, the usual dose is 1,000 µg 2–3 times weekly (Carmel 2008;Watkins et al. 2009). For adolescents and adults with poor dietary cobalamin intake, a cobalamin injection of 30–100 µg/day for 5–10 days is administered, and then changed to 100–200 µg monthly as the maintenance dose with the addition of B_{12} dietary sources (Lee et al. 2008, Watkins et al. 2009). Recently, oral and parenteral cobalamin therapy were compared and found to yield comparable benefits (Butler et al. 2006). Indeed oral therapy with 1 to 2 mg cobalamin daily is cheaper and better tolerated and has become standard treatment in many countries (Watkins et al. 2009). The folic acid dose is 50 mg/day for infants and 1 mg/day for children/adolescents, coupled with dietary counseling, to promote intake of foods containing folic acid.

5.2.6 Treatment

- Treatment requires the identification of the cause of IDA, whether its due to blood loss from intestinal inflammation/malabsorption, surgery, or medications (e.g., chemotherapy, anticonvulsants) and/or lack of adequate iron intake.
- The oral iron dose is 4–6 mg/day elemental iron/kg/day divided bid or tid for children/infants, and 60–120 mg/day for adolescents. Iron preparations should be given with vitamin C-fortified juice or with water because vitamin C promotes iron absorption from the gastrointestinal tract. Iron should not be taken with milk, milk products, or antacids because they interfere with iron absorption.
- Iron-fortified cereal (two or more servings) should be added daily to the diet of the full-term infant, beginning about 4–6 months after birth.
- *Preterm or low birth weight* infants who are exclusively breastfed should take iron drops of 2–4 mg/kg/day beginning 2–3 months after birth until the age of 12 months.
- The use of low-iron milk (cow, goat, or soy) should be discouraged until after the age of 12 months.
- The intake of solid foods that are rich in iron should be encouraged in children, along with a decrease in milk consumption to <16–24 oz daily.
- Dietary counseling regarding the intake of iron-rich foods (e.g., meats, bran, lentils, beans, nuts, and some green leafy vegetables) should be reinforced.
- Iron treatment should be continued until iron stores are replenished (approximately 4–6 months of oral iron therapy after Hgb is normalized). The side effects of iron therapy should be explained to the child and parents; these include gastrointestinal discomfort, constipation, bloating, stained teeth (to prevent, give liquid iron with a straw), and dark/black stools.

Parenteral iron replacement is

- Used when the patient is unable to ingest oral iron or absorb iron from the gastrointestinal tract
- Available in the United States as iron dextran (elemental iron), and administered intramuscularly (IM) using the z-track technique, or intravenously (IV). The preferable route is IV because the IM injection causes pain and skin discoloration
- Composed of iron dextran and contains 50 mg elemental iron per milliliter. The dose of iron (mL) is calculated by 0.0442 × lean body weight(LBW) (kg) × (desired increment Hgb (g/dL) – observed Hb) + (0.26 × LBW) (kg) (Andrews et al. 2009). A peak reticulocytosis will usually occur 10 days after parenteral iron is given, with complete correction of anemia in 3–4 weeks
- Given as a test dose of 12.5–25 mg, with the observation of the patient for 30–60 min after the dose
- Associated with adverse effects such as anaphylaxis, fever, hypotension, rash, myalgias, and arthralgias
- Not recommended for very low birth weight infants (e.g., <1,500 g and premature) for routine use, because it does not have a major impact on transfusion requirements (Stoll 2007)
- Used in conjunction with recombinant human erythropoietin to decrease transfusion requirements in chronic anemias associated with a wide range of diseases (Auerbach 2007).

5.2.7 Transfusion

Depending on whether the child is hemodynamically stable, children with severe anemia (Hgb <5 g/dL) may require red cell transfusion. Common practice is to administer the red cells slowly (2–3 mL/kg/h) in multiple small volumes (aliquots) with careful monitoring of vital signs and fluid balance to prevent pulmonary edema and congestive heart failure (Glader 2007).

5.2.8 Erythropoietin (Epogen)

Recombinant human erythropoietin (rhEPO) may be used as a treatment for mild to moderate anemia to stimulate the proliferation and differentiation of erythroid precursors (Jelkmann 2008). The usual subcutaneous dose is 150–300 IU/kg one to three times a week. Sufficient erythroid precursors must be in the bone marrow with adequate iron stores and protein intake for erythropoietin to be effective (Carley 2003). A common practice is to administer 3 mg/kg/day of supplemental iron concurrently. Erythropoietin has shown efficacy in the treatment of anemia of prematurity and in renal failure, and is being investigated as a treatment for transient bone marrow suppression induced by cancer therapy. Even though there are no proven indications to use rhEPO during cancer therapy, it has been used to decrease the need for transfusion in children with anemia associated with chemotherapy and radiation therapy (Aygun 2005).

5.2.9 Prognosis

Once detected, iron deficiency and other nutritional anemias generally respond positively to supplementation. Follow-up Hgb that fails to show improvement within 4–8 weeks after supplementing with oral iron medication and dietary iron, or an anemia that recurs despite adequate supplementation warrant further investigation (Segel et al. 2002). Further investigation may include examination for disorders such as malignancy, copper deficiency and other anemias, inborn errors of iron metabolism, or other rare disorders.

5.3 Sickle Cell Disease

Sickle cell hemoglobinopathies represent a group of genetic hemolytic anemias that are all related to the presence of Hgb S. SCD consist of two abnormal genes that include several hemoglobin genotypes, such as SS, SC, S-Beta (SB) Thalassemia, and many others. Sickle cell trait with one abnormal gene (Hgb AS) is a benign condition that involves mostly Hgb A with approximately 35–45% of Hgb S. Although complications are rare in Hgb AS, they have been described and include an increased incidence of hematuria and hyposthenuria. Vaso-occlusive crisis has also been reported, especially under hypoxic conditions such as shock, strenuous physical activity,at high elevations,and flying in an unpressurized aircraft.

5.3.1 Epidemiology

SCD has been recognized as a worldwide problem. It is the most common hereditary disorder in the United States with 70,000–100,000 cases reported primarily in African-Americans (Heeney and Ware 2008). SCD affects a variety of nationalities worldwide, including Africans, Hispanics, Arabs, Italians, Native Americans, Caribbeans, Iranians, Turks, and many others.

5.3.2 Etiology

SCD is transmitted as an incomplete autosomal-dominant trait (Karayalcin 2005). When both parents carry the sickle cell trait (heterozygous gene or Hgb AS), there is a 25% chance of producing an infant with SCD with each pregnancy (homozygous gene – Hgb SS or heterozygous Hgb S variant). The incidence of the sickle cell trait is about 8% in African-Americans in the United States, whereas it has been reported to be 40% among West Africans.

5.3.3 Molecular Genetics

The molecular defect in Hgb SS occurs due to the substitution of valine for glutamic acid in the sixth position of chromosome 11 of the β-globin chain. The second most common type of SCD is Hgb SC (heterozygous variant), in which the lysine is substituted for the glutamic acid at the sixth position of the β-chain. Other Hgb S variants include a combination of Hgb S trait and β-thalassemia trait, either producing Hgb SB thalassemia (no normal β-globin production) or Hgb SB^+ thalassemia (decreased β-globin production). Another frequently observed variant is the combination of Hgb SS with α-thalassemia trait (usually two or three functional α-globin genes).

5.3.4 Symptoms/Clinical Signs

The basic pathophysiology of sickle cell is directly related to the abnormal Hgb S that polymerizes when deoxygenated. Sickle cell adhesion to vascular endothelium is the nidus for vaso-occlusion that set in motion the abnormal adhesion–inflammation-increased adhesion of the sickling cycle (Redding-Lallinger and Knoll 2006). Most of the complications of SCD are the result of sickling adhesion–inflammation cycle with entanglement and enmeshing of the sticky, rigid, sickle-shaped cells as they block the

Table 5.2. Diagnostic tests used in SCD

Test	Interval
Baseline CBC, differential, and reticulocyte count, pulse oximetry	Each visit
Red cell minor antigen phenotype	Visit at 6 months of age
Hgb electrophoresis	Confirmatory 2–6 months, 2 years of age, and if needed, at 5 years of age
Renal and hepatitis function tests, amylase, lipase, LDH, liver function tests, urinalysis	Yearly, but more often if abnormal
Human immunodeficiency virus	Yearly posttransfusion
Blood cultures	If febrile ≥38.5°C
Transcranial cerebral ultrasonography	Yearly (start at the age of 2 until 16 years in Hgb SS or comparable sickle hemoglobinopathy)
Pulmonary function tests	Age of 8 and every 2 years unless abnormal
Electrocardiography/echocardiography	Every 2 years unless abnormal
Abdominal ultrasonography	Age of 8–10 or if symptomatic or
Audiogram	Age of 8–10 or if symptomatic
Plain films, MRI of hips/shoulders	Symptomatic
MRI/angiography of brain as needed	Symptomatic
Neuropsychological testing	Age of 6 and repeated as necessary

microcirculation, causing partial to complete vaso-occlusion of vessels. The resultant decreased blood flow to the tissues causes ischemia and infarction which may result in further complications. A thorough history, physical examination, and diagnostic tests tend to identify existing complications (Table 5.2).

5.3.5 Diagnostic Testing

The following descriptions of peripheral blood smears are correlated with the type of SCD:

- The typical Hgb SS smear contains mild to moderate normochromic, normocytic to macrocytic cells with sickled cells and increased anisocytosis and poikilocytosis (Fig. 5.2 slide 4). The average Hgb range is 5–9 g/dL, with an average reticulocytosis from 5 to more than 20%
- The Hgb SC smear contains normochromic, normocytic cells with sickle cells, target cells, and spherocytes (Fig. 5.2 slide 5). The Hgb SC average Hgb range is 9–12 g/dL, with an average reticulocyte count between normal and 10%
- The Hgb SB thalassemia and Hgb SA thalassemia smears contain marked microcytosis, and moderate to marked sickle cells with anisocytosis and poikilocytosis. The average Hgb and reticulocytosis are commensurate with Hgb SS
- The Hgb SB^+ thalassemia smear contains moderate microcytosis, sickle-shaped cells with anisocytosis and poikilocytosis. The average Hgb is 9–12 g/dL with 5–10% reticulocytosis

The differential diagnoses include disorders such as hereditary spherocytosis (HS), G-6PD, pyruvate kinase, thalassemia, leukemia, and juvenile rheumatoid arthritis, which can all be excluded by obtaining the Hgb electrophoresis (Table 5.3).

About 2,000 infants with SCD born yearly in the United States are identified by neonatal screening (AAP 2002). Neonatal screening is included in most

Table 5.3. Neonatal hemoglobin patterns (adapted from DeBaun and Vichinsky 2007, p 462)

Screening phenotype	Confirmed electrophoresis	Possible genotype
FA	Normal newborn pattern	Hgb AA
FAS	Benign sickle cell trait	Hgb AS
FAC	Benign Hgb C trait	Hgb AC
FAA2	Benign β-thalassemia trait	Hgb AA2
FS	Fetal and sickle Hgb S	Homozygous Hgb SS or Hgb SB thalassemia or Hgb SB+ thalassemia
FSC	Hgb S and Hgb C	Hgb SC
FSAA2	Heterozygous Hgb SB+ thalassemia	Hgb SB+ thalassemia
F	Fetal Hgb F or Hgb F with delayed Hgb A	Homozygous β-thalassemia major or homozygous
	Appearance	Hereditary persistence of fetal Hgb F
FA Barts	Fetal Hgb, Hgb A, and Barts Hgb (ranges from 1–2% to 30%)	β-thalassemia silent carrier
		β-thalassemia trait
		Hgb H disease
AF	May indicate prior blood transfusion	Retest 4 months posttransfusion

Hemoglobin variants are reported in the order of decreasing abundance; for example, FA indicates more fetal than adult Hgb. Repeat hemoglobin electrophoresis should be done to confirm original interpretation

state screening programs to identify sickle and thalassemic hemoglobinopathies (Table 5.3).

5.3.6 Complications of SCD

The chronic destruction of the RBCs in SCD results in acute and chronic complications; however, this chapter will focus primarily on the acute complications of SCD. Complications of SCD may occur suddenly and can rapidly become severe; therefore, the medical provider should consult with a hematologist. The most common complication, which is usually not life-threatening, is vaso-occlusive crisis or episode (VOE). Other complications that will be discussed are acute sequestration, aplastic crisis, infection, acute chest syndrome, acute abdominal pain, and acute central nervous system events. Chronic complications associated with SCD include avascular necrosis of the head of the femur/humerus, priapism, retinopathy, and leg ulcers (rare in children).

5.3.6.1 Vaso-Occlusive Crisis/Episode

- Definition: VOE occurs when deoxygenated sticky, rigid sickled-shaped RBCs adhere to vascular endothelium causing inflammation and blockage of microcirculation completely or partially (infarction) causing tissue ischemia or necrosis.
- Signs and symptoms of VOE: Most children with sickle cell anemia experience some degree of acute pain and may express their pain verbally, by crying, grimacing, maintaining a stoic expression, or in a variety of other ways.

Most of the children are able to describe their severity of pain by using self-reporting methods such as the Faces pain scale or the numeric pain scale. Other behavioral indicators may be helpful in the pain assessment of all children, including infants, such as limited movement of a body part, decreased appetite, or increased irritability. The bones and joints are the major pain sites with tenderness, erythema, warmth, and frequent swelling. The initial site of pain in young children and infants is usually the small bones of the hands and feet, called dactylitis or hand/foot syndrome, and may be accompanied by swelling, erythema, and increased warmth. Severe complications may develop after repeated hip/shoulder infarctions (i.e., avascular necrosis of the fibula, femur, or humerus, known as AVN) or repeated skeletal vertebrae infarctions (i.e., lordosis, scoliosis, or kyphosis). Another VOE known as priapism may develop as a painful engorgement of the penis due to sickling in the sinusoids of the corpora cavenosa. Acute multiorgan system failure (AMOF) can also develop during VOE, in which at least two organ systems fail (lungs,kidneys,or liver). AMOF is a widespread vaso-occlusion that can be fatal unless erythrocytaphersis (exchange transfusion) is aggressively implemented.

5.3.6.1.1 Diagnostic Test/Differential Count

A complete blood count, RBC indices, WBC count and differential count, reticulocyte count, renal and liver function tests, and, if needed, bone radiographs are usually carried out during severe VOE. The differential includes VOE vs. osteomyelitis, which is difficult to differentiate because both are associated with erythema and swelling, low-grade fevers, and joint and bone pain. Osteomyelitis may be excluded by clinical observation, blood cultures, and, occasionally, by aspiration of the affected area.

5.3.6.1.2 Treatment

Hydration (oral or IV), opioids and NSAIDS (oral or IV), incentive spirometry, adjuvant therapy (e.g., laxative and antipruritic medications), rest, heat and massage on painful areas, and exercises or diversional activities (school work, friends, meditation, guided imagery) are useful interventions for VOE. Whether VOE is managed by patient-controlled analgesia (PCA) or orally, the pain assessment prior and after treatment should be closely monitored to achieve optimal pain management (Fig. 5.3).

5.3.6.2 Acute Sequestration Crisis

- Definition: Acute splenic sequestration is a sudden, rapid enlargement of the spleen with trapping of a considerable portion of the red cell mass, leading to acute exacerbation of anemia that drops the Hgb level to 2 g/dL or less below the baseline.
- Signs and symptoms: Sudden weakness, dyspnea, rapidly distending abdomen (spleen or liver enlarging), abdominal pain, lethargy, irritability, pallor, vomiting, headache, tachycardia, and tachypnea are manifestations of acute sequestration. Severe cases of splenic sequestration may lead to circulatory collapse (shock) and death.
- Diagnostic tests: The level of Hct may drop to half the patient's usual value. Brisk reticulocytosis with increased nucleated red cells, moderate to severe thrombocytopenia, and leukopenia may be present on the smear.
- Treatment: Volume expansion with a fluid bolus and oxygen supplementation are needed immediately. Immediate yet slow transfusion of small aliquots packed RBCs (PRBCs) to restore the intravascular volume and oxygen-carrying capacity may be instituted. Prevention of further recurrences is achieved by elective splenectomy after the first major or second minor episode of sequestration, preferably in children over 2 years of age.
- Education: Parents should be taught splenic palpation and educated about recognizing the signs and symptoms of splenic sequestration to aid in identifying initial episodes of acute sequestration and preventing recurrent life-threatening episodes.

5.3.6.3 Aplastic Crisis

- Definition: Temporary cessation of erythropoeisis due to suppression by viral or bacterial infection causes a drop in Hct with significant reticulocytopenia. Parvovirus B19 is the most common cause of aplastic crisis (Driscoll 2007).
- Signs/symptoms: Increased pallor, icteric sclera, lethargy, irritability, headache, bone pain, weakness, nausea and vomiting, and dark urine are all manifestations of aplastic crisis.
- Diagnostic tests: The Hct decreases as much as 10–15% per day with no compensatory reticulocytosis.
- Treatment: Isolation precautions with oxygen supplementation may be instituted depending on

the type of infection. Transfusion of PRBCs may be instituted to prevent congestive heart failure. Folic acid should be given in the recovery phase.

5.3.6.4 Infection

- Definition: The major risk factor for increased susceptibility to infection is splenic dysfunction. The ability of the spleen to clear particles from the intravascular space and provide antibody synthesis is impaired in patients with SCD. Insidious progressive fibrosis of the spleen (autosplenectomy) occurs in the Hgb SS child, usually by the age of 6 years. Children with splenic dysfunction are 300–600 times more likely to develop overwhelming pneumococcal or *Haemophilus influenzae* sepsis and meningitis than those without splenic dysfunction (Karayalcin 2005).
- Signs/symptoms: Toxic-appearing children with fever higher than 38.5°C, chills, lethargy, irritability, tachypnea, tachycardia, hypoxia, and history of prior sepsis should be treated promptly with parenteral antibiotics after obtaining a blood culture.
- Diagnostic tests: A CBC with differential, C-reactive protein (CRP), cultures of blood, throat, and urine; chest X-ray, and oxygen saturation should be carried out. If the chest X-ray shows an infiltrate, a sputum culture should be obtained if possible. After obtaining the blood culture, the child should be started on parenteral antibiotics and admitted to the hospital. If osteomyelitis is suspected, an orthopedic specialist should be consulted regarding needle aspiration and culture of the suspected bone site.
- Treatment: A child with SCD and a fever higher than 38.5°C must be considered an emergency case, because of the increased risk of overwhelming sepsis resulting from splenic dysfunction.

Children with SCD who have a low risk of sepsis (no high-risk factors) are treated with outpatient management in most comprehensive sickle cell centers in the United States, with close follow-up care (e.g., return clinic visits or telephone contact) (Driscoll 2007). After obtaining the blood cultures, these children are given long-acting parenteral antibiotics such as ceftriaxone (50–75 mg/kg/dose, with a maximum dose of 2 g). If the child is allergic to cephalosporin, clindamycin 15 mg/kg is given with a maximum dose of 600 mg. These children are monitored in the clinic or emergency center for several hours prior to being discharged with close follow-up care.

A SCD child without high-risk factors (Table 5.4) is discharged on oral antibiotics for 3 days while awaiting blood culture results. The child is prescribed cefprozil 30 mg/kg/day divided twice daily, or Pediazole 40 mg/kg/day three times daily if the child is allergic to cephalosporin. Any positive culture obtained from a child being managed on an outpatient basis requires immediate hospitalization and reevaluation of the child. High-risk factors that prevent children from being eligible for outpatient management are listed in Table 5.4.

- Prevention: Morbidity and mortality rates have decreased dramatically since the advent of established newborn screening programs (United States), widespread penicillin prophylaxis, timely

Table 5.4. High risk factors that require hospital admission

High risk factors
Clinically ill-appearing or toxic-looking
Signs of cardiovascular and/or pulmonary compromise
Age less than 12 months
Temperature ≥40°C
White blood count <5,000/mm^3 or >30,000/mm^3
Platelet count <100,000
Hemoglobin <5 g/dL or reticulocyte count <4%
Dehydration with poor oral fluid intake
Pulmonary infiltrate and/or previous history of acute chest syndrome
Pulse oximetry <92% or 3% below baseline
Central venous catheter
Prior splenectomy
History of previous sepsis
Evidence of acute SCD complications
Prior noncompliance or evidence of inability to comply with outpatient follow-up

administration of immunizations, and parental/caregiver education. Parental/caregiver education is aimed at reducing bacterial septicemia and includes such interventions as immediate medical evaluation of febrile illness (≥38.5°C), twice-daily oral administration of prophylactic antibiotic, and compliance with immunization schedules. In addition to standard immunizations, the SCD patient should also receives the 23-valent pneumococcal vaccine, the meningococcal vaccine at 2 years of age with boosters at 5 and 10 years of age, and recommended yearly influenza virus vaccines at the age of 6 months and older. Prophylactic penicillin is started at 2 months of age and continued until 5 years of age. Continuation of penicillin prophylaxis should be considered for children beyond 5 years of age with a history of pneumococcal sepsis or splenectomy because of to the increased risk of recurrent infection (DeBaun and Vichinsky 2007). Currently, the child with SCD is administered prophylactic penicillin 125 mg twice daily, starting at 2 months of age and increased to 250 mg twice daily at 3 years of age. If the child is allergic to penicillin, then erythromycin is substituted at a dosage of 20 mg/kg orally twice daily (Redding-Lallinger and Knoll 2006, AAP 2002). Benzathinepenicillin G, 300,000 U IM, may be given monthly to the SCD patient with gastrointestinal dysfunction or who is noncompliant with oral antibiotic prophylaxis.

5.3.6.5 Acute Chest Syndrome

- Definition: Acute chest syndrome (ACS) is a common cause of morbidity and mortality in children with SCD and is characterized by a new infiltrate on chest X-ray with fever,pain, and/or respiratory signs and symptoms.
- Signs/symptoms: Clinical manifestations of ACS may include extremity pain, rib or sternal pain, abdominal and chest pain, cough, dyspnea, fever (≥38.5°C), back pain, tachypnea, wheezing, hypoxia (paO_2 <75 mmHg or 3 points of transcutaneous oxygen saturation below baseline), shortness of breath (SOB), dyspnea, dullness (palpation), or normal auscultation (Rackoff et al. 1993, Karayalcin 2005)
- Diagnostic tests: Chest radiography may be clear initially but should be repeated with increasing respiratory distress or hypoxia. Blood cultures, CBC, differential, reticulocyte count, type and crossmatch, and, if possible, sputum cultures and arterial blood gases should be obtained. It is extremely difficult to differentiate between ACS and pneumonia. The most common organism causing ACS or pneumonia is pneumococcus (Vichinsky et al. 2000). Other organisms that cause ACS are *Salmonella*, *Klebsiella*, *Haemophilus influenzae*, and *Mycoplasma pneumoniae*, as well as viruses. Martin and Buonomo (1997) reported that pulmonary infiltrates resolve quickly and dramatically in children with ACS not associated with infection, whereas those with infection have a prolonged radiographic course.
- Treatment: Patients may deteriorate rapidly, with progression to pulmonary failure and death; therefore, all patients with ACS should be treated in the hospital. Early recognition of respiratory distress (cough, chest pain, hypoxia with or without fever) and aggressive treatment with oxygen if hypoxic, analgesics, empiric antibiotics, maintenance of IV hydration (1,500 cc/m²/day), bronchodilators, respiratory treatments, and simple RBC transfusion (10 cc/kg) or exchange transfusion are instituted immediately (Table 5.5).

Table 5.5. Treatment for acute chest syndrome

Treatment for acute chest syndrome
Administer oxygen if hypoxic
Monitor continuous pulse oximetry
Encourage incentive spirometry
Administer empiric antibiotics
Cephalosporin (e.g., cefuroxime 150 mg/kg/day divided every 8 h) Macrolide (e.g., azithromycin 10 mg/kg/day with 5 mg/kg/day on days 2–5)
Administer maintenance IV fluids (1,500 cc/m²/day)
Administer analgesic for pain (see algorithm)
Administer PRBCs if hemoglobin <10 g/dL
Simple transfusion (10 cc/kg) Exchange transfusion

Oxygen treatment is monitored closely by pulse oximetry with an ongoing respiratory assessment of the patient. Incentive spirometry is encouraged every hour while awake, with administered analgesics (Fig. 5.3) to prevent hypoventilation. After obtaining the blood culture, empiric antibiotics are given, which include cephalosporins such as cefuroxime 150 mg/kg/day divided every 8 h (maximum dose 2 g) to eradicate possible pathogens such as pneumococcus. A macrolide such as azithromycin 10 mg/kg on day 1 (maximum dose of 500 mg), followed by 5 mg/kg/day on days 2–5 (maximum of 250 mg) is given to treat possible pathogens, such as *Mycoplasma* or *Chlamydia* (Table 5.5). Hydration at maintenance rate (1,500 cc/m^2/day) is administered to avoid overhydration (e.g., pulmonary edema). Bronchodilators such as albuterol aerosols are a common treatment that is given every 4–6 h to decrease airway hyperreactivity. Transfusion of PRBCs as a simple transfusion of 10 cc/kg may be given. However, if the child's respiratory status continues to deteriorate (worsening hypoxia, anemia, chest pain, and worsening infiltrates on chest radiograph), then an exchange transfusion should be performed (Table 5.5).

- Preventive: Risk factors related to ACS include young age (2–4 years), lower concentration of Hgb F, higher steady-state Hgb concentration, higher steady-state WBC count, and a history of asthma and/or previous ACS, should be assessed to help prevent the development of ACS (Caboot and Allen 2008). Strategies to prevent ACS also include aggressive pain management and the use of incentive spirometry to prevent hypoventilation. Children with recurrent ACS should be evaluated by a pulmonologist to determine early development lung disease and pulmonary hypertension (Caboot and Allen 2008, Driscoll 2007).Transfusion is generally recommended to decrease the concentration of Hgb S and can theoretically prevent ACS and pulmonary hypertension (Kato et al. 2007;Quinn and Buchanan 1999). Hydroxyurea (HU) is an agent that is used to upregulate Hgb F and decrease viscosity and sickling of RBC, which decreases the development of ACS and potentially pulmonary hypertension (Vinchinsky 2008). Hematopoietic stem cell transplant is a therapy only available to approximately 18% of SCD patients but is a known cure of SCD (Bhatia and Walters 2008).

5.3.6.6 Acute Abdominal Pain

- Definition: The etiology of acute abdominal pain is unknown, although mesenteric sickling and vertebral disease with nerve root compression have been suggested (Heeney and Dover 2009).
- Signs/symptoms: Guarding, tenderness, rebound, distended abdomen, fever, jaundice, right upper quadrant pain, and constipation are all manifestations of acute abdominal pain.
- Diagnostic tests: CBC with differential, reticulocyte count, liver enzymes, pancreatic enzymes, hepatitis panel, urinalysis, chest/abdominal films including upright views for perforated viscus, ultrasonography, or biliary scans may be instituted to determine the etiology of acute abdominal pain. Differential diagnoses may include ACS, ileus, pneumonia, constipation, surgical abdomen, pancreatitis, urinary tract infection, intrahepatic and intrasplenic sickling, and cholecystitis.
- Treatment: Maintenance of IV fluids (1,500 cc/m^2/day), analgesics (Fig. 5.3), laxatives if constipated, and a surgical consult to rule out surgical abdomen (i.e., appendicitis) are instituted as soon as possible.

5.3.6.7 Acute Central Nervous System Event

- Definition: An acute central nervous system event develops from chronically injured cerebral vessels in which the lumen is narrowed or completely obliterated by sickled erythrocytes, causing acute cerebral infarction. Approximately 11% of SCD (primarily Hgb SS) patients develop acute cerebral vascular occlusion or stroke, most often between the ages of 2 and 10 years. Cerebral infarction may occur as an isolated event or in combination with such disorders as ACS, pneumonia, aplastic crisis, viral illness, painful crisis, priapism, and dehydration.

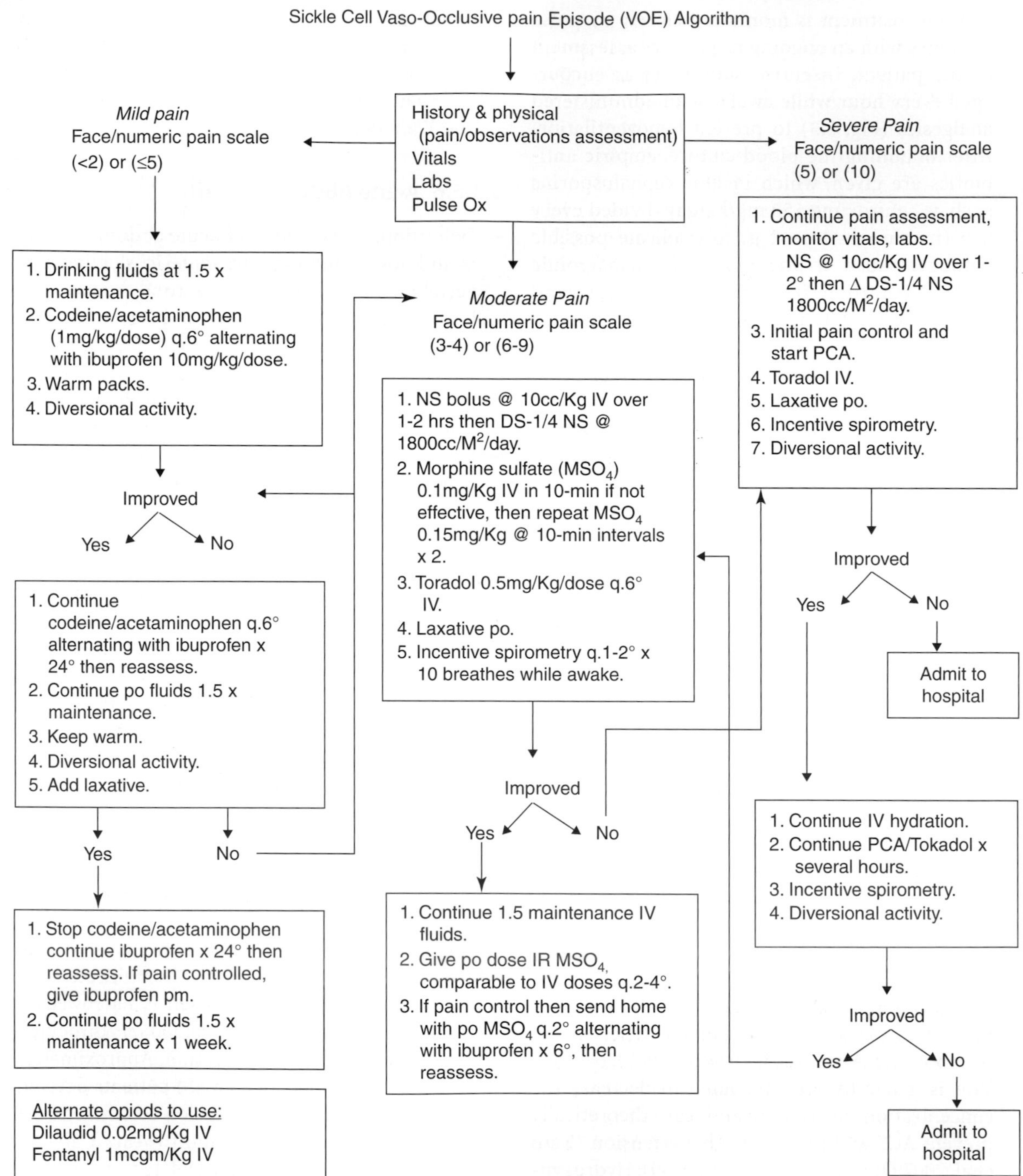

Figure 5.3
Sickle cell VOE algorithm

- Signs/symptoms: Sudden and persistent headache, hemiparesis, hemiplegia, seizures, coma, speech defects, gait dysfunction, visual disturbances, and altered mentation are all manifestations of cerebral infarction.
- Diagnostic test: The initial diagnostic test done is a computed tomography scan (CT scan) of the brain without contrast to identify intracerebral hemorrhage, abscess, tumor, or any other pathology that could explain the symptoms. Magnetic resonance imaging (MRI) and angiography aid in assessment of infarcts associated with obstruction of intracranial vessels (i.e., the anterior and/or middle cerebral vessels), and are usually carried out as soon as possible after CT.
- Treatment: The standard approach to treating a patient with acute cerebral infarction is exchange transfusion (erythrocytapheresis), followed by placement on a maintenance monthly transfusion program. Transfused leukocyte-reduced PRBCs should be sickle-negative and matched for CDE and Kell antigens to reduce alloantibody formation.The transfusion program is designed to maintain the Hgb S level to less than 30%, which lowers the reoccurrence of stroke to 10%. In untreated persons, the mortality rate is approximately 20%, with about 70% of the patients experiencing a recurrence within 3 years of the initial cerebral vascular event (Driscoll 2007; Heeney and Dover 2009). Maintenance monthly transfusion programs are designed to suppress the production of sickle cells, thereby reducing the chance of recurrent strokes. However, multiple transfusions may cause complications such as hemochromatosis, alloimmunization, and infections such as hepatitis, HIV, and West Nile virus. Hemochromatosis is unavoidable with prolong transfusions and is treated with the new oral iron chelator deferasirox or/and parenteral desferrioxamine depending on its severity (Sect. 5.4.6.2)
- Prevention: Transcranial Doppler (TCD) ultrasonography is recommended yearly for children of 2–16 years with severe SCD (e.g., Hgb SS, Hgb SD, HgbS.β Thalassemia). TCD predicts increase risk of stroke in children who have increased abnormal flow velocity (≥200 cm/s) in major cerebral arteries, which is demonstrated on two consecutive TCDs (Adams 2007). In children with abnormal flow velocity, monthly transfusion therapy is recommended owing to the 10% annual risk for developing cerebrovascular accident (Adams et al. 1997, Adams 2007). Neuropsychological testing identifies deficits in intelligence quotient (IQ), which has been instrumental in combination with MRI in discovering SCD children with silent infarcts. Silent infarcts are damage to the brain associated with impaired cognitive abilities secondary to sickling in cerebral vessels without any physical neurological deficits (DeBaun and Vichinsky 2007, Driscoll 2007). Recommendations for the treatment of silent infarcts may include HU therapy, transfusion program, stem cell transplant, or close observation. The best treatment option for silent infarcts is unknown, but the transfusion program is usually recommended as the initial option.

5.3.6.8 Preparation for Surgery

Most children with SCD tolerate chronic anemia well and only require transfusions for severe complications, such as splenic sequestration, CNS infarction/ischemia/hemorrhage, aplastic crisis, severe ACS, and preparation for surgery. As sickling of RBCs is increased during hypoxic periods, it may be necessary to transfuse the patient prior to the surgical procedure that requires anesthesia. If the SCD patient has a history of major complications (e.g., ACS, CNS infarctions, multiple VOE), preoperative transfusion consists of multiple transfusions every 3–4 weeks or exchange transfusion to obtain a goal of less than 30% Hgb S prior to surgery. Exchange transfusion is used to remove sickled cells and replace them with normal cells without increasing blood viscosity. However, if the SCD patient has not sustained any major complications, the patient is transfused to a Hgb of 10 g/dL irrespective of the percentage of Hgb S. A simple transfusion is usually performed 2–5 days prior to the surgical procedure.

5.3.6.9 Hydroxyurea Therapy

- HU is an S-phase-specific cytotoxic agent that upregulates Hgb F, which interferes with Hgb S polymerization and increases the lifespan of the sickled RBCs. HU decreases blood viscosity, has an increase affinity for oxygen, and releases a byproduct known as nitrous oxide that acts as a potent vasodilator. Thus, HU is observed to aid in decreasing sickling and promoting unobstructed circulation.

- Children with SCD complications such as repeated ACS, severe VOE,and neurological deficits are offered HU therapy.
- The initial dose of HU is 15–20 mg/kg/day and is increased to 35 mg/kg/day while monitoring the platelet, neutrophil, and reticulocyte counts (Heeney and Ware 2008, Platt 2008)
- The side effects of HU include neutropenia, leukopenia, reticulocytopenia, elevated liver enzymes, nausea and vomiting, hyperpigmentation, alopecia, and a potential teratogenic, mutagenic and carcinogenic effect. All patients of childbearing age must agree to a contraceptive plan prior to starting HU.

5.3.7 Prognosis

SCD patients without a history of major SCD complications will have lifespans 10–15 years shorter than those without SCD. In an observational study, Miller et al. (2000) found a significant correlation between SCD course and adverse outcomes later in childhood in children who developed dactylitis before the age of 1 year, and had a steady-state of Hgb of less than 7 g/dL and leukocytosis in the absence of infection.

5.3.8 Future Perspectives

- As HU therapy is a lifetime therapy, more studies are needed to determine its long-term safety effects in SCD patients (Heeney and Ware 2008, Steinberg et al. 2003). Ongoing studies will help to answer questions about the proper clinical indications for HU use, its ability to prevent organ damage, preserve organ function, and its long-term safety (Heeney and Ware 2008).
- The allogeneic hematopoietic cell transplantation (HCT), primarily performed in SCD children less than 16 years, from related and compatible donors, have survival rates of more than 90% and event-free survival of 85%(Sonati and Costa 2008). As only a limited number of related umbilical cord blood transplants have been successful, the practice of employing unrelated donors in HCT and umbilical cord blood transplants for SCD is still under investigation (Bhatia and Walters 2008, Pinto and Roberts 2008, Adamkiewicz et al. 2007).
- There are studies focused on gene manipulation to correct and cure the SCD defect. Gene therapy including retroviral vectors that could correct the mutation and integrate permanently with the host genome into the hematopoietic stem cells have been investigated in animal models (Bank 2008).

5.4 Thalassemia

Thalassemia is a group of inherited heterogeneous anemias associated with the absence or decreased production of normal Hgb (Table 5.6). Two broad classifications of thalassemia are the alpha (α) and beta (β) thalassemias, which contain deficits in α- and β-thalassemia globin production, respectively.

5.4.1 Alpha (α)-Thalassemia

5.4.1.1 Epidemiology

The majority of incidences of α-thalassemias are found in Southeast Asia, Malaysia, and Southern China with increasing diagnoses in North America secondary to immigration.

5.4.1.2 Etiology

The deficit in α-globin production is due to the deletion or mutation of one or more of the four α-globin genes located on chromosome 16.

5.4.1.3 Molecular Genetics

More than 30 different mutations affecting α-globin genes have been described (Cunningham 2008, Cunningham et al. 2009):

- Silent carrier has three functional α-globin genes ($-\alpha/\alpha\ \alpha$).

Table 5.6. Classification of thalassemias (adapted from Cunningham et al. 2009)

Syndrome	Phenotypes	Clinical findings
Silent carrier (α- and β-thalassemia)	α: 1–2% Hgb Barts or 1–2% Hgb CS at birth only	Normal or slightly microcytic RBCs; no signs or symptoms
	β: Hgb Az ≥3.5	
	80–90% of Hgb F/Hgb A	
Thalassemia trait (α- and β-thalassemia trait)	α: 5–10% Hgb Barts or 1–2%	Mild anemia to elevated RBCs; microcytosis/ hypochromic
	Hgb CS at birth	
	80–90% Hgb F/Hgb A	
	β: Hgb Az ≥3.5	
	80–90% Hgb F/Hgb A	
Hgb H or Hgb CS (constant spring)	α: 5–30% Hgb Barts or 1–2%	Microcytic/hypochromic anemia (7–10 g/dL); pale, icteric, jaundiced; hepatosplenomegaly
	Hgb CS at birth	
	Hgb F 70–90%	
Hydrops fetalis	α: combination of Hgb Barts, Hgb H	Severe anemia (6.2 g/dL average Hgb); pale, icteric, edematous due to congestive heart
	Hgb Portland usually death in utero failure; hepatosplenomegaly	
Thalassemia inter-media	Hgb Az 2–7%	Anemia (6–10 g/dL) microcytosis
	Hgb F 20–100%	Hypochromic; pale, icteric, and with
	Hgb A 0–80% (depends on phenotype)	Hepatosplenomegaly; rarely transfused
Thalassemia major	Hgb Az 2–7%	Anemia average 6 g/dL with
	Hgb F 20–100%	Microcytic/hypochromia; pale, failure to thrive, frontal bossing, thalassemic facies, short stature, hepatosplenomegaly; transfusion-dependent
	Hgb A 0–80% (depends on phenotype)	

- α-thalassemia trait has two functional α-globin genes (−α/a or α α /−).
- Hemoglobin H disease has one functional α-globin gene (−/−α) and a Hgb H variant = Hgb constant spring (−/α ^{cs} α).
- Hydrops fetalis has no functional α-globin gene (−/−).

5.4.2 Beta Thalassemia (Cooley Anemia)

5.4.2.1 Epidemiology

β-thalassemia mutations are found worldwide in regions including the Mediterranean, Africa, Southeast Asia, India, Italy, Greece, Spain, and North America, but are uncommon in Northern Europe, Korea, and Japan.

5.4.2.2 Etiology

The deficit in β-globin production is due to mutation of the β-globin genes located on chromosome 11.

5.4.2.3 Molecular Genetics

Within the β-globin gene, more than 200 mutations affect the transcription, translation of β-globin messenger, and stability of β-globin product (DeBaun and Vichinsky 2007, Cunningham et al. 2009).

β-thalassemia includes four clinical syndromes (see Table 5.6):

- Silent carrier, which is asymptomatic
- β-thalassemia trait with mild anemia
- Thalassemia intermedia with moderate anemia and usually no transfusion requirement
- Thalassemia major with severe anemia and transfusion-dependent

5.4.3 Diagnostic Testing

Thalassemia testing can be confirmed with Hgb electrophoresis and family studies, or if necessary, DNA analysis can be used to make a definitive diagnosis. In most states of the United States, screening for hemoglobinopathies is performed on newborn infants. Anemias in children who were not screened as newborns but who present with hypochromic, microcytic anemias must be differentiated from iron deficiency (see the following formulas).

Prenatal diagnosis of α-thalassemia may be done by testing the amniotic fluid or obtaining chorionic villus sampling, if there is a suspicion for α-thal trait or a family history of hydrops fetalis. Newborn screen often reports hemoglobin Bart, that is, fast-migrating hemoglobin that appears only in cord and neonatal blood indicating α-globin gene deletion. The typical thalassemia smear contains microcytosis, hypochromia, target cells, teardrops, fragments, and microspherocytes (Fig. 5.2 slide 6). Differentiation between β-thalassemia trait and iron deficiency can be determined by serum ferritin, serum iron, transferrin saturation, hemoglobin A_2 level, and calculated based on a variety of formulas:

Formulas for differentiation of thalassemia trait from iron deficiency (adapted from Cunningham et al. 2009, p 1054 and Beyan et al. 2007, p525) and trait deficiency:

	Thalassemia Trait	Iron deficiency
Mentzer index MCV/RBC	<13	>13
Shine and Lal (MCV)2 ¥ MCH	<1,530	>1,530
Red blood cell distribution index (RDW) £ 14	>14	

5.4.4 Treatment

Supportive therapy includes supplementation with folic acid, avoidance of oxidant drugs and iron salts, prompt treatment of infectious episodes, and judicious use of transfusions. β-thalassemia major patients require regular transfusions to sustain life. Thalassemia intermedia patients are able to maintain Hgb concentration of 6–10 g/dL without transfusions, except during periods of infection, surgery, or other stressors. Splenectomy may be considered in Hgb H, thalassemia intermedia, and β-thalassemia major, if hypersplenism is present with leukopenia, thrombocytopenia, worsening anemia, or the development of increased requirement for transfusion (>200 mL PRBCs/kg/year). Splenectomy reduces the transfusion requirements by eliminating the organ causing the trapping of the RBCs. At least 2 weeks prior to splenectomy, polyvalent pneumococcal and meningococcal vaccines should be given. Following splenectomy, prophylactic penicillin 250 mg orally bid is implemented until adulthood. The importance of seeking medical assistance when the splenectomized patient is febrile is emphasized to the parents and child, to reduce the risk of developing overwhelming infection. Complications of ongoing transfusion therapy regimens are assessed (Sect. 5.2.7) including hemosiderosis.

5.4.5 Treatment of Hemosiderosis (Iron Overload)

Hemosiderosis is the accumulation of iron in organ tissues such as liver, pancreas, and joints as a result of chronic RBC transfusion therapy received by patients with β-thalassemia, Hgb H, sickle cell (e.g., those with a history of cerebrovascular accident, ACS, retractable vaso-occlusive crisis), or bone marrow failure syndromes (Lisowski and Sadelain 2008, Neufeld 2006). Hemosiderosis may also develop in frequently transfused patients receiving myelosuppressive chemotherapy and/or radiation treatments. Chronic hemolysis and increased gut absorption of iron can also result in hemosiderosis. Currently, exchange transfusion, phlebotomy, and chelation therapy are the only methods to manage transfusion-related iron overload.

5.4.6 Chelation Therapy

The objective of chelation therapy is to remove excess intracellular iron and bind free extracellular iron.

5.4.6.1 Initiation of Chelation Therapy

- Liver biopsy is the most accurate measurement of iron load, and hence, if liver iron is 7 mg/g/dry weight or higher, then chelation should be started.
- Ferritin level is helpful, but not reliable because it is an acute-phase reactant. Ferritin levels of more than 1,000 mg/mL are considered to be in steady state, which then start chelation.
- Cumulative transfusions of 120 mL or more PRBCs/kg/year promote hemosiderosis.

5.4.6.2 Chelation Regimens

- Desferrioxamine has been the standard parenteral iron chelator since the 1970s, and is a complex hydroxylamine with a remarkable affinity to iron.
- Desferrioxamine enters the cells, chelates iron, returns iron to serum, and excretes the iron via kidney, liver, and skin.
- Desferrioxamine 20–50 mg/kg/8–12 h is administered every night subcutaneously 5–6 days weekly.
- Desferrioxamine by the IV route accelerates the rate of iron removal.
- Supplemental oral ascorbic acid 100 mg daily enhances the urinary excretion of iron, particularly in vitamin C-deficient patients.

Deferasirox belongs to a new class of oral tridentate chelator, N-substituted bis-Hydroxyphenyltriazoles that penetrate the membranes easily,allowing the removal of potentially toxic iron from the tissues.

Deferasirox was approved in 2005 for children aged 2 years and older by the Food and Drug Administration (FDA) in United States for the dosage of 20–30 mg/kg/day (Vichinsky 2007, Neufeld 2006).

Deferiprone is an oral hydroxypyridineone first used in humans in 1987, and is liscensed in Europe, but is neither approved to be used in the United States nor Canada, although it is currently available on a compassionate-use basis in the United States (Neufeld 2006).

5.4.6.3 Complications of Chelation Medications

- Local erythema at the infusion site characterized by multiple subcutaneous nodules may be suppressed by including 5–10 mg hydrocortisone in the desferrioxamine solution.
- Ototoxicity is a complication of chelation medications; therefore, a hearing test should be done every 6–12 months.
- Ocular toxicity is a complication of chelation medications; therefore, the eyes should be examined every 6–12 months.
- Noncompliance is an ongoing problem, particularly with adolescent patients or parents who dread doing the desferrioxamine subcutaneous injections. However, there tends to be greater compliance with the oral chelator.
- Do not administer chelation medications during infection or fever because the mobilization of iron aids in bacterial growth, particularly *Yersinia enterocolitica.*
- The common side effects of oral chelator include gastrointestinal disturbances, rash, elevation in serum creatinine level, and liver enzyme level.

5.4.7 Clinical Advances (Hemosiderosis)

MRI T2-weighted imaging of the iron content in the liver and heart is available in a few centers within the United States that is comparable with a liver biopsy iron measurement, thereby providing a noninvasive means of measuring iron accumulation in the body. A retrospective cross-sectional study of 66 patients (3–82 years of age) recommended that both the liver and myocardial T2-MRI measurements along with LV ejection fraction be used to make chelation adjustments (Chirnomas et al. 2008).

5.4.8 Prognosis

Bone marrow transplants from human leukocyte antigen (HLA)-identified donors have been successfully performed worldwide on patients with severe β-thalassemia. The most successful transplants were in children younger than 15 years without excessive iron overload (DeBaun and Vichinsky 2007). A marked increase in the survival to the fifth decade of life in well-managed β-thalassemia patients is observed in the developed countries.

5.4.9 Follow-Up

All β-thalassemic major patients should have 3-month interval appointments with the hematologist medical provider to manage therapies and side effects involving hemochromatosis, vision, hearing, enlarged organs, and dental side effects. Other thalassemic patients (β-intermedia, Hgb H) are usually seen every 6 months, provided the patients have not developed any severe complications.

5.4.10 Future Perspectives

The process of bone marrow transplantation with unrelated phenotypically matched donors and in utero transplantation are being investigated. Development of transduction methods and vectors to transfer genes and correct the genetic defect are being researched. A phase I human gene therapy trial for thalassemia and SCD has been initiated in France but the clinical data are not yet available (Cummingham 2008).

5.5. Hemolytic Anemia

Hemolytic anemias comprise a group of disorders that cause destruction of RBCs. The reduced RBCs survival may occur as a result of intracorpuscular defects due to defective intracellular enzymes (e.g., G-6PD deficiency or pyruvate kinase deficiency) or abnormal membrane structural proteins as in HS. The RBC survival is also affected by the extracorpuscular defect of autoimmune hemolytic anemia (AIHA).

5.5.1 Hereditary Spherocytosis

HS is the most common congenital RBC membrane disorder. It is characterized by a deficiency or abnormality of the RBC membrane protein spectrin, one of the major skeletal cell membrane proteins. The HS RBCs are repeatedly trapped by the splenic sinusoids, which causes damage and destruction to the spherocytes.

5.5.1.1 Epidemiology

HS is a common inherited hemolytic anemia, with an estimated incidence of 1–2 in 5,000 individuals in Northern Europe. The majority of patients with HS have European ancestry, but HS also occurs in patients with African-American, Hispanic, and Asian ancestry (Tracy and Rice 2008).

5.5.1.2 Etiology

The primary molecular defects in HS reside in membrane skeletal proteins and is a common inherited hemolytic anemia. Approximately 5–10% of cases of HS are considered new mutations.

5.5.1.3 Molecular Genetics

Microscopically, HS cells show fewer spectrin filaments interconnecting spectrin/actin/protein to junctional complexes, but the overall skeletal architecture is preserved except in the most severe forms of HS (Tracy and Rice 2008, Grace and Lux 2009). Typically, HS is associated with approximately 75% dominant and 25% recessive inheritance (An and Mohandus 2008). The membrane protein defects cause instability of the spectrin, which results in membrane instability, loss of surface area, and abnormal permeability, with the average lifespan of the RBCs being 90 days.

5.5.1.4 Symptoms/Clinical Signs

A thorough history and physical examination may elicit a family history of neonatal hyperbilirubinemia, gallstones, splenomegaly or splenectomy, and intermittent jaundice that typically presents in infancy, but may present at any age. Anemia is the most frequent complaint, accompanied with reticulocytosis, and is manifested primarily by pallor, intermittent jaundice, and splenomegaly. Mild to marked jaundice may be present depending on the rate of hemolysis and the ability of the liver to conjugate and excrete indirect hyperbilirubinemia.

5.5.1.5 Diagnostic Testing

Spherocytes are dense, round, and hyperchromic, and lack central pallor on the peripheral blood smear (Fig. 5.2 slide 7). The laboratory findings of HS vary according to the severity and clinical classification. The trait may have a normal Hgb and normal to slightly elevated reticulocyte count. Mild HS Hgb can be 11–15 g/dL, but with an elevated reticulocyte count of 3–8%. In moderate to moderately severe HS, the Hgb is 8–12 to 6–8 g/dL, respectively, with elevated reticulocyte counts above 8%. Severe HS has a Hgb level of less than 6 mg/dL and a reticulocyte count of greater than 10%. The majority of children with HS suffer from mild to moderate anemia.

Other laboratory findings include anemia (mild to severe) depending on the HS classification, reticulocyte count, and increased osmotic fragility test (the most sensitive test for diagnosing HS). The spherocytes have a decreased surface area to volume ratio, and when placed in the hypotonic solution, the HS cells lose membrane surface area more readily because their membranes are leaky and unstable, resulting in an increase in the osmotic fragility test.

The MCV (mean corpuscular volume) is decreased except during reticulocytosis. The RDW is elevated due to the presence of microspheres in proportion to the degree of hemolysis. The Coombs' test is negative, which excludes AIHA. Several other diagnostic tests used to detect HS include the acidified glycerol lysis test, hypertonic cryohemolysis test, and the autohemolysis test. HS must be differentiated from disorders such as AIHA, G-6PD, pyruvate kinase deficiency, elliptocytosis, and pyropoikilocytosis.

5.5.1.6 Treatment

- As dietary intake of folic acid is inadequate for the increased needs of the erythroid HS bone marrow, the patients should routinely receive folic acid 1 mg/day orally to prevent megaloblastic crisis.
- The parents and child are instructed regarding the signs and symptoms of hemolysis and hypersplenism, such as increased pallor, fatigue, abdominal pain, enlarging spleen, jaundice, and dark urine. The family and child are instructed to avoid trauma to the spleen area and are shown how to monitor spleen size.
- If splenectomy becomes necessary, it is delayed until the child is 5 or 6 years because the increased risk of postsplenic sepsis is very high in infancy and early childhood. The child should have pneumococcal and meningococcal vaccines at least 2 weeks prior to splenectomy. Prior to splenectomy, an abdominal ultrasonography should be done to determine the spleen size and the presence of any accessory spleens and/or cholelithiasis.
- After splenectomy, the child should receive prophylactic penicillin therapy 250 mg orally twice daily until adulthood.

5.5.1.7 Prognosis

Splenectomy laparoscopically eliminates hemolysis, but exposes the patient to life-long risk for lethal infections. Platelet counts tend to increase to more than 1,000 $\times 10^9$/L immediately after splenectomy, but will usually decrease over several weeks without any intervention. Penicillin-resistant strains of *S. pneumoniae* have developed, but the use of prophylactic penicillin supersedes this complication, because of the increase risk of life-threatening infections.

5.5.1.8 Follow-Up

Yearly follow-up is needed for CBC and liver panel, and to reinforce penicillin prophylaxis. The splenectomized HS patient should seek medical attention immediately for febrile illness. Healthcare providers should reinforce with the parents and patient that although hemolysis is eradicated, HS still exists.

5.5.1.9 Future Perspectives

Management of HS by subtotal splenectomy has shown beneficial results in several studies by decreasing hemolysis and maintaining phagocytic function of the spleen (Dutta et al. 2006, Stoehr et al. 2005). Surveillance of the splenic regrowth and correlation with the clinical status of the patient is critical to understand the long-term outcomes of the partial splenectomy(Tracy and Rice 2008).

5.5.2 Autoimmune Hemolytic Anemia

A condition that develops from the interaction between erythrocytes and the immune system is known as AIHA. The most common types are AIHA that is composed of warm-reactive autoantibody, usually immunoglobulin (IgG), that binds with the erythrocyte antigen at 37°C, or cold-reactive autoantibody, usually IgM, that binds to erythrocytes below 37°C (Shah 2004, Ware 2009). These autoantibodies are recognized by the macrophages that lead to the intravascular destruction of the erythrocyte.

5.5.2.1 Epidemiology

AIHA is estimated to occur at an annual incidence of 1 in 80,000 persons of any age, race, or nationality.

5.5.2.2 Etiology

Children tend to develop AIHA after a recent viral illness or systemic illness because of the development of autoantibodies. The autoantibodies bind to the erythrocyte surface membrane, which results in premature RBC destruction, primarily in the spleen.

5.5.2.3 Molecular Genetics

The antierythrocyte antibodies that develop in most patients with AIHA represent a polyclonal B-lymphocyte response that is poorly understood. Case reports suggest that there is an association between AIHA and certain immune response genes.

5.5.2.4 Symptoms/Clinical Signs

Many patients present with signs and symptoms of anemia, such as pallor, weakness, fatigue, and lightheadedness, with a compensated cardiovascular aspect. Occasionally, the patient may develop jaundice, owing to accelerated erythrocyte destruction, and dark urine, reflecting intravascular hemolysis. A thorough history must be obtained, including questions regarding medications and the possibility of underlying systemic illnesses such as any history of newborn jaundice, gallstones, splenomegaly/splenectomy, or episodes of dark urine or yellow sclera. The patient may have a palpable spleen and liver, with tachycardia or a systolic flow murmur manifested on physical examination.

5.5.2.5 Diagnostic Testing

Peripheral blood smear is very useful in establishing the diagnosis of AIHA. It contains numerous small spherocytes, occasional teardrop shapes or schistocytes, polychromasia (common finding), and reticulocytes (Fig. 5.2, slide 8). Bone marrow aspiration is not mandatory but may be helpful to exclude a malignant process, myelodysplasia, or bone marrow failure syndrome. The bone marrow reveals erythroid hyperplasia with myeloid/erythroid ratio.

Elevated lactate dehydrogenase and aspirate aminotransferase levels reflect the release of intraerythrocyte enzymes; in contrast, other hepatic enzymes should not be elevated in AIHA. The serum haptoglobin level is typically low because it acts as a scavenger for free plasma Hgb, but haptoglobin is an acute-phase reactant and is not synthesized well in infants. The unconjugated bilirubin is elevated and reflects accelerated erythrocyte destruction. The most useful laboratory test is the direct antiglobulin test (DAT or Coombs' test), which identifies the antibodies and complement components on the surface of the circulating erythrocytes.

The differential diagnosis includes hereditary spherocytosis, which may be excluded by performing the osmotic fragility test. Other rare disorders such as clostridial sepsis, Wilson's disease, hemolytic-uremic syndrome, thrombotic thrombocytopenic purpura, transient erythroblastopenia of childhood, or acquired AA are excluded by performing a DAT.

5.5.2.6 Treatment

If the patient has severe anemia or decreasing Hgb concentration, then therapy should be instituted. Therapy should begin with close observation and corticosteroid therapy with the judicial use of erythrocyte transfusions. The corticosteroids are widely accepted firstline therapy. Corticosteroids inhibit the Fc receptor-mediated clearance of sensitized erythrocytes and also inhibit autoantibody synthesis. Corticosteroids, prescribed as 1–2 mg/kg of methylprednisolone, administered IV every 6 h for 24–72 h, and then oral prednisone 2 mg/kg/day divided 3 times daily, are given until the patient becomes clinically stable. The prednisone is tapered over 1–3 months based on steroid concentration, reticulocyte count, and DAT.

The second line of therapy includes IV immunoglobulin therapy, with a systemic benefit at high doses of 5 g/kg for 5 days, and may be accompanied by plasma exchange transfusion. Exchange transfusion is reasonable with the large IgM antibodies, which are removed by plasmapheresis, whereas the IgG autoantibodies in the extravascular spaces respond better to splenectomy. Transfusion of RBCs is difficult in the AIHA patient due to the difficulty in obtaining compatible erythrocytes. The transfusion may result in severe hemolysis, and hence, the transfusion is started at a slow rate, checking both plasma and urine for free Hgb. Other therapeutic modalities include cyclosporin A (suppresses cellular immunity), vinblastine (decrease autoantibody production), danazol (decreased IgG production), azathioprine, and cyclophosphamide (both interfere with autoantibody synthesis).

Splenectomy may be considered late in the disease; it removes the major site of autoantibody production, with a response in about 80% of patients. These children should receive pneumococcal/meningococcal immunizations at least 2 weeks prior to splenectomy. Postsplenectomy patients should seek medical attention immediately if they develop a fever higher than 38.5°C, and should take penicillin or erythromycin (if allergic to penicillin) prophylaxis due to the possibility of sepsis.

5.5.2.7 Prognosis

There is a good prognosis for the majority of children who experience acute self-limiting disease, with a mortality rate of less than 10%.

5.5.2.8 Future Perspectives

Rituximab appears to be a useful treatment for refractory AIHA. Rituximab is a humanized murine monoclonal antibody directed against the human CD20 antigen, which is present only on B-lymphocytes (Segal 2007, Ware 2009). Berentsen (2007) hypothesized that rituximab-based combination therapies might show higher efficacy compared with single-agent therapy.

5.5.3 Glucose-6-Phosphate Dehydrogenase Deficiency

G-6PD is the most common RBC enzyme deficiency. As the gene for G-6PD is usually located on the *X* chromosome, males are either fully deficient or of normal phenotype (Maisels 2006). However, females can be deficient fully, heterozygous (trait), or of normal phenotype (Cappellini and Fiorelli 2008, Lanzkowsky 2005).

5.5.3.1 Epidemiology

G-6PD deficiency is a worldwide gender-linked RBC enzyme deficiency. More that 400 million people are affected worldwide, with the highest incidence among Africans, African-Americans, Mediterraneans, Native Americans, Southeast Asians, and Sephardic Jews.

5.5.3.2 Etiology

G-6PD variants may be due to deletions or point mutations affecting transcription and processing or the primary structure. Therefore, G-6PD deficiency may not only be caused by approximately 140 mutations in the coding region and a decreased number of normal molecules, but also by changes in the primary structure by affecting the catalytic function or by decreasing stability of the protein, or both (Cappellini and Fiorelli 2008, Luzzatto and Poggi 2009).

5.5.3.3 Molecular Genetics

As a clone of the G-6PD gene, nearly all the G-6PD variants possess a single amino acid replacement, which is caused by a single missense point mutation (Luzzatto and Poggi 2009). After exposure to an oxidative agent (Table 5.7), the Hgb and other proteins are oxidized. The RBC destruction starts hemolyzing the oldest RBCs with the least G-6PD, and then progresses toward younger RBCs and the denatured Hgb precipitates, causing irreversible damage to the membrane, and subsequently, the RBCs lyse.

Table 5.7. Hemolytic oxidants associated with G-6PD deficiency (adapted from Luzzatto and Poggi 2009)

Analgesics and antipyretics
Acetanilide
Acetylsalicylic acid (large doses)
Para-aminosalicylic acid
Acetophenetidin (phenacetin)
Nitrofurans
Nitrofurazone
Nitrofurantoin
Furaltadone
Furazolidone
Antimalarials
Pentaquine
Pamaquine
Primaquine
Quinocide
Chloroquine
Pyrimethamine
Plasmoquine
Sulfones
Thiazolsulfone
Diaminodiphenylsulfone
Sulfoxone sodium
Sulfonamides
Sulfanilamide
Sulfamethoxazole
Sulfacetamide
Sulfapyridine
Sulfadiazine
Sulfisoxazole
Sulfathiazole
Sulfacetamide
Miscellaneous
Naphthalene (mothballs)
Methylene blue
Chloramphenicol
Probenecid
Quinidine
Fava beans
Phenylhydrazine
Nalidixic acid
Infections
Diabetic acidosis

5.5.3.4 Symptoms/Clinical Signs

A thorough history must be obtained, including the possible precipitant of the acute event. A child with G-6PD deficiency is hematologically normal most of the time until hemolysis occurs secondary to an oxidant (Table 5.7). Within 24–48 h after exposure to an oxidant, the child may develop fever (38°C), nausea, abdominal pain, diarrhea, dark-colored urine, jaundice, pallor, tachycardia, splenomegaly, and possibly hepatomegaly.

5.5.3.5 Diagnostic Testing

The peripheral smear shows moderate to severe normocytic, normochromic anemia, with marked anisocytosis, poikilocytosis, and reticulocytosis with inclusion bodies (Heinz bodies). The diagnosis is confirmed by quantitative spectrophotometric analysis or by a rapid fluorescent spot test, detecting the generation of nicotinamide adenine dinucleotide (NADPH) from NADP in reticulocyte-poor red cells, or by testing RBCs after reticulocytosis resolves (Cappellini and Fiorelli 2008, Ronquist and Theodorsson 2007). Other observations that support the G-6PD diagnosis include a reduced haptoglobin, elevated WBCs (predominance of granulocytes), and elevated unconjugated bilirubin with normal liver enzymes. In addition, urine is positive for blood (free Hgb).

Studies using polymerase chain reaction (PCR) may identify the abnormal gene as well as the biochemical abnormality (Perkins 2001). Direct antiglobulin test will be negative in G-6PD and will exclude antibody-mediated RBC destruction. Other disorders to exclude from the differential include blackwater fever (malarial infection), paroxysmal cold hemoglobinuria, paroxysmal nocturnal hemoglobinuria, and mismatched blood transfusion (ABO mismatch).

5.5.3.6 Treatment

Treatment depends on the extent of the acute hemolysis. Supportive care during the acute event may require transfusion and must definitely include counseling regarding prevention of future events. Healthcare providers should reinforce to the parents and child about the need to avoid the list of oxidants that can possibly trigger hemolysis (Table 5.7). G-6PD hemolysis is commonly acute and intermittent, but can also be chronic (Ronquist and Theodorsson 2007). For those individuals undergoing chronic hemolysis, dietary supplementation with folic acid (1 mg tablet/day) is recommended (Frank 2005).

5.5.3.7 Prognosis

The prognosis is good, provided the patient avoids exposure to the oxidants.

5.6 Bone Marrow Failure Syndromes

Bone marrow failure syndromes are a reduction in the effective production of mature erythrocytes, granulocytes, and platelets by the bone marrow, causing varying degrees of cytopenias. The bone marrow failure syndromes encompass AA, FA, paroxysmal nocturnal hemoglobinuria, Shwachman-Diamond syndrome, dyskeratosis congenita, Diamond-Blackfan syndrome, and many other disorders. This section will focus on AA, which is divided into acquired and inherited classifications.

5.6.1 Aplastic Anemia

AA, a bone marrow failure disorder, may be acquired or inherited. It is characterized by a reduced or absent production of blood cells in the bone marrow and peripheral blood, causing a decrease of two or more cell lines (e.g., RBCs, WBCs, and platelets).

5.6.1.1 Acquired Aplastic Anemia

Acquired AA results from an immunologically mediated, tissue-specific, organ-destructive mechanism.

5.6.1.1.1 Epidemiology

An annual incidence of acquired AA was established as 2/million/year in European studies. The highest mortalities were in Japan, Thailand, and Northern Ireland, with an incidence two or three times higher than in European countries and the United States.

5.6.1.1.2 Etiology

The causative factors of acquired AA include toxins, medications, insecticides, immunologic disorders, irradiation, chemotherapy, and infections (e.g., HIV, CMV, parvovirus, hepatitis); however, most causes are unknown (70% idiopathic). Myelosuppressive drugs such as chemotherapy, antibiotics, insecticides, benzene compounds, and other medications cause dose-related marrow suppression by damaging the DNA and decreasing the numbers of progenitors. Radiation injures the DNA in the actively replicating progenitor cells, which also causes AA.

5.6.1.1.3 Molecular Genetics

Acquired AA is divided into severe and moderate AA. Moderate AA has normal to increased cellular marrow with at least two of the following: granulocyte count more than 500/mL, platelet count more than 20,000/mL, and reticulocyte count more than 1%. Severe AA has an aplastic marrow and at least two of the following: granulocyte count less than 500/mL, platelet count less than 20,000/mL, and reticulocyte count less than 1%.

5.6.1.1.4 Symptoms/Clinical Signs

A detailed history, including medications, infections, radiation exposure, and any family history of AA, should be obtained with a thorough physical examination. Thrombocytopenia and hemorrhagic manifestations are usually the first symptoms and are manifested by petechiae, ecchymoses, epistaxis, or oral mucosal bleeding. Neutropenia causes oral ulcerations, bacterial infections, and fever, which are rarely present early in AA. Erythropenia, manifested by pallor, fatigue, headache, and tachycardia, tends to be a late sign, as red cells live approximately 120 days compared with platelets that live only 10 days and neutrophils that live for 6–12 h.

5.6.1.1.5 Diagnostic Testing

Blood counts are depressed, and blood smear displays a paucity of platelets, leukocytes, and normal to macrocytic red cells with decreased reticulocytes. Increased fetal Hgb (Hgb F) and red cell I antigen may be present secondary to stress hematopoiesis. Bone marrow examination must be done by obtaining an aspirate and biopsy, which demonstrates the conversion of red bone marrow to yellow fatty marrow. There are decreased numbers of blood and marrow progenitor cells due to a microenvironment that fails to support hematopoiesis.

Laboratory findings include the following:

- Normocytic, normochromic anemia with reticulocytopenia, leukopenia, and thrombocytopenia observed on the smear
- Slightly to moderately elevated fetal Hgb noted on Hgb electrophoresis
- Bone marrow denotes marked depression or absence of hematopoietic cells and replacement by fatty tissue containing reticulum cells, lymphocytes, plasma cells, and usually tissue mast cells. Bone marrow biopsy is done to exclude granulomas, myelofibrosis, or leukemia, and a bone marrow chromosomal analysis is done to exclude FA and myelodysplastic syndromes
- Diepoxybutane test (DEB) is performed on peripheral blood to exclude FA
- Sugar-water test, Ham test, and flow cytometry are done to exclude paroxysmal nocturnal hemoglobinuria (PNH)
- Liver function chemistries are done to exclude hepatitis
- Renal function chemistries are done to exclude renal disease
- Viral serology testing: hepatitis A,B,C antibody panel, Epstein–Barr virus antibody panel, parvovirus B19 IgG and IgM antibodies, varicella antibody titer, and cytomegalovirus antibody titer are done to determine etiology
- Quantitative immunoglobulins, C_3, C_4, and complement and antinuclear antibody (ANA), total hemolytic complement (CH50), and Coombs' test are done to exclude systemic diseases
- HLA typing of the patient and nuclear family is done to determine if bone marrow transplantation match is available
- Blood group typing is performed on the patient for possible transfusion
- Clotting profile including prothrombin time (PT), activated partial thromboplastin time (APTT), and fibrinogen is done to determine any clotting dysfunction.

Differential diagnosis for pancytopenia is extensive and includes myelodysplastic syndromes, preleukemias, leukemias, paroxysmal nocturnal hemoglobinuria, myelofibrosis, and some lymphomas. Pancytopenia may occur secondary to systemic diseases such as systemic lupus erythematosus, hypersplenism, vitamin B_{12} or folate deficiencies, alcohol abuse, anorexia nervosa or starvation, and infections such as Sarcoidosis and Legionnaires' disease.

5.6.1.1.6 Treatment

Bone marrow transplant with HLA-matched sibling is the treatment of choice. If no HLA-matched sibling is available and the following indicators are present: bone marrow cellularity less than 30% with at least two of the following findings: absolute neutrophil count less than 500/mm^3, platelet count less than 20,000/mm^3, reticulocyte count less than 1%; then the following immunosuppressive therapy is instituted:

- Antilymphocyte globulin (ALG) or antithymocyte globulin (ATG), which are similar products from either horses or rabbits and mixed with human thoracic duct lymphocytes or thymocytes. ALG and ATG preparations contain mixtures of antibodies to lymphocytes and are immunosuppressive and cytotoxic (T-cell depletion). The recommended dose is 40 mg/kg/day for 4 days. The typical adverse reactions to ATG are thrombocytopenia, headache, myalgia, arthralgia, chills, fever, and serum sickness approximately 7–10 days following ATG administration.
- Methylprednisolone, given as IV boluses on days 1–4 at 10 mg/kg/day, then changed to an oral steroid such as prednisone 1 mg/kg/day until day 30, to prevent serum sickness. The toxicities associated with steroids are hypertension, hyperglycemia, increased susceptibility to fungal infection, potassium wasting, and fluid retention.
- Cyclosporine is a specific T-cell inhibitor with a recommended oral dose of 15 mg/kg/day in children to maintain blood trough levels at 100–250 mg/mL. Toxic effects from cyclosporine include hypertension, azotemia, hirsutism, gingival hypertrophy, and increased serum creatinine levels.
- Hematopoietic growth factors (G-CSF) have shown promise in increasing neutrophil counts. G-CSF are administered subcutaneously at 5–10 mg/kg/day; the side effects include fever, chills, headache, and bone pain.

- Androgens (i.e., methyltestosterone, oxymetholone) no longer have a primary role in the management of AA, unless the therapies discussed earlier are unsuccessful. The androgens increase erythropoietin production and stimulate erythroid stem cells. The oral dose is 2–5 mg/kg/day with side effects such as masculinization (hirsutism, deepening voice, genitalia enlargement), acne, nausea, weight gain, and liver dysfunction.

5.6.1.1.7 Supportive Treatment

- Blood product support should be used sparingly while the family is HLA-typed
- Thrombocytopenic precautions should be implemented:
- Promptly report signs and symptoms of bleeding (e.g., excessive bruising/petechiae, oral purpura, melena, prolonged epistaxis or gingival bleeding or hematuria)
- Avoid contact sports or rough activities (e.g., football, soccer, wrestling, bicycle riding, skating, diving, tree climbing, trampolines)
- Provide a safe environment to prevent trauma (use side rails, gates, helmets, and knee pads and avoid rectal manipulation, including with thermometers, suppositories, and enemas).
- Avoid oral mucosa trauma (use soft toothbrushes and avoid dental floss, electric tooth brush, and sharp food items)
- Add stool softeners and increase fiber and fluids in the diet to prevent constipation.

5.6.1.1.8 Prognosis

With immunosuppressive therapies or bone marrow transplant, the long-term survival for patients with AA has improved to 80%. In the European International Marrow Unrelated Search and Transplant trial, the survival rate from an unrelated donor was about one-half after the conventional transplantation, due to a high rate of graft rejection or failure.

5.6.1.2 Inherited Aplastic Anemia

The most common inherited AA is FA, though several others are also a part of the category (including Diamond-Blackfan anemia, dyskeratosis congenita, and Shwachman-Diamond syndrome). This section will discuss FA.

5.6.1.2.1 Epidemiology

All races and ethnic groups have been reported to present with inherited AA, including American Caucasians, African-Americans, Asians, and Native Americans. The heterozygote frequency may be 1/300 in the United States and in Europe, and 1/100 in South Africa.

5.6.1.2.2 Etiology

The incidence is difficult to ascertain. Approximately 25% of childhood AA occurs in the presence of known marrow failure genes.

5.6.1.2.3 Molecular Genetics

FA is an autosomal recessive trait that has also been associated with *X*-linked recessive disorders and families having consanguineous marriages (Dokal and Vulliamy 2008, D'Souza et al. 2007). Since 1992, when the first FA gene was cloned, there has been approximately 13 subtypes and 12 genes identified (Dufour and Svahn 2008, Levitus et al. 2004).

5.6.1.2.4 Symptoms/Clinical Signs

A detailed history should be obtained including toxin and radiation exposure, medications, and any family history of AA, and a physical examination should focus on the identification of any congenital anomalies. Hemorrhagic manifestations such as petechiae, ecchymoses, epistaxis, and bleeding of oral mucosa are initially observed. Other signs and symptoms such as pallor, fatigue, headache, tachycardia, or infection are also seen.

Classic anomalies are seen in 75% of FA patients and include short stature, absent thumbs or radii, microcephaly, café au lait spots, skin hyperpigmentation, a broad nasal base, epicanthal folds, micrognathia, hyperreflexia, hypogenitalism, strabismus, ptosis, nystagmus, abnormalities of the ears, deafness, mental retardation, and renal and cardiac anomalies.

5.6.1.2.5 Diagnostic Testing

FBC/CBC with RBC indices, WBC count and differential, platelet count, and reticulocyte count should be obtained. Thrombocytopenia and leukopenia develop before pancytopenia, but severe AA develops in most cases. Examination of blood smear shows macrocytic red cells with mild poikilocytosis, anisocytosis, and decreased platelets and leukocytes. The bone marrow is a hypocellular fatty bone marrow with decreased myeloid and erythroid precursors and megakaryocytes. Prenatal diagnosis with chorionic villus biopsy and amniotic fluid cell cultures of FA can be made early in the pregnancy. The following labs and tests are usually obtained:

- ANA and DNA binding titer, Coombs' test, rheumatoid factor, liver function tests
- Viral serology: HIV, EBV, parvovirus, hepatitis A, B, C, and PCR for virus
- Serum vitamin B_{12} and serum folate levels
- Bone marrow aspirate and biopsy
- Cytogenetic studies on blood lymphocytes (i.e., diepoxybutane [DEB] to diagnose FA)
- Cytogenetic studies on bone marrow to exclude FA
- Acid Ham test and sugar-water test to exclude PNH
- Skeletal X-rays, IV pyelogram, chest X-ray to determine congenital anomalies

FA may be differentiated from thrombocytopenia with absent radii (TAR), amegakaryocytic thrombocytopenic purpura, acquired aplastic anemia, and leukemia with a hypoplastic marrow by carrying out the above-mentioned diagnostic tests.

5.6.1.2.6 Treatment

Supportive care includes adherence to thrombocytopenic precautions (Sect. 5.6.1.1.7). Transfusion of PRBCs and/or platelets, growth factors (G-CSF) for neutropenia, erythropoietin, and e-aminocaproic acid (0.1 mg/kg/dose every 6 h orally) may be instituted. Antibiotic and antifungal treatment should be used when clinically indicated. A patient without a matched sibling should be treated with androgens, usually oxymetholone 2–5 mg/kg/day. Oxymetholone in combination with prednisolone 2 mg/kg/day reduces the risk of liver toxicity (Dufour and Svahn 2008).The side effects of androgens are listed in Sect. 5.6.1.1.6. Blood counts, liver function tests, and periodic bone marrow biopsy (to monitor for the development of myelodysplastic syndrome and leukemia) are needed to monitor the patient.

5.6.1.2.7 Prognosis

The prognosis is poor, with projected survival between 20 and 30 years, unless the patient receives HLA-matched nonaffected sibling bone marrow, which offers >70% survival. Almost 6% of FA patients develop myelodysplastic syndrome (dysmyelopoiesis and abnormal megakaryocytes), and almost 10% develop acute myeloid leukemia. With the identification of FA genes combined with the in vitro gene transfer data, gene therapy continues to be an area of active investigation (Dokal and Vulliamy 2008).

References

Adams RJ (2007) Big strokes in small persons. Archives of Neurology 64(11):1567–1574

Adams RJ, Mckie VC, Carl EM, Nichols FT, Perry R, Brock K et al (1997) Long-term stroke risk in children with sickle cell disease screened with transcranial doppler. Annals of Neurology 42(5):699–704

Adamkiewicz TV, Szabolcs P, Haight A, Baker KS, Staba S, Kedar A et al (2007) Unrelated cord blood transplantation in children with sickle cell disease: Review of four-center experience. Pediatric Transplant 11:641–644

American Academy of Pediatrics (AAP) (2002) Health supervision for children with sickle cell disease. Pediatrics 109(3):526–535

An X, Mohandas N (2008) Disorders of red cell membrane. British Journal of Haematology 141:367–375

Andrews NC, Ullrich CK, Fleming MD et al (2009) Disorders of iron metabolism and sideroblastic anemia. In: Orkin SH, Nathan DG, Ginsburg D, Look AT, Fisher DE, Lux SE (eds) Nathan and Oski's Hematology of Infancy and Childhood, pp 521–570. W.B. Saunders, Philadelphia

Auerbach M (2007) Clinical experience with intravenous iron. Transfusion Alternatives in Transfusion Medicine 9:26–30

Aygun B. (2005). Supportive care and management of oncological emergencies. In: Lanzkowsky (ed) Manual of Pediatric Hematology and Oncology, pp 695- 748, San Diego, Elsevier Academic Press

Bank A (2008) On the road to gene therapy for beta-thalassemia and sickle cell anemia. Pediatric and Hematology Oncology 25:1–4

Berentsen S (2007) Rituximab for the treatment of autoimmune cytopenias. Haematologica/The Hematology Journal 92(12):1589–1596

Bessler M, Mason PJ, Link DC, Wilson DB (2009) Inherited bone marrow failure syndromes. In: Orkin SH, Nathan DG, Ginsburg D, Look AT, Fisher DE, Lux SE (eds) Nathan and Oski's hematology of infancy and childhood, W.B.Sanders, Philadelphia, pp 307–395

Beyan C, Kaptan K, Ifan A (2007) Predictive value of discrimination indices in differential diagnosis of iron deficiency anemia and beta-thalassemia trait. European Journal of Haematology 78:524–526

Bhatia M, Walters MC (2008) Hematopoietic cell transplantation for thalassemia and sickle cell disease: past, present and future. Bone Marrow Transplantation 41:109–117

Brugnara C, Schiller B, Moran J (2006) Reticulocyte hemoglobin equivalent (Ret He) and assesment of iron-deficient states. Clinical and Laboratory Haematology 28:303–308

Butler CC, Vidal-Alaball J, Cannings-John R, McCaddon A, Hood K, Papaioannou et al (2006) Oral vitamin B12 versus intramuscular vitamin B12 for vitamin B12 deficiency: a systematic review of randomized controlled trials. Family Practice 23(3):279–285

Caboot JB, Allen JL (2008) Pulmonary complications of sickle cell disease in children. Current Opinion in Pediatrics 20:279–287

Cappellini MD, Fiorelli G (2008) Glucose-6-phosphate dehydrogenase deficiency. Lancet 371:64–74

Carley A (2003) Anemia: when is it not iron deficiency? Pediatric Nursing 29:205–211

Carmel R (2008) How I treat cobalamin (vitamin B12) deficiency. Blood 112:2214–2221

Chirnomas DS, Geukes-Foppen M, Barry K, Braunstein J, Kalish LA, Neufeld EJ et al (2008) Practical implications of liver and heart iron load assessment by T2*-MRI in children and adults with transfusion-dependent anemias. American Journal of Hematology 83(10):781–783

Cunningham MJ (2008) Update on thalassemia: clinical care and complications. Pediatric Clinics of North America 55: 447–460

Cunningham MJ, Sankaran VG, Nathan DG, Orkin SH (2009) The thalassemias. In: Orkin SH, Nathan DG, Ginsburg D, Look AT, Fisher DE, Lux SE (eds) Nathan and Oski's hematology of infancy and childhood. W.B. Saunders, Philadelphia, pp 1015–1106

DeBaun MR, Vichinsky E (2007) Hemoglobinopathies. In: Kliegman RM, Jenson HB, Behrman RE, Stanton BF (eds) Nelson textbook of pediatrics. Philadelphia, Saunders, pp 2025–2037

Dufour C, Svahn J (2008) Fanconi anaemia: new strategies. Bone Marrow Transplantation 41:590–595

Demir A, Yarali N, Fisgin T, Duru F, Kara A (2002) Most reliable indices in differentiation between thalassemia trait and iron deficiency anemia. Pediatrics International 44:612–616

Dokal I, Vulliamy T (2008) Inherited aplastic anaemias/bone marrow failure syndromes. Blood Reviews 22(3):141–53

Driscoll MC (2007) Sickle cell disease. Pediatrics Review 28: 259–268

D'Souza F, Usha MK, Subba Rao SD (2007) Fanconi's anemia in monozygotic twins. Indian Journal of Pediatrics 74(9): 859–861

Dutta S, Price VE, Blanchette V, Langer JC (2006) A laparoscopic approach to partial splenectomy for children with hereditary spherocytosis. Surgical Endoscopy 20:1719–1724

Edison ES, Bajel A, Chandy M (2008) Iron Hemeostatis: new players, newer insights. European Journal of Haematology 9:1–13

Frank JE (2005) Diagnosis and management of G6PD deficiency. American Family Physician 72(7):1277–1282

Glader B (2007) Anemias of inadequate production: iron-deficiency anemia. In: Kliegman RM, Jenson HB, Behrman RE, Stanton BF (eds) Nelson textbook of pediatrics. Philadelphia, Saunders, pp 2006–2018

Grace RF, Lux SE (2009) Disorders of the red cell membrane. In: Orkin SH, Nathan DG, Ginsburg D, Look AT, Fisher DE, Lux SE (eds) Nathan and Oski's hematology of infancy and childhood. W.B. Saunders, pp 659–837

Heeney M, Dover GJ (2009) Sickle cell disease. In: Orkin SH, Nathan DG, Ginsburg D, Look AT, Fisher DE, Lux SE (eds) Nathan and Oski's hematology of infancy and childhood. W.B.Saunders, pp 949–1014

Heeney MM, Ware RE (2008) Hydroxyurea for children with sickle cell disease. Pediatric Clinics of North America 55: 483–501

Jelkmann W (2007) Developments in the therapeutic use of erythropoiesis stimulating agent. British Journal of Haematology 141:287–297

Karayalcin G (2005) Hemolytic anemia. In: Lanzkowsky P (ed) Manual of pediatric hematology and oncology. Elsevier, San Diego, pp 136–198

Kato GJ, Onyekwere OC, Gladwin MT (2007) Pulmonary hypertension in sickle cell disease: relevance to children. Pediatric Hematology and Oncology 24(3):159–70

Kim MH, Ihm CH, Kim HJ (2008) Evaluation of reticulocyte haemoglobin content as marker of iron deficiency and predictor or response to intravenous iron in haemodialysis patients. International Journal of Laboratory Hematology 30:46–52

Lanzkowsky P (2005) Hemolytic anemia. In: Lanzkowsky P (ed) Manual of pediatric hematology and oncology. Elsevier, San Diego, pp 136–198

Lee C, Custer J, Rau R (2008) Drug doses. In: Robertson J, Shilkofski N (eds) The John Hopkins hospital: the harriet lane handbook. Elsevier, Mosby, Philadelphia

Levitus M, Rooimans MA, Steltenpool J, Cool NF, Oostra AB, Mathew CG et al (2004) Heterogeneity in Fanconi anemia: evidence for 2 new genetic subtypes. Blood 103(7): 2498–503

Lisowski L, Sadelain M (2008) Current status of globin gene therapy for the treatment of ß- thalassaemia. Brithish Journal of Haematology 141:335–345

Luzzatto L, Poggi V (2009) Glucose-6-phosphate dehydrogenase deficiency. In: Orkin SH, Nathan DG, Ginsburg D,

Look AT, Fisher DE, Lux SE (eds) Nathan and Oski's hematology of infancy and childhood. W.B. Saunders, Philadelphia, pp 883–907

Maisels MJ (2006) Neonatal jaundice. Pediatrics Review 27: 443–454

Martin L, Buonomo C (1997) Acute chest syndrome of sickle cell disease: radiographic and clinical analysis of 70 cases. Pediatric Radiology 27:637–641

Mateos ME, De-la-Cruz J, López-Laso E, Valdés MD, Nogales A (2008) Reticulocyte hemoglobin content for the diagnosis of iron deficiency. Journal of Pediatric Hematology Oncology 30(7):539–542

Miller ST, Sleeper LA, Pegelow CH, Enos LE, Wang WC, Weiner SJ et al (2000) Prediction of adverse outcomes in children with sickle cell disease. New England Journal of Medicine 342(2):83–89

Nemeth E (2008) Iron regulation and erythropoiesis. Current Option in Hematology 15:1269–175

Neufeld EJ (2006) Oral chelators deferasirox and deferiprone for transfusional iron overload in thalassemia major: new data, new questions. Blood 107(9):3436–3441

Platt OS (2008) Hydroxyurea for the treatment of sickle cell anemia. The New England Journal of Medicine 358(13): 1362–1369

Perkins S (2001) Disorders of hematopoiesis. In: Collins RD, Swerdlow SH (eds) Pediatric hematopathology. Philadelphia, Churchill Livingstone, pp 113–115

Pesce MA (2007) Reference ranges for laboratory tests and procedures. In: Kliegman RM, Jenson HB, Behrman RE, Stanton BF (eds) Nelson textbook of pediatrics. Philadelphia, Saunders, p 2944

Pinto F, Roberts I (2008) Cord blood stem cell transplantation for haemoglobinopathies. British Journal of Haematology 141:309–324

Quinn CT, Buchanan GR (1999) The acute chest syndrome of sickle cell disease. Journal of Pediatrics 135:416–422

Rackoff WR, Kunkel N, Silber JH, Asakura T, Ohene-Frempong K (1993) Pulse oximetry and factors associated with Hgb oxygen desaturation in children with sickle cell disease. Blood 81:3422–3427

Redding-Lallinger R, Knoll C (2006) Sickle cell disease – pathophysiology and treatment. Current Problems in Pediatric and Adolescent Health Care 36:346–376

Richardson M (2007) Microcytic anemia. Pediatrics Review 28:5–14

Ronquist G, Theodorsson E (2007) Inherited, non-spherocytic haemolysis due to deficiency of glucose-6-phosphate dehydrogenase. Scandinavian Journal of Clinical Laboratory Investigation 67:105–111

Segel GB (2007) Hemolytic anemias resulting from extracellular factors. In: Kliegman RM, Jenson HB, Behrman RE, Stanton BF (eds) Nelson textbook of pediatrics. W.B. Saunders, Philadelphia, pp 2042–2044

Segel GB, Hirsh MG, Feig SA (2002) Managing anemia in pediatric office practice: part I. Pediatrics in Review 23:75–83

Shah A (2004) Acquired hemolytic anemia. Indian Journal of Medical Science 58(12):533–536

Sonati Mde F, Costa FF (2008) The genetics of blood disorder: the hereditary hemoglobinopathies. Journal de Pediatria (Rio J) 84(4 suppl):S40–S51

Steinberg MH, Barton F, Castro O, Pegelow CH, Ballas SK, Kutlar A et al (2003) Effect of hydroxyurea on mortality and morbidity in adult sickle cell anemia: risks and benefits up to 9 years of treatment. Journal of American Medical Association 289:1645–1651

Stoehr GA, Sobh JN, Luecken J, Heidemann K, Mittler U, Hilgers R et al (2006) Near-total splenectomy for hereditary spherocytosis: clinical prospects in relation to disease severity. British Journal of Haematology 132:791–793

Stoll BJ (2007) Blood disorders. In: Kliegman RM, Jenson HB, Behrman RE, Stanton BF (eds) Nelson textbook of pediatrics. W.B. Saunders, Philadelphia, pp 766–775

Tracy ET, Rice HE (2008) Partial splenectomy for hereditary spherocytosis. Pediatric Clinics of North America 55:503–519

Vichinsky E (2007) Clinical application of deferasirox: practical patient management. American Journal of Hematology 83:398–402

Vichinsky E (2008) Pulmonary hypertension in sickle cell disease. The New England Journal of Medicine 350(9): 857–859

Vichinsky EP, Neumayr LD, Earles AN, Williams R, Lennette ET, Dean D et al., for National Acute Chest Syndrome Study Group (2000) Causes and outcomes of the acute chest syndrome in sickle cell disease. New England Journal of Medicine 342(25):1855–1865

Ware RE (2009) Autoimmune hemolytic anemia. In: Orkin SH, Nathan DG, Ginsburg D, Look AT, Fisher DE, Lux SE (eds) Nathan and Oski's hematology of infancy and childhood. W.B. Saunders, Philadelphia, pp 613–658

Watkins D, Whitehead VM, Rosenblatt DS (2009) Megablastic anemia. In: Orkin SH, Nathan DG, Ginsburg D, Look AT, Fisher DE, Lux SE (eds) Nathan and Oski's hematology of infancy and childhood. W.B. Saunders, Philadelphia, pp 467–520

Neutropenia

Karyn Brundige

Contents

6.1 Epidemiology 173
6.2 Etiology 174
6.3 Symptoms and Clinical Signs 175
6.4 Diagnostic Testing 175
6.5 Treatment 176
6.6 Prognosis 177
6.7 Follow-Up 178
References 178
Resources 178

6.1 Epidemiology

Neutropenia is a decrease in the number of circulating neutrophil granulocytes, phagocytic white blood cells (WBCs), that can engulf and destroy microorganisms.The absolute neutrophil count (ANC) is calculated by multiplying the WBC count by the total number of bands plus segmented (mature) neutrophils:

ANC = WBC × % neutrophils (bands + segmented forms)

Normal neutrophil counts vary by age and race. Newborn infants usually have an elevated ANC for the first few days of life (range $4.5–13.2 \times 10^3/mm^3$) (Kleigman et al. 2007). Neutropenia is categorized as mild (ANC 1,000–1,500/mm^3), moderate (ANC 500–1,000/mm^3), or severe (ANC <500/mm^3). The risk of bacterial or fungal infection increases with both the duration and the severity of neutropenia (Table 6.1). Patients with severe prolonged neutropenia, especially

Table 6.1. Categories of neutropenia

Category of neutropenia	ANC (mm^3)	Risk of infection
None	>1,500	None
Mild neutropenia	1,000–500	No significant risk of infection
Moderate neutropenia	500–1,000	Some risk of infection
Severe neutropenia	<500	Significant risk of infection

those with an ANC <200/mm^3, are at significant risk for sepsis as well as life-threatening gastrointestinal and pulmonary infections. Patients with neutropenia are not at increased risk for parasitic or viral infection.

6.2 Etiology

Neutrophils are produced by myeloid precursors in the bone marrow. On release into the blood stream, approximately half of the neutrophils circulate freely while the remainder adheres to the vascular surface. The average life span of a neutrophil is only 1–2 days. Neutropenia results from three basic mechanisms: decreased production or ineffective granulopoeisis within the bone marrow, increased consumption (e.g., a shift of circulating granulocytes to the vascular epithelium or tissue pools), or enhanced peripheral destruction (e.g., secondary to severe infection or as a result of immune destruction). Confirmation of one of these mechanisms is difficult to obtain outside of the research laboratory. Therefore, classification of neutropenia is often based on whether the neutropenia is acquired or congenital (Table 6.2).

Table 6.2. Causes of neutropenia

Acquired	Infection Drug-induced Immune-mediated Chronic benign (non-immune) Splenic sequestration Nutritional deficiency Bone marrow disorders (neutropenia usually not isolated)
Congenital	Severe congenital, autosomal recessive (Kostmann syndrome) or autosomal dominant Cyclic neutropenia Shwachman-Diamond syndrome Marrow failure syndromes (Fanconi anemia, Dyskeratosis congenita, Blackfan Diamond syndrome) Immunodeficiency syndromes with associated neutropenia (e.g. Chediak-Higashi syndrome, Reticular dysgenesis)

The most common causes of acquired neutropenia are infections, drugs, and immune disorders. Neutropenia can result from bacterial (typhoid, paratyphoid, tuberculosis, brucellosis), viral (HIV, Epstein–Barr virus [EBV], hepatitis A and B, respiratory syncytial virus [RSV], measles, rubella, varicella), protozoan (malaria), and rickettsial infections. Neutropenia secondary to infection is often mild and acute, rarely resulting in serious secondary infections. Many drugs and chemicals induce neutropenia, including cytotoxic chemotherapy, antibiotics, antithyroid, anti-inflammatory, and cardiovascular agents (Table 6.3). Immune-mediated neutropenia may be autoimmune, isoimmune, or associated with a systemic disorder such as systemic lupus erythematosus (SLE) or Crohn's disease. Autoimmune neutropenia is the most common cause of acquired neutropenia in children aged 6 months through 4 years. Accelerated destruction of neutrophils occurs due to the presence of autoantibodies directed against neutrophil-specific antigens (antineutrophil antibodies). Although neutrophil destruction most commonly occurs in the peripheral blood, targeted granulocytes may also be removed in the bone marrow.

Decreased or ineffective production of neutrophils may occur seconday to a bone marrow disease (aplastic anemia, leukemia) or genetic syndrome (Shwachman–Diamond syndrome, dyskeratosis congenita). Nutritional deficiencies including vitamin B-12, folate, and copper deficiency may also result in neutropenia.

Congenital neutropenias are a heterogeneous group of disorders. Severe congenital neutropenia, also known as Kostmann's syndrome, and cyclic neutropenia are the result of either inherited or sporadic genetic mutations resulting in impaired myeloid differentiation, with few neutrophils in the bone marrow maturing beyond the myelocyte stage ("maturation arrest"). Inherited forms of neutropenia may also be associated with immune defects (e.g., reticular dysgenesis), phenotypic abnormalities (e.g., Shwachman–Diamond syndrome or dyskeratosis congenita) or metabolic disorders (e.g., glycogen storage disease type 1b).

Table 6.3. Common medications that cause neutropenia

Drug group	Examples
Antibiotics	Chloramphenicol Cephalosporins Penicillins Sulfonamides Trimethoprim-sulfamethoxazole Macrolides Vancomycin
Anticonvulsants	Phenytoin Valproic acid Carbamazepine Ethosuximide
Anti-inflammatory agents	Sulfasalazine Nonsteroidal anti-inflammatory drugs Gold salts Phenylbutazone
Cardiovascular agents	Antiarrhythmic agents ACE inhibitors Propranolol Dipyridamole Digoxin Ticlopidine
Psychotropic agents	Clozapine Phenothiazines Tricyclic antidepressants Meprobamate
Antithyroid agents (thionamides)	Methimazole Carbimazole Propylthiouracil

6.3 Symptoms and Clinical Signs

Evaluation of the child with neutropenia should begin with a complete history and physical examination. The review of systems should focus on frequency, duration and severity of infection, and age of onset. Typical signs of infection, such as warmth and swelling, may be absent. History of drug or toxin exposure; family history of chronic infections or sudden death, especially in infancy (may indicate inherited disorder); and maternal medical history (if neonatal neutropenia) will aid in differential diagnosis and direct diagnostic work-up. Previous complete blood count (CBC) results, if available, should be reviewed and may establish chronicity or degree of neutropenia. Physical examination should evaluate for the presence of enlarged or tender lymph nodes (may indicate disseminated infection or malignancy), splenomegaly, upper or lower respiratory tract infection (evidence of chronic or underlying disease), and signs and symptoms of skin and mucous membrane infections (rashes, ulcers, abscesses, thrush, or peridontal disease).

Recurrent infections are the most significant consequence of neutropenia. Localized infections of the mucous membranes, skin, perianal, and genital areas are most common, though with persistent severe neutropenia systemic infections can occur. Common infectious organisms include pyogenic (i.e., *Staphylococcus and Streptococcus*) and enteric (i.e., *Escherichia coli*) bacteria and some fungi. The risk of infection depends on the degree and duration of neutropenia. Patients who have an ANC $<500/mm^3$ due to cytotoxic chemotherapy, bone marrow failure, or bone marrow exhaustion are at increased risk for overwhelming bacterial infection including sepsis, pneumonia, and gastrointestinal infections. In contrast, patients who have chronic benign (nonimmune) neutropenia may frequently have an ANC $<200/mm^3$ without developing serious infections.

6.4 Diagnostic Testing

Diagnostic testing for neutropenia begins with the evaluation of the full/complete blood count (FBC/CBC) and examination of the peripheral smear. WBC differentials that are generated by automatic counters should be repeated manually. If the child is asymptomatic and the neutropenia is of less than 6 weeks duration, serial CBCs should be obtained at least twice a week for a minimum of 6 weeks to assess for a cyclical pattern. A positive viral serology (i.e., cytomegalovirus [CMV], EBV, parvovirus B-19 or RSV) in a patient with recent viral illness supports an infectious etiology, while the presence of antineutrophil antibodies, especially in newborns, suggests immune neutropenia.

If the neutropenia is severe and persists longer than 8 weeks, then referral to a hematologist is indicated. Additional studies may include HIV antibody, quantitative immunoglobulins, C3, C4, CH50, antineutrophil antibody, ANA, anti-DNA, antiphospholipid panel, and a chest radiograph (to check for thymic shadow). A bone marrow aspiration and biopsy may be necessary to identify granulocyte precursors and defects in myeloid maturation. The bone marrow aspiration and biopsy may also help to exclude hematologic malignancies (leukemia, asplatic anemia), tumor infiltration, or fibrosis.

Suggested testing for the child with chronic neutropenia that lasts longer than 6 months includes quantitative T and B subsets, serum immunoglobulins, diepoxybutane (if the patient has dysmorphic features, to rule out Fanconi's anemia), serum B-12, copper and RBC folate levels, radiographs of the long bones, exocrine pancreatic studies (if the patient has a history of diarrhea, short stature, or failure to thrive), CD55/CD59 (for paroxysmal nocturnal hemoglobinuria [PNH]), CBCs of family members, and a leukocyte function test to determine if the patient has chronic granulomatous disease (CGD).

6.5 Treatment

Treatment of neutropenia depends on the etiology, duration, and severity of neutropenia. Nutritional deficiencies if identified should be corrected and, when possible, any causative agents (drugs, chemicals) should be discontinued. Children with neutropenia secondary to malignancy, a genetic syndrome with associated immune defect, or chronic infection should be referred to appropriate specialists (e.g., hematology/oncology or infectious disease).

Myeloid growth factors can be administered to accelerate neutrophil recovery in patients who have received myelosupresssive chemotherapy or stem cell transplant, or in neutropenic patients with life-threatening infection. Filgrastim (Neupogen®) and pegfilgrastim (Neulasta®) are examples of recombinant human granulocyte-colony stimulating factor (G-CSF) which stimulate production of functionally active neutrophils. Following chemotherapy completion, Filgrastim is administered daily intravenously (IV) or subcutaneously (SC) until desired ANC is obtained post the expected chemotherapy-induced neutrophil nadir. Pegfilgrastim, a pegylated formulation with longer half-life, is given as a single SQ injection 24–48 h after completing a cycle of chemotherapy. During the period of neutrophil recovery post stem cell transplant, filgrastim dose is titered to maintain an ANC >1,000/mm^3.

In the setting of neutropenia and serious infection or sepsis, filgrastim is often initiated at a dose of 5 mcg/kg daily until the ANC is >5,000/mm^3 on two occasions. If there is no response after 72 h, the dose of filgrastim may be increased to 10 mcg/kg/day. Although WBCs (granulocytes) can be transfused, cells are difficult to collect and have a short life span. As randomized clinical trials are limited, the clinical benefit of granulocyte transfusion as an adjunct to antibiotic therapy in severely neutropenic patients remains unclear.

Although most forms of chronic neutropenia are responsive to G-CSF therapy, treatment is usually reserved for children with recurrent or severe infection. The dose and frequency of filgrastim required to maintain the ANC >1,000/mm^3 varies widely. Children with severe congenital neutropenia may require doses as high as 120 mcg/kg daily. For patients who do not respond to G-CSF therapy, stem cell transplantation from an HLA-matched sibling has been successful and is the only curative option. Children with cyclic neutropenia often respond to lower doses of filgrastim, typically requiring only 2–3 mcg/kg/day every 1–3 days. The use of G-CSF in cyclic neutropenia does not prevent cycling but reduces infectious complications by shortening both the cycle length and duration of neutropenia. Although G-CSF may be used in patients with autoimmune neutropenia to temporarily increase the ANC for elective surgery or in the setting of severe invasive infection, chronic administration is rarely warranted.

Potential side effects of G-CSF include nausea, bone pain, alopecia, diarrhea, low-grade fever, fatigue, anorexia, rash, and headache. Patients with chronic neutropenia can experience severe osteopenia or osteoporosis that increases the risk of fracture; bone demineralization likely results from underlying disease though may be secondary to G-CSF therapy. Calcium and vitamin D supplementation, weight bearing exercises and pamidronate (biphosphonate) infusions have been used to prevent and reverse the degree of osteopenia in children with chronic neutropenia. A subgroup of children with severe congenital (not cyclic) neutropenia and specific genetic mutations in ELA-2, which encodes for neutrophil elastase ("elastase mutations"), have an increased lifetime risk of developing myeloid malignances such as myelodysplastic syndrome (MDS) or acute myelogenous leukemia (AML). Whether malignancy is secondary to G-CSF therapy or as a complication of their underlying disease process now evidenced due to increased life expectancy remains unknown. Patients requiring chronic therapy with G-CSF should have annual bone marrow examinations, cytogenetic analysis, and measurement of bone density.

Patients with chronic neutropenia should receive regular dental care at least every 6 months to prevent chronic gingivitis and recurrent stomatitis. In the child with neutropenia, measures to prevent infection, such as good general hygience (daily bathing and frequent handwashing) and protection against food-borne illness (avoid raw or undercooked meats, well water, aged cheeses and unpasteurized fruit juices or milk products) should be observed. Children with severe neutropenia should be monitored closely for signs and symptoms of infection, should have frequent evaluation of skin and mucous membranes, and should avoid crowds or contact with individuals known to have serious infections. Routine childhood immunizations are encouraged. Antibiotic prophylaxis, except for recurrent infections such as otitis media and urinary tract infections, is discouraged because of the risk for development of resistant organisms.

Fever in the child with severe neutropenia (ANC <500/mm^3) is a medical emergency requiring prompt assessment and treatment. Fever higher than 38°C may be the only presenting sign of infection; typical signs such as warmth and swelling may be absent. Diagnostic evaluation for febrile neutropenia should include culture of blood and urine, stool culture (if diarrhea), and chest X-ray (if respiratory symptoms or concern for pneumonia). As soon as blood cultures have been obtained, therapy with empiric broad-spectrum parenteral antibiotics should be initiated. Antibiotic selection should provide adequate coverage for both gram-positive and gram-negative organisms. Evidence shows that treatment with a single broad spectrum beta-lactam such as ceftazidime or cefipime (monotherapy) has improved outcomes in cancer patients with febrile neutropenia when compared with narrow spectrum beta-lactam combined with an aminoglycoside (comibination therapy). Adverse events were more frequent with combination therapy, specifically nephrotoxicity and fungal superinfection (Paul et al. 2003). Blood pressure instability or sepsis warrants addition of an aminoglycoside (e.g., gentamicin); vancomycin should be reserved for suspected methicillin-resistant *Staphylococcus aureus* or *Cornybacterium* infections. Antibiotics may be discontinued after 72 h if fever defervesces, cultures remain negative, and the child is clinically stable. Oral antibiotics are unnecessary if there is no known source of infection, such as otitis media or pneumonia, and if all cultures remain negative after 72 h. If fever persists for more than 4–5 days, or if recurrent fever occurs while on broad spectrum antibiotics afer an initial afebrile interval, then empiric antifungal coverage should be initiated with amphotericin B (preferably lipid formulation), a broad spectum azole (e.g., voriconazole), or an echinocandin (e.g., capsofungin). Patients with fever and an ANC >1,000/mm^3 without obvious cause of infection can generally be managed on an outpatient basis with either serial observation or treatment with a beta-lactam antibiotic, such as ceftriaxone, and an oral cephalosporin, such as Cefzil or Ceftin, until all cultures are negative after 72 h. The child who has fever and an ANC between 500/mm^3 and 1,000/mm^3 may be managed on either an inpatient or outpatient basis, depending on other presenting signs and symptoms such as cough, shortness of breath, chills, blood pressure instability, or other signs of infection.

6.6 Prognosis

The prognosis of the child with neutropenia depends on several factors, including the etiology (acquired or congenital), duration (acute or chronic) and severity of the neutropenia, and the rapid recognition and treatment of potentially life-threatening infections. Prior to the use of G-CSF, median survival in children with chronic neutropenia was only 3 years owing to death from sepsis and pneumonia. With improved survival due to G-CSF therapy, myeloid malignancy has emerged as a significant complication in the subset of children with severe chronic neutropenia with ELA-2 mutations; these patients have lower neutrophil counts and require higher doses of G-CSF to achieve clinical response.

6.7 Follow-Up

Follow-up of the child with neutropenia is directed by the etiology, duration and severity of the neutropenia, frequency of severe infections, need for G-CSF therapy, and any underlying immune defects, illnesses, or malignancies.

References

Kleigman RM, Behrman RE, Jenson HB, Stanton BF (2007) Nelson textbook of pediatrics, 18th edn. Saunders Elsevier, Philadelphia

Paul M, Schlesinger A, Grozinsky S, Soares-Weiser K, Leibovici L (2003) Beta-lactam versus beta-lactam-aminoglycoside combination therapy in cancer patients with neutropenia. Cochrane Database Syst Rev (3):CD003038. doi:10.1002/14651858

Resources

The Severe Chronic Neutropenia International Registry (SCNIR) was established in 1994 to collect data to monitor the clinical course, treatments, and disease outcomes for children and adults with severe chronic neutropenia. http://depts.washington.edu/registry/. Retrieved August 2, 2009.

Understanding severe chronic neutropenia: A handbook for patients and their families (written for the SCNIR). http://www.severe-chronic-neutropenia.org/handbooks/handbook_en.pdf. Retrieved August 2, 2009.

The Neutropenia Support Association, Inc. is a charity that was founded in 1989 to increase awareness and understanding of neutropenia; the web site contains links to many articles about neutropenia. http://www.neutropenia.ca/. Retrieved August 2, 2009.

Thrombocytopenia

Karyn Brundige

Contents

7.1 Epidemiology 179
7.2 Etiology 180
7.3 Symptoms and Clinical Signs 180
7.4 Diagnostic Testing 182
7.5 Treatment 182
7.6 Prognosis 184
7.7 Follow-Up 184
7.8 Future Perspectives 184
References 184

7.1 Epidemiology

A normal platelet count in adults and children ranges from 150,000 to 450,000/mm^3. Platelets normally survive for 7–10 days in circulation before being removed by the spleen. Platelets are essential for normal blood clotting. Bleeding can occur if platelets are reduced in number or defective in function. Thrombocytopenia is defined as a platelet count more than two standard deviations below the mean of the general population, or <150,000/mm^3. Clinical bleeding as a result of thrombocytopenia usually does not occur until the platelet count drops below 100,000/mm^3, and bleeding from surgery or trauma is uncommon until the platelet count drops below 50,000/mm^3. Serious sponateous bleeding rarely occurs until the platelet count is less than 10–20,000/mm^3.

The most common cause of thrombocytopenia in children is immune thrombocytopenic purpura (ITP). The incidence of symptomatic ITP is approximately 3–8 per 100,000 children per year. Acute ITP, defined as thrombocytopenia that resolves within 6 months of diagnosis, is more prevalent in children younger than 10 years of age with a peak incidence at 2–5 years of age. Male/female ratio is higher in infants and decreases with age. Spontaneous resolution of thrombocytopenia occurs in at least 65% of patients within 6 month. About 60% of cases are preceded by a viral illness. ITP has also been associated with live measles and varicella vaccination (Steuber 2003).

Chronic ITP, the persistence of thrombocytopenia for more than than 6 months after initial presentation, is more prevalent in adolescents than in younger children and affects females more often than males. The majority of patients with ITP will spontaneously attain remission within 12-18 months from diagnosis. (Kalpatthi and Bussel 2008). A small percentage of patients with persistent thrombocytopenia will have clinical and laboratory evidence of an underlying autoimmune disorder such as systemic lupus erythematous (SLE) or autoimmune thyroid disorder.

Immune thrombocytopenia in the early newborn period may be autoimmune or alloimmune. In autoimmune thrombocytopenia, the mother is thrombocytopenic secondary to ITP or SLE; maternal antiplatelet antibodies cross the placenta and destroy fetal platelets. Neonatal alloimmune thrombocytopenia (NAIT) is a condition that affects 1 in 1,000-5,000 newborns. The mother usually has a normal platelet count. The fetal platelets contain an antigen inherited from the father that the mother lacks resulting in subsequent sensitization and formation of maternal alloantibodies to the fetal platelets. Although both conditions may result in severe thrombocytopenia, the risk of intracranial hemorrhage is greater in alloimmune than in autoimmune thromboytopenia.

7.2 Etiology

The etiology of thrombocytopenia includes disorders of impaired/decreased platelet production, enhanced platelet destruction, and dilutional or distributional thrombocytopenia (Table 7.1). Platelet production within the bone marrow may be suppressed due to a variety of congenital or acquired conditions including malignancy, viral infection, and exposure to certain medications and toxic chemicals. Thrombocytopenia can also result when the bone marrow produces a normal number of platelets but platelet destruction occurs at a faster rate than platelet production. Causes of enhanced platelet destruction include autoimmune diseases such as ITP or lupus, medications, infection, surgery, pregnancy, and thrombotic conditions such as disseminated intravascular clotting (DIC). Dilutional or distributional thrombocytopenia occurs when circulating platelets are trapped or sequestered in the spleen. In these patients, the platelet size and life span are usually normal and clinical bleeding is less common.

7.3 Symptoms and Clinical Signs

Patients with thrombocytopenia may be asymptomatic and only identified when a low platelet count is detected on a routine blood test. The most common symptomatic presentation of thrombocytopenia is mucosal or cutaneous bleeding (Table 7.2). Mucosal bleeding typically manifests as epistaxis, gingival bleeding, or wet purpura on the buccal mucosa; cutaneous bleeding as petechiae, purpura, and ecchymoses. Prolonged and heavy menorrhagia can occur in adolescent females and may result in significant anemia.

Intracranial hemorrhage, though a rare occurrence, is the most common cause of death secondary to severe thrombocytopenia. Bleeding in patients with thrombocytopenia differs from that seen in patients with coagulation disorders; patients with coagulation disorders experience more deep bleeding into joints or muscle, minimal bleeding with superficial injuries, and rarely develop petechiae.

The child with thrombocytopenia warrants a thorough history and physical examination. The history should focus on bleeding symptoms (type, site, severity, and duration); risk factors such as recent live virus immunization, acute or chronic illness, current and recent medications including herbal formulations; other underlying conditions (genetic, autoimmune, hematologic, or oncologic) and family history suggestive of congenital thrombocytopenic or platelet function disorders. The physical examination should concentrate on evidence of bruising or bleeding on the skin or mucosa, especially in dependent areas and in areas of pressure, Lymphadenopathy, hepatosplenomegaly, jaundice, or fever suggest an underlying systemic disorder that may cause or be associated with thrombocytopenia.

Table 7.1. Differential diagnosis of thrombocytopenia

Etiology	Association	Diagnosis
Destructive thrombocytopenias	Immunologic	ITP Drug induced Infection induced Post-transfusion purpura Autoimmune disease Post-transplant Hyperthyroidism Lymphoproliferative disorders
	Nonimmunologic	Microangiopathic disease Hemolytic anemia and thrombocytopenia Hemolytic uremic syndrome Thrombotic thrombocytopenia purpura (TTP)
	Platelet consumption/destruction	Disseminated intravascular coagulation (DIC) Giant hemangiomas Cardiac (prosthetic heart valves, repair of intracardiac defects)
	Neonatal problems	Pulmonary hypertension Polycythemia Respiratory distress syndrome (RDS)/infection (viral, bacterial, protozoal, spirochetal) Sepsis/DIC Prematurity Meconium aspiration Giant hemangioma Neonatal alloimmune Neonatal autoimmune (maternal ITP) Erythroblastosis fetalis (Rh incompatibility)
Impaired production	Congenital and hereditary disorders	Thrombocytopenia-absent radii (TAR) syndrome Fanconi's anemia Bernard–Soulier syndrome Wiskott–Aldrich syndrome Glanzmann's thromboasthenia May–Hegglin anomaly Amegakaryocytosis (congenital) Rubella syndrome
	Associated with chromosomal defect	Trisomy 13 or 18
	Metabolic disorders	Marrow infiltration: malignancies, storage disease, myelofibrosis
	Acquired processes	Aplastic anemia Drug-induced Severe Iron deficiency
Dilutional or distributional	Hypersplenism (portal hypertension, neoplastic, infectious, glycogen storage disease, cyanotic heart disease) Hypothermia	

Adapted from The Children's Hospital Oakland: Hematology/Oncology Handbook (2002)

Table 7.2. Clinical manifestations of thrombocytopenia

Clinical manifestations
Mucosal bleeding
Epistaxis
Gingival bleeding
Wet purpura
Menorrhagia
Hematuria
Melena/Hematochezia
Cutaneous bleeding
Petechiae
Ecchymoses (bruising)

7.4 Diagnostic Testing

Diagnostic testing for thrombocytopenia starts with the evaluation of the full/complete blood count (FBC/CBC). As some automated machines may read clumps of platelets as "one" platelet or count them as other types of cells, the peripheral blood smear should be examined for estimation of platelet numbers, platelet morphology, and the presence or absence of platelet clumping. Congenital disorders associated with thrombocytopenia can often be diagnosed by platelet morphology on the peripheral smear. Platelets that are of normal size (Fig. 7.1) are seen in conditions resulting from decreased platelet production or bone marrow failure. Larger platelets (Fig. 7.2) (increased mean platelet volume or MPV) are more common when the bone marrow increases the rate of platelet production to compensate for increased peripheral destruction. Bone marrow aspiration and biopsy is indicated in patients with unexplained thrombocytopenia or if the peripheral smear is concerning for marrow hypoplasia (pancytopenia) or malignacy (blasts). The presence of normal to increased numbers of megakaryocytes in the bone marrow suggests increased peripheral destruction of platelets. Absent or decreased megakaryocytes in the bone marrow may be the result of a genetic condition, myelodysplastic syndrome, or malignant infiltration. Patients with normal blood smear except for isolated thrombocytopenia, normal physical examination, and negative history including possible drug-induced causes of thrombocytopenia may be presumptively diagnosed as having ITP. These patients do not require bone marrow evaluation unless they are refractory to therapy required to maintain platelet levels in a safe range or if thrombocytopenia persists for longer than 6 months. Additional laboratory evaluation or diagnostic imaging is guided by historical or physical findings (Table 7.3).

Table 7.3. Additional studies to be considered in thrombocytopenic patients

Additional studies
Viral serologies (EBV, CMV, Parvovirus B19)
HIV antibody
Antiplatelet antibody (PAIGG)
Lupus panel
Antiphospholipid antibody
Lupus anticoagulant
C3, C4
Lymphocyte panel
LDH
Direct Coombs
Quantitative immunoglobulins
DEB
PNH
Platelet EMs
X-ray radii
Family members' platelet counts

7.5 Treatment

Treatment for thrombocytopenia depends on the etiology, severity of thrombocytopenia, and risk for bleeding. Bone marrow transplant can be used to treat some disorders of congenital thrombocytopenia, such as Wiskott–Aldrich syndrome and Fanconi's anemia. Thrombocytopenia resulting from decreased platelet production by the bone marrow may be treated by platelet transfusion; transfusion thresholds of 10–20,000/mm3 are usually adequate unless the patient requires invasive procedure or surgery. Although platelet transfusion is generally not indicated to treat thrombocytopenia from immune platelet destruction as the transfused platelets will be rapidly destroyed, transfusion may be used for life- or organ-threatening bleeding.

Management of children with acute ITP is controversial. Because the majority of cases of pediatric ITP will resolve spontaneously, the risk of potential treatment related complications must be balanced against the relatively rare risk of life-threatening hemorrhage. Some patients may also choose treatment due to lifestyle choices, such as travel or desire to participate in specific sports. First-line therapies for acute ITP include intravenous immune globulin (IVIG), corticosteroids, and anti-Rho(D) immune globulin (Table 7.4). The goal of treatment is to transiently increase the platelet count to a safe range, thereby reducing the risk of serious hemorrhage. None of these therapies are curative and duration of response is variable; children may require repeat treatment every 2–8 weeks until thrombctyopenia resolves. For patients refractory to first-line agents, various immunosuppressive therapies may be trialed including vincristine, azathioprine, rituximab, cyclophosphamide, mycophenolate mofetil, and cyclosporine (Blanchette and Bolton-Maggs 2008).

Splenectomy may be considered emergently for patients with refractory acute ITP experiencing life-threatening bleeding. Patients with chronic ITP may benefit from elective splenectomy if thrombocytopenia persists for more than 12 months and requires repeated treatment or interferes significantly with the patient's life style. The potential for spontaneous remission should be balanced against risk of treatment failure and postsplenectomy infection. Splenectomy improves the platelet count in 60–90% of children with chronic ITP; the success of splenectomy is strongly correlated with good response to prior medical therapy (Ramenghi et al. 2006). The risk of overwhelming bacterial sepsis in asplenic patients due to encapsulated organisms limits its safety, especially in patients younger than 5 years of age. For elective procedures, immunization at least 2 weeks prior to splenectomy with polyvalent pneumococal, *Hemophilis Influenza Type b* and

Table 7.4. Comparison of ITP treatments

Treatment	Dose	Advantages	Disadvantages	Side effects
IVIG	0.8-1 g/kg IV per day for 1-2 days	Faster recovery of platelet count	Cost (can be as much as 70 times more expensive than corticosteroids)	Nausea, vomiting, headache, fever, chills Rare: anaphylaxis
Corticosteroids	Prednisone 4 mg/kg/day PO ov IV for 4 days (with or without a taper) or 1-2 mg/kg/day PO for 2–3 weeks, then tapered over 1 week	Oral administration Relatively inexpensive Oral administration	Sharp decrease in platelet count after discontinuation	Weight gain, hypertension, Cushing's syndrome, mood changes, reflux
Anti-Rho(D) immune globulin	75 mcg/kg IV x1 dose	Infusion time less than for IVIG	Must be Rh+ 1–1.5 g/dL or greater fall in hemoglobin as a result of hemolysis (occurs 1–2 weeks after administration)	Fever, chills, headache, anemia Rare: anaphylaxis

quadrivalent meningococcal polysaccharide vaccine is recommended to reduce the incidence of post-splenectomy infection and mortality. Prophylactic antibiotic therapy for asplenic patients remains controversial; patients should wear a MedAlert bracelet and all febrile illnesses require evaluation and initiation of antibiotics until bacterial sepsis is excluded.

Patients with thrombocytopenia should understand signs and symptoms of low platelet counts and serious bleeding, including intracranial hemorrhage. The risk of serious bleeding can be reduced by discouraging participation in contact sports, such as football and wrestling, or activities at high altitudes when there is a chance of falling and sustaining a head injury. Children with thrombocytopenia should avoid medications that can decrease platelet count or impair platelet function (e.g., aspirin, ibuprofen, and other aspirin-containing medications). Preventive care includes adequate intake of fiber and liquids to prevent constipation and the use of lotion, lip balm, and a soft toothbrush to minimize damage to skin and mucous membranes.

The treatment for autoimmune and alloimmune thrombocytopenia in newborns is similar. Both can be treated with IVIG, steroids, platelet transfusions, and exchange transfusions. Platelets should be transfused if the platelet count is <20,000/mm^3, but if the infant is premature or ill, then the transfusion threshold is a platelet count <50,000/mm^3. An adequate platelet count should be maintained for the first 72–96 h to prevent intracranial hemorrhage. Patients with NAIT should receive matched platelet transfusions; if maternal platelets are utilized, they must be processed to remove platelet alloantibodies. In contrast, infants born to mothers with ITP or SLE should not receive platelets from the mother because they contain the antigens responsible for forming platelet autoantibodies.

7.6 Prognosis

The prognosis of the child with thrombocytopenia depends on several factors, including the severity and underlying cause of the thrombocytopenia, the response to treatment, and the frequency and severity of bleeding complications. Prognosis also depends on the incidence, quick recognition, and treatment of life-threatening bleeding complications such as intracranial hemorrhage.

7.7 Follow-Up

Follow-up of the child with thrombocytopenia is determined by the cause and degree of thrombocytopenia, the frequency and severity of bleeding complications, and the response to treatment. The child with chronic ITP with few bleeding complications may be followed in clinic every 3–6 months, whereas the child with congenital thrombocytopenia who requires frequent platelet transfusions to treat bleeding complications may require more frequent follow-up. At each clinic visit or with bleeding episodes, a FBC/CBC should be obtained to monitor the platelet count.

7.8 Future Perspectives

Cytokines to stimulate platelet production are being studied and include interleukin-3 (IL-3), stem cell factor, IL-6, IL-11, and thrombopoietin. The Intercontinental Childhood ITP Study Group (ICIS), a worldwide network of physicians and investigators, was founded in 1997 to clarify questions regarding diagnosis and treatment of ITP and provide long-term concepts for prospective studies.

References

Blanchette V, Bolton-Maggs P (2008) Childhood immune thrombocytopenic purpura: diagnosis and management. Pediatric Clinics of North America 55:393–420

Blanchette VS, Carcao M (2003) Childhood acute immune thrombocytopenic purpura: 20 years later. Seminars in Thrombosis and Hemostasis 29:607–615

Kalpatthi R, Bussel JB (2008) Diagnosis, pathophysiology and management of children with refractory leukemia. Current Opinions in Pediatrics 20:8–16

Ramenghi U, Amendola G, Farinasso L, Giordano P, Loffredo G, Nobili B, Perrotta S, Russo G, Zecca M (2006) Splenectomy in children with chronic ITP: long-term efficacy and relation between its outcome and responses to previous treatment. Pediatric Blood and Cancer 47:742–745

Steuber CP (2003) Idiopathic thrombocytopenic purpura in children. www.uptodate.com. Retrieved 14 Mar 2009

Bleeding Disorders

Joan O'Brien-Shea

Contents

8.1 Hemophilia 187
8.1.1 Epidemiology 187
8.1.2 Etiology 187
8.1.3 Genetics 188
8.1.4 Symptoms and Clinical Signs 188
8.1.5 Diagnostic Testing 190
8.1.6 Treatment 191
8.1.7 Prognosis 194
8.1.8 Follow-Up 194
8.1.9 Future Perspectives 194
8.2 von Willebrand Disease 194
8.2.1 Epidemiology 194
8.2.2 Etiology 195
8.2.3 Genetics 195
8.2.4 Symptoms and Clinical Signs 195
8.2.5 Diagnostic Testing 196
8.2.6 Treatment 199
8.2.7 Prognosis 200
8.2.8 Follow-Up 200
References 201

8.1 Hemophilia

8.1.1 Epidemiology

Hemophilia is a condition characterized by a clotting factor deficiency of the intrinsic or plasma pathway of the coagulation cascade. Over 80% of all individuals with hemophilia have a deficiency in factor VIII, also known as hemophilia A, which occurs in one in every 10,000 men. Hemophilia B (previously called Christmas disease), or a deficiency of factor IX, comprises approximately 20% of those with hemophilia and occurs in one in every 34,000 live male births. A deficiency in either of these coagulation factors results in the delayed formation of fibrin and a consequent tendency to hemorrhage. A factor VIII or IX assay of 0–2%, compared with a normal assay of approximately 50–150%, is classified as severe disease, and these patients can have frequent and significant symptoms. Moderate hemophilia is generally noted as a factor level of 2–5%, and these patients have intermittent symptoms. Mild hemophilia indicates a factor assay of greater than 5%; correspondingly, these patients have less frequent bleeding complications. Hemophilia is reported in all races and ethnicities. Other factor deficiencies are possible and infrequent, but some are associated with bleeding symptoms.

8.1.2 Etiology

Factors VIII and IX are integral parts of the intrinsic coagulation pathway that assists in the formation of a fibrin clot. The pathway of blood coagulation is illustrated in Chap. 19 (Fig. 19.1). Decreased functional amounts of factor VIII or IX hamper clot formation

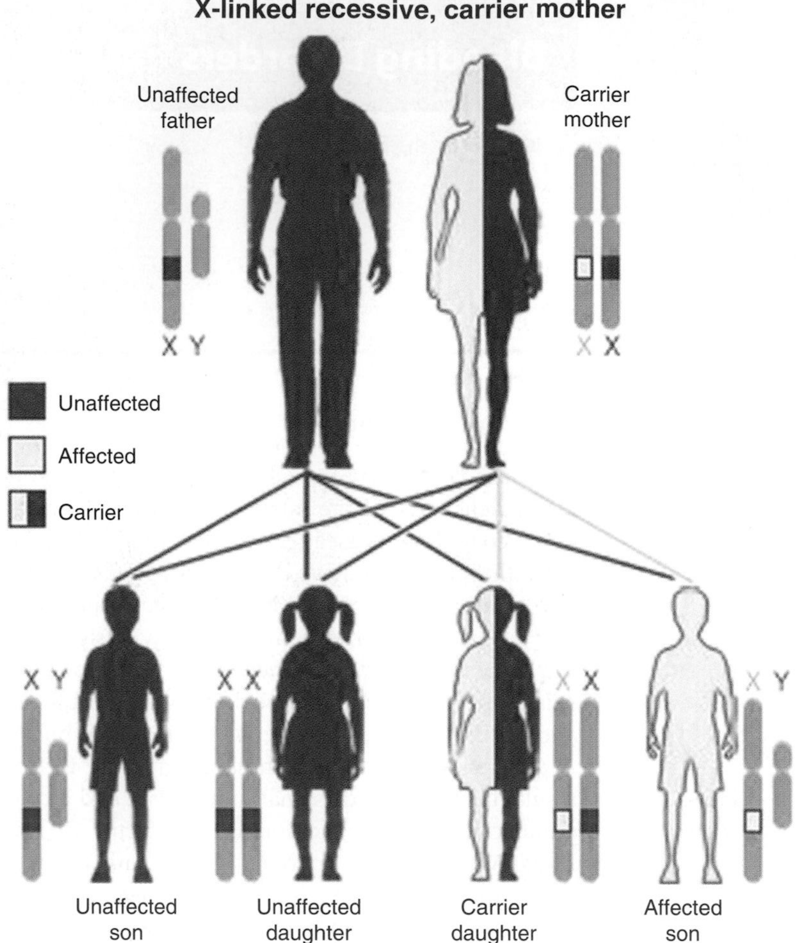

Figure 8.1

Illustration of X-linked recessive gene transfer. Image credit: http://ghr.nlm.nih.gov

and hemostasis. Deficiencies of factor VIII or IX are inherited X-linked diseases. It is now recognized that women, who are generally thought of as carriers of hemophilia, can have significantly low factor assays and be symptomatic due to the effects of lyonization.

8.1.3 Genetics

Hemophilia is a sex-linked recessive disease (Fig. 8.1). The genes for both factor VIII and factor IX are located on the long arm of the X chromosome. Heterozygous women are typically asymptomatic, but can transmit the disease to 50% of their sons and can transmit the carrier state to 50% of their daughters. Random new mutation is possible, although infrequent, and can result in a carrier state in females or a disease state in males. Affected hemizygous males will transmit the gene to all their daughters, making them carriers. It is possible for a woman to have the disease, or symptoms, by lyonization of the carrier state, by new mutation, or as a product of the combination of an affected male and a carrier female.

8.1.4 Symptoms and Clinical Signs

There is no distinguishing clinical difference between hemophilia A and B. Presentation of a patient with hemophilia varies, depending on known family history and severity of the disease. Obviously, if family history is significant for hemophilia, then the patient's diagnosis is typically made prior to any untoward events. Otherwise, patients with severe hemophilia often present within the first year of life. Approximately 5% of these patients present with perinatal intracranial or subgaleal bleeding. Use of forceps, suctioning, or traumatic birth may be associated with intracranial hemorrhage. Prolonged bleeding after circumcision is also a common presenting symptom. Otherwise, infants and children with severe hemophilia typically present with significant and excessive ecchymosis with little or no trauma; abnormal bleeding, especially of the mucous membranes; or hemarthrosis. There may be no associated injury to produce bleeding in these patients, as hemorrhage can be spontaneous.

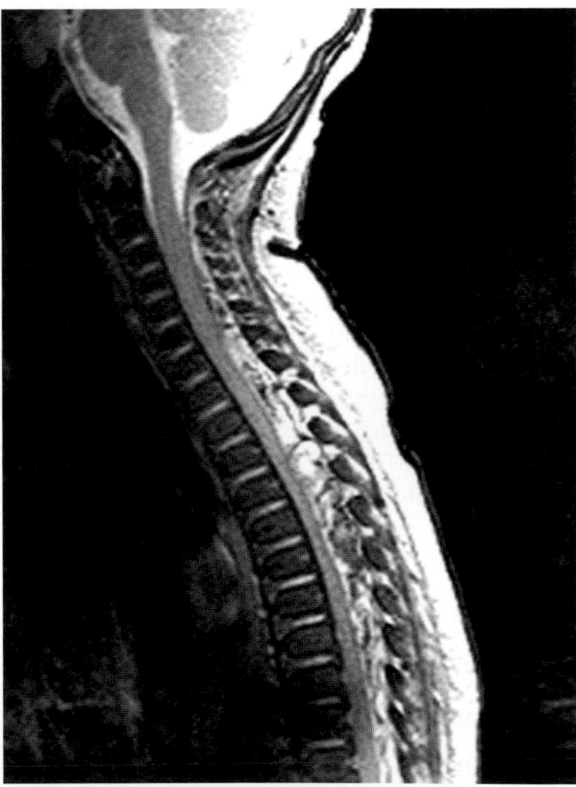

Figure 8.2

CT imaging of a cervical intraspinal epidural hemorrhage in an 8-month-old male with hemophilia A

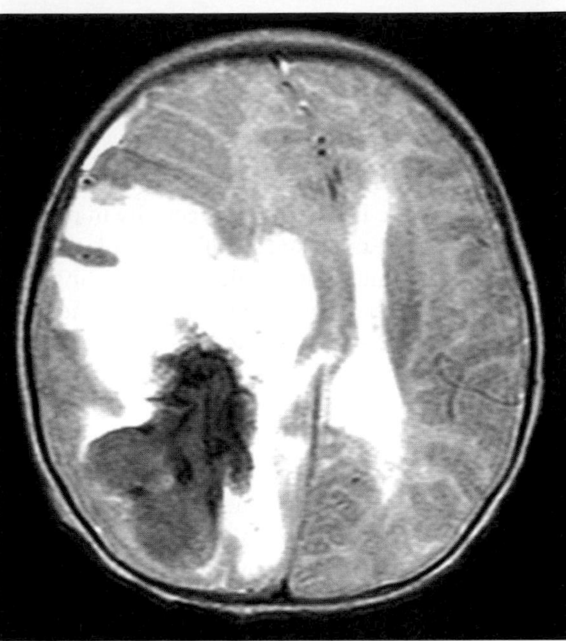

Figure 8.3

CT imaging of a right temporal subdural hemorrhage in a 9-month-old male with hemophilia A

Moderate to mild hemophilia can be associated with bleeding symptoms in later childhood or possibly adulthood. These findings are usually bleeding or bruising thought to be excessive with normal activities or due to some trauma, and hemarthrosis is possible with a significant injuring event. The disease can be so mild that it may not be detected until an adult has an invasive procedure or surgery. It is important to remember that disease genotype does not always accurately correlate with phenotype.

Specific sites of bleeding that are noteworthy include the following:

1. *Central nervous system (CNS)* – Intracranial or spinal hemorrhage can occur spontaneously (Fig. 8.2, 8.3) in those with severe hemophilia, and is possible with injury or trauma in all classes of hemophilia. Typically, presentation includes symptoms of lethargy, headache, and vomiting. Silent hemorrhage is also possible, however. Head or spinal injury is considered a medical emergency; therefore, factor replacement should occur

prior to any diagnostic testing. A CT of the brain is typically performed as it is more immediately available than MRI, but MRI alone may detect some silent intracranial hemorrhages.

2. *Head and neck* – Epitaxis and mouth bleeding after tooth loss, eruption, or trauma is not uncommon in hemophilia. The fibrinolytic activity in mucous membrane areas makes stabilization of clot formation difficult, and prolonged bleeding can occur. Retropharyngeal bleeding, considered a medical emergency because of the possibility of airway obstruction, can be caused by pharyngitis, coughing, vomiting, or trauma to the neck area.
3. *Musculoskeletal system* – Hematoma development within the muscle causes pain, swelling, and possible decreased muscle function. When bleeding occurs in an extremity, compartment syndrome is possible, and consequent damage to peripheral nerves, vasculature, and tissue can be permanent. Pseudotumor, or encapsulated hematoma, can occur when a muscle hematoma is left untreated, and once developed it is difficult to treat and often recurs. Bleeding into a joint area, or hemarthrosis, is more common in patients with severe disease, but can occur in any patient. Joint swelling, warmth, pain, stiffness, and limp or limited movement are common symptoms of this event. Irritability and refusal to use the affected area may be the only symptoms in infants and small children. Recurrent hemarthrosis to a target joint can culminate in significant chronic arthropathy.
4. *Genitourinary system* – Hematuria can be spontaneous in severe hemophilia or due to trauma in all types of hemophilia. The patient most often has no symptoms other than the noted hematuria, but pain can indicate clotting in the ureter or renal pelvis. Other diagnoses must be ruled out. Hematoma to the penis can result in urinary obstruction, and testicular hematoma is significant as this may lead to infertility.
5. *Posttraumatic bleeding* – Most patients, whether with severe or mild disease, will not have significant bleeding after venipuncture. Bleeding post-trauma is related to the trauma itself and the severity of hemophilia. Bleeding can be delayed, occurring hours after the injury or procedure.

Other complications that may occur in a patient with hemophilia include infections due to exposure to blood products or factor replacement and the development of inhibitors. Prior to 1990, a number of children receiving factor concentrates became infected with hepatitis C and/or HIV. Infections are extremely rare now owing to the advent of virucidal treatments such as pasteurization, solvent-detergents, and through current screening techniques (Lefrere and Hewitt 2009). Despite treatments and screening, it is still possible for parvovirus B19 to be transmitted, and the latest concern is the possible transmission of Creutzfeldt–Jakob disease (CJD), a transmissible spongiform encephalopathy. There have been no known transmissions of CJD, but there are no current screening tests or treatments for this disease (Allain et al. 2009).

The development of inhibitors, or antibodies, to factor VIII or IX is a significant complication that occurs in approximately 25% of those with severe hemophilia A and up to 5% of those with severe hemophilia B. Inhibitor development in mild or moderate disease states is possible, but not common. Routine testing for the presence of inhibitors is recommended in all patients with hemophilia who have received factor replacement; testing should be annual or semiannual, or more frequently in high-titer patients. The inhibitor, measured in Bethesda units (BU), removes infused factor replacement at a rate directly proportional to the level of the inhibitor, thus making bleeding episodes difficult to treat. A low-titer inhibitor, or low responder, is usually classified as less than 5 BU, and a high-titer inhibitor, or high responder, as greater than 5 BU. It may be possible to overwhelm a low-titer inhibitor with a high dose of factor replacement, but this is not usually possible with high titers. There is a significant risk, as high as 26%, that those with hemophilia B who develop inhibitors will have anaphylactic reactions to factor IX replacement.

8.1.5 Diagnostic Testing

Initial evaluation should include:

1. Platelet count should be within normal limits
2. Prothrombin time (PT) should be within normal limits

3. Activated partial prothrombin time (aPTT) – aPTT, as a test of the intrinsic clotting pathway, will be prolonged in most patients with hemophilia (with the exception of some patients with mild factor IX deficiency)

Further testing may require:

4. Factor VIII or IX assays will indicate the deficiency state. Several types of factor assays are available. The one-stage clotting assays are commonly used, but two-stage assays are less influenced by variables; the chromogenic assay is very specific but technically complicated. Factor VIII levels can be low in several types of vWD, and therefore it is important to distinguish between the two diseases.
5. A von Willebrand panel, to include the ristocetin cofactor assay, von Willebrand factor (vWF) antigen assay, and multimer analysis, should be done. In addition, the type 2N (Normandy) vWD panel, or factor VIII binding assay, will distinguish mild hemophilia A type from 2N vWD. In patients with 2N vWD, the factor VIII assay is low, but the von Willebrand panel may be normal. Prenatal diagnosis is availble to known carriers through DNA analysis.

8.1.6 Treatment

There are several options for Factor VIII replacement. The safety and efficacy of recombinant factor VIII (rFVIII) has been well established and is the recommended first-line treatment in Hemophilia A (Musso 2008). rFVIII is a genetically engineered product, as this has the least known risk of viral contamination, but these products are among the most costly treatments available. First-generation recombinant products contain human albumin, which is used to stabilize the factor VIII protein, but the second-generation products have little or no albumin and are stabilized in sucrose. Plasma-derived factor VIII products are less expensive than recombinant products and are most commonly used by those who have previously been exposed to this type of product, or when cost or availability are issues. One unit of factor VIII, either recombinant or plasma-derived, is equal to 2% of factor activity in vitro. The half-life of plasma-derived or recombinant factor VIII is between 8 and 12 h. Dosing is reviewed in Table 8.1.

Recombinant factor IX used to treat Hemophilia B is also available and recommended as a first-line therapy. It is a DNA-synthesized product that has no added albumin; therfore, the risk of viral contamination is virtually nonexistant. Plasma-derived factor IX is less expensive than recombinant factor IX but carries some risk of viral contamination. Factor IX is dosed in units per kg of body weight; one unit of plasma-derived factor IX is equal to 1% factor IX activity in vitro, but one unit of recombinant factor IX is equal to about 0.8% activity in vitro. The half-life of plasma-derived or recombinant factor IX is approximately 16 h.

In emergency situations when factor replacement is not available, fresh frozen plasma can be used for those with hemophilia A or B. Cryoprecipitate can be used for factor VIII-deficient patients. Both these products are typically available through local blood banks, and although the risk is small, possible viral contamination is always a concern for patients and families. For dosing recommendations, see Chap. 31.

Prophylaxis is used in hemophilia A and B to decrease the risk of bleeding and involves a strategy of routine administration of factor replacement. Primary prophylaxis refers to the initiation of regular long-term factor replacement therapy before the age of 2 years and/or after no more than one joint bleed. Several studies have demonstrated significant reductions in the risk of chronic arthropathy in the future (Panicker et al. 2003; Shapiro 2003). Recent studies have shown that primary prophylaxis may also prevent the development of inhibitors (Mancuso et al. 2009). Primary prophylaxis is the recommended standard treatment for severe hemophiliacs in both Europe and North America (Coppola et al. 2008).

Secondary prophylaxis refers to regular long-term factor replacement therapy started any other time beyond the primary prophylaxis criteria. Retrospective studies have demonstraed slower progression of arthropathy in children but issues surrounding dosing and duration of secondary prophylaxis remain unresolved (Tagliaferri et al. 2008).

Several therapies other than factor replacement can be utilized for adjuvant therapy for bleeding in the patient with hemophilia. Desmopressin, or DDAVP, is

Table 8.1. Intravenous treatment guidelines for factor VIII and IX deficiency

Hemarthrosis, any joint prednisone	40–50 U/kg x1 (80–100), followed by 25–50 U/kg (50–100) q12–24 h for 2–5 days	25–50 U/kg x1 (25–50), followed by 25–50 U/kg (25–50) q24 h for 1–3 days	Apply ice/cold pack, immobilize x48 h, then light ambulation; increase dose prn worsening symptoms; consider 1–2 mg/kg/day
Hematoma, soft tissue	25–35 U/kg x1 (50–70), followed by 25 U/kg (50) q.d. x2	20–30 U/kg x1 (20–30), followed by 30 U/kg (30) q.d. x2	Ice/cold pack
Hematuria	35 U/kg x1 (70), followed by 25 U/kg (50) q12–24 h x2–7 days	25–50 U/kg x1 (25–50), followed by 30 U/kg (30) q24 h x2–7 days	Hydration is helpful; may use prednisone 1–2 mg/kg/day x7–14 days; consider differential diagnosis; do not use antifibrinolytic (risk of thrombosis)
Gastrointestinal	35–50 U/kg x1 (70–100), followed by 35 U/kg (70) q12 h x2–7 days	50–100 U/kg x1 (50–100), followed by 50–100 U/kg (50–100) q.d. x2–7 days	Determine cause/extent; monitor CBC; potentially life-threatening
Mucosal	35–50 U/kg x1 (70–100), followed by 25–35 U/kg (50–70) q24 h x1–2 days	25–50 U/kg x1 (25–50), followed by 25–50 U/kg (25–50) q12–24 h x1–2 days	Ice/ cold pack; use antifibrinolytic
Head trauma	50 U/kg x1 (100), followed by 35 U/kg (70) q12 h x7–10 days	100 U/kg x1 (100), followed by 50–100 U/kg (50–100) q12 h x7–10 days	First dose to be given immediately, then CT, etc.; maintain trough >50% activity
Major surgery	50 U/kg x1 (100), followed by 35 U/kg (70) q12 h x3–8 days	50–100 U/kg x1 (50–100), followed by 50–100 U/kg (50–100) q24 h x7–10 days	Monitor factor activity, trough >50%
Dental extraction	50 U/kg x1(100), followed by 35 U/kg (70) q12 h x3 days	25–50 U/kg x1 (25–50), followed by 25–50 U/kg (25–50) q24 h x 2–7 days	Use antifibrinolytic
Prophylaxis	25–35 U/kg (50–70) three times per week	25–40 U/kg twice per week	
Immune tolerance	50–100 U/kg q24–48 h	Risk of anaphylaxis	

Table 8.2. Desmopressin challenge

DDAVP IV or SQ	0.3 mg/kg in 50 mL of normal saline IV over ~20 min, or same dose for SQ injection
Stimate (150 mg/mL)	<50 kg; one puff intranasally or >50 kg two puffs intranasally, q12–24 h

DDAVP IV may elicit a stronger response than intranasal dosing. An increase in factor VIII levels can be expected in approximately 30 minutes.
Challenge instructions: Draw factor VIII assay just before dose is given, and repeat 1 h after dose. A threefold increase is considered a good response

a synthetic antidiuretic hormone and can increase available factor VIII levels for 12 and up to 24 h by stimulating release of factor VIII from storage sites in the endothelial cells. This is typically effective only in those with mild factor VIII deficiency, but it does not work on each individual; therefore, a trial dose (DDAVP challenge) should be given to determine efficacy (Table 8.2). This medication is available in IV form or as a nasal formulation, Stimate (150 mg/mL). Common side effects include flushing, tachycardia, and headache, and uncommonly, hyper- or hypotension. A decreased infusion rate may diminish these effects. Overuse of DDAVP can lead to the antidiuretic

Table 8.3. Antifibrinolytic medications

Aminocaproic acid (Amicar)	50–100 mg/kg/dose q6 h (maximum 3–4 doses) IV or PO
Tranexamic acid (Cyklokapron)	25 mg/kg/dose q6–8 h IV or PO

These drugs cannot be used with PCCs or APCC replacement products

effects of this medication, including fluid retention and sodium depletion. Giving more than three doses of DDAVP requires fluid restriction and sodium monitoring. Repeated doses will lead to depletion of stored factor VIII and decreased drug efficacy.

Antifibrinolytic therapies are available for mucous membrane bleeding. Aminocaproic acid (Amicar) and tranexamic acid (Cyklokapron) inhibit the action of fibrinolysis that occurs at mucous membrane sites. Both these medications stabilize clot formation and are typically used in conjunction with factor replacement, but they may be effective when used alone for minor bleeding in a patient with mild hemophilia. To avoid thrombotic risk, these drugs should not be used concomitantly with prothrombin complex concentrate (Table 8.3). Fibrin sealants and platelet gels have been successfully used to promote clotting in dental and orthopedic surgery and with circumcision in patients with hemophilia (Burnouf et al. 2004).

Currently, the most serious complication in hemophilia is the development of inhibitors (Haya et al. 2007). Inhibitors are antibodies to the proteins in infused FVIII. The first clinical sign of inhibitor development is often continued bleeding despite factor replacement treatment. The Bethesda assay test is used to quantify inhibitors. The inhibitor may be bypassed by using activated prothrombin complex concentrates (APCCs) for factor VIII inhibitors, and recombinant factor VIIa for factor VIII or IX inhibitors. Large doses of APCCs are associated with some risk of thrombosis, and there is no in vitro assay to monitor efficacy of APCCs. Porcine factor VIII concentrate can be used to bypass the factor VIII inhibitor and is typically a treatment option for those with high-titer inhibitors. There is the possibility of cross-reactivity between porcine and human factor inhibitor development; therefore, a porcine factor VIII inhibitor assay must be evaluated prior to any treatment with this product. Hypersensitivity is also an issue with porcine factor VIII.

Immune tolerance (IT) strategies or desensitization is used to overwhelm factor inhibitor production in hopes of eliminating the inhibitor. Studies report that this works best if the inhibitor is at low titer levels at the initiation of IT. IT therapy involves repeated exposure to Factor VIII sometimes over years until tolerance is achieved by antigen acceptance. There are several protocols for IT therapy using multiple products. The cost of IT treatment is high but is currently still less expensive than long-term treatment with bypassing agents (Kruse-Jarres et al. 2008).

The use of immunoadsorption, cyclosporin, and Rituximab in IT therapy has been reported but currently there are no reported successful clinical trials (Kruse-Jarres et al. 2008). Continued research is necessary for those inhibitor patients who do not respond to IT treatments.

The therapeutic management of hemophilias A and B are similar and will be reviewed together. Tables 8.1 and 8.4 provide general guidelines for treatment of typical bleeding. Each patient's plan of care must be individualized to reflect any special

Table 8.4. Treatment for acute bleeding in patients with factor inhibitors

FEIBA (factor VII inhibitor bypass activity) or autoplex	Effective for factor VIII inhibitors	75–100 U/kg IV q12–24 h	Monitor fibrinogen and D-dimers after third dose due to thrombosis risk; not to be used with antifibrinolytic drugs
Recombinant factor VIIa (NovoSeven)	Effective for factor VIII or factor IX inhibitors	~90 mg/kg IV q2 h, weaning to larger intervals as bleeding stabilizes; larger doses may be necessary in some patients	

circumstances or conditions that may require more or less intervention. The patient's dose should be rounded to the nearest vial whenever possible. It is important to note that doses of recombinant factor IX must be adjusted upward by a factor of 1.2 (1 unit = 0.8% activity) to achieve the desired factor IX in vitro percent activity goal.

Supportive treatments are beneficial and include application of an ice or cold pack to the injured area when possible, pressure (local pressure or Ace wrap, if applicable), elevation of the extremity, and rest or immobilization of the affected extremity. Use of nonsteroidal anti-inflammatory drugs should be avoided because they typically diminish platelet function.

8.1.7 Prognosis

Hemophilia is a genetic condition, and as such is a lifelong, chronic condition. Currently, there is no cure. In countries where treatment is readily available, individuals with hemophilia typically have normal lifespans, with heart disease as the leading cause of death. Dangers of morbidity and mortality are more significant in those with severe hemophilia.

8.1.8 Follow-Up

The chronicity and multisystem effects of hemophilia lend themselves well to the care provided at a multidisciplinary comprehensive center. Routine surveillance visits to a hemophilia specialist are recommended every 3–6 months for more severe disease and annually for mild hemophilia. Prevention of complications is the key to the care of the individual with hemophilia, and prompt treatment when bleeding or injury occurs is paramount. Management of disease complications and health maintenance are additional aspects of care.

Home care for these patients is an integral aspect of care, as prompt treatment can be given in the home. Additionally, home care can help facilitate the goal of self-infusion, which is especially important in the patient with severe disease. Routine immunizations are necessary; the deep subcutaneous injection route is preferred to intramuscular injections. Hepatitis B vaccinations are advised due to possible contamination of factor concentrates. Routine surveillance of blood-borne infections should be done in those exposed to factor concentrates. Regular dental care is important, with a focus on preventing caries, infection, and extraction. Dental procedures should be discussed in advance with the treatment team because extraction and, in some cases, cleaning can cause bleeding that would require treatment. Physical therapy evaluation and treatment are required for those with affected joints or musculoskeletal complications. Certainly, education regarding hemophilia, treatment options, and safety precautions must be provided to the patient and family. Exercise is encouraged, but contact sports should be avoided. Genetic counseling should be offered to all parents and patients.

8.1.9 Future Perspectives

The search for a cure for hemophilia continues, and there are several human phase 1 trials currently in progress. Progress in gene therapy is encouraging. The goal of gene therapy is to convert severe factor deficiency to mild, or greater than 5% activity, but one of the difficulties has been to incorporate the normal gene; viral and plasmid vectors are showing great promise (Viiala et al. 2009).

8.2 von Willebrand Disease

vWD was first described in 1926 by Finnish pediatrician, Erik Adolf von Willebrand (Geil 2009).

8.2.1 Epidemiology

vWF is an important component of the clotting system because it acts as a carrier and stabilizer for factor VIII and adhesively binds platelets to subendothelial cells at the site of injury. vWD is a group of bleeding diatheses in which there is a quantitative deficiency or qualitative defect in one of the functions of vWF. vWD is thought to be the most common bleeding disorder worldwide, affecting up to 1% of the population. Spread over a continuum of mild to severe disease manifestations, vWD classification includes type

Table 8.5. Classifications of von Willebrand disease

Type	Pathology	Frequency (%)
Type 1	Partial quantitative deficiency of vWF	70–80
Type 2A	Absence of hwm and associated decrease in platelet binding functions	10–12
Type 2B	Increased affinity for platelet complex	3–5
Type 2M	Decrease in platelet binding functions	<1
Type 2N	Significantly decreased affinity for factor VIII	<1
Type 3	Almost complete absence of vWF	<1
Pseudo platelet-type	Intrinsic abnormality of the platelets, leading to loss of hwm*	<1

**hwm* high-weight multimers

1, type 2 (with several variants), type 3, and pseudo platelet-type. Type 1 vWD is the most common variant; the frequencies of the other types are identified in Table 8.5. This is typically a relatively mild bleeding disorder, and can be so mild as to go undiagnosed until late in life. In a few patients, vWD is severe, leading to symptoms comparable with those of severe hemophilia. This is a genetic condition passed on through inheritance, but random mutation is possible. vWD affects males and females equally and is not associated with a specific ethnicity.

8.2.2 Etiology

vWF is a high-molecular-weight adhesive protein (or multimer) that is produced in the endothelial cells of the vasculature and in small amounts in the megakaryocytes. Disease classification is based on the qualitative and/or quantitative defect present in the vWF (Table 8.5).

vWF is an acute phase reactant; therefore, vWF levels rise in individuals during stress, inflammatory processes, pregnancy, exercise, and adrenergic stimulation.

Acquired vWD is possible and is associated with several diseases. Most frequently, acquired vWD occurs in individuals with clonal lymphoproliferative or autoimmune diseases who have formed an antibody to vWF. Other associated causes include absorption of vWF into tumor cells (e.g., Wilms' tumor), destruction by proteolytic enzymes during accelerated fibrinolysis (e.g., pancreatitis), reduced production in hypothyroidism, and associated decreases with certain pharmacological agents (e.g., valproic acid, dextrans, hetastarch).

8.2.3 Genetics

The genetic code for vWF is located on the short arm of chromosome 12 and is a complex single-copy gene. This gene has been sequenced and, more recently, most mutations have been identified. Most types of vWD are autosomal dominant (Fig. 8.4); however, type 2A can be either dominant or recessive, and type 2N and type 3 are autosomal recessive (Fig. 8.5).

8.2.4 Symptoms and Clinical Signs

Logically, symptoms of vWD vary depending on the severity of the disease. The most common symptoms overall are easy bruising and mucous membrane bleeding. However, the patient with type 1 vWD may have no symptoms at all until an untoward event causes significant injury or until surgery is required. Symptoms of bleeding early in life, hemarthrosis, and significant bruising with normal activities or minor trauma can occur with type 3 vWD. Patients with type 2N vWD can also exhibit more serious bleeding difficulties, such as soft tissue and urinary bleeding, as it is associated with low factor VIII levels and can mimic hemophilia (Table 8.6).

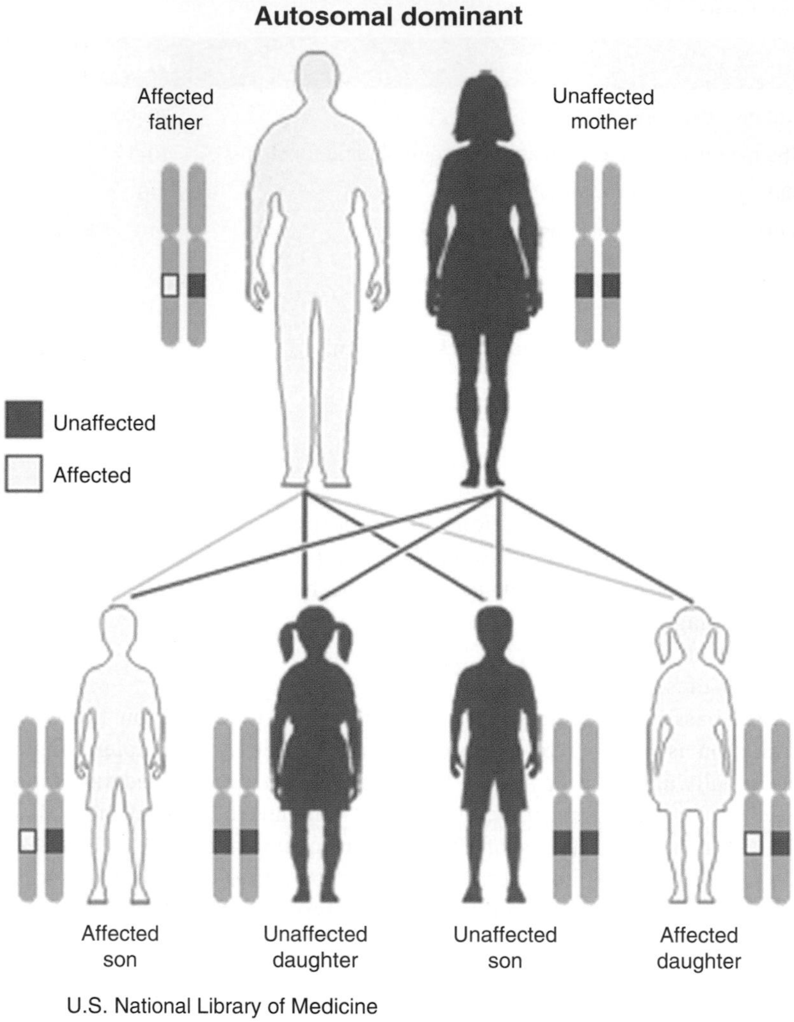

Autosomal dominant

Affected father

Unaffected mother

Unaffected

Affected

Affected son

Unaffected daughter

Unaffected son

Affected daughter

U.S. National Library of Medicine

Figure 8.4

Illustration of autosomal dominant gene transfer. Image credit: http://ghr.nlm.nih.gov

8.2.5 Diagnostic Testing

Diagnostic testing should be done in those who present with clinical symptoms suspicious for a bleeding disorder. The following laboratory tests are common screening tests for vWD: activated partial thromboplastin time (aPTT); a von Willebrand panel, including vWF antigen (vWf:Ag), vWF ristocetin cofactor (vWF activity or functional assay; vWf:RCo), vWF multimers; and factor VIII assay. During screening for bleeding disorders, a PT is often done, the results of which should be normal in the patient with vWD. The aPTT, part of the routine screening for bleeding disorders, serves as a measure of the intrinsic pathway. It may be prolonged in an individual with vWD, but if the disease is quite mild, it may be normal. Some centers use a bleeding time (BT) to assist with screening, but this test has fallen out of favor due to variable results and poor correlation with disease. The platelet function analyzer assay, or PFA 100, is a relatively new screening test that identifies patients with poor platelet aggregation, which if noted would place a high index of suspicion on vWD. The PFA 100 appears to be replacing the BT as a screening test. A platelet count is also routinely done and may be abnormally low in those with type 2B, type 2M, type 3, and pseudo platelet-type vWD.

Figure 8.5

Illustration of autosomal recessive gene transfer. Image credit: http://ghr.nlm.nih.gov

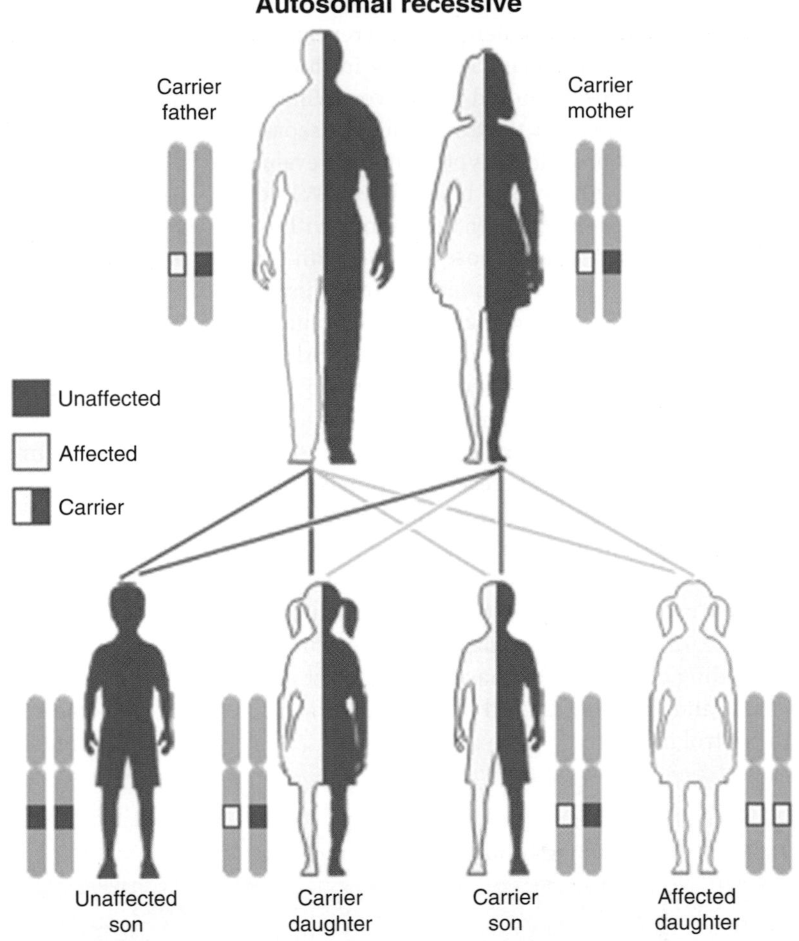

Table 8.6. Signs and symptoms of von Willebrand disease

Easy bruising or hematomas	Recurrent epistaxis
Mouth or gum bleeding	Excessive bleeding postdental extractions
Menorrhagia	Hematuria
Gastrointestinal bleeding	Bleeding with IM injections
Hemarthrosis	Mild thrombocytopenia
Prolonged oozing from minor wound	Postoperative hemorrhage

The acute phase reactant qualities of vWF make laboratory evaluation challenging, and repeated testing is commonly necessary, especially in those with mild vWD or type 1. Should repeat von Willebrand panel testing be needed, the tests should be separated by 4 weeks or more. Blood type should be evaluated because those with type O blood have vWF levels approximately 25–30% lower than those with other blood types. Therefore, in those patients with type O blood and no significant personal or family history of bleeding, and with low normal von Willebrand panel assay results, vWD can likely be excluded. Also confounding laboratory evaluation is the issue of vWF (both antigen and ristocetin cofactor) as an acute phase reactant. Consequently, physical stressors such as illness and exercise, and even emotional stressors, can elevate vWF levels; a low normal von Willebrand panel may indeed indicate that disease is present but not demonstrated on that particular day. Estrogen therapy can increase vWF levels, making it another complicating factor, as women sent for evaluation of a bleeding diathesis often have symptoms of menorrhagia and are being treated with oral contraceptives to control menses.

Ristocetin platelet aggregation (RIPA) testing is typically used to determine subtypes of vWD after initial von Willebrand panel testing has been abnormal. vWD type 2B and platelet-type vWD both have increased sensitivity to low doses of ristocetin; a low-dose RIPA is performed if either type of vWD is suspected (Table 8.7).

In emergency situations when vWF replacement is not available, cryoprecipitate can be used. Platelet transfusions are the appropriate treatment for pseudo platelet-type vWD. Both these products are typically available through local blood banks, and although the risk is small, possible viral contamination is always a concern for patients and families. For dosing recommendations, see Chap. 31.

Factors beyond laboratory testing should assist in determining diagnosis. The personal and family history has significant relevance in the patient being evaluated for a bleeding disorder. Patients with vWD may experience easy bruising; bleeding or oozing of blood after dental or surgical procedures, especially tonsillectomy; menorrhagia; or epistaxis. Family history is often remarkable for the same complaints or events. Some female relatives may have undergone

Table 8.7. Diagnostic testing for von Willebrand disease

Test	Type 1	Type 2A	Type 2B	Type 2M	Type 2N	Type 3	Platelet-type pseudo
vW ristocetin factor	Normal or decreased	Decreased	Normal or decreased	Normal or decreased	Normal	Decreased or absent	Normal
vWF antigen	Normal or decreased	Decreased	Normal or decreased	Decreased	Normal	Decreased or absent	Normal
Multimer	Normal	Absent hwm and iwm, increased lwm	Absent hwm	Normal	Normal	Absent	Absent hwm
Factor VIII	Normal or decreased	Normal or decreased	Normal or decreased	Normal or decreased	Decreased	Decreased or absent	Normal
Ristocetin-induced platelet aggregation	Poor	Poor	Poor			Poor	Hyperresponsive at low dose
Platelet Count	Normal	Normal	Decreased	Decreased	Normal	Decreased	Decreased

hwm high-weight multimers; *iwm* intermediate-weight multimers; *lwm* low-weight multimers

hysterectomy for uncontrolled uterine bleeding but were never diagnosed with vWD. It should be noted that any history of family members as being "free bleeders" or even as having hemophilia should alert the provider to the possibility of vWD. The individual's personal and family history is utilized in conjunction with laboratory reports to determine diagnosis. Should family and personal history be unremarkable, the possibility of acquired vWD should be considered.

8.2.6 Treatment

Treatment of vWD is based on the pathophysiology of the specific variant or type of vWD. Several treatment strategies are available to control bleeding events. Desmopressin, or DDAVP, is a synthetic antidiuretic hormone and can increase available vWF levels for 12 and up to 24 h by stimulating release of vWF from storage sites in the endothelial cells. Desmopressin is usually most effective in those with type 1 vWD and is somewhat effective in types 2A, 2M, and 2N, but it does not work on every individual; therefore, a trial dose should be given to determine efficacy (DDAVP challenge, Table 8.8). DDAVP should not be used in those with type 2B vWD, as the vWF high-molecular-weight multimers have an increased affinity for platelets; thus, increasing the endogenous vWF may cause thrombocytopenia and possibly worsen bleeding.

Once the degree of efficacy is established, DDAVP can be used for minor bleeding events, and for those who respond very well, it may be used for some of the more serious events (epistaxis, menorrhagia, etc.). DDAVP should be used in conjunction with vWF replacement therapy for life-threatening injury or when repeated dosing is likely. This medication is available in IV or subcutaneous form or as Stimate, a nasal formulation (150 mg/mL). A lower-concentration nasal spray and pill forms are also available but are not useful for this diagnosis. Common side effects include flushing, tachycardia, and headache, and uncommonly, hyper- or hypotension. A decreased infusion rate may diminish these effects. Overuse of DDAVP can lead to the antidiuretic effects of this medication, including fluid retention and sodium depletion. Giving more than three doses of DDAVP requires fluid restriction

Table 8.8. Desmopressin dosing guidelines

DDAVP IV or SQ	0.3 mg/kg in 50 mL of normal saline IV over ~20 min, or same dose for SQ injection
Stimate (150 mg/mL)	<50 kg; one puff intranasally or >50 kg two puffs intranasally, q12–24 h

DDAVP IV may elicit a stronger response than intranasal dosing. Increase in vWF levels can be expected in ~30 minutes
Challenge instructions: Draw factor VIII assay, ristocetin cofactor, and vWF antigen just before dose is given, and repeat 1 h after dose. A threefold increase is considered a good response

and sodium monitoring. Repeated doses of desmopressin will lead to tachyphylaxis (Table 8.8).

Humate-P® is considered replacement therapy for vWD, as it contains plasma-derived vWF. This is a pasteurized, solvent-treated product, and the risk of viral transmission is considered low. It is typically dosed in ristocetin cofactor units; dosing recommendations and indications are outlined in Table 8.9 (Behring 2007). These recommendations are general guidelines for treatment of typical bleeding. Each patient's plan of care must be individualized to reflect any special circumstances or conditions that may require more or less intervention. The patient's dose should be rounded to the nearest vial whenever possible. Other similar products are available in the United Kingdom and Europe.

Antifibrinolytic therapies are available for mucous membrane bleeding. Aminocaproic acid (Amicar®) and tranexamic acid (Cyklokapron®) inhibit the action of fibrinolysis that occurs at mucous membrane sites. Antifibrinolytics do appear to be effective for menorrhagia and are also used to prepare for dental procedures and oral surgery. Both these medications stabilize clot formation and are typically used in conjunction with factor replacement, but may also be effective when used alone for minor bleeding in a patient with mild or type 1 vWD (Table 8.10).

Supportive treatments are beneficial and include application of an ice or cold pack to the injured area when possible, pressure (e.g., local pressure or Ace wrap) if needed, elevation of the extremity, and rest or

Table 8.9. Humate-P dosing guidelines

Type	Event	Dosage (IU vWf:RCo/kg)
Type 1 Mild	Serious event Severe epistaxis GI bleeding CNS trauma Traumatic hemorrhage	Loading dose 40–60 U/kg Then 40–50 U/kg q8–12 h for 3 days to keep nadir >50% Then 40–50 U/kg q.d. for ~7 days of treatment
Moderate to severe	Minor event Mucous membrane bleeding Menorrhagia	40–50 U/kg, 1–2 doses
	Serious event Severe epistaxis GI bleeding CNS trauma Traumatic hemorrhage	Loading dose 50–75 U/kg Then 40–60 U/kg q8–12 h for 3 days to keep nadir >50% Then 40–60 U/kg q.d. for ~7 days of treatment
Type 2 (all variants) and 3	Minor event Mucous membrane bleeding Menorrhagia	40–50 U/kg, 1–2 doses
	Serious event Severe epistaxis GI bleeding CNS trauma Traumatic hemorrhage	Loading dose 60–80 U/kg Then 40–60 U/kg q8–12 h for 3 days to keep nadir >50% Then 40–60 U/kg q.d. for ~7 days of treatment

immobilization of the affected extremity. Use of nonsteroidal anti-inflammatory drugs should be avoided because they typically diminish platelet function.

8.2.7 Prognosis

The prognosis for the patient with vWD is excellent. Most patients have very mild symptoms except at times of significant trauma or surgery. Those with type 3 vWD can have more serious symptoms and sequelae, similar to the patient with moderate to severe hemophilia.

Table 8.10. Antifibrinolytic medications

Aminocaproic acid 50–100 mg/kg/dose q6 h	(Amicar) (maximum 3–4 doses) IV or PO
Tranexamic acid 25 mg/kg/dose q6–8 h IV or PO	(Cyklokapron)

These drugs work best if continued for an additional 3–4 days after bleeding stops

8.2.8 Follow-Up

Individuals with vWD should be seen at regular intervals by a hematologist who is familiar with vWD management. Routine surveillance visits are recommended every 6–12 months or more frequently for severe disease. Prevention of complications depends on prevention prior to anticipated bleeding events and to prompt treatment when bleeding or injury does occur. Routine immunizations are necessary; in those with more severe types of vWD, the deep subcutaneous injection route is preferred to intramuscular injections. Hepatitis A and B vaccinations are advised because these viruses are possible contaminates of factor concentrates. Routine surveillance of bloodborne infections should be done in those exposed to factor concentrates. Regular dental care is important, with a focus on preventing caries, infection, and extraction. Dental procedures should be discussed in advance with the treatment team because extraction and, in some cases, cleaning can cause bleeding that would require treatment. Home care may be useful for patients with more severe variants, as prompt treatment with Humate-P can be given in the home. Physical therapy evaluation and treatment are required for those with severe disease and those with affected joints or musculoskeletal complications. Certainly, education regarding vWD, treatment options, and safety precautions must be provided to the patient and family. Exercise is encouraged, but contact sports should be avoided. Genetic counseling should be offered to all parents and patients (Ludlam et al. 2005).

References

Allain JP et al (2009) Transfusion transmitted infectious diseases. Biologicals 37:71–77

Behring CSL (2007) Dosing schedule for the treatment of bleeding episodes in von Willebrand disease. CSL Behring, King of Prussia, PA

Burnouf T, Radosevich M, Goubran HA (2004) Local hemostatic blood products: fibrin sealant and platelet gel. World Federation of Haemophilia, Technical Report, Treatment of Hemophilia 36, pp 1-10

Coppola A, Di Capua M, De Simone C (2008) Primary prophylaxis in children with haemophilia. Blood Transfusion 6(Suppl 2):s4–s11

Geil JD (2009) Von Willebrand Disease. http://emedicine.medscape.com/article/959825-overview. Retrieved 13 April 2009

Haya S, Moret A, Cid AR, Cortina V, Casana P, Cabrera N et al (2007) Inhibitors in haemophilia A: current management and open issues. Haemophilia 13(Suppl 5):52–60

Kruse-Jarres R, Barnett B, Leissinger C (2008) Immune tolerance induction for the eradication of inhibitors in patients with hemophilia A. Expert Opinion on Bilogical Therapy 8:1885–1896

Lefrere JJ, Hewitt P (2009) From mad cows to sensible blood transfusion: the risk of prior transmission by labile blood components in the United Kingdom and France. Transfusion 49:797–812

Ludlam CA, Pasi KJ, Bolton-Maggs P, Collins PW, Cumming AM, Dolan G et al (2005) A framework for genetic service provision for haemophilia and other inherited bleeding disorders. Haemophilia 11(2):145

Mancuso ME, Graca L, Auerswald G, Santagostino E (2009) Haemophilia care in children–benefits of early prophylaxis for inhibitor prevention. Haemophilia 15:8–14

Musso R (2008) Efficacy and safety of recominant factor VIII products in patients with hemophilia A. Drugs Today 44: 735–750

Panicker J, Warrier I, Thomas R, Lusher J (2003) The overall effectiveness of prophylaxis in severe haemophilia. Haemophilia 9:272–278

Tagliaferri A, Di Perna C, Franca-Rivolta G (2008) Secondary prophylaxis in adolescent and adult haemophiliacs. Blood Transfusion 6(Suppl 2):s17–s120

Shapiro A (2003) A global view on prophylaxis: possibilities and consequences. Haemophilia 9(Suppl 1):10–18

Viiala NO, Larsen SR, Rasko JE (2009) Gene therapy for Hemophilia: clinical trials and technical tribulations. Seminars in Thrombosis and Hemostasis 35:81–92

PART III

Chapter 9

Chemotherapy

Christine Chordas • Kristen Graham

Contents

9.1 Introduction . . . 204
9.2 Cancer Cell Characteristics . . . 204
9.2.1 The Cell Cycle . . . 204
9.2.2 Cell Cycle Control . . . 205
9.3 Chemotherapy . . . 206
9.3.1 Principles . . . 206
9.3.2 Resistance . . . 206
9.3.3 The Principles of Pharmacokinetics, Pharmacodynamics, and Pharmacogenomics . . . 206
9.3.4 Chemotherapy Techniques . . . 207
9.4 Clinical Trials . . . 207
9.4.1 Phase I Clinical Trials . . . 208
9.4.2 Phase II Clinical Trials . . . 208
9.4.3 Phase III Clinical Trials . . . 208
9.4.4 Phase IV Clinical Trials . . . 208
9.5 Chemotherapy Agents . . . 208
9.5.1 Antimetabolites . . . 211
9.5.1.1 Mechanism of Action . . . 211
9.5.1.2 Side Effects . . . 211
9.5.1.3 Long-Term Effects . . . 216
9.5.2 Alkylating Agents . . . 216
9.5.2.1 Mechanism of Action . . . 216
9.5.2.2 Side Effects . . . 217
9.5.2.3 Long-Term Effects . . . 217
9.5.3 Antitumor Antibiotics . . . 217
9.5.3.1 Mechanism of Action . . . 217
9.5.3.2 Side Effects . . . 218
9.5.3.3 Long-Term Effects . . . 218
9.5.4 Anthracycline Antibiotics . . . 218
9.5.4.1 Mechanism of Action . . . 218
9.5.4.2 Side Effects . . . 218
9.5.4.3 Long-Term Effects . . . 218
9.5.5 Plant Derivatives . . . 218
9.5.5.1 Mechanism of Action . . . 218
9.5.5.2 Side Effects . . . 219
9.5.5.3 Long-Term Effects . . . 219
9.5.6 Antiangiogenic Agents . . . 219
9.5.6.1 Mechanism of Action . . . 219
9.5.6.2 Side Effects . . . 220
9.5.7 Miscellaneous Agents . . . 220
9.5.7.1 Corticosteroids . . . 220
9.5.7.1.1 Mechanism of Action . . . 220
9.5.7.1.2 Side Effects . . . 220
9.5.7.1.3 Long-Term Effects . . . 220
9.5.7.2 Enzymes: Asparaginase . . . 220
9.5.7.3 Targeted Growth Inhibitors . . . 220
9.5.7.4 Differentiating Agents . . . 220
9.6 Chemotherapy Protectants . . . 221
9.6.1 Allopurinol (Zyloprim) . . . 221
9.6.2 Amifostine (Ethyol) . . . 221
9.6.3 Dexrazoxane (Zinecard) . . . 221
9.6.4 Leucovorin Calcium (LCV, Wellcovorin, Citovorum Factor, Folic Acid) . . . 221
9.6.5 Mesna (Mesnex) . . . 221
9.6.6 Palifermin . . . 222
9.7 Administration of Chemotherapy Agents . . . 222
9.7.1 Preparation . . . 222
9.7.2 Administration and Practice Considerations . . . 223
9.7.2.1 Documentation . . . 224
9.8 Professional Guidelines to Minimize the Risk of Medication Errors . . . 224
9.8.1 Prescribing Errors . . . 224
9.8.1.1 Compounding . . . 224
9.8.1.2 Dispensing . . . 224
9.8.1.3 Administration . . . 224
9.9 Safe Practice Considerations . . . 224
9.9.1 Mixing Chemotherapeutic Agents . . . 225
9.9.2 Transporting Cytotoxic Agents . . . 225
9.9.3 Safe Handling After Chemotherapy . . . 225
9.9.4 Disposal of Cytotoxic Materials . . . 225
9.9.5 Spill Management . . . 226
9.9.6 Procedures Following Accidental Exposure . . . 226
9.9.7 Storage . . . 226
9.9.8 Medical Management . . . 226
9.10 Administration of Chemotherapy in the Home . . . 226
9.11 Immediate Complications of Chemotherapy Administration . . . 226
9.11.1 Extravasation . . . 227

9.11.1.1 Pathophysiology of Extravasation 227
9.11.1.2 Risk Factors of Extravasation. . 227
9.11.1.3 Assessment and Treatment of Extravasation 227
9.11.1.4 Signs and Symptoms of Extravasation 227
9.11.1.5 Treatment for Extravasation . 227
9.11.2 Acute Hypersensitivity Reactions (HSRs) to Chemotherapy 230
9.11.3 Risk Factors for Hypersensitivity, Flare Reactions, or Anaphylaxis 230
9.11.4 Recommended Steps to Prevent HSRs . 230
9.11.5 Emergency Management of HSR/Anaphylaxis 230
9.12 Summary 231
References 231

9.1 Introduction

In the 1940s, following the effects of mustard gas during World War I, nitrogen mustard was introduced as part of the treatment for childhood cancer. Prior to this time, surgery and radiation therapy were the only treatments available. Rapid anticancer drug development followed and continues into the twenty-first century. Since the introduction of chemotherapy, overall 5-year survival rate for childhood cancers has increased from near 0% to near 90% in some childhood malignancies (Ries et al. 2008). Success is in part due to refinement of the existing chemotherapy agents and administration guidelines coupled with advancement in surgical, radiotherapy, and imaging techniques. Today, targeted therapy is at the forefront of preclinical and clinical investigations. While advancement in all areas pushes survivorship curves upward, challenges continue to drive investigators to find a cure for all childhood cancers with minimal acute and long-term toxicity.

9.2 Cancer Cell Characteristics

9.2.1 The Cell Cycle

All nonmalignant and malignant cells during their lifespan move through four phases ofthe reproductive cell cycle from resting to active/growing and then to mitosis/dividing (Fig. 9.1). It is during the active phases that most chemotherapy agents exert their effects.

Malignant and nonmalignant cells in the resting phase (G0) are not dividing and are more resistant to the effects of chemotherapy. Cells stay in the resting phase for hours to years carrying out various functions they are involved with (e.g., stem cells). In the first gap phase (G1), genes direct the synthesis of ribonucleic acid (RNA) and proteins. The length of time cells spend in G1 is variable. Later in the G1 phase the cells pass a certain point (restriction point R) committing to a path of replication. During the synthesis phase (S), all 46 chromosomes containing genetic deoxyribonucleic acid (DNA) are copied, so both new cells that are formed will have matching DNA. This process takes 10–20 h. In the second gap phase

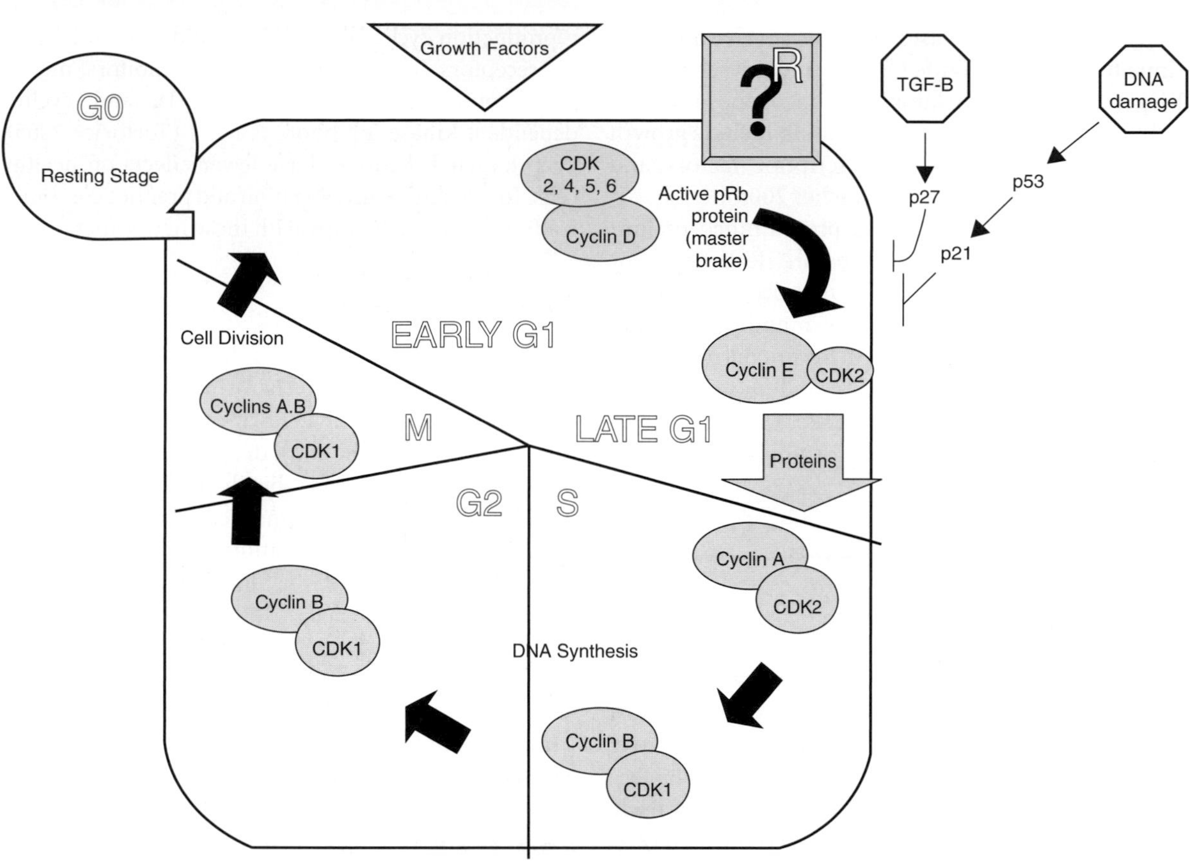

Figure 9.1

The reproductive cell cycle. From Merkle and Loescher (2005). Reprinted with permission

(G2), DNA chromatin is condensed to form rod-like chromosomes as the cell prepares to divide into two cells during mitosis (M). Mitosis is characterized by chromosomes passing through phases of change (cytokinesis) to form two genetically identical cells. The phases include prophase (spindle cells formation), metaphase (chromosomes assemble), anaphase (identical halves separate), and telophase (envelopment of the two cells) (Merkle and Loescher 2005).

9.2.2 Cell Cycle Control

Progression through the cell cycle is regulated by complexes of proteins called cyclins and associated enzymes called cyclin-dependent kinases (CDK). These complexes respond to signals at specific points in the cell cycle to control progression through each phase. Checkpoints ensure that the cycle proceeds in the correct sequence with completion of each phase before proceeding. The restricton point (R) in late G1 phase acts as a checkpoint when cells decide whether conditions are satisfactory for chromosome replication. Malignant cells have lost function of these checkpoints; therefore, genetically damaged cells continue to move through the cycle and proliferate. The retinoblastoma protein (Rb) and the p53 protein are examples that act as checkpoints for healthy cells; however, when damaged or lost as in some cancers, genetic stability decreases and cells survive and continue to grow and divide (Merkle and Loescher 2005; Rieger 2004). Other examples of oncogenes involved in the control of cellular proliferation include growth factors, tyrosine kinases, transcription factors, and RAS proteins (Merkle and Loescher 2005).

Nonmalignant cells have a programmed or limited number of cell divisions before death. Apoptosis is the process of cell dealth that occurs naturally via signals causing cell breakdown and/or cell lysis. Malignant cells characterized by uncontrolled cell division have lost the ability to undergo aptoptosis and therefore continue to replicate. Death of malignant cells results from external signals like chemotherapy or necrosis.

9.3 Chemotherapy

9.3.1 Principles

Chemotherapy is drug therapy that is cytotoxic and that prevents malignant cell division and spread. Most chemotherapy agents kill malignant cells in the active/dividing phases of the cycle (G1, S, G2, M) by damaging the RNA or DNA that tell the cell how to copy itself. Nonmalignant cells that undergo rapid division (e.g., hematopoietic, mucosal, and gastrointestinal cells) are not spared, as demonstrated by some of the common side effects exhibited (e.g., bone marrow suppression, mucositis) with chemotherapy administration.

Tumors/cancer cells initially grow exponentially, with a large number of cells dividing at one time (high growth fraction) and having a short time to multiply (short doubling time), making them most susceptible to chemotherapy agents. The cell kill hypothesis applies to all actively dividing cells and predicts the number of cells killed based on a given chemotherapy dose. This hypothesis assumes that all cells are dividing with a constant growth rate and therefore chemotherapy always kills a constant fraction of cells. The Gompertian model explains tumor growth decreasing over time (Tortorice 2005). When the growth of the tumor is higher there is increased response from chemotherapy agents.

Today, newer treatments target mechanisms of tumor growth and protein pathways rather than a cell's reproduction cycle. These include epidural growth factor receptors (EGFR), angiogenesis inhibitors, matrix metalloproteinase inhibitors (MMPI), and cyclin-dependent kinase inhibitors (CDKI) (Tortorice 2005). Such targeted therapies have fewer effects on healthy cells. Today, clinical investigation and practice combines traditional chemotherapy with these newer therapies.

9.3.2 Resistance

Some malignant cells demonstrate resistance to chemotherapeutic agents. The mechanisms of drug resistance can be explained by changes in patient factors (e.g., toxicity, organ dysfunction), drug metabolism, alterations in cytotoxic targets, biochemical modification, increased DNA repair systems, decreased or increased intracellular drug concentration, dysfunction in cell cycle checkpoints, and the development of genetic mutations (Tortorice 2005). To overcome resistance, a combination of drugs are given early in the treatment to decrease the total number of cells. Resistance may be temporary and be overcome by altering dose or administration technique. Premanent resistance results from a genetic mutation (Tortorice 2005).

9.3.3 The Principles of Pharmacokinetics, Pharmacodynamics, and Pharmacogenomics

Optimization of drug dose and effective and timely scheduling and administration of drugs is crucial to achieve maximum cell death. How the body processes a specific drug and how the specific drug affects the body, and an individual's genetic variables are the basic principles intregal in the development of drugs for specific cancers. Physiologic and cellular factors, including concomitant agents, side effects, age, gender, nutritional status, organ function, environmental exposures, and genetic factors may affect these principles (Tortorice 2005). Treatments are designed and modified using the principles of pharmokinetics, pharmocodynamics, and pharmacogenomics.

Pharmacokinetics is the drug's absorption, distribution, metabolism, and excretion pattern as it moves through the body. Nurses are often involved in obtaining blood samples at sequential time points to determine a drug's metabolism and action. Pharmokinetic principles

Table 9.1. Key terms related to the pharmacokinetics of drugs

Term	Definition
Bioavailability	Rate and extent of absorption
Biotransformation	Metabolism of a drug
Clearance	Rate of drug elimination
Half-life	Time to reduce a concentration by 50%
Area under curve (AUC)	Exposure to drug over time
Excretion	Elimination pattern

include bioavailability, biotransformation, clearance, half-life, area under the curve (AUC), and elimination (Table 9.1) (Tortorice 2005).

Pharmacodynamics is the relationship between the concentration of the drug at receptor sites or targets in the body and how the concentration produces a response or an intended or unintended effect.

Pharmacogenomics is the response to chemotherapy considering an individual's genetic composition (e.g., polymorphisms, chromosomal abnormalities, gene amplificaiton, loss of heterozygosity) (Adamson et al. 2005). Drug effect and treatment response affected by one's genetic make-up can be used in the development of individualized approaches to anticancer treament (Walters 2007).

9.3.4 Chemotherapy Techniques

Chemotherapy is used across the treatment continuum, alone or in combination with other treatment modalities.

- *Multimodality treatment* includes chemotherapy in combination with surgery, radiation, immunotherapy, and stem cell transplant.
- *Neoadjuvant chemotherapy* is given prior to surgery or radiation to reduce tumor burden.
- *Adjuvant chemotherapy* is given to eliminate micrometastatic tumor cells after surgery and/or radiation.
- Chemotherapy used concurrently with radiation as a *radiation sensitizer* is thought to make cells more vulnerable to treatment.
- *Sanctuary therapy* is chemotherapy administered to areas not readily accessible by systemic treatment (intrathecal (i.t.) chemotherapy).
- *Palliative chemotherapy* is administered in low tolerated doses with limited side effects when cure is not possible.
- *High-dose chemotherapy with stem cell transplant* uses high doses of chemotherapy to destroy cells in the bone morrow followed by infusion of one's stem cells to help recovery. May offer higher potential for cure in some childhood malignancies.
- *Metronomic chemotherapy* uses low steady doses of chemotherapy drugs to attack the vasculature matrix (*angiogenesis*) that supports cancer cell growth. The effects are enhanced when given in combination with *antiangiogenic agents* (Stempak et al. 2006).

9.4 Clinical Trials

Clinical trials in cancer research have improved the survival and well-being of children and continue to identify the most current successful and evidenced-based treatments available. More than 70% of children who are diagnosed with cancer currently enter national or international phase III clinical trials in most western European countries (Pritchard-Jones et al. 2008). While some institutions conduct in-house clinical trials, participation in a cooperative group allows higher accrual targets. Therefore, many countries have developed national childhood cancer study groups, which have designed tumor-specific committees to create and carry out clinical trials. Examples include the Children's Oncology Group (COG), United Kingdom Children's Cancer Study Group (UKCCSG), and the International Society of Pediatric Oncology (SIOP) (Chap. 16).

Clinical trials are conducted to determine the safety and effectiveness of treatments and ultimately to identify the best treatment. Trials are regulated by intra-institutional review boards and the credited national sponsor to ensure scientific validity (Bond and Pritchard 2006). Specific eligibility criteria, laboratory and diagnostic testing and thorough documentation is required.

Initially, drugs are tested in vitro. Preclinical studies are then performed in animals to determine toxic effects and safe doses to start clinical trials in human subjects. Investigational new drugs (INDs) are next given to adult subjects in three phases of clinical trials. Only a small fraction of these are evaluated in children with cancer. Pediatric phase I studies usually follow adult phase I studies, starting at 80% of the adult maximum tolerated dosage (MTD). Current directions include testing of new agents for children during the initial stages of drug development using preclinical models as predictors of clinical benefit.

Trials are statistically designed to recruit eligible patients to answer the objectives of the trial to ultimately improve outcome with better treatments. Accrual to any clinical trial first involves approval by an institutional review board (IRB) or research and ethics board (REB) to ensure the safety and welfare of participants. Board approved informed consent must be signed by the patient (assent or consent based on age) and their parent or legal guardian. The contents of the informed consent outline the purpose, length of participation and procedures involved, participant rights, possible benefits, probable risks, alternative therapies, a confidentiality statement, and a statement indicating voluntary participation and right to withdraw. The consent process continues throughout the entire length of treament and after completion of treatment. Nurses may be involved in the entire consenting process from educating patients and famililes about the diagnosis and recommended treatment to ensuring that all questions related to the consent are appropriately answered.

9.4.1 Phase I Clinical Trials

- The goal of Phase I clinical trials is to establish the MTD by administering increasing dosages of the drug or combination of drugs on a recommended schedule. Initial dosages are low and increased until unacceptable side effects are observed. The MTD is the highest dose able to be given without unacceptable side effects.
- A dose-limiting toxicity may be scored according to the common toxicity criteria for adverse events (CTCAE) scoring system defined by the National Cancer Institute. CTCAE reporting is part of all US clinical trials.
- Pharmacokinetics are often required on phase I trials to identify how the drug is metabolized.
- Phase I clinical trials are offered to children with advanced disease resistant to standard therapies. All participants must meet specified disease and organ criteria outlined in the trial.

9.4.2 Phase II Clinical Trials

- One goal of Phase II trials is to determine efficacy of a drug in a particular type of cancer.
- Another goal is to further define the safety and toxicity profile of the drug.
- Phase II clinical trials are offered to children who have shown little or no response to previous treatment. All participants must meet specified disease and organ criteria outlined in the trial and have a reasonable life expectancy and functional status.

9.4.3 Phase III Clinical Trials

- The goal of Phase III clinical trials is to determine the effectiveness of the new treatment compared with the existing standard treatment via randomized clinical trials.
- Phase III clinical trials are offered to newly diagnosed children. A large number of children are recruited to these studies and evaluated over a long period of time.
- These trials look at overall response, toxicity, survival, and quality of life.

9.4.4 Phase IV Clinical Trials

- The goal of Phase IV clinical trials is to evaluate the agent's therapeutic profile following FDA approval for use, or conduct further studies to obtain approval for another indication.

9.5 Chemotherapy Agents

There are many types of chemotherapy agents classified by chemical and biological profiles and mechanisms of action. The section that follows is an overview of common agents, therapeutic uses in childhood cancer, and acute (Table 9.2) and long-term toxicities (Table 9.3).

Table 9.2. Examples of acute side effects after chemotherapy

Gastrointestinal: nausea, vomiting, mucositis	Most drugs
Highly emetic	Cisplatin, lomustine, mechlorethamine, busulfan, cyclophsophamide, cytarabine, dacarbazine, dactinomycin, procarbazine
Moderately emetic	Carboplatin, carmustine, daunorubicin, doxorubicin, etoposide, ifosfamide, imatinib, melphalan, oxaliplatin, premetrexed, temozolomide
Diarrhea	Topotecan, irinotecan
Constipation	Vincristine, thalidomide
Mucositis	Methotrexate, mercaptopurine, fluorouracil
Hematologic: pancytopenia	Most drugs
Skin: Alopecia, darkening, nail changes, rash	Most drugs
Vesicant	Cisplatin, Dactinomycin, anthracyclines, mechlorethamine, vinca alkoids
Irritant	Carboplatin, carmustine, cyclophosphamide, dacarbaxine, etoposide, fluorouracil, ifosfamide, melphalan, paclitaxel, teniposide, thiotepa
Ototoxicity: high frequency loss	Platinum agents
Ocular toxicity	Cytarabine (conjunctivitis)
Pulmonary: HSRs	Asparaginase, platinum agents, dacarbazine, fludarabine, etoposide, teniposide taxanes
Pneumonitis	Bleomycin, fludarabine, lomustine
Nephrotoxicity	Platinum agents
Electrolyte disturbances	Cisplatin (Mg wasting)
Hyperglycemia	Corticosteroids
SIADH	Vincristine
Hemorrhagic cystitis	Cyclophosphamide, ifosfamide
Cardiac: arrythmia, pericarditis, myocarditis, left ventricular changes	Antracyclines, cyclophosphamide
Hypotension	Etoposide, teniposide
Neurologic: neuropathy	Vincristine, thalidomide, platinum agents, taxanes
Somnolence	Thalidomide
Leukoencephalopathy	Methotrexate (IT)
Hepatic: elevated LFTs	Most agents
Acute pancreatitis	Asparaginase

Table 9.3. Examples of late effects after chemotherapy

Chemotherapy agent	Late effect
Alkylating agents	Infertility Hypogonadism
Cisplatin, carbplatin (less)	Sensorineural high-frequency hearing loss, tinnitus Nephropathy Neuropathy Dyslipidemia
Cyclophosphamide, ifosfamide	Cystitis
6-Mercaptopurine, methotrexate, thioguanine	Cirrhosis
High-dose methotrexate, high-dose cytarabine, IT methotrexate or cytarabine	Neurocognitive deficits
Vincristine	Neuropathy
Bleomycin Lomustine, carmustine	Fibrosis Pneumonitis
Doxorubicin Daunorubicin Idarubicin Epirubicin Mitoxantrone	Left ventricular dysfunction Cardiomyopathy Arrhythmias Leukemia
Corticosteroids	Cataracts, osteopenia, osteoporosis, avascular necrosis
Etoposide/teniposide cyclophosphamide/ifosfamide	Second malignancies (*t*-AML/MDS) bladder cancer

With the clinical application of drugs, the severity of unfavorable and unintended symptoms or blood results is often graded by descriptive terminology according to the NCI Common Terminology Criteria for Adverse Events (CTCAE) (NCI 2006). A grading system (1-mild, 2-moderate, 3-severe, 4-life-threatening, 5-death) is available for all pathophysiologic categories (i.e., auditory, cardiac) and potential adverse events (i.e., tinnitus, hypotension) (http://ctep.cancer.gov/protocolDevelopment/electronic_applications/docs/ctcaev3.pdf). For clinical monitoring of late effects, guidelines are available at http://www.curesearch.org (Table 9.4).

Chemotherapy may be classified according to the point in the cell cycle individual agents act.

Cell Cycle Specific Agents

- Kill actively dividing cells only during a specific reproductive/dividing phase (mostly S and M phases).
- Arrest or inhibit mitosis; interfere with nucleic acids necessary for DNA replication, and inhibit protein synthesis. Most effective in tumors with a a lot of cells dividing at one time (high growth fraction).
- Typical administration is in small divided doses given at repeated intervals or by continuous infusion to target cells during active phases of reproduction.
- Types of chemotherapy agents include plant alkaloids and antimetabolites

Cell Cycle Nonspecific Agents

- Kill cells actively dividing during all phases of the reproductive cycle.
- Mechanism of action: disrupt DNA replication; inhibit DNA and RNA synthesis repair and recombination and interfere with nucleic acid synthesis.
- Most effective in tumors with a few number of cells dividing at one time (low growth fraction).
- Typical administration is via single intravenous (IV) bolus dose.
- Types of chemotherapy agents include alkylating agents, antitumor antibiotics, nitrosoureas, topoisomerase I inhibitors, Asparaginase, heavy metals

9.5.1 Antimetabolites

9.5.1.1 Mechanism of Action

Antimetabolites are similar in structure (analogs) to normal cellular metabolites. When cells incorporate these substances into the cellular metabolism, they are unable to divide. Drugs are cell cycle specific, active during the S phase. These drugs require metabolic activation in the target cell to have cytotoxic effects and are classified according to the substances with which they interfere:

- Folic acid antagonist: methotrexate
- Pyrimidine antagonist: 5-fluorouracil, cytarabine, capecitabine, gemcitabine
- Purine antagonist: 6-mercaptopurine and 6-thioguanine
- Adenosine deaminase inhibitor: cladribine, fludarabine
- Ribonucleotide reductase inhibitor: hydroxyurea, clofarabine

Methotrexate and mercaptopurine are most widely used in the treatment of leukemias, non-Hodgkin's lymphoma (NHL), the histiocytoses, and osteosarcoma. Thioguanine is used in gliomas. Cytarabine is often used in combination treatment for ALL and lymphoma. DepoCyte is a liposomal encapsulated form of cytarabine for i.t. use under investigation in brain tumors and for meningeal relapse of ALL (Parasole et al. 2008). Fluorouracil and gemcitabine are used in childhood germ cell tumors and hepatic tumors.

Antimetabolites with varying degrees of activity in childhood leukemias include: fludarabine, cladribine, and clofarabine. Nelarabine has shown activity in T-cell malignancies. The role of capecitabine and gemcitabine in the treatment of childhood cancer is currently being defined (Adamson et al. 2005).

9.5.1.2 Side Effects

Myelosuppression, mucositis, nausea, and vomiting, and alopecia are the most common side effects

Table 9.4. Chemotherapy agents and administration considerations

Classification (drug/names/trade names)	Administration considerations
Antimetabolites	Cell cycle specific agents
Folic acid antagonist	
Methotrexate (amethopterin, methotrexate sodium, MTX, Rheumatrex®, Trexall®)	IV, IM, PO, IT; yellow substance Administer leucovorin with doses >1,000 mg/m^2 Ensure adequate hydration and alkalinization Avoid sunburn, vitamins/food with folic acid Hold TMP-sulfa, ASA, NSAIDS Monitor liver function tests
Pyrimidine antagonist	
Capecitabine (Xeloda®)	PO; do not crush, chew, or dissolve; administer with food
Cytarabine (Ara-C, arabinosylcytosine, Cytosar-U®)	IM, IV push, IV infusion, SQ, IT Highly emetic; provide antiemetics Conjunctivitis with high dose; administer steroid eye drops Monitor liver function tests
Fluorouracil (Adrucil®, 5-fluorouracil, 5-FU)	IV, PO; dilute in water or carbonated beverage; administer on an empty stomach Limit sun exposure Skin irritant
Gemcitabine (Gemzar®)	IV <60 min to decrease toxicity Dermatologic toxicity

Table 9.4. (Continued)

Classification (drug/names/trade names)	Administration considerations
Purine antagonist	
Mercaptopurine (Purinethol®)	PO; solution can be prepared by pharmacy; administer on an empty stomach; milk and grapefruit juice decrease absorption Dose reduce 75% if given with allopurinol Avoid use of the abbreviations, 6-MP; 6-mercaptopurine as overdoses have been reported sixfold
Thioguanine (6-TG, , Tabloid®, Lanvis®)	PO; administer on an empty stomach; milk decreases absorption Teratogenic
Adenosine deaminase inhibitor	
Cladribine (Leustatin®)	IV; dilute in normal saline Monitor for tumor lysis syndrome
Fludarabine (Fludara®)	IV; administer allopurinol, and hydration, alkalinization if tumor burden high Pulmonary function tests recommended prior, during, and after treatment
Nelarabine (Arranon®)	IV; ensure adequate hydration Monitor for neurologic toxicity and acute tumor lysis syndrome
Ribonucleotide reductase inhibitor	
Hydroxyurea (Droxia®, Hydrea®, Mylocel®)	PO; capsules can be opened; administer on an empty stomach
Clofarabine (Clolar®, Clofarex®)	IV; administer with continuous fluids Monitor blood pressure, cardiac, and respiratory status and for tumor lysis, systemic inflammatory response, and capillary leak syndrome (may use prophylactic steroids)
Alkylating agents	Cell cycle nonspecific agents
Mustard gas derivatives	
Mechlorethamine (nitrogen mustard, mustine, mechlorethamine hydrochloride, Mustargen®)	IV Vesicant Inhalation can cause irritation of nasal and bronchial mucous membranes and eyes Highly emetic; provide antiemetics
Melphalan (Alkeran®)	IV, PO; administer on an empty stomach Administer hydration with i.v. form; maintain adequate urinary output Skin irritant
Cyclophosphamide (Cytoxan®, Neosar®)	IV slow infusion, p.o.; elixir can be prepared Hemorrhagic cystitis; encourage hydration and frequent voiding; administer mesna with doses >1 g/m^2/day; monitor specific gravity and heme before and during administration Highly emetic; provide antiemetics; skin irritant

Table 9.4. (Continued)

Classification (drug/names/trade names)	Administration considerations
Ifosfamide (Ifex®)	IV infusion Administer pre- and post-hydration with mesna Monitor specific gravity and heme before and during administration Skin irritant
Ethylenimines	
Thiotepa (Thioplex®)	IV, IM, PO, IT; intratumor Skin irritant Bathe patients 3–4 times/day during and for 24 h after infusion/avoid creams and lotions Change diapers Q2h, change linens with each bath, avoid occlusive dressings Avoid all skin contact
Alkylsulfonates	
Busulfan (Busulfex®, Myleran®)_	IV, PO; can crush or mix; elixir can be prepared
Hydrazines and Triazines	
Procarbazine (Matulane®)	PO; administer on an empty stomach Avoid foods with tyramine (aged cheese, bananas, yogurt, chocolate) Late nadir Highly emetic; provide antiemetics
Dacarbazine (DTIC, DTIC-Dome®)	IV Skin irritant Risk for acute hypersensitivity reaction (HSR)
Temozolomide (Temodar®)	PO; administer on an empty stomach; capsules can be opened and mixed in apple juice/sauce; round dose to nearest 5 mg
Nitrosureas	
Carmustine (BCNU, BiCNU, Gliadel®)	IV slow infusion; use glass containers and polyethylene lined administration sets Skin irritant
Lomustine (CCNU, CeeNu®)	PO; capsules can be dissolved; administer with fluid on empty stomach Recommend baseline and routine PFTs Highly emetic; provide antiemetics
Metal salts	Avoid aluminum needle or administration sets Dose modified based on serial GFR or creatinine clearance and audiometric tests
Carboplatin	Renal and audiometric tests recommended prior to, during, and after treatment IV infusion over 15 min to 1 h; i.v. continuous Skin irritant Maintain adequate hydration

Table 9.4. (Continued)

Classification (drug/names/trade names)	Administration considerations
Cisplatin (CDDP, Platinol®-AQ)	Renal and audiometric tests recommended prior to, during, and after treatment Risk for acute HSR; may pre medicate; desensitization may be tried with mild reactions IV infusion Administer hydration with mannitol; maintain urine output ≥2 c/kg/h Administer magnesium supplements Intensifies aminoglycoside toxicity; use caution with concurrent administration
Oxaliplatin (Eloxatin™)	Highly emetic; provide antiemetics; risk for acute HSR IV; do not mix with sodium chloride; flush line before and after with dextrose Risk for acute HSR
Antibiotics	Cell cycle nonspecific agents
Bleomycin (Blenoxane®)	IV, IM, SQ Administer i.m. test dose of 1–2 U; monitor vital signs every 15 min; wait a minimum of 1 h before administering remainder of dose Administer i.v. slowly over at least 10 min (≥1 U/min) at a concentration not to exceed 3 U/mL Pulmonary function tests recommended prior, during, and after treatment
Dactinomycin (actinomycin-D, Cosmegen®)	IV push; protect from light Vesicant Highly emetic; provide antiemetics
Anthracyline agents	Cell cycle nonspecific agents
Daunorubicin (daunomycin, Cerubidine®) Doxorubicin (Adriamycin®, Rubex®) Idarubicin (Idamycin®, Idamycin PFS®)	IV infusion; protect from light Vesicants Do not give with radiation Monitor cumulative dose Cardiac studies recommended prior, during, and after treatment looking at left ventricular ejection fraction
Anthracenedione	
Mitoxantrone (DHAD, Novantrone®)	Discolors urine pink/red; mitroxantrone discolors urine green/blue
Plant derivatives	Cell cycle specific agents
Vinca alkaloids	Fatal if given intrathecally
Vincristine (vincristine sulfate, VCR, Oncovin®, Vincasar PFS®)	IV push; IV infusion (vinorelbine only) Vesicants
Vinblastine (vinblastine sulfate, vincaleukoblastine, VLB, velban, alkaban AQ)	Maximum single dose for vincristine is 2 mg Prescribe stool softeners
Vinorelbine (vinorelbine tartrate, Navelbine®)	Neurologic toxicity (peripheral neuropathy)
Taxanes	IV; use non-PVC bag or tubing
Paclitaxel (Taxol®, Onxol®)	Skin irritants

Table 9.4. (Continued)

Classification (drug/names/trade names)	Administration considerations
Docetaxel (Taxotere®)	Risk for acute HSR; premedicate with corticosteroids, antihistamines, and an H2 receptor antagonist 24 h before, during, and 24 h following administration
Podophyllotoxins	Topoisomerase II inhibitors
Etoposide (VP-16, etoposide phosphate 16, Toposar®, VePesid®, Etopophos®) Teniposide (VM-26, Vumon®)	IV over 1 h, PO (etoposide); refrigerate capsules Use non-PVC bag/tubing; etoposide can crack plastic tubing; teniposide can precipitate in lines Skin irritant; eye irritant Hypotension with rapid infusion; monitor blood pressure Risk for acute HSR
Camptothecan analogs	Topoisomerase I inhibitors (cell cycle nonspecific)
Irinotecan (camptothecin-11, CPT-11, Camptosar ®)	IV Provide supportive care for diarrhea Encourage oral hydration
Topotecan (Hycamtin ®)	IV infusion, IT over 5 min, p.o. daily × 5 days Skin irritant Premedicate with deacadron for i.t. use
Antiangiogenic agents	
Thalidomide (Thalamid ®) In clinical trial Bevacizumab (avastin, Angiostatin®) Endostatin	PO, dose escalation; administer 1–2 h after food at bedtime, Blister packs prescribed intact Prescriber must register with Celgene Corporation (STEPS); monthly authorization required via a prescriber and patient/caregiver telephone survey Obtain pregnancy test prior to initiating and then monthly on all females of childbearing potential Teratogenic; educate females of childbearing potential on safe handling and administration; ensure contraception at least 4 weeks before, during, and 4 weeks after taking
Miscellaneous agents	
Glucocorticoids	
Prednisone Dexamethasone Hydrocortisone Methylprednisolone	IV over 20–30 min, IT, PO; administer with food; recom mend concurrent histamine H2-receptor antagonist (ranitidine) Monitor for hypoglycemia Taper after long-term use Recommend monitoring bone mineral density
Enzymes	Cell cycle nonspecific agents
Asparaginase (l-asparaginase, Elspar®, Kindrolase®) Erwinia asparaginase PEG-asparagase (PEG-l-asparaginase, Oncaspar®)	IV, IM.; larger dose can be divided into two syringes High risk for acute HSR with i.v. form; skin test first dose; observe patient for 60 min after administration; have emergency equipment and drugs readily available If reaction to Erwinia can switch to another form Monitor glucose and coagulation factors

Classification (drug/names/trade names)	Administration considerations
Target-specific inhibitors	
Erlotinib (Tarceva®) Imatinib mesylate (STI 571, Gleevac™) Gefitinib (Iressa®) Bevacizumab (avastin) Sunitinib (sutenta)	PO; administer on an empty stomach except for Imatinib; tablets can be dissolved Monitor for fluid retention
Retinoids	
Isotretinoin (13-*cis*-retinoic acid; Accutane®) Tretinoin (ATRA, all-*trans* retinoic acid, Vesanoid®)	PO daily; capsules can be chewed; contents can be removed from capsule and put in high fat food Avoid excessive exposure to sunlight and excessive vitamin A intake Monitor for dry/peeling skin, cracked lips and dry eyes; recommend vitamin E moisturizers and lipsalves Obtain pregnancy test prior to initiating treatment on all females of childbearing potential
Differentiating agent	
Arsenic trioxide (Trisenox®)	IV; monitor blood counts, electrolytes and symptoms of acute premyelocytic leukemia (fever, weight gain, shortness of breath, musculoskeletal pain) Moderate to highly emetic; provide antiemetics

following administration of antimetabolites. Other rare effects include dermatitis (characterized by erythema and desquamation), acral erythema characterized by painful erythema of the palms and soles (Varela et al. 2007), allergic reactions, acute pneumonitis, osteopathy, and neurotoxicity.

Methotrexate has been associated with acute (elevated liver function tests) and potentially fatal hepatotoxicity. Central system abnormalities are seen as changes on imaging or with clinical manifestations such as aseptic meningitis, transverse myelopathy, stroke-like syndrome, and acute or chronic encephalopathy (Keime-Guibert et al. 1998). High-dose methotreatate (1000–33000mg/m^2) is given in combination with leucovorin te reduce associated side effects (Widemann et al. 2004).

A syndrome of high fever, malaise, myalgias, joint or bone pain, rash, conjunctivitis, and chest pain has been reported with standard doses of IT cytarabine. Acute neurotoxic effects including cerebellar dysfunction (Nathan et al. 2007) and peripheral neuropathy are also associated.

In patients with long-term use of thioguanine, liver toxicity has been reported. Some of the most common reported side effects with capecitibine in adults include the common effects listed above and hand and foot syndrome (also reported with fluorouracil), diarrhea, and hepatotoxicity.

9.5.1.3 Long-Term Effects

IT administration of methotrexate and i.v. administration of high doses of methotrexate may worsen cognitve deficits induced by chemotherapy and radiation (Riva et al. 2002), and contribute to deficits in attention and visual motor control. Triple IT chemotherapy with methotrexate, cytarabine, and corticosteroids increases the risk of late neurotoxicity (Nathan et al. 2007).

9.5.2 Alkylating Agents

9.5.2.1 Mechanism of Action

Alkylating agents act through the bonding of saturated carbon atoms to cellular molecules, causing intracellular alteration in transcription and replication of DNA and ultimately cell death. These agents are cell cycle nonspecific. There are several types:

- Mustard gas derivatives: mechlorethamine, cyclophosphamide, melphalan, ifosfamide
- Ethylenimines: thiotepa
- Alkylsulfonates: busulfan
- Hydrazine and triazines: procarbazine, dacarbazine, temozolomide
- Nitrosureas: carmustine, lomustine
- Metal salts: carboplatin, cisplatin, oxaliplatin

Several of the alkylating agents are widely used today as part of multiagent regimens for acute leukemia, a variety of solid tumors, brain tumors, germ cell tumors, Wilms' tumor, and neuroblastoma. Melphalan appears to be active against rhabdomyosarcoma. The nitrosoureas have been used primarily to treat patients with brain tumors or lymphomas, and high-dose carmustine has been incorporated into transplant preparative regimens.

9.5.2.2 Side Effects

While myelosuppression is the primary dose-limiting side effect for most of the alkylating agents, other common toxicities include nausea, vomiting, anorexia, diarrhea, constipation, mucositis, alopecia, allergic and cutaneous reactions, elevated liver function tests, and gastrointestinal and neurological toxicity (Adamson et al. 2005).

Hemorrhagic cystitis or bladder epithelial damage and bleeding is a toxicity of cyclophosfamide and ifosfamide. It can range from mild dysuria and frequency to severe hemorrhage. Mesna is a bladder protectant administered to decrease effects.

Kidney damage is a major dose-limiting side effect of cisplatin and to a lesser extent with carboplatin and oxaliplatin (Tortorice 2005). Treatment guidelines may reduce or omit cisplatin if GFR is less than 60 mL/min/1.73 m^2 (Jones et al. 2008). Cisplatin also causes magnesium wasting and patients may need magnesium supplementation. Sensorineural, high-frequency hearing loss is reported after use with cisplatin and in fewer instances with carboplatin. It is most often observed at cumulative doses approaching 400 mg/m^2 (Bertolini et al. 2004) and at higher doses may be irreversible. Risk of acute hypersensitivity reaction (HSR) can occur with carboplatin and may be an indication for the administration of antihistamines and/or steroids with future use. Cisplatin, carboplatin, and oxaliplatin can cause varying degrees of peripheral neuropathy.

Side effects seen with procarbazine include the common toxicities above, and a flu-like syndrome. Rare effects include peripheral neuropathy, nightmares, hallucinations, depression, insomnia, convulsions, coma, pruritis, hypertension, and hemolytic anemia. Carmustine can cause early-onset alveolitis and fibrosis.

9.5.2.3 Long-Term Effects

Most alkylating agents are carcinogenic, mutagenic, and teratogenic causing treatment-related acute myelogenous leukemia/myelodysplastic syndrome (t-AML/MDS) (Bhatia 2004). The risk increases with increasing doses of alkylating agents and age at treatment. Testicular or ovarian dose related damage permanently affecting reproductive function can occur particularly with busulfan, procarbazine, and mechlorethamine. Men treated with cumulative doses of cyclophosphamide >7.5 g/m^2 are at highest risk for infertility (Afify et al. 2000). Nitrogen mustard, busulfan, cyclophosphamide, and carmustine have been linked to pulmonary fibrosis (Meadors et al. 2006) and delayed-onset fibrosis has been described up to 17 years after treatment with carmustine (O'Driscoll et al. 1990). Nephrotoxicity occurring after treatment with cisplatin, and ifosfamide can permanently damage renal function, and hemorrhagic cystitis can be a chronic recurring problem as long as 20 years after completion of therapy (Heyn et al. 1992).

9.5.3 Antitumor Antibiotics

9.5.3.1 Mechanism of Action

Antitumor antibiotics interfere with cellular metabolism by binding to DNA through a process called intercalation in which a part of the drug inserts between the base pairs of the DNA helix . These drugs are cell cycle nonspecific, active in multiple phases of the cell cycle (i.e., bleomycin and dactinomycin). The anthracyclines (Sect. 9.5.4) are a subgroup of this class.

Bleomycin is used in Hodgkin's disease, lymphomas, and testicular cancer and other germ cell tumors (Green 2008). Although used less often, dactinomycin is used to treat in Wilm's tumor and rhabdomyosarcoma and brain tumors.

9.5.3.2 Side Effects

Bleomycin can cause thrombocytopenia. Primary side effects include skin and fingernail hyperpigmentation, stomatitis, acral erythema, hypotension, nausea, vomiting, alopecia, anorexia, mucositis, and fever. There is a high risk of acute HSRs with administration and may develop into inflammatory interstitial pneumonitis (Meadors et al. 2006).

Myelosuppression can be seen with dactinomycin as well as mucositis, and nausea and vomiting. Veno-occlusive disease is a rare, potentially fatal toxicity manifested as fever, hepatomegaly, ascites, weight gain, jaundice, elevated liver function tests, and thrombocytopenia. Dactinomycin can also cause a radiation recall effect. It is a vesicant and extravasation can cause local tissues damage and ulceration.

9.5.3.3 Long-Term Effects

Late pulmonary toxicity from bleomycin includes pulmonary fibrosis, restrictive-obstructive lung disease, and delayed interstitial pneumonia. The risk of pulmonary fibrosis more commonly occurs with cumulative doses greater than 400–500 units (Meadors et al. 2006).

9.5.4 Anthracycline Antibiotics

9.5.4.1 Mechanism of Action

Anthracyclines disrupt DNA binding resulting in the formation of free radicals that attack DNA and the cell membrane. The cells of the heart muscle lack enzymes to detoxify radicals and thus cardiac toxicities are a high risk (Shankar et al. 2008). Anthracyclines also inhibit topoisomerase II action by preventing the rejoining of DNA strands and by inducing breaks in DNA. Common anthracyclines include daunorubicin, doxorubicin, and idarubicin. Mitoxantrone is a synthetic anthracenedione that has the topoisomerase II actions similar to anthracylines but lacks the ability to form free radicals and therefore may have fewer cardiac toxicities (Shankar et al. 2008). Agents are cell cycle nonspecific.

Doxorubicin is used in acute leukemia, lymphoma, sarcomas of soft tissue and bone, Wilm's tumor, neuroblastoma, and hepatoblastoma. Daunomycin and idarubicin use is limited to leukemia. Mitoxantrone has similar uses.

9.5.4.2 Side Effects

Acute toxicities include myelosuppression, mucositis, nausea, vomiting, diarrhea, and alopecia. If extravasated cause local tissue damage and ulceration. Can enhance radiation effects in tissues and organs and therefore should not be given with radiation. Acute cardiac toxicity can manifest usually within the first year of treatment as transient arrhythmias, pericarditis, or myocarditis, or left ventricular failure. Acute cardiac effects are generally reversible (Shankar et al. 2008), but their use may be limited by the risk of cumulative cardiac toxicity. Encapsulating anthracyclines in liposomes may reduce cardiac toxicity and possibly increase drug availability to tumors. Pegylated-liposomal doxorubicin is being investigated in children with resistant solid tumors (Lowis et al. 2006) and relapsed high-grade malignant brain tumors (Wagner et al. 2008).

9.5.4.3 Long-Term Effects

Chronic cardiotoxicity, ranging from benign arrhythmias to potentially fatal myocardial ischemia or infarction and heart failure, has been associated with anthracycline use (Viale and Yamamoto 2008). Cardiomyopathy is dose-dependent with increase reports at >400 mg/m^2 of doxorubicin (Youssef and Links 2005), although cardiac toxicity at lower doses can be seen.

9.5.5 Plant Derivatives

9.5.5.1 Mechanism of Action

Plant derivatives are obtained from plant material or manufactured from plant extracts. They are cell-cycle-specific causing arrest during mitosis.

- Vinca alkaloids (periwinkle plant): vincristine, vinblastine, vinorelbine
- Taxanes (Pacific Yew tree bark): paclitaxel, docetaxel
- Podophyllotoxins (May apple plant): etoposide, teniposide
- Camptothecan analogs (Asian Happy tree): irinotecan, topotecan

Podophyllotoxins and camptothecan analogs are also known as topoisomerase inhibitors. They act by interfering with the function of topoisomerase enzymes, which are responsible for DNA arrangement and rearrangement and cell growth and replication. Inhibitors stop cell growth and cause cell death.

- Topoisomerase I inhibitors: irinotecan, topotecan
- Topoisomerse II inhibitors: etoposide, teniposide

Vincristine is used in the treatment of ALL, Hodgkin's and non-Hodgkin's lymphomas, rhabdomyosarcoma, Ewing's sarcoma, Wilms' tumor, brain tumors, and neuroblastoma. Vinblastine is used to treat histiocytosis, testicular cancer, and Hodgkin's disease and brain tumors. Vinorelbine is being evaluated in childhood cancers.

The podophyllotoxins are used to treat ALL, Hodgkin's and non-Hodgkin's lymphoma, neuroblastoma, rhabdomyosarcoma, Ewing's sarcoma, germ cell tumors, and brain tumors.

Topotecan may have some activity in neuroblastoma, rhabdomyosarcoma, and brain tumors. Oral and IT use is currently being investigated in phase II trials in neoplastic meningitis, gliomas, and medulloblastomas.

In children, the taxanes are under investigation in relapsed ALL and AML and brain tumors.

9.5.5.2 Side Effects

Extravasation of the vinca alkaloids can cause local tissue damage and ulceration. Peripheral neuropathy, greatest with vincristine, includes decreased or absent deep tendon reflexes, paresthesias, sensory symptoms, motor weakness, paralytic ileus, and cranial neuropathies (Hausheer et al. 2006) also seen with paclitaxel, docetaxel, and to a lesser extent with etoposide. IT *administration of all vinca alkaloids is lethal.* SIADH, hypotension, and seizures can occur with vincristine. Myelosuppression is the dose-limiting toxicity with vinblastine and vinorelbine. These agents have a low emetic potential. Acute HSRs can occur with etoposide, teniposide, and the taxanes.

Myelosuppression and diarrhea are the most common toxicities of topotecan and irinotecan. Other toxicities include nausea, vomiting, alopecia, mucositis, fatigue, elevated hepatic transaminases, and rash. Malaise and electrolyte abnormalities have been observed. IT administration of topotecan can cause nausea, vomiting, headache, fever, back pain, leukoencephalopathy, seizures, or paralysis. Symtpoms mitigated with decadron.

Myelosuppression is the dose-limiting toxicity of etoposide and teniposide. Other side effects include alopecia, nausea, vomiting, phlebitis, peripheral neuropathy, elevation of liver function tests, diarrhea, mucositis, and acute HSRs. The taxanes can enhance acute cardiac toxicity if given with anthracyclines.

9.5.5.3 Long-Term Effects

The podophyllotoxins (etoposide, teniposide) have been reported to cause a distinct type of secondary acute leukemia/myelodysplastic syndrome (t-AML/MDS) characterized by a short time to presentation, chromosomal translocation of the MLL gene at 11q23, and M4 or M5 classification (Bhatia 2004).

9.5.6 Antiangiogenic Agents

9.5.6.1 Mechanism of Action

Antiangiogenic agents limit tumor growth and development by interfering with proliferating microvessels, a process called angiogenesis. Unlike the classical chemotherapy agents, antiangiogenic agents limit further tumor growth and metastases by preventing growth of new blood vessels via direct inhibition of endothelial cells, interruption of the angiogenesis messaging process, and prevention of the breakdown of the tissue (Muehlbauer 2003). Many antiangiogenic agents inhibit the vascular endothelial growth factor (VEGF)pathway preventing the VEGF protein from binding with a receptor to signal blood vessel growth. An example is thalidomide. Bevacizumab is an anti-VEGF monoclonal antibody that blocks activators of angiogenesis. Other examples include endostatin, VEGF-Trap, AZD2171, sunitinib, celengitide, and lenalidolimide under clinical investigation in childhood cancer.

Thalidomide was initially used as a sedative in the early 1960s; however, it was withdrawn from the market secondary to associated severe birth defects. It was found to have a therapeutic benefit in the treatment of recurrent myeloma and is now used in the treatment of some recurrent childhood cancers (brain tumors, neuroblastoma) but remains under strict guidelines for prescribing. Celgene Corporation has developed a program called STEPS ("system for thalidomide education and prescribing safety") for controlling and monitoring access to thalidomide (Muehlbauer 2003).

9.5.6.2 Side Effects

Side effects include birth defects constipation, somnolence, fatigue, skin rash, and peripheral neuropathy.

9.5.7 Miscellaneous Agents

Miscellaneous agents include those with a wide range of actions that do not fit into a particular class.

9.5.7.1 Corticosteroids

9.5.7.1.1 Mechanism of Action

Corticosteroids interfere with protein synthesis and cellular metabolism by binding with intracellular glucocorticoid receptors. Saturation of receptors induces apoptosis. Corticosteroids primarily used in pediatrics include prednisone and dexamethasone. Corticosteroids have a role in treatment regimens for acute leukemia, lymphoma, Hodgkin's disease, histiocytoses, and brain tumors. They may also be used to control disease symptoms and side effects (e.g., nausea, vomiting, increased intracranial pressure).

9.5.7.1.2 Side Effects

Side effects include increased appetite, centripetal obesity, immunosuppression, myopathy, stomach upset, hypertension, hyperglycemia, acne, impaired wound healing, pituitary-adrenal axis suppression, and atrophy of subcutaneous tissue. Dexamethasone can adversely alter sleep and fatigue (Hinds et al. 2007). Rarer effects include psychiatric disorders, gastrointestinal bleeding/ulceration, increased intraocular pressure, hypertension, aseptic necrosis of the femoral head, growth retardation, osteoporosis, and osteopenia.

9.5.7.1.3 Long-Term Effects

Skeletal damage may be associated with steroid use manifested as osteopenia, osteoporosis, avascular necrosis, spinal deformities, and other changes (Nandagopal et al. 2008). Steroid use may also contribute to late obesity and cataracts.

9.5.7.2 Enzymes: Asparaginase

Used in the treatment of acute leukemia and lymphomas, asparaginase has a unique mechanism of action of relative selectivity with regard to the metabolism of malignant cells. Its unique antitumor effect results from the depletion of asparagine, an amino acid essential to leukemic cells (but not found in nonmalignant cells), and subsequent inhibition of protein synthesis (Fu and Sakamoto 2007). Acute HSRs ranging from erythema to bronchospasm or anaphylaxis can occur. Patients who develop HSRs may receive a different form. PEG-asparaginase is a form of *Escherichia coli* l-asparaginase covalently linked to polyethylene glycol. PEG-asparaginase was synthesized to decrease immunogenicity of the enzyme, thereby reducing hypersensitivity reactions, and to prolong its half-life (Fu and Sakamoto 2007). Hepatic toxicity, coagulopathies, encephalopathy, and acute pancreatitis are potential side effects.

9.5.7.3 Targeted Growth Inhibitors

Targeted therapies disrupt the process of carcinogenesis by blocking cellular signals and enzymes and proteins necessary for continued growth. For example some tumors overexpress epidermal growth factor receptors (EGFR). Inhibition of the EGFR pathway with iressa causes cell cycle arrest at G1 and cell death. Imatinib (Gleevac) inhibits the tyrosine kinase activity of BCR-ABL gene expressed by the Philadelphia chromosome in chronic myelogenous leukemia (Tortorice 2005). Targeted cancer therapies are designed to kill cancer cells with little damage to normal, healthy cells.

9.5.7.4 Differentiating Agents

Retinoids, derivatives of vitamin A, signal cell effects through different receptors that lead to changes in gene expression. An example is Isotretinoin (*cis*-retinoic acid) and tretinoin (all-*trans* retinoic acid, ATRA). Isotretinoin is used in neuroblastoma unresponsive to conventional chemotherapy and is under investigation in brain tumors. Tretinoin is used in acute promyelocytic leukemia induction and maintenance phases of therapy.

Arsenic trioxide is another targeted drug used in the treatment of refractory acute promyelocytic leukemia.

Side effects of these agents include hematological toxicity, mild skin toxicity and chelitis, hypercalcemia (Veal et al. 2007), conjunctivitis, dry mouth, xerosis, pruritus, headache, bone and joint pain, epistaxis, and fatigue. Retinoids are teratogenic. Retinoid acid syndrome manifests with weight gain, respiratory distress, effusion, and cardiac and renal failure. Arsenic trioxide is associated with fatigue, lightheadedness, and a maculopapular rash.

9.6 Chemotherapy Protectants

Protectant drugs minimize the adverse effects of some chemotherapy agents and have no effect on overall survival, disease-free survival, progression-free survival, or local control rate. Agents are given simultaneously or in a sequential pattern before or after administration of the chemotherapy drug. The American Society of Clinical Oncology publishes evidence-based clinical guidelines for chemotherapy protectants and the following are guidelines from an update committee (Hensley et al. 2008):

9.6.1 Allopurinol (Zyloprim)

Reduces uric acid, associated with tumor cell lysis, thus protecting organs from damage. Use requires hydration and dose reduction in renal impairment.

9.6.2 Amifostine (Ethyol)

Reduces cisplatin-associated nephrotoxicity. Insufficient evidence exists to recommend use as a neurologic or otologic protectant. Monitor administration, can cause hypotension.

9.6.3 Dexrazoxane (Zinecard)

Reduces cardiac toxicity associated with doxorubicin by chelating intracellular iron, thus inhibiting the production of free radicals responsible for cardiac damage. Insufficient data exists to recommend use in pediatric malignancies; however, it has been used in some clinical trials. Recommended for consideration in patients who receive >300 mg/m^2 of doxorubicin with a ratio of dexrazoxane to doxorubicin 10:1. It is given 15–30 min before doxorubicin administration. There are ongoing studies looking at using an encapsulated form of doxorubicin to reduce toxicity.

9.6.4 Leucovorin Calcium (LCV, Wellcovorin, Citovorum Factor, Folic Acid)

Reduces bone marrow and digestive tract toxicities associated with methotrexate. Serial administration is initiated 24 h after the completion of systemic methotrexate or as a single dose after IT use.

9.6.5 Mesna (Mesnex)

Reduces hemorrhagic cystitis associated with ifosfamide and cyclophosphamide.

- Administration with standard-dose ifosfamide
  - Dose equals 60% of the total daily dose of ifosfamide, given as three boluses over 15 min pre- and at 4 and 8 h after
  - With doses less than 2.5 g/m^2/day given as a short infusion
  - With continuous ifosfamide infusion dose equals 20% of the total ifosfamide dose followed by a continuous infusion of mesna equal to 40% of the ifosfamide dose, continuing for 12–24 h
- Administration with high dose ifosfamide
  - Insufficient evidence for recommendations with ifosfamide doses >2.5 g/m^2/day; more frequent and prolonged dosing may be necessary
- Administration with oral ifosfamide
  - Dose equals 20% of ifosfamide given as an IV bolus at time of ifosfamide administration
  - Mesna tablets can be given orally with dose equal to 40% of the ifosfamide dose at 2 and 6 h after ifosfamide infusion
  - Total daily dose of mesna is 100%
- Repeat oral dose or administer IV if emesis within 2 h
- Administration with cyclophosphamide
- Doses ≤1,000 mg/m^2/day may not need mesna
- Administration with high-dose cyclophosphamide requires mesna as repeated boluses or continuous infusion post-cyclophosphan infusion and aggressive hydration

9.6.6 Palifermin

Palifermin is a growth factor for epithelial cells. It has been showed to reduce the incidence of severe mucositis in patients undergoing autologous stem cell transplant with total body radiation conditioning but further studies are required to identify the potential beneficial effects of this drug (Blazar et al. 2006).

9.7 Administration of Chemotherapy Agents

Chemotherapy handling and administration is not without risks and a thorough understanding by the pediatric oncology nurse is pertinent for safety of the patient, caregiver, and oncology nurse. Table 9.4 lists drugs by classification and highlights nursing considerations for safe handling and administration of specific drugs. Please refer to your institutional guidelines and pharmacy as well as a drug's package insert and the therapeutic protocol using the drug for a more comprehensive description regarding safe handling and administration and prescriptive recommendations.

9.7.1 Preparation

Safety of the patient, caregiver, and healthcare provider is essential throughout all phases of treatment and begins with preparation of the pediatric oncology nurse. The Association of Pediatric Hematology Oncology Nurses (APHON) offers a chemotherapy and biotherapy provider course for certification in chemotherapy administration. Additionally, most institutions require education and validation of knowledge and skills at time of hire and then annually. These competency requirements ensure that healthcare providers and patients are protected from harmful exposures and undue toxicities (Saca-Hazbourn 2008). Beyond demonstrated competency, treating a child safely requires a thorough comprehension of an institution's policies and procedures regarding chemotherapy handling and administration.

In the clinical context, knowledge of the treatment plan prescribed for each child is essential. Children are treated on a study protocol or according to a protocol. Knowing the basics about the child's plan of care by reviewing the chart, the protocol, and the information regarding the drugs to be given ensures accuracy in drug administration. Clinical and laboratory/diagnostic criteria are outlined in the plan and serve as initial checkpoints that must be verified before proceeding with drug administration. Preparation of patients and families involves clarifying information provided by the physician, answering questions, and providing teaching opportunities and educational materials prior to any treatment.

Institutions should have policies outlining the necessary checkpoints that nurses are required to take to ensure safe and accurate administration of agents. Steps recommended for all nurses to take include the following (Roll 2007):

- Verify chemotherapy orders and compare with the protocol the patient is being treated on or according to. Most institutions have two nurses to verify chemotherapy orders for accuracy.
- Assess the patient's prior experience with chemotherapy to provide additional premedications or fluids with the current course if needed.
- Review lab values and associated diagnostic tests required prior to specific types of chemotherapy (i.e., Audiogram) to assure that all criteria are met before drug administration.
- Calculate drug dosages. Review the patient's height and weight and double-check the body surface area (BSA). The BSA is determined by a BSA calculator or nomogram or by calculating the square root of the height (cm) multiplied by weight (kg) divided by 3,600. In obese patients, some institutions use the ideal body weight (IBW) to calculate the BSA. Know your institution's policy regarding the administration of chemotherapy to obese patients. Ascites or edema may affect a patient's weight. Evaluate the prefluid retention weight as a possible basis for dosage calculations. The AUC is used in patients receiving carboplatin. This dose is calculated based on the GFR or the creatinine clearance.
- Assess the records for any dose modifications. Doses are reduced if there has been severe toxicity with prior treatments. Many protocols or treatment regimens outline how the dose reduction is to be done. Patients may have an increase in the medication if they have tolerated treatment very well.

- Before administering drugs, verify correct patient, identify yourself to the patient/caregiver, explain your role, review the plan for chemotherapy administration, describe side effects that may be expected, offer supportive care, and answer all questions.
- Wash hands and don appropriate protective clothing

9.7.2 Administration and Practice Considerations

Chemotherapy can be administered by the topical, oral, i.v., intramuscular, subcutaneous, and i.t. routes (Table 9.5). Intraperitoneal and intraarterial routes are rarely used in children. With all routes, prepare

Table 9.5. Routes of administration and practice considerations (adapted from Sievers et al. 2007)

Route	Practice considerations
Topical	Instruct on application to the affected area Avoid mucous membranes Observe for adverse reactions (i.e., burning, rash)
Oral (PO)	Evaluate developmental level/ability for liquid or pill Follow dietary and medication restrictions and interactions Provide calendars or pill boxes to encourage compliance
Intramuscular (IM)	Never administer vesicant via i.m. route Never give a sleeping child an injection Inject into large muscles: anterior or lateral aspect middle third of thigh, deltoid, dorsogluteal Recommended volumes for age: Children/adolescents: deltoid (0.5–1 mL), vastus lateralis (2 mL), rectus femoris (2 mL), dorsogluteal (2 mL) Infants: vastus lateralis (0.5 mL), ventrogluteal (0.5 mL) Alternate sites to avoid fibrosis and contractures Decrease pain with ethyl chloride or a topical anesthetic; administer two injections simultaneously with two nurses Maintain increased pressure at site if platelets <50,000
Subcutaneous (SQ)	NEVER administer vesicants via SQ route Teach caregiver technique for daily SQ medications (i.e., GCSF) Decrease pain using correct technique; alternate sites Maintain increased pressure at site if platelets <50,000 Routes: peripheral, peripheral inserted central catheter (PICC), central venous catheter (portacatheter, broviac) Assess for blood return and patency Use central venous catheters for administration of vesicants
Intravenous (IV)	Peripheral access: Celgene Corporation (STEPS). Avoid dominant hand or foot veins in children who are learning to walk or are already walking. Choose a site that restricts movement as little as possible. For veins in the extremities, it is best to start with the most distal site. Avoid using veins in the antecubital fossa for chemotherapy administration. Use of scalp veins for nonvesicant chemotherapy is acceptable in children younger than 12 months. Secure site; maintain visualization so infiltration can be identified early. Start a new line if existing peripheral i.v. is older than 24 h, especially with vesicants or irritants. Vesicant administration greater than 1 h should never be done via a peripheral i.v.
Intrathecal (IT)/ intraventricular	Routes: lumbar, ommaya reservoir (a quarter size dome shaped device placed surgically between the scalp and the skull with a catheter providing access to the ventricles) Conscious sedation or general anesthesia may be required Apply a topical anesthetic Have the child lie flat for 30 min to an hour to facilitate drug distribution throughout the central nervous system and to potentially minimize headache Separate i.t. and i.v. medications. Accidental administration could be fatal

the child and caregiver. Assessment of a child's developmental level and education of the patient and family of potential side effects before giving any drug helps ensure safety and compliance. Use medical play, child life or psychosocial support or distraction techniques to assist with compliance. For drug preparation and administration, always use personal protective equipment (PPE): gowns, latex gloves, and chemical splash goggles or equivalent safety glasses, and *NIOSH (National Institute for Occupational Safety and Health) approved respirators when administering aerosolized drugs* (NIOSH (2004), www.cdc.gov/niosh/topics/antineoplastic).

9.7.2.1 Documentation

Documentation of all encounters is key to safety and should include the following:

- Patient's name, date, and time
- Site, needle gauge, and length or type of central line
- Site assessment prior to infusion
- Presence of blood return before, during, and after the infusion
- Amount and type of flush used
- Chemotherapy agent, route, dose, and duration of infusion

Doses/timing of supportive drugs and hydration.

- Patient's response to infusion/side effects/adverse reactions
- Patient education
- Follow-up care required (Sievers et al. 2007)

9.8 Professional Guidelines to Minimize the Risk of Medication Errors

9.8.1 Prescribing Errors

- Only a healthcare provider responsible for the care of the patient and most familiar with the chemotherapy regimen should write the orders.
- Use preprinted or computer generated order sheets, or if these are not available, the generic drug name should be written clearly and in its entirety.
- Avoid using abbreviations.
- Indicate the name of the agent, the dose in mg/m2, the dose to be given, the total daily dose, and the total number of days that the dose is to be given on the order sheet.
- Avoid using "0.0" to avoid tenfold dosing errors.

9.8.1.1 Compounding

- Compounding should be performed by a well-trained pharmacist.
- In most settings, computer-generated labels are used. Make sure all information on the label is accurate: the child's name, name of medication, amount of drug, and the amount and type of solution the drug is mixed in.
- Label medications with warning labels as needed; (e.g., "Do not give intrathecally," "Chemotherapy – Handle with care," or "For oral use only").

9.8.1.2 Dispensing

- Dispense a patient's drugs on trays or in plastic zip-locked bags.
- Do not combine more than one patient's drugs in the bags or on the tray.

9.8.1.3 Administration

- Administer in a safe, nonhurried environment.
- Double-check the treatment plan, medication, and orders prior to administration.
- Verify patient with two patient identifiers (e.g., name, date of birth, medical record number)
- Perform hand hygiene and don personal protective equipment (PPE).

9.9 Safe Practice Considerations

The Occupational Safety and Health Administration (OSHA) requires that healthcare institutions provide safe working conditions for those under their employment. Institutions are required to develop policies based on OSHA's guidelines for the safe handling of cytotoxic agents. These guidelines are to assist healthcare personnel who may be exposed to cytotoxic drugs through inhalation, skin absorption, or trauma. The guidelines listed are based on OSHA recommendations (http://www.osha.gov/dts/osta/otm/otm_vi/otm_vi_2.html#3).

9.9.1 Mixing Chemotherapeutic Agents

- Chemotherapy is usually prepared by pharmacy personnel, but in some hospitals and small physicians' offices, chemotherapy may be prepared by physicians and nursing staff. Refer to OSHA guidelines.
- Chemotherapy should be prepared under a biological safety cabinet (BSC) in an area that is well ventilated. Crush oral medications under the BSC cabinet.
- PPE should be worn, and hands should be washed prior to donning equipment. A double layer of gloves should be used if it does not interfere with technique and changed immediately if torn or punctured. A protective gown made of lint-free low-permeability fabric with a closed front, long sleeves, and elastic cuffs must be worn. Surgical masks do not protect against the breathing of aerosolized agents and if worn a plastic face shield or splash goggles should also be worn. An eyewash fountain should be available. All PPE and disposable materials should be disposed of according to the institution's toxic waste procedures.
- Cytotoxic agents should be prepared in one centralized area, and have a closable, puncture-resistant, shatterproof container for disposing of contaminated sharps and breakable materials.
- Syringe bottles and i.v. bottles should be labeled with the patient's name and room number (if applicable), drug name and quantity per total volume, route of administration, date and time prepared, dose, expiration date, and storage requirements (if the drug is not to be transported immediately). All syringes, IV bags, and bottles containing cytotoxic drugs should be labeled with a distinctive warning label such as "Chemotherapy – handle with gloves – dispose of properly."
- Wash hands immediately after handling cytotoxic agents.
- Avoid eating, drinking, smoking, chewing of gum or tobacco, application of cosmetics, or food storage in areas where antineoplastic agents are prepared.

9.9.2 Transporting Cytotoxic Agents

- Securely cap or seal and package drugs for transport.
- Educate and train personnel involved in transporting should a spill occur.
- Lablel all drugs with a warning label and clearly identify as a cytotoxic agent.
- Avoid transport methods that may harm contents (e.g., pneumatic tubes).

9.9.3 Safe Handling After Chemotherapy

- Institute universal precautions and wear PPE when handling the blood, emesis, excreta, or linen soiled with bodily fluids of a patient who has received chemotherapy within 48 h.
- For children who are incontinent of urine, clean the skin with each diaper change and apply a barrier ointment.
- Flush the toilet with the lid down at least twice with each void for 48 h after receiving chemotherapy.
- Wash contaminated bed linens twice without other items in hot water.
- Place bed linens in the hospital into a plastic contamination bag.

9.9.4 Disposal of Cytotoxic Materials

- Place chemotherapy in a sealable leak-proof plastic bag.
- Use puncture-proof containers for sharps and breakable items.
- Do not break or recap needles.
- Wear gloves when disconnecting chemotherapy.
- Dispose of the chemotherapy bag and tubing as an intact unit and cap the end of the infusion tubing after disconnecting it from the patient.

9.9.5 Spill Management

- Locate spill kits in preparation and administration areas.
- Know your institution's policy regarding spill management
- In the event of a chemotherapy spill, notify the institutional safety officer and post a sign or have a person available to warn others of the spill. Don protective clothing. Use the items in the spill kit to prevent the spill from contaminating other areas. Seal and double-bag all contaminated materials for disposal. Clean the spill according to the type of spill and the location.
- Report and document spill according to institutional policy.

9.9.6 Procedures Following Accidental Exposure

- Seek attention immediately.
- If direct skin exposure occurs, rinse immediately with water.
- For eye exposure, rinse with an eye wash solution for at least 5 min.
- Report all episodes of exposure to employee health.

9.9.7 Storage

- Store chemotherapy drug containers in a location with appropriate safety regulations.
- Label all drug containers to indicate hazardous materials.
- Provide instructions to handle accidental exposure (e.g., Material Safety Data Sheets).
- Ensure that packaging is intact before removing chemotherapy drug containers.

9.9.8 Medical Management

- Employees who are pregnant or planning to become pregnant, who are breastfeeding, or who have a reason to limit exposure to cytotoxic agents (e.g., HSRs) should be offered work in areas where exposure is not likely.

9.10 Administration of Chemotherapy in the Home

Advances in equipment and supportive measures have attributed to the increased use of accredited and licensed home health agencies. They can provide i.v. hydration, administer some chemotherapeutic agents, and administer symptom management drugs. The administration of chemotherapy in the home provides an alternative to hospitalizations and numerous outpatient visits and can result in reduced expenses, reduced loss of income for parents, and improved patient and family satisfaction (Kandsberger 2007).

When selecting a home health agency, assuring safe chemotherpy administration in the home is mandatory. Competency programs for pharmacists, compounding technicians, and pediatric nurses demonstrating skill with central venous access devices (CVADs) and chemotherapy certification should be required, including safe administration of vesicants and management of side effects. Written policies and procedures that address the handling and safe administration of chemotherapy and documentation must be in place.

Selection of patients for home therapy involves evaluation of the patient and family, the home environment, and the appropriateness for home chemotherapy. Any chemotherapy drugs that are known for acute HSRs have a high risk of anaphylaxis or previously caused an adverse reaction in the patient should not be administered in the home. Education of the patient and family should be initiated early in the preparation phase and include the safe handling and storing and disposal of drugs, review of treatment schedule and administration considerations, management of potential side effects, and provision of emergency contact information. Continuous collaboration among the pediatric oncology treatment team, the home care agency, and the family is essential for successful treatment at home.

9.11 Immediate Complications of Chemotherapy Administration

Although most immediate complications from chemotherapy are rare, it is important that the pediatric oncology nurse be knowledgeable on how to recognize and manage acute adverse events that can be potentially damaging or life-threatening.

9.11.1 Extravasation

Extravasation occurs when there is leakage during the administration of a chemotherapeutic agent into the tissue surrounding the vein. Extravasation of a vesicant can result in blistering, local and/or extensive tissue damage. Extravasation of an irritant may result in local inflammation, burning sensation, and pain. Flare reactions present themselves as immediate painless red streaks, wheals with or without pruritis at the site of injection. The degree of tissue damage is dependent on the agent and the concentration and quantity of drug extravasated and can include significant tissue damage, altered limb function, and can effect emotional health and well-being (Schulmeister 2007).

9.11.1.1 Pathophysiology of Extravasation

Two major mechanisms are thought to cause tissue damage. Some agents (e.g., anthracyclines, alkylating agents) are absorbed by local cells in the tissue and bind to DNA, causing cell death. The agent is then released into the surrounding tissue, causing further cell death. Healing is inhibited when the process repeats itself and the drug is absorbed by other cells (Schulmeister 2007).

Other agents (e.g., vinca alkaloids, taxanes) do not bind to cellular DNA but indirectly affect the cells in healthy tissue. Non-DNA binding vesicants are neutralized more easily (Ener et al. 2004) and injuries are more localized improving over time (Schulmeister 2007).

Flare reactions are a result of a histamine release and patients exhibiting this reaction to the chemotherapeutic agent will often be premedicated with antihistamines or steroids.

9.11.1.2 Risk Factors of Extravasation

Although the use of central venous access devices CVADs in the pediatric oncology population has improved the ease and safety of chemotherapy administration, especially for continuous infusions of vesicants, the risk for extravasation still exists.

Risk factors may include, but are not limited to, the following:

- Anatomic issues, including the access site, venous integrity, vessel size, and blood flow
- Duration of tissue exposure and the amount of infiltrate
- Types and sizes of i.v. catheters
- Needle dislodgement, incorrect needle length, and incomplete or improper access technique
- Rupture or tear in the catheter or port tubing. Fibrin sheath formation at the catheter tip; thrombosis
- Persistent inability to draw blood but able to flush the line without difficulty or "positional blood draws" (Sauerland et al. 2006)

9.11.1.3 Assessment and Treatment of Extravasation

9.11.1.4 Signs and Symptoms of Extravasation

It is important that anyone who administers vesicant agents be aware of the signs and symptoms of extravasation so that quick and appropriate intervention can limit damage (Table 9.6). Many of these signs and symptoms are noticeable immediately after the event, but some may occur over several weeks or months. Continued monitoring of the affected site is necessary.

9.11.1.5 Treatment for Extravasation

Knowledge and understanding of the appropriate actions (Table 9.7) to take in the event of an extravasation may limit its long-term effects. Individual vesicants require immediate and specific actions to limit extent of damage. Several cooperative groups and associations provide guidelines for the identification and management of extravasation including the Children's Oncology Group (http:// www.curesearch.org), the Oncology Nursing Society, and the

Table 9.6. Nursing considerations and management for peripheral and central administration of vesicants (adapted from Sievers et al. 2007)

Site	Administration considerations	Extravasation management
Peripheral intravenous access (PIV)	Nurses skilled at venipuncture and assessment and intervention should administer vesicant agents Use a new PIV site, if possible Use large veins in the nondominant upper extremity when possible, avoiding the dorsum of the hand and foot and the antecubital fossa Avoid repeated to place the catheter below the original i.v. site Select appropriate catheter. Small-gauge catheters (0–3 gauge) are recommended Short, single dose infusions can be safely administered through a butterfly catheter, longer infusions should be administered through polyethylene or Teflon catheters Use two-syringe method, one to inject the vesicant and the other syringe to check blood return and patency Give over less than 3 min checking blood return after every 1–2 mL of drug administered Avoid using syringe pumps	Stop infusion at the first sign of infiltration or at first report of pain, burning, swelling, color change, change in sensation, or lack of blood return Notify the physician or nurse practitioner Remove syringe with vesicant agent from tubing, but leave the PIV in place Aspirate residual drug Administer appropriate antidote (Table 9.7) Elevate affected area and apply warm or cool compresses as indicated (Table 9.7) For subcutaneous administration of the antidote, discontinue the PIV catheter attempting to aspirate as much medication as possible. Use a 25–30 gauge needle to inject the antidote into the surrounding subcutaneous tissue. Apply heat or cold to the site as appropriate. Instruct the patient and family to rest the site for 48 h. Provide instructions not to break blisters Apply a nonocclusive dressing if necessary Monitor site at 24, 48 h , and then 7 days post extravasation Consult plastic surgery depending on the extent of tissue damage or/and functional limitation
Central venous access (CVA)	Use CVA devices for continuous infusions Use appropriate size, non-coring needle Note a brisk blood return immediately before starting administration Monito and document blood return least every 4 h or even more with continuous infusions and every 1–2 mL with i.v. push administration Assess site for signs of inflammation and extravasation after every 10 mL or every hour during the infusion Administer altetplase if persistent withdrawal occlusion occurs, per institutional policy Obtain radiographic studies if alteplase unsuccessful	Stop infusion at first report of pain, burning, swelling, color change, change in sensation, or lack of blood return Notify the physician or nurse practitioner. Assess needle placement with portacatheters Aspirate residual drug Administer appropriate antidote (Table 9.7): For IV administration instill into CVA device; for SQ administration remove port needle attempting to withdraw as much agent as possible and then inject the antidote into the surrounding tissue using a 26–30 gauge needle Obtain radiographic studies if necessary Monitor site at 24, 48 h, and then 7 days post extravasation Consult plastic surgery depending on the extent of tissue damage or/and functional limitation

Table 9.7. Antidotes for extravasations of chemotherapy vesicants (V) and irritants (I)

Agents	Antidote	Local Care	Comments
Dactinomycin(V)	None	Elevate affected extremity; apply ice	Consult plastic surgery as necessary
Anthracyclines(V)	Dexrazoxane (Totect™)-a metal iron chelator that protects against free radical toxicity	Apply cool packs for 15 min every 3–4 h as tolerated for 24–48 h Administer within 6 h of extravasation; discontinue ice for 15 min; administer Dexrazoxane over 15 min; reapply ice 15 min; repeat at 24 and then 48 h after event	Consult surgery as necessary with evidence of tissue damage; doxorubicin can produce prolonged tissue necrosis
Mechlorethamine (V)	Sodium thiosulfate	Inject through existing PIV/CVAD line or SQ at site	Heat and/or ice not proven to be effective
Vinca alkoids (V)	Hyaluronidase	Inject antidote through existing PIV/CVAD line or SQ at site Apply warm compresses 15–20 min at least four times a day for 24–48 h.	Antidote not commercially available; however, it is still being used at some institutions; Applying heat increases local blood flow, which enhances absorption and removal of the drug from the site; Cooling area is not recommended
Carboplatin (I) Carmustine (I) Dacarbazine (I) Etoposide (I) Ifosfamide (I) Paclitaxel Teniposide (I)	None	Apply cold packs to site and along irritated vein; Warm packs are recommended for Etoposide	Slowing the rate of infusion may decrease the amount of local irritation
Taxanes (I)	Hylauronidase	Inject SQ at the site	Conflicting literature on warm vs. cool applications

European Oncology Nursing Society (EOS) (http://www.cancerworld.org/CancerWorld/getStaticModFile.aspx?id=2340). Refer to your individual institution's policies and procedures.

With any event, documentation of extravasation verifies that care met standard of practice (Sauerland et al. 2006). Documentation should and include:

- Date and time of occurrence
- Size and type of needle/type of CVAD
- Needle insertion site
- Number of previous venipuncture attempts and sites if using peripheral access
- Sequence of chemotherapy agent administration
- Drug administration technique
- Patient complaints/statements/activities
- Appearance of site
- Approximate amount of drug administered
- Physician or nurse practitioner notification
- Nursing interventions at time of the incident
- Follow-up measures
- Patient education provided

9.11.2 Acute Hypersensitivity Reactions (HSRs) to Chemotherapy

Although HSRs to chemotherapy are rare, with an incidence of ≤5% (Lenz 2007) it is important for the pediatric oncology nurse to recognize agents that may have a higher incidence of causing them. These include l-asparaginase, taxanes, platinum compounds, and the podophyllotoxins. HSRs range from a localized immune response that is mild and short to systemic anaphylaxis severe in nature, and may lead to shock and death (Table 9.8).

Reactions to platinum compounds are consistent with type 1 hypersensitivity caused by the IgE-mediated release of histamines, leukotrienes, and prostaglandins from mast cells in tissue and basophils in peripheral blood while taxanes produce similar reactions via direct effects on immune cells (Zanotti and Markman 2001). The exact mechanism for reactions to monoclonal antibodies is not known. The timing of HSRs is consistent with the mechanism. Reactions to platinum compounds generally occur after multiple treatments while reactions to taxanes are more immediate, occurring during the first minutes of the first or second treament and most monoclonal antibody reactions are delayed occurring late in treatment (Lenz 2007). Intervention may involve temporary or permanent interruption of the infusion, reduction of the infusion rate, and symptom management.

Table 9.8. Clinical manifestions of HSRs

Symptom
Urticaria (hives, welts, wheals)
Shortness of breath, with or without wheezing
Cough
Periorbital edema or facial edema
Tightness in the chest
Chills
Localized or generalized itching
Uneasiness or agitation
Lightheadedness or dizziness
Headache
Abdominal cramping nausea/vomiting
Hypotension, hypertension
Tachycardia
Drug fever

9.11.3 Risk Factors for Hypersensitivity, Flare Reactions, or Anaphylaxis

Factors identified to increase the risk of experiencing a type 1 HSR include (Ream and Tunison 2001):

- History of allergies, particularly drug allergies.
- Receiving a drug known to cause HSR (e.g., carboplatin, cisplatin, oxaliplatin, l-asparingase, paclitaxel, docetaxel, etoposide, teniposide).
- Repeated exposure to the agent.
- Failure to receive known effective prophylactic premedications.
- Intraveous administration of agent.

9.11.4 Recommended Steps to Prevent HSRs

- Obtain BCLS and PALS certification.
- Identify and locate emergency equipment and medication.
- Obtain orders for anaphylaxis prior to drug administration.
- Obtain and document vital signs before, during, and after the infusion.
- Review patient's allergy and hypersensitivity history.
- Administer premedications when necessary.
- Educate the patient and family on signs and symptoms of HSR.
- Administer a test dose before giving the drug. Observe patient for any local or systemic reaction for at least 20 min and if no sign of hypersensitivity, proceed with initial dosing.
- Infuse the drug slowly and observe the patient for signs and symptoms of hypersensitivity.

9.11.5 Emergency Management of HSR/Anaphylaxis

Prompt recognition of a reaction is essential for the safety of the patient. Review your institution's policy outlining emergency management of HSRs.

The following steps are recommended with the first signs or report of symptoms (Sievers et al. 2007):

- Stop the chemotherapy infusion immediately.
- Stay with the patient; call for help and emergency equipment.
- Assess airway, breathing, and circulation.
- Maintain an IV line with normal saline; place patient in supine position.
- Monitor vital signs every 2 min until stable, then every 5 min for 30 min, then every 15 min.
- Administer emergency medications as necessary.
- Provide emotional support for the patient and family.
- Re-challenge (attempting to give the drug a second time following HSR) is generally discouraged in severe initial reaction (grade 3 and 4) but may be attempted in mild to moderate reactions (grade 1 and 2) using a slower infusion time and appropriate premedications.
- Document intervention and patient's response.

9.12 Summary

Chemotherapy is essential in most treatment plans for childhood cancers. Chemotherapy use and the risks related to exposure compounded by the impact of a diagnosis of cancer can contribute to feelings of anxiety and fear for the patient and family. Confident and knowledgeable pediatric nursing care provided in a supportive and competency-based environment helps ensure safe practice and ultimately good clinical care.

References

Adamson PC, Balis FM, Berg W, Blaney SM (2005) General principles of chemotherapy. In: Pizzo PA (ed) Principles and practice of pediatric oncology, 5th edn. Lippincott Williams & Wilkins, Philadelphia, PA, pp 290–365

Afify A, Shaw PJ, Clavano-Harding A, Cowell CT (2000) Growth and endocrine function in children with acute myeloid leukaemia after bone marrow transplantation using busulfan/cyclophosphamide. Bone Marrow Transplantation 25(10): 1087–1092

Bertolini P, Lassalle M, Mercier G, Raquin MA, Izzi G, Corradini N, Hartmann O (2004) Platinum comound-related ototoxicity in children: long-term follow-up reveals continuous worsening of hearing loss. Journal of Pediatric Hematology/Oncology 26:649–655

Bhatia W (2004) Epidemiology. In: Wallace WH, Green DM (eds) Late effects of childhood cancer. Arnold, London, United Kingdom, pp 57–69

Blazar BR, Weisdorf DJ, DeFor T, Goldman A, Braun T, Silver S, Ferrara JLM (2006) Phase 1/2 randomized placebo controlled trial of palifermin to prevent graft versus host disease (GVHD) after allogeneic hematopoietic stem cell transplantation. Blood 108(9):3216–3222

Bond MC, Pritchard S (2006) Understanding clinical trials in childhood cancer. Paediatrics & Child Health 11(3):148–150

Ener RA, Meglathery SB, Styler M (2004) Extravasation of systemic hemato-oncological therapies. Annals of Oncology 15:858–862

Fu CH, Sakamoto KM (2007) PEG-asparaginase. Expert Opinion on Pharmacotherapy 8(12):1977–1984

Green DM (2008) Chemotherapy for the treatment of children and adolescents with malignant germ cell tumors. Journal of Clinical Oncology 26(20):3297–3298

Hensley ML, Hagerty KL, Kewalramani T, Green DM, Meropol NJ, Wasserman TH, Cohen GI, Emami B, Gradishar WJ, Mitchell RB, Thigpen JT, Trotti A, vonHoff D. Schuchter LM (2008) American society of clinical oncology 2008 clinical practice guideline update: use of chemotherapy and radiation therapy protectants. Journal of Clinical Oncology. http://jco.ascopubs.org/cgi/doi/10.1200/JCO.2008/17/2627. Retrieved 21 Mar 2009 from

Heyn R, Raney RB, Hays DM, Tefft M, Gehan E, Webggber B, Maurer HM (1992) Late effects of therapy in patients with paratesticular rhabdomyosarcoma. Intergroup rhabdomyosarcoma study committee. Journal of Clinical Oncology 10:614–623

Hinds PS, Hockenberry MJ, Gattuso JS, Srivastava DK, Tong X, Jones H, West N, McCarthy KS, Sadeh A, Ash M, Fernandez C, Pui C (2007) Dexamethasone alters sleep and fatigue in pediatric patients with acute lymphoblastic leukemia. Cancer 110(10):2321–2330

Jones DP, Spunt SL, Green D, Springate JE (2008) Renal late effects in patients treated for cancer in childhood: a report from the children's oncology group. Pediatric Blood & Cancer 54(6):724–731

Kandsberger D (2007) Factors influencing the successful utilization of home health care in the treatment of children and adolescents with cancer. Home Health Care Management & Practice 19(6):450–455

Keime-Guibert F, Napolitano M, Delattre JY (1998) Neurological complications of radiotherapy and chemotherapy. Journal of Neurology 245:695–708

Lenz H (2007) Management and preparedness for infusion and hypersensitivity reactions. The Oncologist 12:601–609

Lowis S, Lewis I, Elsworth A, Weston C, Doz F, Vassal G et al (2006) A phase I study of intravenous liposomal daunorubicin (DaunoXome) in paediatric patients with relapsed or resistant solid tumours. British Journal of Cancer 95(5):571

Ma R, Tunison D (2001) Hypersensitivity reactions. In: Yaski JM (ed) Nursing management of symptoms associated with chemotherapy. Meniscus health Care, Bala Cynwyd, PA, pp 213–224

Meadors M, Floyd J, Perry MC (2006) Pulmonary toxicity of chemotherapy. Seminars in Oncology 33(1):98–105

Merkle CJ, Loescher LJ (2005) Biology of cancer. In: Yarbo CH, Frogge MH, Goodman M (eds) Cancer nursing, principles and practice, 6th edn. Jones and Bartlett, Boston, pp 3–26

Muehlbauer PM (2003) Antiangiogenesis in cancer therapy. Seminars in Oncology Nursing 19(3):180–192

Nandagopal R, Laverdiere C, Mulrooney D, Hudson MM, Meacham L (2008) Endocrine late effects of childhood cancer therapy: a report from the children's oncology group. Hormone Research 69:65–74

Nathan PC, Patel SK, Dilley K, Goldsby R, Harvey J, Jacobsen C, Kadan-Lottick N, McKinley K, Millham AK, Moore I, Okcu F, Woodman CL, Brouwers P, Armstrong FD (2007) Guidelines for identification of, advocacy for, and intervention in neurocognitive problems in survivors of childhood cancer. Archives of Pediatrics and Adolescent Medicine 161(8):798–806

National Cancer Institute (2006) Common Terminology Criteria for Adverse events v3.0, (CTCAE). Available at http://ctep.cancer.gov/protocolDevelopment/electronic_applications/docs/ctcaev3.pdf. Accessed 15 Mar 2009

National Institute for Occupational Safety and Health (NIOSH) (2004) Preventing occupational exposure to antineoplastic and other haardous drugs in health care settings. http://www.cdc.gov/niosh/topics/antineoplastic/. Retrieved on 17 Dec 2008

O'Driscoll BR, Hasleton PS, Taylor PM, Poulter LW, Gattameni HR, Woodcock AA (1990) Active lung fibrosis up to 17 years after chemotherapy with carmustine (BCNU) in childhood. The New England Journal of Medicine 323(6):378–382

Parasole R, Menna G, Marra N, Petruzziello F, Locatelli F, Mangione A, Misuraca A, Buffardi S, Di Cesare-Merlone A, Poggi V (2008) Efficacy and safety of intrathecal liposomal cytarabine for the treatment of meningeal relapse in acute lymphoblastic leukemia: experience of two pediatric institutions. Leukaemia & Lymphoma 49(8):1553–1559

Pritchard-Jones K, Dixon-Woods M, Naafs-Wilstra M, Valsecchi MG (2008) Improving recruitment to clinical trials for cancer in childhood. The Lancet Oncology 9:392–399

Rieger PT (2004) The biology of cancer genetics. Seminars in Oncology Nursing 20(3):145–154

Ries LAG, Melbert D, Krapcho M, Stinchcomb DG, Howlader N, Horner MJ, Mariotto A, Miller BA, Feuer EJ, Altekruse SF, Lewis DR, Clegg L, Eisner MP, Reichman M, Edwards BK (eds) (2008) SEER cancer statistics, 1975–2005. National Cancer Institute, Bethesda, MD. http://seer.cancer.gov/csr/1975_2005/. Retrieved on 15 Mar 2009

Riva D, Giorgi C, Nichelli F, Bulgheroni S, Massimino M, Cefalo G, Gandola L, Giannotta M, Bagnasco I, Saletti V, Pantaleoni C (2002) Intrathecal methotrexate affects cognitive function in children with medulloblastoma. Neurology 59:48–53

Roll L (2007) Preadministration considerations. In: Kline NE (ed) The pediatric chemotherapy and biotherapy curriculum, 2nd edn. Association of Pediatric Hematolology/Oncology Nurses, Glenview, pp 65–67

Saca-Hazbourn H (2008) Safe handling of chemotherapy. ONS Connect 23(8):10–14

Sauerland C, Engelking C, Wickham R, Corbi D (2006) Vesicant extravasation part 1; mechanisms, pathogenesis, and nursing care to reduce risk. Oncology Nursing Forum 33(6):1134–1141

Schulmeister L (2007) Totect™: a new agent for treating anthracycline extravasation. Clinical journal of oncology nursing 11(3):387–395

Shankar SM, Marina N, Hudson MM, Hodgson DC, Adams J, Landier W, Bhatia S, Meeske K, Chen MH, Kinahan KE, Steinberger J, Rosenthal D (2008) Monitoring for cardiovascular disease in survivors of childhood cancer: report from the cardiovascular disease task force of the children's oncology group. Pediatrics 121(2):387–395

Sievers TD, Andam R, Madsen L (2007) Chemotherapy administration and immediate postadministration issues. In: Kline NE (ed) The pediatric chemotherapy and biotherapy curriculum, 2nd edn. Association of Pediatric Hematolology/Oncology Nurses, Glenview, pp 68–85

Stempak D, Seely D, Baruchel S (2006) Metronomic dosing of chemotherapy: applications in pediatric oncology. Cancer Investigation 24(4):432–443

Tortorice PV (2005) Biology of cancer. In: Yarbo CH, Frogge MH, Goodman M (eds) Cancer nursing, principles and practice, 6th edn. Jones and Bartlett, Boston, pp 315–351

Varela CR, McNamara J, Antaya RJ (2007) Acral erythema with oral methotrexate in a child. Pediatric Dermatology 24(5):541–546

Veal GJ, Cole M, Errington J, Pearson ADJ, Foot ABM, Whyman G, Boddy AV (2007) Pharmacokinetics and metabolism of 13-cis-retinoic acid (isotretinoin) in children with high-risk neuroblastoma- a study of the Untied Kingdom children's cancer study group. British Journal of Cancer 96:424–431

Viale PH, Yamamoto DS (2008) Cardiovascular toxicity associated with cancer treatment. Clinical journal of oncology nursing 12(4):627–638

Wagner S, Peters O, Fels C, Janssen G, Liebeskind A, Sauerbrey A et al (2008) Pegylated-liposomal doxorubicin and oral topotecan in eight children with relapsed high-grade malignant brain tumors. Journal of Neurooncology 86(2):175

Walters LA, Walters LA (2007) Pharmacokinetics and pharmacogenetics. In: Kline NE (ed) The pediatric chemotherapy and biotherapy curriculum, 2nd edn. Association of Pediatric Hematolology/Oncology Nurses, Glenview, p 27

Widemann BC, Balis FM, Kempf-Bielack B, Bielack S, Pratt CB, Ferrari S, Bacci G, Craft AW, Adamson PC (2004) High-dose methotrexate-induced nephrotoicity in patients with osteosarcoms. Cancer 100:2222–2232

Youssef G, Links M (2005) The prevention and management of cardiovascular complications of chemotherapy in patients with cancer. American Journal of Cardiovascular Drugs 5(4):233–243

Zanotti KM, Markman M (2001) Prevention and management of antineoplastic induced hypesensitivity reactions. Drug Safety 24:767–779Table 9.2 Examples of acute side effects after chemotherapy

Radiotherapy

Irene Loch • Jane Khorrami

Contents

10.1 Introduction 233
10.2 Radiation 233
10.3 Principles of Treatment 234
10.4 Treatment Planning 234
10.4.1 CT Simulation 234
10.4.2 Simulation 234
10.5 Treatment Methods 235
10.5.1 External Beam Radiotherapy (Teletherapy) 235
10.5.1.1 Ensuring Accuracy of Treatment Delivery 235
10.5.1.2 Marking 235
10.5.1.3 Patient Immobilization 236
10.5.2 Fractionation 237
10.5.3 Total Body Irradiation (TBI) 237
10.5.4 Brachytherapy 237
10.5.5 Sealed Sources 237
10.5.6 Unsealed Sources 237
10.6 Side Effects of Radiotherapy 238
10.6.1 Acute Effects 238
10.7 Special Considerations 240
10.7.1 Preparation of Children and Young People 240
10.8 Future Perspectives 240
10.8.1 Image-Guided Radiotherapy 240
10.8.2 Intra-Operative Radiotherapy 240
10.8.3 Proton Radiotherapy (PRT) 240
References 241

10.1 Introduction

Radiotherapy is the use of ionizing radiation to treat malignant disease. Generally, radiotherapy has a diminishing role in the treatment of childhood cancers due to very effective chemotherapy regimens and also the recognition of the late effects of radiotherapy, which is of particular significance to the pediatric patient still in the process of growth and development.

However, radiotherapy is still required for approximately 20% of children and young people with cancer. It is the main mode of treatment for brain tumors and it plays a significant role in the palliation of symptoms.

The aim of radiotherapy is to achieve local tumor control while minimizing long-term effects; therefore, it has an important role in the management of children with cancer.

10.2 Radiation

There are two types of radiation:

- Particle radiation, e.g. alpha and beta particles, consists of low energy and is limited to a few millimeters of penetration. Electrons, protons, and neutrons will penetrate to a depth of several centimeters depending on their energy and beam modulation. Electrons are most commonly used to treat superficial areas located a few centimeters beneath the skin.
- Ionizing electromagnetic radiation, e.g. X-rays, which include gamma rays have a much higher energy level and are deeply penetrating.

The use of X-rays is currently the most common form of radiotherapy. These X-rays are artificially generated in a linear accelerator as a stream of electrons bombard tungsten metal targets, releasing energy.

Cobalt machines are different and are still used in some parts of the world. Cobalt emits gamma radiation as part of its radioactive decay process. It requires concrete or lead to absorb the radiation (Byrne 2006).

In radiotherapy, the unit of radiation dose used is the Gray (Gy), which is a measure of absorbed energy (1 Gy=1 J as absorbed by 1 kg of body tissue). This unit has replaced the rad.
For example:

1 Gy=100 centigray (cGy) or rads

1 cGy=1 rad

10.3 Principles of Treatment

Radiotherapy causes damage to the tissues that are in the path of the radiation. Tumor cell DNA is the main target of radiotherapy and the damage done occurs directly and indirectly through the production of toxic free-radicals from the interaction of radiation with water within the cell. Single- and double-strand breaks occur in the DNA, and if repair does not take place, reproductive cell death occurs when the cell attempts to replicate (Neal and Hoskin 2003; Tarbell and Kooy 2002).

Radiosensitivity is closely related to cell proliferation activity. Although malignant cells are the target of radiotherapy, healthy rapidly dividing cells of normal tissue (e.g. skin, epithelium of the gastrointestinal and urinary tract, gonads and bone marrow) are also sensitive to radiation damage resulting in the side effects of radiotherapy (Byrne 2006).

Hypoxic cells are considered radioresistant. To compensate for this, treatment is delivered in small daily doses or fractions (fractionated radiotherapy). This type of treatment allows time for re-oxygenation to occur, enhancing radiosensitivity. To optimize oxygenation, the child's hemoglobin should be maintained at a minimum of 10 g/dL.

Radiation treatment can be classified as follows:

- Radical – treatment with curative intent. Usually, high doses of radiation are given daily for 3–7 weeks. This is the main treatment for brain tumors.
- Adjuvant – added to other treatment (i.e. surgery or chemotherapy) With certain diseases, there may be a residual tumor mass following chemotherapy (i.e. neuroblastoma).
- Palliative – treatment aimed at symptom control with few acute side-effects. This may involve either a single treatment or fractions given daily over 1–2 weeks. The treatment may be used to relieve pain by shrinking the tumor and releasing pressure or obstruction. If the tumor is life-threatening or impeding organ function, palliative radiotherapy can often quickly improve the progression of the symptoms (i.e. spinal cord or airway compression). If given in a timely fashion, radiotherapy can make a significant difference to morbidity and quality of life.

10.4 Treatment Planning

Accuracy and quality assurance in planning radiation therapy is of paramount importance to patient outcome. With external beam radiotherapy, once the plan is complete, it is tested by simulation (Aistars 2007).

10.4.1 CT Simulation

Information obtained from computerized tomography (CT) and magnetic resonance imaging (MRI) is transferred to the treatment planning system and the treatment volume is then calculated.

Vital structures can be identified and avoided or protected during treatment. A physics plan (Fig. 10.1) will be produced defining the treatment fields and the number and angle of the beams targeting the tumor site.

10.4.2 Simulation

Once the plan is agreed and finalized, a simulator X-ray film using diagnostic radiographic imaging

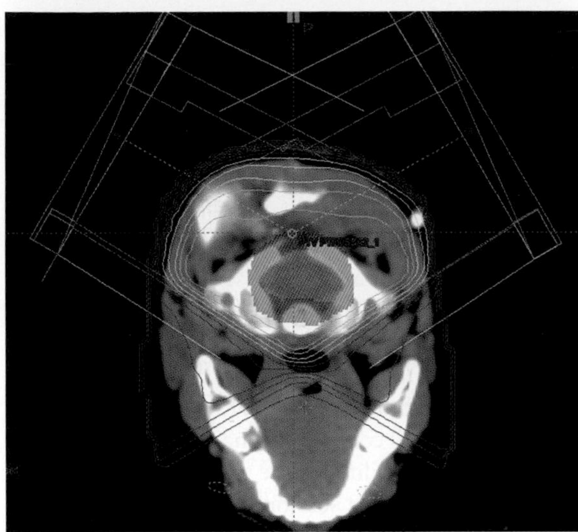

Figure 10.1

A physics plan defining treatment fields and beam angles

will then be taken to verify the size of the treatment field and the shape and placing of the proposed treatment beams (Coyler 2003). The treatment prescription will then be completed by the physician.

10.5 Treatment Methods

10.5.1 External Beam Radiotherapy (Teletherapy)

External beam therapy accounts for more than 95% of all radiotherapy delivered to cancer patients.

Linear accelerators form the mainstay of clinical radiotherapy and are described as megavoltage units producing high-energy X-ray beams. Units containing the radioactive source Cobalt-60 also produce megavoltage radiation, but have been virtually discontinued in favor of linear accelerators. This is due to the presence of the radioactive source, the safeguards required to protect staff, and the increased time necessary to deliver treatment.

Treatment is now usually delivered using three-dimensional (3-D), conformal, and intensity-modulated radiotherapy (IMRT).

- Three dimensional conformal radiotherapy is planned using the information from CT and MRI to provide a 3-D image of the tumor. Integrated computer software shapes the radiation beam using the multi-leaf collimator in the head of the treatment machine. This device uses a series of finger-like processes projected into the beam, which can be adjusted to the shape of the tumor. The healthy tissue around the tumor is spared using this technique and higher doses of radiation can be used (Munro 2008).
- IMRT is a further type of 3-D conformal radiotherapy that uses radiation beams of varying intensities to deliver different doses of radiation to small areas of tissue at the same time. The intensity of the beam can be altered or modulated to provide more flexibility in shaping the dose to the target volume, which is particularly valuable in treating tumors that may be surrounding a vital structure such as the spinal cord (Munro 2008).
- Stereotactic radiation can be performed as radiosurgery, where multiple beams converge at a point to deliver high dose of radiation to a small area of tumor. This is done as a one-time treatment and produces a high degree of tumor necrosis. Tumors must be well circumscribed, <4 cm in size, and not involve critical structures (e.g. brain stem). For treatment of brain tumors, a fixed frame is secured to the head to ensure precise delivery of the radiation beam. Stereotactic radiotherapy is similar to radiosurgery, but is carried out over multiple fractions and can treat larger tumor volumes.

10.5.1.1 Ensuring Accuracy of Treatment Delivery

10.5.1.2 Marking

Once the treatment plan has been verified and the clinician is satisfied with the final simulator film, external markings and a tattoo mark is applied to the skin to indicate the treatment site. These should not be removed. If the marks fade, the radiographers will renew them during a scheduled visit. Occasionally, a transparent dressing such as Op-site may be used to prevent marks being rubbed off.

The tattoo is a permanent identifying mark of the treatment field. This is helpful in the future, should the child require further radiotherapy near the original treatment site.

10.5.1.3 Patient Immobilization

The detail and accuracy involved in the planning phase ensures correct positioning of the patient for each treatment. Daily reproducibility of body position is essential to ensure that the treatment beams reach the intended target area. There are various methods used to help the child stay immobile throughout the treatment.

For treatment to the brain or head and neck area, a shell is made for individual use. This may be made from:

(a) A clear plastic material (e.g. perspex), which is heated and molded over a plaster of Paris cast impression of the patient's head or
(b) A thermoplastic mesh, which can be molded easily and quickly by immersing in warm water and placing over the contours of the area to be treated (see Fig. 10.2). As the mesh cools, it will conform to the shape of the physical area. It can then be fitted with devices to secure it to the treatment table. Often a duplicate of the mask will be made, so the child can take it home to "play" allowing them to become familiar with the idea, texture, and "feel" of the mask, to help reduce their anxiety.

- Vacuum bag with Styrofoam beads

These vacuum bags are often used when treating the thorax or abdomen. They are normally flaccid but are shaped around the child while in the optimum position for treatment. During simulation the air is removed and the bag becomes solid providing support for the child. The bag will continue to maintain its shape aiding the reproducibility of the position for the child during each treatment session (see Fig. 10.3).

- Sedation and general anesthesia

Some children, because of young age or delayed developmental status etc., may require general anesthetic to assist immobilization throughout simulation and treatment. In recent years, the use of propofol has become the standard of anesthetic care for radiotherapy in children, because of its rapid and predictable induction of anesthesia, minimal need for airway manipulation, and rapid recovery of the patient (Anghelescu et al. 2008).

A central venous catheter is often inserted to provide access for daily anesthesia.

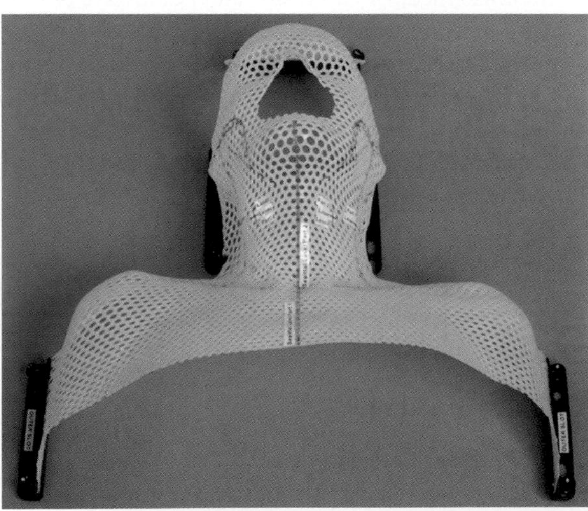

Figure 10.2
A thermoplastic shell

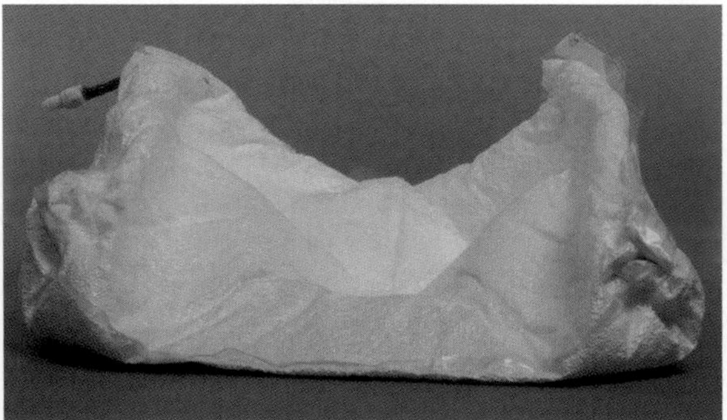

Figure 10.3
Vacuum bag with air removed to maintain shape

The services of an anesthetist/anesthesiologist or Certified Registered Nurse Anesthetist (CRNA) and support staff need to be available and the child's cardiovascular and respiratory status monitored throughout the duration of anesthesia, usually from a remote location outside the radiotherapy treatment room.

Children requiring anesthesia need to be treated early in the day to avoid prolonged daily fasting and their fluid and nutritional intake closely monitored.

On occasion when other procedures need to be carried out, such as lumbar puncture or dressing and nasogastric tube changes, these can often be arranged to be done while the child is under anesthesia to minimize anxiety and trauma for the child.

Some centers may still use sedation ranging from a mild antianxiolytic such as midazolam to conscious sedation.

10.5.2 Fractionation

Fractionation is a technique where the radiotherapy dose is given in small daily doses.

Fractionation provides better tumor control, for a given level of normal tissue toxicity, than a single large dose.

Fractionation spares the normal tissues due to:

- The repair of sub-lethal damage to the cells between fractions
- Cellular repopulation

Tumor damage is increased because of:

- Re-oxygenation of hypoxic cells.
- Re-distribution of cells within the tumor so that more of them are in the radiosensitive phases of the cell cycle (Faithfull 2008).

Hyperfractionation divides the daily dose into two or three fractions, usually with 6–8 h between treatments. Theoretically, higher doses may be given with less toxicity and greater tumor cell kill.

10.5.3 Total Body Irradiation (TBI)

TBI is used to prepare the bone marrow site for bone marrow or stem cell transplantation. It clears the bone marrow of malignant cells to allow for normal cellular growth. It may also be used to eradicate chemotherapy-resistant tissues and sanctuary sites. It has an anti-leukemic/anti-tumor effect. All organ systems are at risk of side effects as the whole body is within the radiation field.

TBI is usually given in fractionated doses twice a day for 4–5 days.

10.5.4 Brachytherapy

Brachy means "near" and this treatment is delivered using:

(a) Solid radioactive sealed sources placed near or in the tumor site or
(b) Radioactive unsealed source in fluid form given intravenously or orally

10.5.5 Sealed Sources

Sealed radioactive implants may come in the form of seeds or pellets and are placed on to or into a site near the tumor. They provide a high dose of radiation to a localized area, while causing minimal damage to normal tissue. These implants may be (a) intracavitary (as required in pelvic rhabdomyosarcoma where the radioactive source cesium-137 is contained in a small mold (Fig. 10.4) and inserted into the vagina for a prescribed period of time) or (b) interstitial and placed directly into the tissues of the target area, usually in the form of radioactive iridium wires.

This type of treatment must be delivered in a facility designed for radiation safety and where radiation protocols are strictly adhered to.

10.5.6 Unsealed Sources

Children with Stage IV neuroblastoma may require radiotherapy using an unsealed source (i.e. meta-iodobenzylguanidine (MIBG)). MIBG resembles noradrenaline and therefore localizes in andrenergic tissue. It is used for diagnostic and therapeutic purposes in a variety of neuroendocrine tumors. It is labelled with the isotope, radioiodine I-131. As there is some release of free iodide, which is normally taken up by the thyroid gland, the thyroid must be

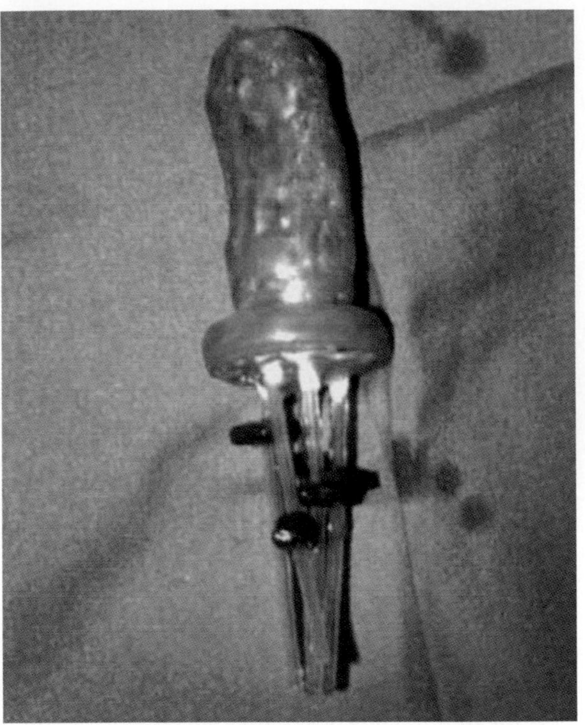

Figure 10.4
Vaginal mould containing sealed sources

protected by giving the patient potassium iodate, which effectively blocks the thyroid and is continued for 2 weeks after treatment.

This radiation treatment must be carried out in a facility designed for radiation safety, using radiation protection protocols determined by the facility. Children and their parents are encouraged to visit the facility, prior to admission date, to familiarize themselves to the area and the room where the child will spend their time following administration of the I-131 MIBG. The principles of radiation protection must be clearly explained to the parents.

The MIBG is given systemically via an intravenous central line following hydration, which is continued for 24 h. Adequate intravenous hydration is necessary to eliminate the radioactive isotope from the body as soon as possible to minimize the effect of the radiation on the other body tissues. The child will need to have vital signs monitored every 10 min throughout the process as MIBG administration may cause a dramatic increase in blood pressure.

It is safe for adults to be with the child for up to a total of 1 h/day. Where possible, there should be a distance of approximately 4 feet between the child and adult and a lead screen used as a barrier. They must also wear gloves and gowns if entering the room and carry a small dosimeter to measure any radiation dose they may receive. This will be monitored closely by radiation physics staff.

The radioiodine is excreted mainly in the urine and to a lesser degree in sweat. Therefore, all body fluids must be treated as radioactive. Local radiation protection protocols must be followed when dealing with spills and used laundry.

Other children and pregnant women should not be permitted to visit, even once the child is home, until it is clear that the radiation levels have fallen to an acceptable level. It is unlikely that these precautions will be required for more than 2 weeks.

10.6 Side Effects of Radiotherapy

The sensitivity of specific tissues to radiation will determine the side effects of the treatment.

The side effects of radiotherapy falls into two distinct groups: early or acute effects (during and within 3 months of radiotherapy) and late or delayed effects (which occur 3–12 months after radiotherapy) (Faithfull 2008).

The severity of these effects will be related to the total treatment dose and fractionation, treatment site, age of the child, and adjuvant chemotherapy.

10.6.1 Acute Effects

- General – patients receiving radiotherapy often display symptoms of tiredness and fatigue during the course of treatment and for a few weeks afterwards. Children may require more sleep and naps than usual.
- Specific – radiotherapy is a localized, targeted treatment; therefore, areas outside the treatment field should not be affected. Tissue made up of rapidly

dividing cells, such as skin and mucosa, will be affected more quickly than tissue comprising cells with a longer cell replication rate.

- Skin

Skin reaction usually starts approximately 10 days after treatment begins and may occur in three stages, including

1. Erythema – reddening of the skin that may feel warm to the touch
2. Dry desquamation – dry, flaky skin, which may be very itchy
3. Moist desquamation – flaking or peeling of the skin exposing the moist dermal layer

It is important to protect the treatment area and optimize the integrity of the skin by gentle cleansing and moisturizing the area using an emollient cream recommended by the radiotherapy staff (e.g. an aqueous preparation). Friction to the area must be avoided and loose fitting clothing in a natural fabric, such as cotton, will assist in keeping the child comfortable.

For erythema and dry desquamation, often this is all that is required. If pruritis becomes a problem, a steroid cream such as 1% hydrocortisone, used sparingly twice a day, is often helpful. If moist desquamation has occurred, the principles of moist wound healing apply. The use of hydrogels in gel or sheet form is recommended to occlude the painful area and promote wound healing (NHS QIS 2004).

- Head and Neck Area

Hair Loss – hair loss will occur 2–3 weeks after treatment starts. This may be temporary or permanent depending on the total dose of radiation. Generally, a radical course of radiotherapy given with curative intent will result in permanent hair loss while a palliative, shorter course of treatment will not. Hats and caps appropriate for the child's age and gender may be useful.

Cerebral edema – children being treated for brain tumors may show signs of raised intracranial pressure within the first week of radiotherapy as the radiation may cause some initial cerebral edema. Steroid medication may need to be carefully adjusted. Several weeks following cranial radiotherapy, some neurological changes may occur leading to somnolence syndrome. This lasts for a few days to a few weeks and is characterized by extreme sleepiness and occasionally nausea, vomiting, and headache, in fact, mimicking many of the symptoms of the original disease. Education and support is vital to the child and parents at this time.

Oral effects – every effort will be made to avoid and protect the oral cavity from the effects of radiotherapy. However, where this cannot be avoided, there may be significant issues for the child and parent. Xerostomia or dry mouth may result from the salivary glands being included within the treatment field. The reduction in the volume of saliva may lead to dental caries, taste alteration, and opportunistic infections (e.g. *Candida albicans*). Mucositis may also be a problem resulting in pain, infection, and poor oral intake. Meticulous oral care is paramount with the provision of extra fluids, antibacterial or antifungal preparations, analgesics and continuous oral assessment.

Abnormal or blunted tooth roots may develop as the child continues to grow. Careful, on-going dental care is extremely important to prevent early permanent tooth loss (McGuire Cullen et al. 2002, Byrne 2006).

- Thorax

esophagitis may occur if the esophagus lies within the treatment field. Encourage the use of dairy products to help ease the discomfort and some antacid treatments, such as ranitidine or omeprazole, may be helpful (McGuire Cullen et al. 2002).

- Abdomen and pelvis

Nausea and vomiting may be a sequelae of treatment and the use of the antiemetics (e.g. ondansetron, granesetron) can be very effective.

Diarrhea may a problem necessitating the use of a low residue diet, eliminating or reducing dairy products and increasing fluid intake. Antidiarrheal medication may be prescribed. Inspection of the perianal skin is important, and gentle, frequent cleansing of the area should be carried out and a barrier cream, e.g. zinc cream, applied. Care should be taken that the cream does not contain any metal, as this will accentuate skin reaction if radiation therapy is ongoing.

Cystitis can occur. If symptomatic (i.e. hematuria, pain on mictuition), urine samples should be taken for urinalysis and culture to confirm if there is any underlying infection. If this is confirmed, antibiotic treatment should be commenced (McGuire Cullen et al. 2002).

- Bone Marrow

Children with large areas of bone marrow in the radiation field (e.g. pelvis, long bones) may develop myelosuppression. It is important that they have full blood counts on a weekly basis and red blood cell transfusions given as appropriate (McGuire Cullen et al. 2002).

10.7 Special Considerations

10.7.1 Preparation of Children and Young People

Radiotherapy can be a frightening process. There is evidence that preparation and information is vital to reduce anxiety (Aistars 2007). It also helps to familiarize the child with the environment and new staff that will be encountered during the forthcoming weeks.

The role of the Play Specialist (i.e. child life specialist) can be vital in this preparation. Their knowledge of the radiotherapy department, equipment, and positioning for treatment helps them to assist the child in becoming familiar and comfortable with their radiotherapy experience. These professionals can also enlist the help of parents and siblings in the preparation of the child. Games such as playing "statues," once the treatment position is known, can help the child considerably to maintain their treatment position.

Visits to the radiation therapy department with their parents prior to the commencement of treatment can be arranged. This non-threatening experience may help when the child has to return to begin simulation for treatment.

10.8 Future Perspectives

10.8.1 Image-Guided Radiotherapy

Image-guided radiotherapy is a further advancement among the latest techniques available in delivering radiotherapy. As target volumes become smaller, minor movements within the tissues become important (i.e. peristalsis in the intestines, respiratory effort in the lungs). If the target area moves beyond the treatment field, the tumor will not be treated. This new technology can more accurately determine the target and if it moves out of the treatment field, it will automatically adjust once the target moves back into field again. The time taken to carry out the treatment will be increased, which may make this form of treatment impractical in a busy department (Faithfull 2008).

10.8.2 Intra-Operative Radiotherapy

Intra-operative radiotherapy (IORT) is now a potential option where radiation is delivered to the tumor site during surgery. Feasibility has been shown in a phase 1 clinical trial involving IORT and children have been carried out in children with recurrent brain tumors (Kalapurakal et al. 2006). Recently, a portable source of therapeutic X-rays has been developed allowing it to be used in the operating theater for microscopic residual disease without having to move the patient. This is currently being evaluated in the conservative treatment of breast cancer (Munro 2008). Other patient groups being treated with IORT include gastric, pancreatic, colorectal, cervical, and retroperitoneal sarcomas (Aistars 2007).

10.8.3 Proton Radiotherapy (PRT)

To attain the highest probability of cure with the least morbidity is the greatest challenge in the treatment of children with cancer. Proton radiotherapy (PRT) is the latest advancement in radiation technology and has the advantage over conventional radiotherapy because of its ability to confine high dose treatment to the tumor volume and minimize the radiation dose to the surrounding tissue. With PRT, the volume of normal tissue irradiated is dramatically reduced, thus reducing the potential for future treatment related complications. To date, there are only a few centers in the world that have the facility to treat with proton therapy. The cost to update to this new equipment may limit the availability of the new technology. However, as research reveals that PRT is shown to reduce treatment-induced complications while having improved local tumor control, proton therapy may largely replace conventional radiotherapy in pediatric oncology (Wilson et al. 2005).

References

Anghelescu DL, Burgoyne LL, Lui W, Hankins G, Cheng C, Beckham PA, Shearer J, Norris AL, Kun L, Bikhazi GB (2008) Safe sedation for radiotherapy in pediatric oncology: St. Jude children's research hospital experience, 2004–2006. International Journal of Radiation Oncology Biology Physics 71(2):491–497

Aistars J (2007) Radiation therapy. In: Langhorne ME, Fulton JS, Otto SE (eds) Oncology nursing, 5th edn. Mosby, Elsevier, St. Louis, Amsterdam, pp 346–361

Byrne B (2006) Radiotherapy. In: Alexander MF, Fawcett JN, Runciman PJ (eds) Nursing practice: hospital and home, 3rd edn. Churchill, Edinburgh, pp 1029–1052

Coyler H (2003) The context of radiotherapy care. In: Faithfull S, Wells M (eds) Supportive care in radiotherapy. Churchill Livingstone, Edinburgh, pp 1–16

Faithfull S (2008) Radiotherapy. In: Corner J, Bailey C (eds) Cancer nursing: care in context, 2nd edn. Blackwell, Oxford, pp 317–359

Kalapurakal JA, Goldman S, Stellpflug W, Curran J, Sathiaseelan V, Marymont MH, Tomita T (2006) Phase I study of intraoperative radiotherapy with photon radiosurgery system in children with recurrent brain tumors: preliminary report of first dose level (10 Gy). International Journal of Radiation Oncology Biology Physics 65(3): 800–808

McGuire Cullen P, Derrickson JD, Potter JA (2002) Radiation therapy. In: Rasco Baggott C, Patterson Kelly K, Fochtman D, Foley GV (eds) Nursing care of children and adolescents with cancer. Saunders, Philadelphia, pp 116–132

Munro A (2008) Developments in the management of cancer. In: Corner J, Bailey C (eds) Cancer nursing: care in context, 2nd edn. Blackwell, Oxford, pp 94–95

National Health Service Quality Improvement Scotland (2004) Best practice statement – skincare for patients receiving radiotherapy. http://www.nhshealthquality.org/nhsqis/files/20373%20NHSQIS%20Best%20Practice.pdf. Accessed 8 December 2008

Neal AJ, Hoskin PJ (2003) Principles of radiotherapy. In: Koster J, Rabson J (eds) Clinical oncology: basis principles and practice, 3rd edn. Arnold, London, pp 32–38

Tarbell NJ, Kooy HM (2002) General principles of radiation oncology. In: Pizzo PA, Poplack DG (eds) Principles and practice of pediatric oncology, 4th edn. Lippencott Williams & Wilkins, Philadelphia, pp 369–380

Wilson VC, McDonough J, Tochner Z (2005) Proton beam irradiation in pediatric oncology: an overview. Journal of Pediatric Hematology/Oncology 27(8):444–448

of normal tissue irradiated is dramatically reduced, thus reducing the potential for acute treatment-related complications. To date, there are only a few centers in the world that have the facility to treat with proton therapy. The cost to update to this new equipment may limit the availability of the new technology. However, as research reveals that PBT is able to reduce treatment-induced complications while having improved local tumor control ... may largely replace conventional ... pediatric oncology (Wilson et al. ...

Hematopoietic Stem Cell Transplantation

Robbie Norville • Deborah Tomlinson

Contents

11.1 Principles of Treatment . . . 243
11.2 Stem Cell Collection (Harvest) . . . 244
11.2.1 Bone Marrow Stem Cells . . . 244
11.2.2 Peripheral Blood Stem Cells . . . 246
11.2.3 Umbilical Cord Blood Stem Cells . . . 246
11.3 Donor Stem Cell Typing/Tissue Typing . . . 247
11.4 Donor Stem Cell Sources . . . 248
11.5 Stem Cell Processing and Infusion . . . 249
11.5.1 ABO Mismatch . . . 249
11.5.2 Graft vs. Leukemia . . . 251
11.6 Description of Treatment . . . 251
11.7 Potential Side Effects . . . 253
11.7.1 Early Side Effects . . . 253
11.7.1.1 Hematologic Complications . 253
11.7.1.2 Gastrointestinal Complications . . . 254
11.7.1.3 Cutaneous Complications . . . 254
11.7.1.4 Infectious Complications . . . 254
11.7.1.5 Urologic and Renal Complications . . . 255
11.7.1.6 Pulmonary Complications . . . 255
11.7.1.7 Hepatic Complications . . . 257
11.7.1.8 Nervous System Complications . . . 257
11.7.2 Intermediate Side Effects . . . 257
11.7.2.1 Infectious Complications . . . 257
11.7.2.2 Graft vs. Host Disease . . . 258
11.7.2.3 Graft Failure . . . 259
11.7.2.4 Pulmonary Complications . . . 259
11.7.3 Late Side Effects . . . 261
11.7.3.1 Immunosuppression . . . 261
11.7.3.2 Graft vs. Host Disease . . . 261
11.7.3.3 Pulmonary Complications . . . 262
11.7.3.4 Endocrine Complications . . . 262
11.7.3.5 Cataracts . . . 262
11.7.3.6 Disease Recurrence and Secondary Malignancies . . . 262
11.8 Special Considerations . . . 263
11.9 Future Perspectives . . . 264
References . . . 265

11.1 Principles of Treatment

The purpose of hematopoietic stem cell transplantation (HSCT) is to replace diseased, damaged, or absent hematopoietic stem cells (HSCs) with healthy HSCs. In general, allogeneic transplants are used when the hematopoietic stem cells are diseased (e.g., leukemia), damaged (e.g., sickle cell disease), or absent (e.g., severe immunodeficiency disease). Autologous transplants are used to provide stem cell rescue after higher doses of chemotherapy or radiation therapy, for example, in the treatment of solid tumors.

Malignant and nonmalignant diseases treated with HSCT are listed in Table 11.1.

Higher doses of chemotherapy and radiation therapy can cause dose-limiting myelosuppression. Infusing healthy stem cells allows the bone marrow (BM) to recover after intensive therapy. In the allogeneic setting, the new immune system from the donor may be effective in preventing disease recurrence by providing a graft vs. tumor effect.

HSCT is an important treatment modality for children with aggressive malignancies in first remission or those who have recurrent disease.

Types of HSCT include the following:

- Autologous: Stem cells are collected (or harvested) from the recipient, and are usually cryopreserved to be used at a later date. Autologous transplantation is a much different procedure than allogeneic transplants as the transplant is part of consolidation therapy. Autologous transplants are used more frequently for children with solid tumors [e.g., neuroblastoma, medullablastoma, sarcomas,

Table 11.1. Diseases for which HSCT is a treatment option

Disease	Rationale for HSCT
Leukemias, lymphomas	Chemotherapy, with or without total body irradiation, is used to eradicate tumor cells and to make room for engraftment of healthy cells. Irradiation is often used in mismatched and unrelated transplants
Solid tumors: neuroblastoma, sarcoma, brain tumors rhabdomyosarcoma, retinoblastoma	High doses of chemotherapy or radiation therapy are given to kill tumor cells. An autologous "rescue" is given to prevent prolonged myelosuppression
Hemoglobinopathies: thalassemia, sickle-cell disease	Chemotherapy is given to eradicate cells in the BM and to make space for engraftment of healthy allogeneic cells. The new donor cells will produce normal white cells, red cells, and platelets
Acquired marrow failure: severe aplastic anemia	As above
Congenital marrow failure: Fanconi's anemia	As above
Genetic/metabolic disorders: Hurler's syndrome	As above
Immunodeficiency diseases: Wiskott–Aldrich syndrome, severe combined immunodeficiency syndrome (SCIDS), cartilage-hair hypoplasia	Chemotherapy is given to eradicate cells in the BM and to make space for engraftment of healthy allogeneic cells. In the case of SCIDS, chemotherapy may not always be used
Genetic diseases: adrenoleukodystrophy, metachromatic leukodystrophy, Hurler's syndrome	Chemotherapy is given to eradicate cells in the BM. Donor cells, which will eventually produce the deficient enzyme, are infused

(Gratwohl et al. 2004; Meyers 2004; Dallorso et al. 2008)], when intense chemotherapy regimens are required and the child's own HSCs will not have a high risk of disease involvement.

- Allogeneic: Stem cells are collected from someone other than the recipient. A human leucocyte antigen (HLA)-matched donor is ideal for an allogeneic transplant (see Sect. 11.2.4). This procedure is more complex than autologous transplantation, and it results in greater toxicity from conditioning regimens and BM aplasia. Stem cells from a full HLA-matched sibling are generally considered to be the ideal for HSCT, with studies showing reduced graft versus host disease (GVHD) in these recipients (Ringdén et al. 2009).
- Syngeneic: This is a particular type of allogeneic transplant where stem cells are collected from a donor who is an identical twin of the recipient. This transplant is comparable with an autologous transplant.

Advantages and disadvantages of the various types of HSCT are listed in Table 11.2.

11.2 Stem Cell Collection (Harvest)

HSCs are immature progenitor cells that mature in the BM space. After differentiation and maturation, they are released into the peripheral circulation as mature erythrocytes, lymphocytes, and thrombocytes. Stem cells can be obtained from the BM, peripheral circulation, and umbilical cord blood (UCB).

11.2.1 Bone Marrow Stem Cells

The stem cells are collected directly from the BM space, with the posterior iliac crest being the most common harvest site. The collection is done in the operating room, and the donor will usually receive general anesthesia for the procedure. The cells are

Table 11.2. Comparison of the advantages and disadvantages of different types of HSCT and different donor sources

Types of HSCT	Advantages	Disadvantages
Allogenic		
Matched related	Healthy source of cells Easy access to donor Lower risk of infection Lower risk of cytomegalovirus reactivation Lower risk of mortality	Some risk of GvHD Only 30% likelihood of sibling match
Matched unrelated	Healthy source of cells	Risk of GvHD 3–6 month waiting period for donor procurement Limited ethnic minority donor Expensive donor charges
Mismatched unrelated	Healthy source of cells Easy access to donor Availability of donor for most patients	Greater risk of GvHD Risk of graft failure Reduced overall survival
Autologous	Easy access to donor No GvHD	No graft versus tumor effect Possible tumor contamination
Synergenic	Healthy source of cells	Little graft versus leukemia effect Greater risk of relpase
Donor source		
Bone marrow	Well-tested collection method	General anesthesia risks Pain at harvest site
Peripheral blood	Possible faster engraftment	Venous access Volunteer donor must receive G-CSF
Cord blood	Easy procurement of cells Decreased chance of viral transmission May be successfully performed with one or two HLA mismatches Banked CB is available within 1–2 weeks Minimal donor attrition	Limited number of cells per unit Slower engraftment leading to increased hospitalization, increased risk of viral infections Potential transmission of genetic diseases Costs for cryopreservation and storage Limited ability for donor lymphocyte infusions or retransplantation for poor graft function or graft failure

placed in a sterile collection system, mixed with heparin, and filtered to remove bone spicules, fat globules, and blood clots.

Stem cells collected from any donor source can be frozen and infused at a later time. In general, frozen stem cells are most often used for autologous transplants, as the collection will require to be carried out prior to administration of conditioning therapy. To minimize the destruction of stem cells during the freezing and thawing processes, a preservative (dimethyl sulfoxide, DMSO) is added to the stem cell product. DMSO has a garlic-like odor which is excreted from the lungs of the recipient for 24–48 h after the stem cell infusion. DMSO infusion can cause transient cardiac arrhythmias, most commonly bradycardia, and hypertension. For this reason, many institutions require cardiac monitoring during and immediately after the infusion. Once the product is thawed, a rapid intravenous (IV) infusion is recommended.

11.2.2 Peripheral Blood Stem Cells

If peripheral blood is used, the stem cells are collected by pheresis, usually in an outpatient setting (see Fig. 11.1). Temporary pheresis catheters may be placed prior to the procedure when venous access is difficult.

Stem cells are mobilized into the peripheral circulation using granulocyte colony-stimulating factor (G-CSF) or chemotherapy (for autologous HSCT). Using a pheresis machine and large venous catheters, the desired stem cells are selected and removed from the peripheral blood, based on weight. The remaining cells (red cells, platelets, and plasma) are then reinfused into the donor. The cells are placed in a sterile collection system, mixed with heparin, filtered, and mixed with a preservative prior to being cryopreserved.

Mobilized peripheral blood stem cells (PBSCs) engraft more rapidly than BM-derived stem cells. However, if a BM donor was treated with G-CSF before harvesting, as the PBSC donor would be treated before leukapheresis, the engraftment times would be comparable (Elfenbein et al. 2004). Therefore, it is considered that the mobilization of PBSCs produces more rapid engraftment (Elfenbein 2005; Chiang et al. 2007).

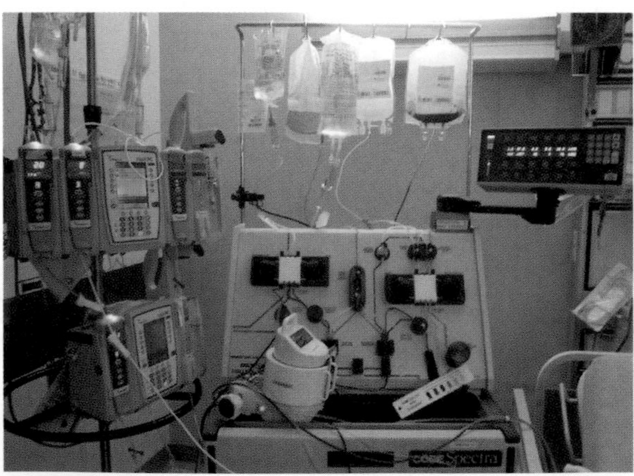

Figure 11.1
Pheresis machine that uses centrifugation to remove the fraction of blood-containing stem cells

Healthy donor volunteers of PBSCs must receive G-CSF to ensure mobilization of the stem cells. However, potential long-term effects of repeated. In addition to its known mobilizing role for peripheral blood progenitor cells, G-CSF can mobilize dendritic and endothelial progenitor cells also. It has a known activating role on neutrophil kinetics and functional status, and G-CSF administration can affect monocytes, lymphocytes, and the hemostatic system (Anderlini 2009). Clinically, G-CSF-related life-threatening adverse events (e.g. splenic rupture) remain rare. Common side effects include bone pain, fever and malaise. There have been a few reports of previously healthy volunteers who have developed hematological malignancies after receiving hematopoietic growth factors (Bennett et al. 2006; Hsia et al. 2008; Makita et al. 2004).

G-CSF effects in healthy volunteers, although normally transient and self-limiting, are now considered to be more complex than previously thought. Although G-CSF administration to healthy volunteers continues to have a favorable risk–benefit profile (Anderlini and Champlin 2008), these new findings have implications for safeguarding the safety of normal individuals. Long-term follow-up among healthy individuals who receive hematopoietic growth factors is needed (Bennett et al. 2006).

11.2.3 Umbilical Cord Blood Stem Cells

Stem cells may also be collected directly from the umbilical cord at the time of birth. These cells are then cryopreserved (frozen) and stored for use at a later time. UCB transplant has extended the availability of allogeneic HSCT to patients who would not otherwise be eligible for this curative therapy (Gluckman and Rocha 2009).

The first successful UCB transplant was carried out in 1989, in a boy with Fanconi's anemia with the

HLA-matched UCB from his sister (Gluckman et al. 1989). The first unrelated cord blood (CB) transplant was performed in 1993 (Kurtzberg et al. 1996), with the first adult to undergo UCBT in 1996 (Laporte et al. 1996). Since the first UCB transplant in 1989, more than 20,000 UCB transplants have been performed in children and in adults (Gluckman and Rocha 2009). Although acceptable as an alternative to PBSC and BM transplant, lower engraftment and delayed hematopoietic recovery with UCB transplant has been reported (Cohen and Nagler 2004). However, there are also reduced complications of graft vs. host disease (GvHD), while graft vs. leukemia (GvL) effect is preserved with UCB transplants (Kurtzberg 2009). Reduced GvHD might be explained by the lower number and slightly immature CB-derived T-cells, and the preserved GvL effect might be due to the higher numbers and unique properties of natural killer (NK) cells in the CB grafts (Stanevsky et al. 2009). The advantages and disadvantages of the different types of HSCT are listed in Table 11.2.

The umbilical cord is clamped within 1 min after delivery of the infant; a sample of CB (10–15 mL) is collected from the umbilical vein in a syringe within approximately 3 min of the delivery, or collected in a standard blood donor bag by free flow. This is transferred into a container with preservative-free heparin. A similar volume of CB may be collected after delivery of the placenta (Bornstein et al. 2005); there may however be risk of collapse of the umbilical vein. Guidelines now recommend that collection of CB should be performed after the delivery of the infant, but before delivery of the placenta, using a closed collection system and procedures that minimize the risk of bacterial and maternal fluid contamination (Armson et al. 2005). Samples may be analyzed by flow cytometry, progenitor cell assay, and examined for the presence of macroscopic clots. Removal of red blood cells from the CB may be carried out by centrifugation or by gelatin (or similar) sedimentation. Informed parental consent is obtained for the CB collection. International guidelines have been created and all aspects are detailed in the last version of the Netcord-FACT Standards (www.factwebsite.org) (Gluckman and Rocha 2009).

While public UCB banks have been established to support transplant programs, parents also have the option of storing their child's UCB in a private commercial UCB bank for personal or family use. CB donation should be encouraged for public programs, while informing parents that this may not be accessible for private use (AAP et al. 2007) and encouraged for parents of children with transplant treatable diseases. If UCB prove to be beneficial for tissue repair or replacement in the management of degenerative disorders, such as diabetes and Parkinson's disease, then a stronger case may be made in support of commercial banking of UCB for personal use. This could then have a major impact on public UCB programs (Samuel et al. 2008).

11.3 Donor Stem Cell Typing/Tissue Typing

Polymorphic proteins encoded by certain genes, found on the surface of almost every cell, are known as antigens. HLA make up the major histocompatibility complex (MHC) in humans. The major HLA antigens are essential elements in immune function by helping the body recognize foreign proteins and cells. These genes are expressed on chromosome 6, and encodes cell-surface antigen-presenting proteins and many other genes. Different classes have different functions:

HLA Class I antigens (A, B, C) present peptides which come from degraded cellular proteins (including viral peptides, if present). Foreign antigens attract killer T-cells (also called CD8-positive cells) that destroy infected cells. At least 17 Class I antigens have been identified; however, HLA-A, B, and C are of prime concern in HSCT.

HLA Class II antigens (DR, DP, DQ, DN, DO) present peptides that come from processing extracellular proteins. These particular antigens stimulate T-helper cells to reproduce, and these T-helper cells then stimulate antibody-producing B-cells. HLA-DR is the most important Class II antigen in the context of HSCT.

The full HLA complex on each chromosome are known as the "haplo-type." There are two sets of HLA antigens in each individual. Thus, a child can inherit two haplo-type combinations from the parents (Trivedi et al. 2007). An example of HLA transfer from parents to children is shown in Fig. 11.2.

They are the most important antigens when considering the human genomic variations that affect GvHD, GvL reaction, or graft rejection in the course of HSCT (Nowak 2008). HLAs are used for donor–recipient matching. The current standard of HLA typing is at A, B, C, DRBI, and DQBI genetic loci (Nowak 2008). HLA typing is carried out by polymerase chain reaction (PCR).

11.4 Donor Stem Cell Sources

Donor stem cells can be obtained from a variety of donor sources:

- Matched related donor: This is a family member, usually a sibling, with a 6/6 antigen match. This is the most optimal HSCT donor who is identical in both copies of the HLA-A, B, and DRB1 loci.This donor is available in 15–30% of patients, depending on the number of siblings (Nowak 2008). The typing of HLAs in siblings is usually not extended beyond both alleles on these three antigens, because invariably, there will be matching with the others due to the haploid transfer of genes. Low-resolution (two-digit) typing is carried out for the class 1 (A and B) antigens and high-resolution (four-digit) typing is performed for the class 2 (DRBI) antigen.
- Matched unrelated donor: This donor is one who is not genetically related to the recipient. Typing is normally carried out on five antigens using high resolution. A perfect (10/10) matched unrelated donor is available in about 30–70% of patients (Nowak 2008). Donor stem cells for HSCT recipients of nonmalignant disease will usually have four-digit typing carried out on all five HLAs, as the recipient would not benefit from any degree of GvHD (see Sect. 11.2.6).
- Mismatched donor: All the remaining patients (15–50%) thus require alternative donors with various degrees of HLA incompatability:
  - Haploidentical family donors (5 to 9/10 alleles match). One set of antigens is inherited from each parent; therefore, a biological parent will be at least a 5/10 match for a child.
  - Partially mismatched unrelated CB units (3 to 6/6 alleles matched in the A, B, and DRB1 loci).
  - Partially mismtached unrelated donors (7 to 9/10 alleles matched) (Nowak 2008).

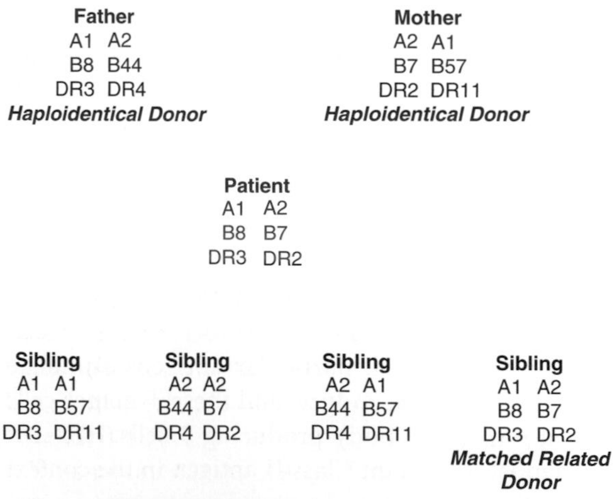

Figure 11.2
Example of HLA typing

High-resolution typing may be considered for HLA-A, B, C, DRB1, and DQ as mismatch can have adverse clinical effect on survival (Flomenberg et al. 2004; Lee et al. 2007; Tiercy et al. 2007). An 8/8 HLA-matched donor would assist in maximizing the success of an unrealted donor (Lee et al. 2007). A lack of any significant impact of DQB1 on survival means that if a mismatch is unavoidable, it may be acceptable to have a mismatch for HLA-DQB1 (Flomenberg et al. 2004). A 10/10 HLA match would remain to be the ideal.

The greater disparity that exists between the donor and the recipient, the greater is the risk of GvHD and graft failure. However, in allogeneic transplants for malignant diseases, a small degree of GvHD is often desirable to provide a GvL effect (Ringdén et al. 2009) (see Sect. 11.2.6).

When a perfectly HLA-matched donor is not available, donor stem cells with an alternative one allele/antigen mismatch (9/10) may be just as benefical as a perfectly matched stem cells. The possible use of the mismatch and the resulting outcome depends on: the potential adverse effect of the HLA mismatch; the urgency of transplantation; the type of disease to be treated; the desirable GvL effect; the child's age and gender, the cytomegalovirus (CMV) status, and the potential efficacy of the alternative treatment options for the child (Anasetti 2008; Lee et al. 2007; Nowak 2008; Rocha and Locatelli 2008; Tiercy et al. 2007; Gluckman et al. 2004). In most cases, the adverse consequences of using HLA-mismatched donor stem cells are less serious than proceeding to HSCT with more advanced disease, and this may offer better outcomes than any other treatments that are available (Lee et al. 2007).

Consideration must be given to physical and psychological support required by sibling donors, regardless of the outcome for the recipient (Macleod et al. 2003). Pain and anxiety are issues for donors of either BM or peripheral stem cells (Fortanier et al. 2002; Bredeson et al. 2004). If the HSCT is unsuccessful, the sibling may experience feelings of guilt and distress (Macleod et al. 2003; Packman et al. 2004; Wiener et al. 2007). Educational and psychosocial interventions should be provided for sibling donors.

11.5 Stem Cell Processing and Infusion

Stem cell processing can include buffy-coating to deplete volume, or erythrocyte contamination and purging to remove any remaining tumor cells. This process includes density gradient centrifugation to obtain the part of an anticoagulated blood sample after density gradient centrifugation which contains most of the white blood cells and platelets, i.e., the buffy coat. The layer that is drawn off is usually whitish in color and the technician can compare the layers with a color-coded chart to help ensure the most appropriate fraction.

T-cell depletion and CD34^{+} selection (collection of specific progenitor cells) are techniques used to reduce the number of T-lymphocytes in the final product. In vitro T-cell depletion in pediatric patients is usually reserved for those with transplants from partially matched family donors or unrelated volunteers. This is generally carried out to prevent donor-derived alloreactive T-cells contained in the graft, from attacking non-shared recipient antigens on target tissues, which causes GvHD (Locatelli and De Stefano 2005). However, major drawbacks of T-cell depletion include an enhanced risk of graft rejection and leukemia relapse, as well as delayed immune reconstitution, with a consequent increased risk of viral and fungal infections, and lymphoproliferative disorders associated with Epstein–Barr virus (Locatelli and De Stefano 2005). These complications reduce the advantage offered by T-cell depletion, and hence, a better outcome in patients given a T-cell-depleted allograft has not been consistently reported (Wagner et al. 2005; Huang et al. 2008).

Stem cell infusion is similar to a blood product transfusion, although the process may often wrongly be assumed to be comparable with organ transplant involving surgery. Stem cells are infused through a central line and should not be filtered or irradiated. The side effects associated with stem cell infusions are listed in Table 11.3.

Fresh stem cell products are most often used for allogeneic transplants, which are generally infused within 48 h of collection. The stem cell product is infused over 2–4 h, as a slow intravenous (IV) infusion. Red cell depletion or volume reduction prior to infusion is dependent on the donor and recipient's ABO status and the volume of the donor cells collected, compared to the recipient's body weight.

11.5.1 ABO Mismatch

The donor blood group may be different from that of the recipient. Delayed red cell engraftment and/or hemolysis have been documented in association with ABO incompatibility between the donor and the recipient in patients undergoing HSCT (Helming et al. 2007). In the pediatric setting, ABO major and/or minor mismatch between the donor and the recipient did not significantly influence the outcome of HSCT (Helming et al. 2007). Therefore,the choice of donor should be determined by the degree of HLA match

Table 11.3. Common side effects of hematopoietic stem cell infusions

Type of product	Side effect	Nursing assessment	Nursing interventions
Fresh stem cells	Allergic reaction	Obtain baseline vital signs (VS) and breath sounds	Premedicate with antihistamine, corticosteroid, and antipyretic
		Assess skin for evidence of flushing, itching, and urticaria	Monitor VS and breath sounds frequently during and immediately after infusion according to institutional policy
	Hemolytic transfusion reaction	Assess ABO compatibility of donor and recipient	Administer pre and post hydration fluids for ABO incompatibility
			Administer diuretic
			Maintain brisk urine output (1–2 mL/kg/h) for 24 h after infusion
			Monitor for fever, chills, chest or back pain, dark urine, dyspnea, tachycardia, hypotension, shock
	Fluid overload	Assess baseline weight and fluid status	Monitor fluid status during and immediately after infusion
		Assess baseline breath sounds and pulse oximetry	Monitor for cough, dyspnea, decreased oxygen saturation, hypertension, tachycardia, edema
			Administer diuretic
			Maintain brisk urine output (1–2 mL/kg/h) for 24 h after infusion
	Micropulmonary emboli	Assess preinfusion VS, breath sounds, and pulse oximetry	Monitor respiratory rate and pulse oximetry during infusion
			Monitor for dyspnea, decreased oxygen saturation, sudden severe headache, or chest pain
	Infection	Assess baseline VS, including temperature	Monitor temperature frequently during infusion
			Administer antipyretic for elevated temperature
			Obtain sample of product and blood sample from the patient for cultures
Preserved stem cells	Bad taste in mouth (due to DMSO)		Administer antiemetics prior to infusion
			Offer hard candy or chewing gum if patient not sedated
	Nausea and vomiting		
	Arrhythmia and hypertension	Assess baseline VS and EKG	Monitor VS and EKG during and immediately after infusion
			Administer antihypertensive and diuretic
	Hemoglobinuria		Administer pre and post hydration fluids
			Administer diuretic
			Maintain brisk urine output (1–2 mL/kg/h) for 24 h after infusion

Table 11.3. (Continued)

Type of product	Side effect	Nursing assessment	Nursing interventions
	Allergic reaction	Obtain baseline VS and breath sounds	Premedicate with antihistamine, corticosteroid and antipyretic
		Assess skin for evidence of flushing, itching, and urticaria	Monitor VS and breath sounds frequently during and immediately after infusion according to institutional policy
	Fluid overload	Assess baseline weight and fluid status	Monitor fluid status during and immediately after infusion
		Assess baseline breath sounds and pulse oximetry	Monitor for cough, dyspnea, decreased oxygen saturation, hypertension, tachycardia, edema
			Administer diuretic
			Maintain brisk urine output (1–2 mL/kg/h) for 24 h after infusion
	Micropulmonary emboli	Assess preinfusion VS, breath sounds, and pulse oximetry	Monitor respiratory rate and pulse oximetry during infusion
			Monitor for dyspnea, decreased oxygen saturation, sudden severe headache, or chest pain
	Infection	Assess baseline VS, including temperature	Monitor temperature frequently during infusion
			Obtain sample of product and blood sample from the patient for cultures
			Administer antipyretic for elevated temperature

and CMV status in preference to the ABO blood group compatibility (Helming et al. 2007). However, acute renal failure due to hemolysis is a risk.

Note: The donor blood group will change to the recipient blood group. Parents and child (if appropriate) must be made aware that this conversion will occur.

11.5.2 Graft vs. Leukemia

Patients with GvHD, especially chronic GvHD, have a lower risk of relapse compared with patients without GvHD (Ringdén et al. 2009). Allogeneic lymphocytes can produce a strong GvL effect, but this beneficial effect is limited by GvHD. Furthermore, identical twins undergoing HSCT run a higher risk of relapse than recipients of grafts from HLA-identical sibling donors. This increased risk of relapse is due to lack of GVL because there is less disparity between recipient and donor. T-cell depletion of stem cell grafts, which may effectively prevent severe GvHD, can decrease any GvL effect, which increases the risk of relapse (Ringdén et al. 2009).More effective immunosuppression, for instance, by combining cyclosporine and methotrexate, may be more effective than monotherapy to prevent GvHD (Ringdén et al. 2009).

Delayed transfusion of donor lymphocytes after T cell-depleted stem cell transplantation produces a GvL effect without necessarily producing GvHD (Kolb 2008; Pérez et al. 2008).

11.6 Description of Treatment

HSCT can be divided into three phases:

- Pretransplant: The pretransplant phase includes donor and recipient evaluation, and administration of a conditioning regimen (chemotherapy agents selected for specific activity).

- Transplant: Day 0, the day of stem cell infusion, constitutes the transplant phase. Donor stem cells collected on this day are administered as a fresh product infusion. Donor cells collected prior to the initiation of conditioning are cryopreserved for infusion on Day 0.
- Post transplant/engraftment: During the post transplant or engraftment phase, the recipient is monitored for side effects of the conditioning regimen, complications of the transplant, and engraftment, which is the term used to indicate that the donor cells have migrated to and are repopulating the BM space.

Pretransplant evaluation of the donor assures healthy stem cells and a donor who is able to tolerate the collection procedure. The age range of donors varies from infancy (3–4 months) to 65 years. The donor evaluation should include physical examination, complete health history for genetic disorders, and serological testing that includes CBC with differential, confirmatory HLA typing, ABO cross-matching, chemistry profile, coagulation screen, infectious disease testing, and a pregnancy test (if appropriate). Donors may be offered an opportunity to donate, if needed, an autologous unit of blood prior to collection of stem cells for autotransfusion.

The donor should have an opportunity to discuss issues such as testing procedures, health risks, and psychosocial sequelae with appropriate healthcare providers. These issues are especially important in the case of child donors. Consultation with child-life specialists, social workers, and clergy may be beneficial and make the procedure less stressful and easier to tolerate.

The purpose of the recipient evaluation is to determine the disease status and identify any underlying medical issues, such as organ dysfunction or infections that could pose additional risks to the recipient. The recipient will have a more extensive evaluation than the donor. In addition to the studies listed earlier, the evaluation should include an assessment of the recipient's disease status, which will depend on the type of disease and the areas of previous involvement or treatment. These studies may include diagnostic scans (e.g., CT, MRI) as well as BM aspirate/biopsy and lumbar puncture. Studies useful in evaluating organ dysfunction include chest X-ray, echocardiogram, pulmonary function tests (PFTs) (if age-appropriate), creatinine clearance or glomerular filtration rate, and dental examination. An audiogram may be ordered for patients who have a history of hearing loss or have previously received ototoxic agents. An ophthalmology examination may be done if the recipient is to receive total body irradiation (TBI).

Baseline monitoring for late effects might include baseline neuropsychological testing, endocrine function studies, and bone scans. A central venous access device will be placed, and information regarding sperm banking and egg harvesting should be provided to age-appropriate patients.

Conditioning (preparative) regimens are used to:

- Prepare the BM space for the incoming graft
- Immunosuppress the recipient to prevent GvHD
- Eradicate tumor cells when treating a malignant disease

In general, the conditioning regimen is given for 4–10 days prior to the stem cell infusion. The conditioning regimen selection depends on the disease being treated and the type of HSCT. Conditioning regimens can include chemotherapy, radiation therapy, and immunotherapy. Chemotherapy is the primary component of the conditioning regimen and is used for most HSCT.

The commonly used agents include cyclophosphamide, busulfan, cytarabine, melphalan, thiotepa, cisplatin, carboplatin, and etoposide. Radiation therapy in the form of TBI provides immunosuppression as well as treatment for sanctuary sites (central nervous system and testes). TBI is usually delivered in fractionated doses twice a day for 4–5 days. Local control radiation therapy may be given before or after transplant to patients with a history of central nervous system disease. Immunotherapy includes agents such as antithymocyte globulin (ATG) and monoclonal antibodies, such as alemtuzumab (Campath) and anti CD45 antibody. These agents are usually given once a day for 3–4 days and are used to bind with and destroy recipient circulating T-lymphocytes in an attempt to decrease the risk of nonengraftment and GvHD, or relapse (Shah et al. 2007).

11.7 Potential Side Effects

Side effects and complications associated with HSCT can occur at any time during the transplant process (Table 11.4). The side effects commonly associated with the conditioning regimen and time period to engraftment tend to occur early, within the first few weeks of transplant. Intermediate side effects that occur from the time of engraftment and during the first 100 days thereafter, usually result from the conditioning regimen, prolonged immunosuppression, or early engraftment. Complications occurring 100 days or more after transplant are categorized as late effects.

11.7.1 Early Side Effects

Early side effects of the conditioning regimen can include BM suppression, nausea, vomiting, diarrhea, anorexia, mucositis, parotitis, skin erythema, infections, capillary leak syndrome, diffuse alveolar hemorrhage, engraftment syndrome (ES), acute renal insufficiency, sinusoidal obstructive syndrome, and seizures.

11.7.1.1 Hematologic Complications

BM suppression typically occurs 7–10 days after the conditioning regimen begins. Fully ablative conditioning regimens will eradicate all cell lines in the BM, causing anemia, thrombocytopenia, and neutropenia, with an absolute neutrophil count (ANC) of 0. BM suppression is prolonged and will continue until engraftment occurs. The timing of engraftment is affected by the conditioning regimen administered, the stem cell source, manipulation of the cells, the recipient's past history of prior chemotherapy, and the recipient's clinical condition. An ANC of 500/mm^3 for 3 consecutive days and a platelet count of 20,000 mm^2 without transfusions indicate engraftment. The average time to engraftment is, in general, 14–28 days. Typically, platelets are the last cell line to become self-sustaining. As red cells engraft, the recipient's blood type will change to that of the donor when ABO differences are present.

Table 11.4. Timing of potential complications associated with HSCT (adapted from Norville 2008)

Early (conditioning to engraftment)	Intermediate (engraftment to first 100 days)	Late (after 100 days)
BM suppression	Infections	Immunosuppression
Nausea, vomiting, diarrhea, anorexia, mucositis	Acute GvHD (AGvHD)	Chronic GvHD
Parotitis	Graft failure	Infections
Infections	Idiopathic pneumonia syndrome	Bronchiolitis obliterans
Skin erythema	Pulmonary veno-occlusive disease	Endocrine dysfunction
Capillary leak syndrome	Bronchiolitis obliterans-organizing pneumonia	Cataracts
Diffuse alveolar hemorrhage		Disease recurrence
Engraftment syndrome		Secondary malignancies
Acute renal insufficiency		
Hemorrhagic cystitis		
Sinusoidal obstructive syndrome		
Seizures		

Transfusions of leukocyte-depleted and irradiated red blood cells are often administered when hemoglobin levels fall below 8 g/dL. Leukocyte depletion minimizes the risk of viral contamination, particularly, CMV. Irradiation reduces the risk of GvHD from the transfused blood products by rendering the immunocompetent lymphocytes in the product inactive, without compromising the functional qualities of the red cells. There is a potential for cardiac and respiratory compromise associated with hemoglobin levels less than 7 g/dL.

The side effects of anemia include fatigue, irritability, pallor, tachycardia, shortness of breath (SOB), and dizziness. The administration of blood products or supplemental oxygen may be required. During transfusion, one should monitor for signs and symptoms of adverse effects (Chap. 19).

The risk of bleeding is increased when the platelet count is less than 20,000 mm^2. The nurses must assess for signs and symptoms of bleeding or blood loss, including bruising, petechiae, epistaxis, or oozing from the gums or central venous line. If transfusion is required, platelet products should be leukocyte-depleted and irradiated.

When the ANC falls below $500/mm^3$, the patients are at a significantly increased risk of infection. Physical examination should include detailed inspection of the mouth, perirectal area, IV sites, and all wounds for evidence of infection. Symptoms including dysuria, sore throat, cough, and rectal pain are particularly worrisome in the neutropenic patient (Chap. 19).

11.7.1.2 Gastrointestinal Complications

Gastrointestinal (GI) complications in the form of nausea and vomiting can begin within the first 24 h of starting the conditioning regimen, and can continue for several days after the transplant. Antibiotics, infections, and mucositis can exacerbate vomiting. Diarrhea can occur anytime during the conditioning regimen and can last as long as 2 weeks after the transplant. Although chemotherapy is the usual cause of diarrhea during this time period, an infectious cause must be excluded. Mucositis usually peaks 7–14 days after the start of the conditioning regimen and resolves as engraftment (return of white blood cells) occurs. Anorexia often accompanies nausea, vomiting, diarrhea, and mucositis, and can continue for several months after the transplant, especially in adolescent and young adult patients (Chap. 18).

Supportive care for GI symptoms includes administering antiemetics on a scheduled basis, as well as nutritional supplements, fluids, and total parenteral nutrition. Meticulous oral hygiene, perirectal hygiene, and skin care to prevent skin breakdown and secondary infections are necessary. Blood and stool cultures may be needed to isolate infectious agents. Pain assessment must be performed during each shift, and more often if the child is experiencing pain. Oral or IV analgesics, preferably patient-controlled analgesia, may be required for mucositis pain.

Parotitis, or inflammation of the parotid gland, usually occurs after the first or second dose of TBI. Common complaints are bilateral swelling and pain in the jaws. This side effect is self-limited, often lasting only a day or two. Applying warm compresses externally to the jaw and administering mild analgesics will usually provide relief.

11.7.1.3 Cutaneous Complications

Skin erythema, darkening, and dryness is not uncommon after TBI. This condition is most often mild and typically responds to moisturizing lotions, creams, and gels. A head-to-toe skin assessment is required daily. To prevent additional skin damage, patients need to be instructed not to use oil-based skin products while receiving TBI (Chap. 25).

11.7.1.4 Infectious Complications

Infections during the early phase of transplant are a result of neutropenia, immunosuppression, and alterations in mucosal integrity and indwelling central lines. Patients are susceptible to bacterial, viral, and fungal infections. Common bacterial pathogens are *E. coli*, *Klebsiella*, *Pseudomonas*, *Staphylococcus aureus*, and coagulase-negative *Staphylococcus*. Reactivation of herpes simplex virus (HSV) is the predominant viral pathogen complicating mucositis during this time period. *Candida* spp. can infect the GI tract, complicate toxicities, and secondarily infect other wounds and IV sites.

Prevention of infections is multifactorial and includes handwashing, limits on the number of visitors, high-energy particulate air (HEPA) filter systems, prophylactic antimicrobials, and administration of CMV-negative blood products to CMV-seronegative recipients. A combination of broad-spectrum antibiotics is given from initiation of the conditioning regimen until engraftment as the common prophylaxis against bacterial infections. Acyclovir or valacyclovir prophylaxis can reduce the risk of HSV reactivation. Fluconazole, voriconazole, or low-dose amphotericin is considered to be an effective prophylaxis against fungal infections. Although benefits are controversial, intravenous immunoglobulin (IVIG) therapy may be administered every 2–4 weeks to provide passive immunity (Raanani et al. 2009).

Other interventions include monitoring the patient for fever and other signs of infection, obtaining blood and urine cultures at the onset of fever before starting antibiotics, drawing blood cultures daily for subsequent fevers, and obtaining other diagnostic studies (e.g., chest X-ray, CT) as appropriate. Patients who continue to be febrile after 3–5 days should receive treatment doses of amphotericin.

11.7.1.5 Urologic and Renal Complications

Hemorrhagic cystitis can occur within 24 h of administration of chemotherapy and as late as several months after HSCT (Leung et al. 2002). The primary causes of hemorrhagic cystitis include cyclophosphamide, radiation therapy, and viruses. The active metabolite of cyclophosphamide, when allowed to remain in contact with the bladder mucosa, will cause irritation and bleeding. Viruses that can cause this complication include adenovirus, CMV, and BK virus. Signs and symptoms of hemorrhagic cystitis include hematuria (microscopic or gross), urinary frequency, dysuria, suprapubic pain, and bladder spasms. A bladder ultrasound and urine cultures for bacteria and viruses are used for the diagnosis. Management includes pre and post hydration fluids, and mesna for cyclophosphamide administration, placement of a Foley catheter with or without continuous bladder irrigation, as well as platelet transfusions. If a urinary catheter has not been placed, the child must void at least every 1–2 h during, and for 24 h after, each dose of cyclophosphamide. Strict measuring of intake and output must be done, in addition to platelet counts, coagulation studies, and close monitoring for microscopic hematuria. Administering blood products and providing pain control are other necessary supportive care measures (Chap. 21).

Acute renal failure and nephritis are frequent complications after HSCT. Radiation therapy, immunosuppressive agents, and virus and bacterial toxins can cause nephritis. Acute renal failure can result from nephrotoxic drugs, infection, and inadequate renal perfusion. Common symptoms of renal toxicity include increased weight, edema, decreased urine output, hypertension, elevated creatinine and blood urea nitrogen (BUN), and altered sensorium.

Medical management includes administration of diuretics, antihypertensives, vasopressors, and dialysis. Blood chemistries need to be monitored daily, and blood levels of nephrotoxic medications (e.g., cyclosporine, tacrolimus, vancomycin, gentamicin) must be checked frequently until the appropriate dose level is reached, and then routinely monitored. Dose and frequency of nephrotoxic medications need to be adjusted as ordered, and renal doses of dopamine are given to promote renal perfusion.

11.7.1.6 Pulmonary Complications

Noninfectious pulmonary complications are responsible for an increasing percentage of complications and morbidity in pediatric HSCT patients. The symptoms of many of these complications mimic infectious processes; consequently, astute clinical assessment and accurate diagnosis is essential. Table 11.5 provides a comparison of pulmonary complications. Capillary leak syndrome, a shift of intravascular fluid into the extravascular space, often occurs 7–14 days after HSCT. Tissue damage from the conditioning regimen causes the release of cytokines that cause a capillary permeability. This permeability can lead

Table 11.5. Pulmonary complications associated with HSCT

	DAH	ES	IPS	PVOD	BOOP	BO
Definition	Progressively bloodier BAL	Clinical entity of fever, rash, diffuse pulmonary infiltrates, and generalized noncardiogenic capillary leak	Alveolar injury without infection	Pulmonary venules and small vein fibrosis, vascular obstruction	Restrictive lung disease without infectious cause	Obstructive lung disease without infectious cause
Incidence	5%	7–11%	6–8%	Rare	Unknown	2–20%
Risk actors	TBI, presence of high fever, severe mucositis, renal insufficiency	Allogeneic HSCT	High-intensity conditioning regimen, GvHD		GvHD	GvHD
Etiology	Conditioning regimen, RT, occult infection	Release of proinflammatory cytokines	Chemoradiation damage, occult CMV infection, GvHD	Chemotherapy, radiation therapy, viral infections	Multifactorial	Immune-mediated process; direct attack of bronchiolar epithelium by T-lymphocytes
Diagnosis	BAL	Clinical assessment	BAL	Right-heart catheterization, angiography	Surgical lung biopsy	Surgical lung biopsy; PFT
Histology	Diffuse alveolar damage		Interstitial pneumonia, diffuse alveolar damage	Increased pulmonary artery pressures with normal artery wedge pressures	Granulation tissue plugs filling lumen of distal airways; chronic interstitial inflammation	Fibrous obliteration of lumen of respiratory & membranous bronchioles
Clinical features	Dyspnea, fever, cough, hemoptysis	Fever, cough, SOB	Dyspnea, fever, cough, increasing oxygen requirement	Dyspnea, fatigue, hypoxemia, resting tachycardia	Dyspnea, fever, nonproductive cough	Cough, dyspnea, SOB, wheezing
Treatment	Mechanical ventilation, corticosteroids	Corticosteroids	Corticosteroids, TNF	Corticosteroids	Corticosteroids	Corticosteroids, immunosuppressive agents

DAH diffuse alveolar hemorrhage; *ES* engraftment syndrome; *IPS* idiopathic pneumonia syndrome; *PVOD* pulmonary veno-occlusive disease; *BOOP* bronchiolitis obliterans-organizing pneumonia; *BO* bronchiolitis obliterans; *TBI* total body irradiation; *RT* radiation therapy; *BAL* bronchoalveolar lavage; *SOB* shortness of breath; *GvHD* graft vs. host disease; *TNF* tumor necrosis factor; *PFT* pulmonary function tests

to weight gain, fluid retention, ascites, cough, SOB, and pulmonary edema. The child must be assessed for signs and symptoms of fluid overload, including weight gain, hypertension, abnormal breath sounds, and intake that is greater than output.

Diffuse alveolar hemorrage (DAH) is a syndrome of progressively bloodier return from a broncho-alveolar lavage (BAL), and has an incidence of 5% after stem cell transplant. Risk factors include older patients, TBI-based conditioning regimens, and presence of high fevers, severe mucositis, and renal insufficiency. Conditioning regimen, radiation therapy, and occult infections are the causes of DAH. Clincial symptoms include dyspnea, fever, cough, and hemoptysis. Treatment includes mechanical ventilation and corticosteroids (Watkins et al. 2005; Gower et al. 2006). Patients should be assessed for tachypnea, tachycardia, SOB, oxygen saturation, and decreased hemoglobin levels.

ES is a clinical entity comprising fever, erythrodermatous skin rash, diffuse pulmonary infiltrates, and generalized noncardiogenic capillary leak syndrome. This pulmonary complication typically occurs around the time of neutrophil recovery with an incidence of approximately 7–11%. The increased capillary permeability of ES is thought to be secondary to the release of proinflammatory cytokines during engraftment.Treament includes supportive care and corticosteriods (Watkins et al. 2005; Gower et al. 2006). The nurse should assess the child for fever, rash, dyspnea, and oxygen saturation.

11.7.1.7 Hepatic Complications

Sinusoidal obstructive syndrome, previously called veno-occlusive disease (VOD), is caused by endothelial damage to the hepatic sinusoids and small hepatic venules from high-dose chemotherapy and radiation therapy administered during the conditioning regimen. The small vessels and central vein of the liver become occluded, causing congestion, venous outflow obstruction, and eventual hepatocyte damage. The onset is usually within the first 30 days after transplant. The clinical features of sinusoidal obstructive syndrome include weight gain, right upper quadrant pain, hepatomegaly, elevated serum bilirubin, ascites, and encephalopathy. Management includes maintaining fluid and electrolyte balance by strictly monitoring intake and output, obtaining accurate daily weights and measuring abdominal girth every shift, minimizing the adverse effects of ascites by restricting oral and IV fluids and administering diuretics and pain medications, adjusting medications to reflect hepatic and renal function, avoiding compounding encephalopathy with medications that alter mental status, and preventing bleeding.

11.7.1.8 Nervous System Complications

Neurotoxicity can occur anytime during the transplant process. Seizures can result from medication toxicity, infection, hemorrhage, hypertension, and electrolyte abnormalities. In the early phase of transplant, high levels of chemotherapeutic agents (busulfan) and immunosuppressive agents (cyclosporine, tacrolimus) can cause seizures. Cyclosporine and tacrolimus can also cause tremors and peripheral neuropathy. Monitoring blood levels and adjusting doses can prevent and minimize these side effects.

11.7.2 Intermediate Side Effects

Intermediate side effects and complications of HSCT can include infections, graft failure, acute GvHD (AGvHD), idiopathic pneumonia syndrome (IPS), pulmonary VOD, and bronchiolitis obliterans-organizing pneumonia (BOOP).

11.7.2.1 Infectious Complications

Infections during this phase are more common and more severe for allogencic patients than autologous patients, as a result of impaired cell-mediated and humoral immunity, immunosuppressive therapy to prevent GvHD, and the presence of indwelling lines. Common pathogens include gram-negative bacteria (*E. coli*, *Klebsiella*, *Pseudomonas*, *Enterobacter*), gram-positive bacteria (*Staphylococcus aureus*, coagulase-negative *Staphylococcus, Streptococcus pneumoniae*), fungus (*Candida, Aspergillus*), and viruses (adenovirus, CMV).

Predisposing factors associated with infections during this period include neutropenia, central venous lines, immunosuppressive therapy, and GvHD. Strategies to prevent or minimize the risk of infections include handwashing, HEPA filtration, low-bacterial diets, avoidance of crowded places, and antibacterial, antifungal, and antiviral prophylaxis. Antibacterial and antifungal (fluconazole, low-dose amphotericin B) prophylaxis continues until engraftment (defined as an ANC >500/mm^3 for3 consecutive days).

CMV infection is a life-threatening infection that usually occurs within the first 2 months post transplantation. Most centers will provide some form of prophylaxis when the recipient or donor is CMV-seropositive before transplantation, either administering ganciclovir IV from engraftment through 100 days post transplantation, or CMV antigenemia monitored with ganciclovir treatment when the virus is detected. Additional strategies to prevent CMV infection include administration of leukocyte-depleted blood products and CMV-seronegative blood products to seronegative recipients. IVIG may also be given to provide passive immunity during this phase of HSCT.

Treatment of infections is aimed at the specific pathogens causing infections. Initial treatment usually includes broad-spectrum antibiotics, followed by specific antimicrobials based on culture and sensitivity results. Treatment of CMV infection can include ganciclovir and IVIG, foscarnet, and cidofovir.

11.7.2.2 Graft vs. Host Disease

AGvHD is an immune-mediated response in which the immunocompetent donor T-cells recognize the host (recipient) antigens as foreign and mount an attack. It is the consequence of alloreactivity between the donor and recipient. The immunocompetent donor T-cells recognize the alloantigens (major and minor histocompatibility antigens) of the recipient and become activated, which leads to further expansion of alloreactive T-cells. This leads to the release of cytokines, recruitment of other immune system effector cells, and eventual tissue damage (Goker et al. 2001).

Incidence and severity depend on the type of transplant and the degree of HLA disparity between the donor and recipient. The recipient's age, the number of T-cells transfused, and the GvHD prophylaxis used are additional risk factors. The onset of AGvHD usually coincides with engraftment and occurs within the first 100 days of transplantation.

Clinical presentation typically involves one of three targeted organs: the skin, liver, or gut. Diagnosis can be made clinically based on the symptoms and laboratory values. However, tissue biopsy is required for definitive diagnosis. Individual organ involvement is staged for severity, and an overall grade is assigned based on severity and combined organ involvement. Skin AGvHD is the most common initial presenting manifestation (Chap. 25). The rash begins as a macular erythematous rash of the palms and soles. It can progress to a maculopapular erythematous rash on the trunk and extremities to bullae and generalized desquamation. Pruritus and pain are common associated symptoms (Table 11.6).

Liver AGvHD causes degeneration of mucosa and small bile ducts and results in hepatitis-like symptoms (fatigue, abnormal liver function tests, right upper quadrant pain, hepatomegaly, jaundice, and pruritus). Increased bilirubin and alkaline phosphatase levels are the earliest and most common abnormalities noted.

GI AGvHD is characterized by diarrhea and abdominal cramping, which can progress to severe ileus. Degeneration of the mucosal lining of the GI tract results in green, watery, guaiac-positive diarrhea, abdominal discomfort, nausea, vomiting, anorexia, malabsorption, and ascites. Both the upper and lower GI tract can be involved.

Prevention remains the key to effective management of AGvHD. Prevention strategies are aimed at preventing the activation of T-cells and depleting mature alloreactive T-cells from donor grafts. Cyclosporine, used in combination with other immunosuppressive agents, has been the standard GvHD prophylaxis; however, tacrolimus is being used instead of cyclosporine for unrelated and mismatched transplants because it has proven to be superior to cyclosporine in this group of patients. New monoclonal antibodies, such as alemtuzumab (Campath)

Table 11.6. AGvHD stage and grading systems

Staging of individual organ system(s)		
Organ	**Stage**	**Description**
Skin	+1	Maculopapular (M-P) eruption over <25% of body area
	+2	Maculopapular eruption over 25–50% of body area
	+3	Generalized erythroderma
	+4	Generalized erythroderma with bullous formation and often with desquamation
Liver	+1	Bilirubin, 2.0–3.0 mg/dL; SGOT, 150–750 IU
	+2	Bilirubin, 3.1–6.0 mg/dL
	+3	Bilirubin, 6.1–15.0 mg/dL
	+4	Bilirubin, >15.0 mg/dL
Gut	+1	Diarrhea, >30 mL/kg or >500 mL/day
	+2	Diarrhea, >60 mL/kg or >1,000 mL/day
	+3	Diarrhea, >90 mL/kg or >1,500 mL/day
	+4	Diarrhea, >90 mL/kg or >2,000 mL/day; or severe abdominal pain and bleeding with or without ileus

Overall grading of AGvHD				
Grade	**Skin staging**	**Liver staging**		**Gut staging**
I	+1 to +2	0		0
II	+1 to +3	+1	And/or	+1
III	+2 to +3	+2 to +4	And/or	+2 to +3
IV	+2 to +4	+2 to +4	And/or	+2 to +4

and anti CD45 antibody, are being incorporated into conditioning regimens as GvHD prophylaxis. T-cell depletion, monoclonal antibodies, and $CD34^+$ selection are successful strategies to deplete alloreactive T-cells from donor grafts.

Treatment consists of adding corticosteroids and continuing cyclosporine or tacrolimus (Table 11.7). ATG and newer monoclonal antibodies are added in cases of steroid-resistant or severe AGvHD.

11.7.2.3 Graft Failure

Graft failure or rejection occurs when the donor graft is not sustained in the recipient. This complication is relatively uncommon after fully ablative allogeneic HSCT, with an incidence of approximately 1% with HLA-matched sibling donors and 5% with mismatched donors (Bollard et al. 2006). Graft failure can occur when the stem cell dose is too low, the recipient marrow is not completely ablated, or the immunosuppression is inadequate. Infections and tumor recurrence can also cause graft failure. Treatment may include increased immunosuppression or infusion of donor T-lymphocytes.

11.7.2.4 Pulmonary Complications

IPS is a clinical syndrome described as widespread alveolar injury in the absence of active lower

Table 11.7. Agents used to prevent and treat

	Mechanism	Toxicities
Cyclosporine (Sandimmune)	Blocks synthesis of IL-2, suppresses development of cytotoxic T-lymphocytes	Renal toxicity, hypertension, magnesium wasting, hyperkalemia, tremors, seizures, gingival hypertrophy, hirsutism, cortical blindness
FK506 (Prograf)	Is similar to cyclosporine	Are similar to those associated with cyclosporine, hyperglycemia
Methotrexate (Mexate)	Inhibits DNA synthesis by competitively binding with dihydrofolate reductase	Renal toxicity, liver toxicity, mucositis
Glucocorticoids	Prevents production and release of IL-1 from macrophages	Myelosuppression, mood swings, hypertension, hyperglycemia, GI bleeding, osteoporosis, acne, cushingoid syndrome
Antithymocyte globulin (ATG) (an immune globulin)	Acts against human thymocytes	Fever, chills, rash, anaphylaxis, serum sickness
OKT3 (Orthoclone) (a monoclonal antibody)	Is specific for circulating CD3 T-cells	First-dose reaction: fever, chills, diarrhea, dizziness, chest pain, wheezing, tremor
Thalidomide	Decreases the number of helper T-cells and increases the number of suppressor T-cells	Peripheral neuropathies, constipation, sedation
Hydroxychloroquine (Plaquenil)	Reduces secretion of IL-1, IL-6, and tumor necrosis factor	Ocular toxicity, nausea, diarrhea, rash, photosensitivity

respiratory tract infection. Previously known as idiopathic interstital pneumonia, it is the leading cause of respiratory failure in HSCT patients; IPS often follows engraftment, strongly suggesting an immunologic response involved in the process. The incidence is approximately 6–8% after HSCT. Risk factors and etiology include high-intensity conditioning regimens, GvHD, and occult infection. Clinical features of IPS are dyspnea, fever, nonproductive cough, and an increasing oxygen requirement. Chest X-ray indicates diffuse infiltrates and the BAL reveals difuse alveolar injury without infection. The mortality rate for this complication is extremely high despite aggressive treatment with antimicrobials, blood products, steroids, and ventilatory support. There are limited reports suggesting that tumor necrosis factor may be useful in addition to standard immunosuppression (Michelson et al. 2007; Gower et al. 2006).

Although rare, pulmonary veno-occlusive disease (PVOD) is almost always a fatal complication. It usually presents with an incidious onset of dyspnea, fatique, cardiomegaly, pulmonary hypertension, and pulmonary infiltrates on chest X-ray. PVOD typically occurs 3–4 months after transplant and has been associated with hepatic sinusodial obstructive syndrome. The etiology is unclear but may be related to the pretransplant conditioning regimens. PVOD is characterized by fibrosis of the pulmonary venules and small veins which leads to progressive vascular obstruction and increased pulmonary and capillary pressures. Right-heart catheterization and angiography show elevated pulmonary artery pressures with normal pulmonary artery wedge pressures. Again, the etiolgy is thought to be chemotherapy, radiation therapy, and viral infections. Treatment is supportive and responses to high-dose corticosteroids and defibrotide have been reported (Michelson et al. 2007; Gower et al. 2006).

BOOP is defined as a restrictive lung disease after HSCT, in the absence of an infectious cause. GvHD has been reported as a risk factor and the etiology is multifactorial. The clinical manifestations include dyspnea, fever, and nonproductive cough. Chest X-ray often shows an alveolar or nodular pattern; whereas, chest CT reveals nodular, patchy infiltrates bilaterally. A surgical lung biopsy is required for definitive diagnosis. Tissue histology demonstrates granulated tissue plugs filling the distal airway lumen in a patchy distribution along with chronic interstitial inflammation. The treatment consists of supportive care, steroids, and antimicrobials (Gower et al. 2006).

Astute nursing assessment of the child's respiratory status and prompt treatment of symptoms and supportive care is essential to minimize symptoms, promote comfort, and accurately treat these critical pulmonary complications.

11.7.3 Late Side Effects

Late side effects and complications can include immunosuppression and infections, chronic GvHD, bronchiolitis obliterans, endocrine dysfunction, cataracts, disease recurrence, and secondary malignancies.

11.7.3.1 Immunosuppression

Immunosuppression and infections remain a risk during this time, despite neutrophil engraftment. Both cellular and humoral immunity remain depressed until full immune reconstitution occurs. This delayed immune recovery can lead to acute and chronic infections and nutritional deficits. Several factors contribute to this protracted impaired immunity: patient and donor age, conditioning regimen used, degree of HLA disparity between the donor and the recipient, presence of GvHD, presence of infection, and type of post transplant immunosuppression used (Chap. 19)

Common post transplant infections include *Pneumocystis jiroveci* (formerly called *Pneumocystis carinii*), varicella-zoster, CMV, adenovirus, and Epstein–Barr virus lymphoproliferative disease. Management includes *Pneumocystis jiroveci* prophylaxis for 1 year post transplant (Table 11.8) and frequent monitoring for evidence of infections and immune recovery.

11.7.3.2 Graft vs. Host Disease

Chronic GvHD (CGvHD) is a chronic autoimmune syndrome that resembles collagen vascular diseases, such as scleroderma and systemic lupus erythematosus. The primary effect of CGvHD is the epithelial cell damage to tissue that can lead to fibrosis and atrophy. CGvHD targets the same organs as AGvHD – the skin, liver, and gut – however, it may affect others as well, such as the eyes and lungs. The secondary effect of marked immunosuppression has a significant impact on morbidity and mortality post transplant.

The risk factors for CGvHD include prior AGvHD, donor and recipient HLA disparity, and increasing patient age. The decreased incidence over the last decade can be attributed to improved HLA matching and effective AGvHD prevention. CGvHD can occur as the progression of AGvHD, follow a period of quiescence after AGvHD, or occur as a de novo disease. Historically, GvHD that occurs 100 days after transplant is considered chronic. The increased

Table 11.8. Prophylaxis for PCP

Age	Primary recommendation	Second
Infants (1–12 months)	[a]TMP-SMZ (150/750 mg/m^2) orally, twice daily for 3 consecutive days	Dapsone (infants >1 month) 2 mg/kg, orally, daily
Children (>12 months)	TMP-SMZ (150/750 mg/m^2) orally, twice daily for 3 consecutive days	Dapsone 2 mg/kg, orally, daily, maximum of 100 mg, orally, daily
Adolescents	TPM-SMZ (160/800 mg) orally, three times a week	Dapsone 100 mg, orally, daily

[a] Prophylaxis – sulfomethoxazole/trimethoprim/co-trimoxazole

use of donor T-lymphocytes in the post transplant period requires careful assessment and diagnosis of GvHD symptoms.

Clinical presentation is remarkable for sicca syndrome, extreme dryness of mucous membranes and tissues, and infections (Table 11.9). Diagnosis can be made clinically, based on symptoms and laboratory values (Chap. 25). However, tissue biopsy is required for definitive diagnosis. CGvHD is graded as limited or extensive: limited is described as localized skin involvement and/or hepatic dysfunction, and extensive is described as generalized skin involvement with multiorgan involvement.

Treatment consists of immunosuppression with many of the same agents used to treat AGvHD (Table 11.7). Initial treatment usually includes cyclosporine or tacrolimus and steroids that are slowly tapered over several months. Several newer agents are now available. For severe CGvHD of the skin, both psoralen and ultraviolet radiation (PUVA) and extracorporeal photopheresis have been beneficial.

11.7.3.3 Pulmonary Complications

Bronchiolitis obliterans (BO) is described as an obstructive lung disease following HSCT in the absence of an infectious cause. The exact incidence in pediatrics is unknown but estimates range from 2 to 20%. The most consistent risk factor is GvHD; consequently, the etiology when associated with GvHD involves T-lymphocytes directly attacking bronchiolar epithelium. Aspiration due to esophageal GvHD, ciliary dysfunction, occult infection, and medication toxicies have also been implicated. Surgical lung biopsy reveals partial or complete obstruction of small airways due to inflammation and fibrosis. The classic presentation is chronic, irreversible, obstructive lung disease. Patients may be asymptomatic or report cough and SOB. Chest X-ray shows hyperinflation, and chest CT demonstrates hypoattenuation and expiratory air trapping. Treatment includes corticosteriods and immunosuppressive agents. BO is assocatiated with a very high mortality rate (Gower et al. 2006; Michelson et al. 2007; Soubani and Uberti 2007) (Chap. 20).

11.7.3.4 Endocrine Complications

Endocrine dysfunction may present as growth failure, thyroid dysfunction, ovarian dysfunction, or testicular dysfunction. The risk factors include TBI and long-term steroid therapy, although fractionated TBI has decreased the incidence of hypothyroidism to 10–28% (Chemaitilly et al. 2006). Treatment includes thyroid replacement therapy and growth hormone therapy, respectively, for thyroid dysfunction and growth delays. Females who undergo chemotherapy after puberty have more permanent infertility and menopausal symptoms, than those treated before puberty. Testicular dysfunction includes sterility, azoospermia, and premature ejaculation in males treated with TBI. Regardless of age, TBI may result in primary gonadal failure in both the genders. Treatment may include hormone replacement therapy (Chap. 26).

11.7.3.5 Cataracts

Cataracts, usually posterior and bilateral, can occur several years post transplant in patients who have received TBI (Fahnehjelm et al. 2007). Fractionated TBI has significantly reduced the incidence. Treatment includes the surgical removal of the cataracts (Chap. 28).

11.7.3.6 Disease Recurrence and Secondary Malignancies

Disease recurrence remains the primary cause of treatment failure after autologous and allogeneic HSCT (Ringdén et al. 2009). Patients at increased risk for relapse include those with high-risk diseases, poor response to initial therapy, unfavorable cytogenetic abnormalities, and significant disease/tumor burden at the time of transplant. Treatment can include donor lymphocyte infusions, second transplants, and discontinuing immunosuppressive therapy.

Secondary malignancies can occur for both autologous and allogeneic transplant recipients. HSCT recipients have a four- to sevenfold increased risk of developing a secondary malignancy (Forrest et al. 2003). High-dose chemotherapy, TBI, and immunosuppression are the primary etiologies.

Table 11.9. Chronic GvHD: clinical effects and nursing interventions

Organ/ system involved	Clinical effects	Nursing interventions
Skin	Itching, burning, scleroderma, ulcerations, hyperpigmentation, erythema, dryness	Teach patient to use skin moisturizers and nondrying, nonabrasive soaps
	Erythema can be activated by sun exposure	Teach patient to protect skin from sunlight and avoid prolonged sun exposure; emphasize the need to use sunscreens
	Alopecia, nail ridging, joint contractures	Apply topical steroid creams to relieve itching and/or burning
		Provide range of motion exercises
		Practice specific exercise regimens recommended by PT/OT to prevent contractures
Liver	Obstructive jaundice	Monitor liver function tests
	Cirrhosis with esophageal varices and hepatic failure	Teach patient about low-fat diet, if indicated
GI tract	Xerostomia, stomatitis, ulcerations, lichen planus-like striae and plaques, taste changes, dysphagia, retrosternal pain, diarrhea, malabsorption	Promote oral hygiene and regular dental follow-up
		Encourage use of artificial saliva or alkaline-saline mouthwash to relieve oral dryness
		Provide lanolin for lip moisturizing
		Provide nutritional counseling and dietary referral
		Monitor weights
Eyes	Decreased tear production	Promote regular ophthalmology exams
	Burning, photophobia, itching, sensation of grittiness in eyes	Provide artificial tears to relieve ocular dryness
		Suggest use of sunglasses to decrease discomfort of photophobia
Lungs	Obstructive and restrictive lung changes	Provide chest PT and incentive spirometer, if indicated
	Cough, dyspnea, pneumothorax	Monitor pulmonary function tests on a regular basis
Immunosuppression	Increased risk of infection	Maintain measures to prevent infections
	Slowed immune recovery	Promote good general hygiene
		Administer immunosuppressive therapy and monitor for side effects
		Monitor compliance with infection prophylaxis medications

Myelodysplastic syndrome and leukemia are most common after autologous transplant. Patients receiving an allogeneic transplant are at risk of developing post transplant lymphoproliferative disease, which can occur within 6 months after transplant, and a variety of solid tumors (Bollard et al. 2006).

11.8 Special Considerations

Discharge planning and teaching become focused once engraftment begins. Discharge can be anticipated once engraftment has occurred. Engraftment is generally defined as an ANC greater than 500/mm^3 for

3 consecutive days. In general, patients are required to remain in close proximity to the transplant center for the first 100 days after allogeneic transplant. Autologous transplant patients may be referred to their primary physician once engraftment has occurred and HSCT complications have resolved.

General discharge criteria include the following:

- ANC greater than 500/mm^3
- Afebrile for 24 h
- Able to take oral medications
- Oral intake of calories and fluids is 50% of nutritional needs
- Patient is on total parenteral nutrition or nasogastric feedings
- Any transplant complications are resolved or controlled
- Primary caregiver is able to care for central venous line and provide any nutritional support that is needed

Instructions to patient and caregiver should include the following topics:

- Infection control practices: handwashing, social isolation, face masks, temperature monitoring, and avoidance of new pets and plants
- Activities of daily living: diet, personal hygiene, mouth care, sun exposure, exercise, and school reentry
- Central line care and parenteral medication administration
- Importance of oral medication compliance
- Reportable signs and symptoms: fever, cough, rash, vomiting, diarrhea, bleeding, pain, and inability to take oral medications

Outpatient follow-up will be tailored to the patient's needs. The frequency of clinic appointments is based on the type of transplant, engraftment status, and unresolved complications. Regular monitoring will include physical assessment, routine blood counts, serum chemistries and medication levels (cyclosporine and tacrolimus), symptom and toxicity management, medication compliance, and nutritional assessment.

Annual evaluations of recipients of allogeneic transplants are required for monitoring engraftment status and assessing for late effects. Typical tests performed on an annual basis include:

- Complete blood count with differential count
- Serum chemistries
- Immunoglobulin levels
- Immune function tests
- Endocrine function tests
- Pulmonary function tests
- Cardiac function tests
- Ophthalmologic examination
- Renal function tests
- Neuropsychological evaluation

Psychosocial issues faced by patients and their families are numerous, with different issues presenting during each phase of transplant. Some of these include prolonged hospitalization, emotional isolation from family and friends, role changes within the family dynamics, invasive medical procedures, treatment-related side effects and complications, fear of relapse, and financial concerns. All these can have a significant impact on the quality of life experienced by the patient and the entire family. Consequently, a diverse multidisciplinary team of healthcare providers is required to assist the patient and family in successfully dealing with these issues.

11.9 Future Perspectives

Future direction in HSCT should consist of optimizing GvL effects, minimizing toxicity, engineering more precise grafts, moving to outpatient procedures, and combining stem cell transplantation with gene therapy. GvL is an immune response to donor cells against recipient leukemia. There is evidence for GvL effect with the infusion of unmanipulated donor lymphocytes on relapsed patients after allogeneic HSCT (Xia et al. 2006). The future holds identification of minor antigens and their roles in GvL and GvHD. Molecular typing for some of the newly identified minor antigens is becoming available (Bollard et al. 2006).

Minimizing regimen-related toxicity would broaden the use of HSCT to nontraditional disorders, such as autoimmune and degenerative diseases, and improve long-term survival of transplant recipients. Monoclonal antibodies, such as the CD52 antibody, alemtuzumab (Campath), anti CD45, and anti CD20 (Rituxan) antibodies, are being incorporated into conditioning regimens to substitute partly or completely the traditional cytotoxic and immunosuppressive drugs currently used (Abutalib and Tallman 2006; Barfield et al. 2008). Many centers are developing submyeloablative conditioning regimens with less toxic chemotherapy. The use of adoptive immunotherapy in the form of cytotoxic T-lymphocytes has been demonstrated to prevent and treat transplant infections and post transplant lymphoproliferative disorders (Mackinnon et al. 2008; Leen & Heslop 2008; Myers et al. 2007).

T-cell depletion and $CD34^+$ selection are examples of more precise graft engineering to reduce complications such as graft failure and GvHD. Further identification of minor antigens could lead to more selective T-cell depletion techniques that might allow GvHD prevention without significant loss of GvL effect (Qasim et al. 2005).

Several centers are exploring the possibility of providing stem cell transplants in the outpatient arena. This could have a significant impact on the length of hospitalization and financial costs of HSCT in the future. As technology and basic science advance, HSCT will be combined with gene therapy as a vehicle for gene insertion (Alderuccio et al. 2006), which will enhance the applicability of stem cell transplantation, provide less toxic therapy, and improve survival.

References

Abutalib SA, Tallman MS (2006) Monoclonal antibodies for the treatment of acute myeloid leukemia. Current Pharmaceutical Biotechnology 7(5):343–369

Alderuccio F, Siatskas C, Chan J, Field J, Murphy K, Nasa Z, Toh BH (2006) Haematopoietic stem cell gene therapy to treat autoimmune disease. Current Stem Cell Research and Therapy 1(3):279–287

American Academy of Pediatrics Section on Hematology/Oncology, American Academy of Pediatrics Section on Allergy/Immunology, Lubin BH, Shearer WT (2007) Cord blood banking for potential future transplantation. Pediatrics 119(1):165–170

Anasetti C (2008) What are the most important donor and recipient factors affecting the outcome of related and unrelated allogeneic transplantation? Best Practice and Research. Clinical Haematology 21(4):691–697

Anderlini P (2009) Effects and safety of granulocyte colony-stimulating factor in healthy volunteers. Current Opinion in Hematology 16(1):35–40

Anderlini P, Champlin RE (2008) Biologic and molecular effects of granulocyte colony-stimulating factor in healthy individuals: recent findings and current challenges. Blood 11(4):1767–1772

Armson BA, Maternal/Fetal Medicine Committee, Society of Obstetricians and Gynaecologists of Canada (2005) Umbilical cord blood banking: implications for perinatal care providers. Journal of Obstetrics and Gynaecology Canada 27(3):263–290

Barfield RC, Kasow KA, Hale GA (2008) Advances in pediatric hematopoietic stem cell transplantation. Cancer Biology and Therapy 7(10):1533–1539

Bennett CL, Evens AM, Andritsos LA, Balasubramanian L, Mai M, Fisher MJ, Kuzel TM, Angelotta C, McKoy JM, Vose JM, Bierman PJ, Kuter DJ, Trifilio SM, Devine SM, Tallman MS (2006) Haematological malignancies developing in previously healthy individuals who received haematopoietic growth factors: report from the Research on Adverse Drug Events and Reports (RADAR) project. British Journal of Haematology 135(5):642–650

Bredeson C, Leger C, Couban S, Simpson D, Huebsch L, Walker I, Shore T, Howson-Jan K, Panzarella T, Messner H, Barnett M, Lipton J (2004) An evaluation of the donor experience in the canadian multicenter randomized trial of bone marrow versus peripheral blood allografting. Biology of Blood Marrow Transplantation 10(6):405–414

Bollard CM, Krance RA, Heslop HE (2006) Hematopoietic stem cell transplantation in pediatric oncology. In: Pizzo PA, Poplack DG (eds) Principles and practice of pediatric oncology. Lippincott Williams & Wilkins, Philadelphia, pp 476–500

Bornstein R, Flores AI, Montalbán MA, del Rey MJ, de la Serna J, Gilsanz F (2005) A modified cord blood collection method achieves sufficient cell levels for transplantation in most adult patients. Stem Cells. 23(3):324-34

Chemaitilly W, Boulad F, Sklar C (2006) Endocrine complications of childhood hematopoietic stem-cell transplantation. In: Kline RM (ed) Pediatric hematopoietic stem cell transplantation. Informa Healthcare, New York, pp 287–298

Chiang KY, Haight A, Horan J, Olson E, Gartner A, Hartman D, Youssef S, Worthington-White D (2007) Clinical outcomes and graft characteristics in pediatric matched sibling donor transplants using granulocyte colony-stimulating factor-primed bone marrow and steady-state bone marrow. Pediatric Transplantation 11(3):279–285

Cohen Y, Nagler A (2004) Umbilical cord blood transplantation–how, when and for whom? Blood Reviews 18(3):167–179

Dallorso S, Dini G, Faraci M, Spreafico F, EBMT Paediatric Working Party (2008) SCT for Wilms' tumour. Bone Marrow Transplantation 41(Suppl 2):S128–S130

Elfenbein GJ, Sackstein R, Oblon DJ (2004) Do G-CSF mobilized, peripheral blood-derived stem cells from healthy, HLA-identical donors really engraft more rapidly than do G-CSF primed, bone marrow-derived stem cells? No! Blood Cells Mol Dis. 32(1):106-11

Elfenbein GJ (2005) Granulocyte-colony stimulating factor primed bone marrow and granulocyte-colony stimulating factor mobilized peripheral blood stem cells are equivalent for engraftment: which to choose? Pediatric Transplantation 9(Suppl 7):37–47

Fahnehjelm KT, Törnquist AL, Olsson M, Winiarski J (2007) Visual outcome and cataract development after allogenic stem cell transplantation in children. Acta Opthalmologica Scandinavica 85(7):724–733

Flomenberg N, Baxter-Lowe LA, Confer D, Fernandez-Vina M, Filipovich A, Horowitz M, Hurley C, Kollman C, Anasetti C, Noreen H, Begovich A, Hildebrand W, Petersdorf E, Schmeckpeper B, Setterholm M, Trachtenberg E, Williams T, Yunis E, Weisdorf D (2004) Impact of HLA class I and class II high-resolution matching on outcomes of unrelated donor bone marrow transplantation: HLA-C mismatching is associated with a strong adverse effect on transplantation outcome. Blood 104(7):1923–1930

Forrest DL, Nevill TJ, Naiman SC, Le A, Brockington DA, Barnett MJ, Lavoie JC, Nantel SH, Song KW, Shepherd JD, Sutherland HJ, Toze CL, Davis JH, Hogge DE (2003) Second malignancy following high-dose therapy and autologous stem cell transplantation: incidence and risk factor analysis. Bone Marrow Transplantation 32(9):915–923

Fortanier C, Kuentz M, Sutton L, Milpied N, Michalet M, Macquart-Moulin G, Faucher C, Le Corroller AG, Moatti JP, Blaise D (2002) Healthy sibling donor anxiety and pain during bone marrow or peripheral blood stem cell harvesting for allogeneic transplantation: results of a randomized study. Bone Marrow Transplantation 29(2):145–149

Gluckman E, Broxmeyer HA, Auerbach AD, Friedman HS, Douglas GW, Devergie A, Esperou H, Thierry D, Socie G, Lehn P et al (1989) Hematopoietic reconstitution in a patient with Fanconi's anemia by means of umbilical-cord blood from an HLA-identical sibling. New England Journal of Medicine 321(17):1174–1178

Gluckman E, Rocha V (2009) Cord blood transplantation: state of the art. Haematologica 94(4):451–454

Gluckman E, Rocha V, Arcese W, Michel G, Sanz G, Chan KW, Takahashi TA, Ortega J, Filipovich A, Locatelli F, Asano S, Fagioli F, Vowels M, Sirvent A, Laporte JP, Tiedemann K, Amadori S, Abecassis M, Bordigoni P, Diez B, Shaw PJ, Vora A, Caniglia M, Garnier F, Ionescu I, Garcia J, Koegler G, Rebulla P, Chevret S, Eurocord Group (2004) Factors associated with outcomes of unrelated cord blood transplant: guidelines for donor choice. Experimental Hematology 32(4):397–407

Goker H, Haznedaroglu IC, Chao NJ (2001) Acute graft-vs-host disease: pathobiology and management. Experimental Hematology 29(3):259–277

Gower WA, Collaco JM, Mogayzel PJ (2006) Pulmonary dysfunction in pediatric hematopoietic stem cell transplant patients: non-infectious and long-term complications. Pediatric Blood and Cancer 49:225–233

Gratwohl A, Baldomero H, Demirer T, Rosti G, Dini G, Ladenstein R, Urbano-Ispizua A; Accreditation Committee, European Group for Blood and Marrow Transplantation; Working Party on Pediatric Diseases; Working Party on Solid Tumors. (2004) Hematopoetic stem cell transplantation for solid tumors in Europe. Ann Oncol. 15(4):653-60

Helming AM, Brand A, Wolterbeek R, van Tol MJ, Egeler RM, Ball LM (2007) ABO incompatible stem cell transplantation in children does not influence outcome. Pediatr Blood and Cancer 49(3):313–317

Hsia CC, Linenberger M, Howson-Jan K, Mangel J, Chin-Yee IH, Collins S, Xenocostas A (2008) Acute myeloid leukemia in a healthy hematopoietic stem cell donor following past exposure to a short course of G-CSF. Bone Marrow Transplantation 42(6):431–432

Huang X, Liu D, Liu K, Xu L, Chen H, Han W, Chen Y, Wang Y, Zhang X (2008) Haploidentical hematopoietic stem cell transplantation without in vitro T cell depletion for treatment of hematologic malignancies in children. Biology of Blood Marrow Transplantation 15(1 Suppl):91–94

Kolb HJ (2008) Graft-versus-leukemia effects of transplantation and donor lymphocytes. Blood 112(12):4371–4383

Kurtzberg J (2009) Update on umbilical cord blood transplantation. Current Opinion in Pediatrics 21(1):22–29

Kurtzberg J, Laughlin M, Graham ML, Smith C, Olson JF, Halperin EC, Ciocci G, Carrier C, Stevens CE, Rubinstein P (1996) Placental blood as a source of hematopoietic stem cells for transplantation into unrelated recipients. New England Journal of Medicine 335(3):157–166

Laporte JP, Gorin NC, Rubinstein P, Lesage S, Portnoi MF, Barbu V, Lopez M, Douay L, Najman A (1996) Cord-blood transplantation from an unrelated donor in an adult with chronic myelogenous leukemia. New England Journal of Medicine 335(3):167–170

Lee SJ, Klein J, Haagenson M, Baxter-Lowe LA, Confer DL, Eapen M, Fernandez-Vina M, Flomenberg N, Horowitz M, Hurley CK, Noreen H, Oudshoorn M, Petersdorf E, Setterholm M, Spellman S, Weisdorf D, Williams TM, Anasetti C (2007) High-resolution donor-recipient HLA matching contributes to the success of unrelated donor marrow transplantation. Blood 110(13):4576–4583

Leen AM, Heslop HE (2008) Cytotoxic T lymphocytes as immune-therapy in haematological practice. British Journal of Haematology 143(2):169-179

Leung AY, Mak R, Lie AK, Yuen KY, Cheng VC, Liang R, Kwong YL (2002) Clinicopathological features and risk factors of clinically overt haemorrhagic cystitis complicating bone marrow transplantation. Bone Marrow Transplantation 29(6):509–513

Locatelli F, De Stefano P (2005) T-cell depletion to prevent GVHD after unrelated-donor marrow transplantation. Lancet 366(9487):692–694

Mackinnon S, Thomson K, Verfuerth S, Peggs K, Lowdell M (2008) Adoptive cellular therapy for cytomegalovirus infection following allogeneic stem cell transplantation using virus-specific T cells. Blood Cells, Molecular Diseases 40(1):63–67

MacLeod KD, Whitsett SF, Mash EJ, Pelletier W (2003) Pediatric sibling donors of successful and unsuccessful hematopoietic stem cell transplants (HSCT): a qualitative study of their psychosocial experience. Journal of Pediatric Psychology 28(4):223–230

Makita K, Ohta K, Mugitani A, Hagihara K, Ohta T, Yamane T, Hino M (2004) Acute myelogenous leukemia in a donor after granulocyte colony-stimulating factor-primed peripheral blood stem cell harvest. Bone Marrow Transplantation 33(6):661–665

Meyers PA (2004) High-dose therapy with autologous stem cell rescue for pediatric sarcomas. Curr Opin Oncol. 16(2):120-5

Michelson PH, Goyal R, Kurland G (2007) Pulmonary complications of haematopoietic cell transplantation in children. Paediatric Respiratory Reviews 8:46–61

Myers GD, Bollard CM, Wu M-F, Weiss H, Rooney CM, Heslop HE, Leen AM (2007) Reconstitution of adenovirus-specific cell-mediated immunity in pediatric patients after hematopoietic stem cell transplantation. Bone Marrow Transplantation 39(11):677-686

Norville R (2008) Hematopoietic stem cell transplantation. In: Kline NE (ed) Essentials of pediatric hematology/oncology nursing: a core curriculum, 3rd edn. Association of Pediatric Hematology/Oncology Nurses, Glenview, IL, pp 98–108

Nowak J (2008) Role of HLA in hematopoietic SCT. Bone Marrow Transplant.;42 Suppl 2:S71-6

Packman W, Gong K, VanZutphen K, Shaffer T, Crittenden M (2004) Psychosocial adjustment of adolescent siblings of hematopoietic stem cell transplant patients. Journal of Pediatric Oncology Nursing 21(4):233–248

Pérez A, González-Vicent M, Ramirez M, Sevilla J, Madero L, Díaz MA (2008) Intentional induction of mixed haematopoietic chimerism as platform for cellular therapy after HLA-matched allogeneic stem cell transplantation in childhood leukaemia patients. British Journal of Haematology 140(3):340–343

Qasim W, Gaspar HB, Thrasher AJ (2005) T cell suicide gene therapy to aid haematopoietic stem cell transplantation. Current Gene Therapy 5(1):121–132

Raanani P, Gafter-Gvili A, Paul M, Ben-Bassat I, Leibovici L, Shpilberg O (2009) Immunoglobulin prophylaxis in hematopoietic stem cell transplantation: systematic review and meta-analysis. Journal of Clinical Oncology 27(5):770–781

Ringdén O, Pavletic SZ, Anasetti C, Barrett AJ, Wang T, Wang D, Antin JH, Di Bartolomeo P, Bolwell BJ, Bredeson C, Cairo MS, Gale RP, Gupta V, Hahn T, Hale GA, Halter J, Jagasia M, Litzow MR, Locatelli F, Marks DI, McCarthy PL, Cowan MJ, Petersdorf EW, Russell JA, Schiller GJ, Schouten H, Spellman S, Verdonck LF, Wingard JR, Horowitz MM, Arora M (2009) The graft-versus-leukemia effect using matched unrelated donors is not superior to HLA-identical siblings for hematopoietic stem cell transplantation. Blood 113(13):3110–3118

Rocha V, Locatelli F (2008) Searching for alternative hematopoietic stem cell donors for pediatric patients. Bone Marrow Transplantation 41(2):207–214

Samuel GN, Kerridge IH, O'Brien TA (2008) Umbilical cord blood banking: public good or private benefit? Medical Journal of Australia 188(9):533–535

Shah AJ, Kapoor N, Crooks GM, Weinberg KI, Azim HA, Killen R, Kuo L, Rushing T, Kohn DB, Parkman R (2007) The effects of Campath 1H upon graft-versus-host disease, infection, relapse, and immune reconstitution in recipients of pediatric unrelated transplants. Biology of Blood Marrow Transplantation 13(5):584–593

Soubani AO, Uberti JP (2007) Bronchiolitis obliterans following haematopoietic stem cell transplantaion. European Respiratory Journal 29:1007–1019

Thornley I, Eapen M, Sung L, Lee SJ, Davies SM, Joffe S (2009) Private cord blood banking: experiences and views of pediatric hematopoietic cell transplantation physicians. Pediatrics 123(3):1011–1017

Tiercy JM, Nicoloso G, Passweg J, Schanz U, Seger R, Chalandon Y, Heim D, Güngör T, Schneider P, Schwabe R, Gratwohl A (2007) The probability of identifying a 10/10 HLA allele-matched unrelated donor is highly predictable. Bone Marrow Transplant. 40(6):515-22

Trivedi VB, Dave AP, Dave JM, Patel BC (2007) Human leukocyte antigen and its role in transplantation biology. Transplantation Proceedings 39(3):688–693

Wagner JE, Thompson JS, Carter SL, Kernan NA; Unrelated Donor Marrow Transplantation Trial (2005) Effect of graft-versus-host disease prophylaxis on 3-year disease-free survival in recipients of unrelated donor bone marrow (T-cell depletion trial): a multi-centre, randomised phase II-III trial. Lancet 366(9487):733–741

Watkins TR, Chien JW, Crawford SW (2005) Graft versus host-associated pulmonary disease and other idiopathic pulmonary complications after hematopoietic stem cell transplant. Seminars in Respiratory and Critical Care Medicine 26:482–489

Wiener LS, Steffen-Smith E, Fry T, Wayne AS (2007) Hematopoietic stem cell donation in children: a review of the sibling donor experience. Journal of Psychosocial Oncology 25(1):45–66

Xia G, Truitt RL, Johnson BD (2006) Graft-versus-leukemia and graft-versus-host reactions after donor lymphocyte infusion are initiated by host-type antigen-presenting cells and regulated by regulatory T cells in early and long-term chimeras. Biology of Blood Marrow Transplant 12(4): 397–407

Surgical Approaches to Childhood Cancer

Carol L. Rossetto

Contents

12.1 Principles of Treatment 269
12.2 Method of Delivery 270
12.2.1 Preoperative Evaluation. 270
12.2.2 Postoperative Nursing Care 271
12.3 Potential Side Effects. 271
12.3.1 Complications of Medical Therapy Requiring Surgical Evaluation 271
12.3.2 Complications Arising from Surgical Management of Solid Tumors. 272
12.4 Special Considerations. 273
12.4.1 Vascular Access Devices. 273
12.5 Future Perspectives. 274
12.5.1 New Surgical Techniques and Directions for Future Research . . . 274
References 275

12.1 Principles of Treatment

A local and regional determination of the extent of disease, or staging, is performed at diagnosis and relapse (Leonard 2002). A system of staging exists for many pediatric tumors and helps one to determine both prognosis and treatment. It is based on the premise that cancer of similar histologic features and sites of origin grows and metastasizes in a similar manner. All treatment protocols are based on the stage of the tumor, which determines such factors as use of radiotherapy and intensity of chemotherapy. Correct staging allows the medical team to minimize therapy and yet maximize cure. This further provides the opportunity to limit therapy to minimize the long-term sequelae of different treatments.

Similar to staging of the disease, use of the correct biopsy technique is critical to the childhood cancer patient. The diagnosis of childhood cancer requires meticulous tumor analysis carefully planned before the biopsy by the pediatric oncologist, pathologist, and surgeon. In particular, molecular studies should be well planned prior to tumor sampling. Biopsy is best performed in a pediatric cancer center because optimal use of the surgical specimen can be performed only in specialized childhood cancer centers. Considerations when selecting the method and type of incision include the creation of an incision that may be incorporated in the future incision used for resection, the need to avoid contaminating an uninvolved body cavity, the need to avoid contaminating otherwise uninvolved lymphatic drainage, and adequate staging at the time of biopsy if the child is to receive preoperative chemotherapy. Common

Table 12.1. Common surgical techniques for management of childhood malignancies

Procedure	Description
Biopsies, including fine needle aspiration, core biopsy, and incisional/open or excisional biopsy	Biopsies include taking a sample of the desired tissue by means of a needle aspiration, a core biopsy for larger specimens, and open procedures to remove entire sections of tumor and/or lymph nodes
Staging and second-look surgery	Staging is used when treatment depends on the location of the cancer and the extent of disease involvement. "Second-look" procedures are used to assess response to nonsurgical treatment
Debulking	Debulking involves removing a portion of the tumor mass when it is not possible to remove the entire mass. This may be done as first-line therapy or after receiving chemotherapy or radiation
Management of metastasis	Provides pathologic confirmation of metastasis via biopsy and can include staging and/or debulking efforts
Supportive care surgery	Surgeries necessary for placement of central venous access devices/ catheters or feeding tubes vital to supportive care measures
Palliative surgery	Palliative surgery is done to relieve the symptoms caused by tumors that have been unresponsive to medical therapy. It may also be done to relieve pain and bleeding

surgical techniques in the management of childhood malignancies include, but are not limited to, those listed in Table 12.1.

12.2 Method of Delivery

12.2.1 Preoperative Evaluation

The pediatric oncology patient undergoing surgery warrants detailed consideration with regard to perioperative and anesthetic management. Clinically, this includes coagulation and transfusion evaluation and support, evaluation of the airway in patients with an anterior mediastinal mass, and immunization of those patients undergoing splenectomy. For patients already treated with chemotherapy, assessment of cardiac, pulmonary, renal, and electrolyte status is also critical, since various systems can be affected by previous chemotherapy or radiation therapy. Close coordination between services will avoid duplication of studies and decrease the need for repeated sedation for procedures or diagnostic tests.

A complete blood count, including hemoglobin, white blood cell count, platelet count, and coagulation studies, is necessary prior to surgery. Low blood counts can be corrected using granulocyte colony-stimulating factor and red blood cell and/or platelet transfusions when indicated. It is difficult to discern, however, particularly in the leukemic patient, whether neutropenia may be functional or a result of a bone marrow "packed" with leukemic cells. The clinical situation will mandate the need for transfusion support of the oncologic surgical patient. Immunodeficient patients should receive irradiated and leukocyte-reduced blood products.

Most often, elevations in prothrombin time (PT) and partial thromboplastin time (PTT) are acquired defects. For the patient with a normal platelet count and fibrinogen, administration of vitamin K – or for immediate correction, fresh frozen plasma – can correct these abnormalities. For the patient with other associated abnormal laboratory values (e.g., fibrinogen), disseminated intravascular coagulation (DIC) or liver disease should be considered (Table 12.2).

A child with a mediastinal mass is at risk for respiratory collapse due to airway compression during induction of general anesthesia. Anterior mediastinal masses may also compress the superior vena cava, causing some or all manifestations of superior vena cava syndrome. These symptoms include orthopnea,

Table 12.2. "Ideal" blood counts prior to surgical procedure

Platelets >50,000/mm^3
Hemoglobin >6–8 g/dL
Absolute neutrophils >1,000/mm^3
Normal coagulation studies (including prothrombin time, partial thromboplastin time, fibrinogen and INR international normalized ratio)

headache, dizziness, fainting, plethoric facial swelling, jugular venous distension, papilledema, and pulsus paradoxus. Computed tomography (CT) with intravenous contrast material is helpful to evaluate the airway and obtain further anatomic information (La Quaglia and Su 2006). Pulmonary function testing can also be important in evaluating this type of patient. It is generally very important to obtain a diagnosis of a mediastinal mass prior to therapy as chemotherapy, radiation, or steroids may obliterate the tumor architecture and prevent the final diagnosis from being established. In patients with significant airway compression, biopsy under conscious sedation, or even local anesthesia may be required. A child needs to be immunized at least 2 weeks before undergoing a splenectomy. The spleen contains macrophages, which provide defense against infections. Necessary vaccines include *Haemophilus influenzae* type B (Hib), pneumococcal vaccine, and meningococcal vaccine.

Patients who have a history of receiving bleomycin, anthracycline agents, or radiation therapy will be assessed differently prior to surgery than those children who have not been exposed to these treatments. Pulmonary fibrosis with a loss of lung volume, compliance, and diffusing capacity can occur as a result of bleomycin, BCNU, or radiation therapy to the lung; therefore, these patients need to be identified to the anesthesiologist as high-risk. All patients who have a history of receiving anthracycline agents (cardiotoxic) or mediastinal radiation will also need further preoperative evaluation, which can include an echocardiogram (ECHO) and/or multigated angiography (MUGA).

Preparation of the patient and his or her family cannot be overemphasized as a vital part of preoperative nursing management. Besides ensuring adequate nutrition, confirming no evidence of infection, and checking that laboratory criteria are met or within normal limits, the child and family will need education to support them. Play therapy is often used to help prepare children for surgery. This may include allowing the child to handle medical equipment, providing developmentally appropriate explanations, and giving a tour of the operating room if time permits; these measures can positively influence the operative experience. Assessing the patient and family's learning needs is an important part of this preparation phase before surgery.

12.2.2 Postoperative Nursing Care

The child with cancer is often a high-risk surgical patient. Postoperative care of these patients must include attention to the following areas: prevention of infection, airway maintenance and oxygenation, fluid and electrolyte balance, pain control, nutritional support, and wound care.

12.3 Potential Side Effects

Immunosuppression related to cancer therapy presents the increased potential for complications due to infectious causes. A secondary problem related to this is that signs and symptoms of infection are often delayed in these patients because of their immune suppression. Therefore, surgical oncology patients require close monitoring postoperatively.

12.3.1 Complications of Medical Therapy Requiring Surgical Evaluation

Bowel obstruction can be partial or complete and may be caused by tumors, adhesions, constipation, or ileus as a result of narcotics, vincristine, or graft-vs.-host disease in hematopoietic stem cell transplant patients. Perforation and necrosis are rare but can occur. Treatment usually includes hydration, antibiotics, and laxatives for first-line therapy. A nasogastric tube is inserted to relieve pressure, and subsequent surgery is used if the obstruction persists despite the previous interventions.

Pancreatitis is an inflammation of the pancreas. Symptoms are nausea, vomiting, and right-sided tenderness, and the diagnosis is confirmed by physical examination and elevated lipase and amylase. CT or ultrasound shows an enlarged and inflamed pancreas. The cause may be due to tumor lysis and/or chemotherapy (asparaginase or, less frequently, steroids). Treatment includes stopping the causative agent and restricting the diet. Necrotizing pancreatitis may require surgical debridement in extreme cases. Maintenance of nothing-by-mouth status with total parenteral nutrition until symptoms resolve is the usual first-line therapy, with a subsequent low-fat diet prescribed.

In neutropenic children, inflammation of the cecum (typhlitis) can occur postoperatively and can progress rapidly to gangrene or perforation of the bowel. Symptoms include abdominal pain in the right lower quadrant, fever, distention, diarrhea, and vomiting. An X-ray can demonstrate bowel wall thickening, and a CT scan confirms inflammation and its extent. Treatment includes antibiotics and bowel rest. Laparotomy is a surgical intervention to remove the diseased bowel if there is clinical deterioration, persistent gastrointestinal bleeding, uncontrolled sepsis, or evidence of perforation.

Different types of infections can occur and are not uncommon in the immunosuppressed pediatric oncology patient. Surgical site infections are the leading type of infection among hospitalized patients. Infections of the surgical wound/site or the central line site often can be treated with antibiotics without having to remove the newly planted central venous access device. Symptoms of wound infection are tenderness, erythema, fever, and wound drainage. Wound infections usually occur after 5–7 days postoperatively. Other than antibiotics, wound infection treatment may also include incision and drainage, particularly when symptoms of cellulitis are present. The surgeon may debride a wound when infection interferes with healing. Temporary drains are used to remove fluid accumulation.

Currently, clinical practice standards for the prevention of surgical site infections have been derived from guidelines prepared by the American College of Surgeons and the Centers for Disease Control (CDC) (Nichols 2000). These guidelines include educational preparation of the patient/family; antisepsis of the surgical team; management of infected surgical personnel; antimicrobial prophylaxis; intraoperative ventilation; intraoperative cleaning and disinfection; microbiologic sampling; sterilization of surgical instruments, surgical attire, and drapes; and asepsis and sterile technique, incision care, and surveillance.

Incision care is defined per the aforementioned guidelines as following recommendations during the postoperative phase to prevent surgical site infections. Specifically, these recommendations include the following:

- Protect incision with sterile dressing 24–48 h postoperatively
- Wash hands before and after any contact with the surgical site
- Use sterile technique when changing dressing
- Educate patient and family regarding proper incision care, symptoms of an infection, and the need to report these symptoms.

Pneumothorax is the collapse of a lung and can be spontaneous, a presenting symptom of metastatic lung disease, or a direct result of an invasive procedure (e.g., thoracotomy, central venous line insertion). The most common symptoms of pneumothorax are shortness of breath and chest pain. A chest X-ray revealing lung collapse will confirm the diagnosis. Symptoms can develop within 24 h postoperatively. The treatment includes lung expansion via insertion of a chest tube. The tube is left in place until the X-rays and the clinical condition of the patient show that the lung has re-expanded. For patients who have an asymptomatic pneumothorax, supplemental oxygen is administered to accelerate spontaneous resolution (Zierold et al. 2000).

12.3.2 Complications Arising from Surgical Management of Solid Tumors

Operations for solid tumors can present risks unique to the type of tumor being approached. Specific tumor considerations include, but are not limited to, neuroblastoma and Wilms' tumor. Surgery is the mainstay for children with resectable localized neuroblastoma with favorable biologic and genetic characteristics

(Grosfeld 2006). In the more advanced stages of neuroblastoma, following a biopsy, chemotherapy is given followed by an extended resection. Injury to the major vessels can occur with the most common intraoperative complication is the need for nephrectomy. In addition, extensive dissection of renal vessels can lead to ultimate damage that may not become apparent until the postoperative period. Renal impairment is evidenced by an abnormal renal scan evaluating function or anuria/oliguria.

In children with Wilms' tumor, the standard treatment is surgery followed by chemotherapy and in some cases radiation therapy (Cotton et al. 2009; Green 2004). Risk factors for the development of surgical complications in patients with Wilms' tumor include advanced local tumor at the time of diagnosis, intravascular tumor extension, and resection of other organs at the time of nephrectomy. The most common complication is intestinal obstruction, followed by hemorrhage, wound infection, and vascular injury. Furthermore, two risk factors related to local recurrence of Wilms' tumor are directly related to the type of surgical resection performed: The presence of microscopic tumor at the margin of the surgical resection and intraoperative tumor spill are both factors that can predict disease recurrence. Other childhood cancers that are benefiting from advances in surgical techniques and coordination with multimodality treatment regimens include rhabdomyosarcoma, Ewing's sarcoma, desmoplastic small round blue cell tumors, germ cell tumors, and hepatoblastoma.

12.4 Special Considerations

12.4.1 Vascular Access Devices

Vascular access devices (VADs) are vital in managing and treating childhood cancer. Central venous catheters (CVCs) provide for the long-term delivery of prolonged courses of chemotherapy as well as parenteral nutrition, blood products, intravenous fluids, antibiotics, pain medications, and other agents. Furthermore, they are useful devices for repeated blood sampling. There are three types of devices most commonly used in the pediatric cancer population: peripherally inserted central venous catheters (PICCs), tunneled and nontunneled external CVCs, and the implanted vascular access device or port-a-catheter. The tunneled CVC uses a flexible silicone tube placed in a central vein that exits through a subcutaneous tunnel. The CVC has historically been placed surgically, but is also being inserted by the interventional radiology service with the use of ultrasound image guidance. Totally implanted devices or ports consist of a reservoir implanted in a subcutaneous pocket connected to a silicone catheter placed in a central vein.

Despite the fact that the central VAD has greatly improved the quality of care received by pediatric oncology patients, these devices are not without the potential for complications, including pneumothorax, hemothorax, arterial perforation, air embolism, nerve injury, catheter malposition, infection, and occlusion or thrombosis.

The most common complications of these devices are infection and occlusion. The incidence of intravascular catheter infection varies considerably by type of catheter, frequency of catheter manipulation, and patient-related factors (e.g., underlying disease and acuity of illness). The majority of serious catheter-related infections are associated with CVCs (O'Grady et al. 2002). Migration of organisms from the patient's skin or from the hub or port of the catheter into the intravascular part of the catheter are the most common cause of catheter-related blood stream infections (CR-BSI) (Crnich and Maki 2002; Raad et al. 2007). Organisms that frequently cause CR-BSI are coagulase-negative staphylococci followed by enterococci. Antibiotic ointments (e.g., bacitracin, mupirocin, neomycin, and polymixin) should not be applied to catheter insertion sites, as they have the potential to promote fungal infections and antimicrobial resistance (Zakrzewska-Bode et al. 1995). Indicators that reduce the incidence of catheter-related bloodstream infections are:

1. Implementation of educational programs that include didactic and interactive components for those who insert and maintain catheters
2. Use of maximal sterile barrier precautions during catheter placement
3. Use of chlorhexidine for skin antisepsis

4. Removal of the catheter when it is no longer required for treatment (O'Grady et al. 2002)
5. Heparin-coated or antibiotic-impregnated CVCs (Gilbert and Harden 2008) (However, a large randomized controlled clinical trial needs to be done to determine which of these are more effective.)
6. Antibiotic impregnated biopatches have also been effective in reducing CR-BSI

Catheter occlusions can be intermittent, sluggish, partial, or complete/total and can result from several different mechanisms. Patency may be affected by anatomical obstruction due to compression of the catheter between the first rib and clavicle or by improper catheter tip placement. Occlusion may also result from precipitation caused by the administration of incompatible drugs or infusates; however, this is a less common cause.

The most common cause of catheter occlusion is thrombus formation within the lumen of the catheter, in the portal reservoir, or at the catheter tip. There are many factors that put patients at risk for catheter-related thrombosis. Improper catheter tip placement, site of insertion, and suboptimal catheter care as well as diseases such as malignancies, infections, diabetes, and end-stage renal failure have been associated with increased risk of thrombus formation (Yacopetti 2008). Venous stasis, hypercoagulability, and local trauma of the intima of the vein wall are also contributing factors to the development of catheter thrombosis. The majority of thrombi causing central catheter occlusion develop without symptoms. Warning signs of catheter malfunction are most often recognized by an experienced clinician. The incidence of catheter thrombosis has been reported as high as 31% despite routine flushing with heparin or saline (Bagnall et al. 1989). Catheter occlusions due to the formation of a thrombus are treated by instilling a thrombolytic agent. Currently, recombinant tissue plasminogen activator (rt-PA) or alteplase is used to restore patency to occluded catheters. Rt-PA is a fibrin-specific thrombolytic agent produced through recombinant DNA technology. The optimal rt-PA dose, solution volume, and dwell time for the clearance of thrombosed CVCs is using a 1 mg/mL concentration and instilling a volume equal to the internal volume of the catheter. The dwell time is 60–120 min. The rt-PA should be aspirated out of catheter. For the persistent occlusion, this dose may be repeated once. Clinical experience has demonstrated that increasing the dwell time (e.g., allowing the rt-PA to remain in the catheter overnight) has also had success for persistent occlusions.

Two common complications associated with the use of VADs, infection and occlusion, can be diminished by adhering to institutional protocols for catheter insertion, catheter site dressings, and drug and fluid administration. However, compliance with catheter care regimens also needs to occur in the home care setting. Standardization of line care between the treating institution and the home care agency is key to reducing confusion and anxiety in the child and family. Teaching is based on the educational level of the child and parents as well as on their preferred methods of learning.

12.5 Future Perspectives

12.5.1 New Surgical Techniques and Directions for Future Research

The past decade has brought significant changes to the surgical management of the child with cancer. Currently, pediatric surgical oncology has become extremely complex, requiring advanced technical skills using newly developed equipment. Minimally invasive surgery (MIS) is an example of one of the most recent additions to the surgical armamentarium. MIS is used for a variety of abdominal and thoracic procedures and describes a surgical procedure accomplished with instruments directed through cannulas. The advantages of MIS for certain types of operations include smaller wound size, less tissue exposure, and minimal tissue and organ manipulation. Because the body's response to MIS is different from its response to open surgical procedures, there is less stress imposed on the body, postoperative pain is decreased, and respiratory management and activity restrictions are also decreased. Examples of MIS include, but are not limited to, fundoplication, colon pull-through for Hirschsprung's disease, splenectomy, and thoracoscopic procedures.

The surgical oncology team now includes not only physicians and nurses but also scientists, computer specialists, and bioengineers. This is critical as new surgical procedures and devices are directed by computer technology, which includes robotics. This type of procedure allows surgeons to control robotic instruments through remote computer consoles. Several types of surgical robotic systems have been developed that allow the performance of surgery with a higher degree of accuracy than that capable by human hands (Bagnall-Reeb and Perry 2002). For pediatric surgical oncology, the implications of this new technology are immense. Robotic surgery offers the prospect of performing complex resections with much less tissue trauma. Similarly, surgeons who are specialists in a particular tumor type will be able to perform surgical procedures from afar.

Radiofrequency ablation (RFA) is another example of minimally invasive treatment aimed at heating and destroying cancer cells. Imaging techniques such as ultrasound, CT scan, and magnetic resonance imaging (MRI) are used to help guide a needle electrode into a cancerous tumor. High-frequency electrical currents are passed through the electrode providing ionic vibration and heat in the surrounding tissues to destroy abnormal cells. RFA is not intended to replace surgery, chemotherapy, or radiation therapy, but may be effective for the patient who is a poor surgical candidate or for quality of life issues.

Today, the surgeon administers vital services in the care of children and adolescents with malignant disease. Managing vascular access and its complications, as well as providing supportive care and appropriate intervention for medical complications of chemotherapy, have become the standards for the modern pediatric surgical oncologist. Advances in surgical devices and technology have given pediatric nurses an active role and opportunity to manage these complex patients.

References

Bagnall-Reeb H, Perry S (2002) Surgery. In: Rasco Baggott C, Patterson Kelly K, Fochtman D, Foley GV (eds) Nursing care of children and adolescents with cancer, 3rd edn. Saunders, Philadelphia, pp 91–115

Bagnall HA, Gomperts E, Atkinson JB (1989) Continuous infusion of low-dose urokinase in the treatment of central venous catheter thrombosis in infants and children. Pediatrics 83(6):963–966

Cotton CA, Peterson S, Norkool PA, Takashima J, Grigoriev Y, Breslow NE (2009) Early and late mortality after diagnosis of Wilms tumor. Journal of Clinical Oncology 27(8):1304–1309

Crnich CJ, Maki DG (2002) The promise of novel technology for the prevention of intravascular device-related bloodstream infection. II. Long-term devices. Clinical Infectious Diseases 34(10):1362–1368

Gilbert RE, Harden M (2008) Effectiveness of impregnated central venous catheters for catheter related blood stream infection: a systematic review. Current Opinion in Infectious Diseases 21(3):235–245

Green DM (2004) The treatment of stages I-IV favorable histology Wilms' tumor. Journal of Clinical Oncology 22(8):1366–1372

Grosfeld JL (2006) Neuroblastoma. In: Grosfeld JL, O'Neill JA, Fonkalsrud EW, Coran AG (eds) Pediatric surgery, vol 1. Mosby, Elsevier, Philadelphia, pp 467–494

La Quaglia MP, Su WT (2006) Hodgkin's disease and non-hodgkin's lymphoma. In: Grosfeld JL, O'Neill JA, Fonkalsrud EW, Coran AG (eds) Pediatric surgery, vol 1. Mosby, Elsevier, Philadelphia, pp 575–592

Leonard M (2002) Diagnostic evaluations and staging procedures. In: Rasco Baggott C, Patterson Kelly K, Fochtman D, Foley GV (eds) Nursing care of children and adolescents with cancer, 3rd edn. Saunders, Philadelphia, pp 66–89

Nichols R (2000) Guideline for prevention of surgical site infection. Bulletin of the American College of Surgeons 85(7):23–29

O'Grady NP, Alexander M, Dellinger EP, Gerberding JL, Heard SO, Maki DG et al (2002) Guidelines for the prevention of intravascular catheter-related infections. The Hospital Infection Control Practices Advisory Committee, Center for Disese Control and Prevention, U.S. Pediatrics 110(5):e51

Raad I, Hanna H, Maki D (2007) Intravascular catheter-related infections: advances in diagnosis, prevention, and management. The Lancet Infectious Diseases 7(10):645–657

Yacopetti N (2008) Central venous catheter-related thrombosis: a systematic review. Journal of Infusion Nursing 31(4):241–248

Zakrzewska-Bode A, Muytjens HL, Liem KD, Hoogkamp-Korstanje JA (1995) Mupirocin resistance in coagulase-negative staphylococci, after topical prophylaxis for the reduction of colonization of central venous catheters. Journal of Hospital Infection 31(3):189–193

Zierold D, Lee SL, Subramanian S, DuBois JJ (2000) Supplemental oxygen improves resolution of injury-induced pneumothorax. Journal of Pediatric Surgery 35(6):998–1001

Cell and Gene Therapy

Robbie Norville

Contents

13.1 Introduction 277
13.2 Principles of Treatment 278
13.2.1 Genetic Deficit Repair 278
13.2.2 Viral-Mediated Gene Transfer 278
13.2.3 Drug-Resistant Genes 278
13.2.4 Angiogenetics Inhibitors 279
13.2.5 Gene Marking 279
13.2.6 Cell Therapy 279
13.3 Method of Delivery 279
13.3.1 Viral Vectors 280
13.3.2 Plasmid Vectors 280
13.4 Potential Side Effects 280
13.5 Special Considerations 281
13.6 Future Perspectives 281
References 281

13.1 Introduction

Cell and Gene therapies are novel additions to the current multimodal approach of chemotherapy, radiation, surgery, and hematopoietic stem cell transplant (HSCT) for the treatment of pediatric cancers. The manipulation of genes and the immune system can treat cancer and prevent genetic diseases as well as increase the body's ability to receive intense treatment that would be impossible otherwise. Humans have between 30,000 and 40,000 genes (National Cancer Institute 2009). A gene is a stretch of the DNA molecule and is the basic unit of heredity. Genes determine traits such as height, hair, and eye color. Genes also carry the instructions that allow cells to produce specific proteins that have certain functions in the body. The pattern of active and inactive genes in a cell and the resulting protein composition determine the type of cell and its capabilities. Genes that protect against cancer are referred to as tumor suppressor genes. Mutated genes that are capable of causing cancer when expressed at the wrong sequence are known as oncogenes.

Although the last 50 years of cancer-directed therapy (i.e., radiation and chemotherapy) have targeted cells that divide, it has become apparent that cancer therapy may be more effective if therapy is directed at the abnormal, mutated genes and their signaling pathways. The first gene therapy clinical trial was conducted in 1990 on two children with adenosine deaminase (ADA) deficiency (Blaese 1993). Gene therapy is being evaluated with the hope of curing a host of monogenic diseases (e.g., cystic fibrosis, severe combined immunodeficiency, muscular dystrophy, and hemophilia) and multigenic diseases (e.g., cancer, cardiovascular disease, chronic granulomatous disease, and multiple sclerosis) (Rubanyi 2001). One of the major goals of gene therapy is to supply cells with healthy copies of missing or altered genes or proteins. Even though more than 1,000 clinical protocols for gene therapy have been approved, it remains an experimental therapy, with limited success thus far. Therapeutic applications of gene therapy include gene transfer (repair), prodrug metabolizing enzyme gene therapy, drug-resistance gene therapy, angiogenesis, gene marking, and immunotherapy (Gottschalk et al 2006).

Cell therapy involves the administration of autologous or allogeneic cells for a therapeutic effect. These therapies include stem cell transplantation and strategies for manipulating or modulating the patients' immune status, such as vaccines, and adoptive transfer of modified T-cells (Gottschalk et al. 2006).

13.2 Principles of Treatment

There are multiple strategies used for incorporating cell and gene therapy into cancer treatment.

13.2.1 Genetic Deficit Repair

The tumor cell itself can be modified, either by repairing one or more of the genetic defects associated with the malignant process or by introducing a gene that triggers an antitumor response. An example of genetic defect repair includes reintroducing key regulatory genes that have become dysfunctional in the tumor, such as p53, whose normal function is to prevent abnormal (cancer) cells from dividing. Another approach is downregulating oncogenes that typically stimulate tumor formation by inserting genetic material that blocks the transcription, processing, or translation of RNA from the oncogene, thus disrupting tumor growth. This strategy is hindered by the polyclonal nature of most pediatric cancers since transducing the majority of tumor cells is not possible with the vectors currently available (High and Brenner 2005).

13.2.2 Viral-Mediated Gene Transfer

The tumor can be injected with a suicide gene encoded to kill tumor cells when instructed. This transfer of a pro-drug metabolizing enzyme therapy involves the insertion of genes into tumor cells that encode enzymes able to convert harmless prodrugs into lethal cytotoxins. In this approach, the tumor is injected directly with a vector carrying the herpes simplex virus-1 thymidine kinase (TK). Ganciclovir, a nucleoside analog, is then administered intravenously to the patient and the expressed TK phosphorylates the ganciclovir within the tumor cells. The resulting nucleotide analog is a potent inhibitor of deoxyribonucleic acid (DNA) synthesis and causes the death of the dividing tumor cells. Normal cells exposed to ganciclovir will not be affected as TK expression is required for activation. However, "bystander effect" can occur when neighboring tumor cells that have not taken up the transgene are also killed. This effect likely occurs when channels between cells, known as gap junctions, allow the toxic metabolite to spread to neighboring cells, thus destroying them. This approach has been used in phase I therapies for patients with retinoblastoma and supratentorial brain tumors (High and Brenner 2005; Wilson 2002).

13.2.3 Drug-Resistant Genes

To enhance chemotherapy, modification of the drug sensitivity of normal host tissue allows delivery of cytotoxic drug-resistant genes to marrow progenitor cells. The most widely known drug-resistant gene is the multidrug-resistant-1 gene (High and Brenner 2005). Once inserted, this gene acts as a drug-efflux pump and prevents the accumulation of small toxic molecules, including a range of cytotoxic drugs. The transfer of drug-resistant genes into hematopoietic progenitor cells exerts a protective effect by attenuating drug-induced myelosuppression. Other drug-resistant genes are being investigated, including dihydrofolate reductase, which rescues patients from toxicity following methotrexate, and the bacterial nitroreductase, which protects patients from side effects related to thiotepa (High and Brenner 2005; Gottschalk et al. 2006).

13.2.4 Angiogenetics Inhibitors

Angiogenesis, the formation of new blood vessels supplying needed nutrients and oxygen, is required for tumor growth and metastasis. A number of antiangiogenic proteins have been found that block new blood vessel formation, thus inhibiting tumor growth. Several agents currently under study that could produce antiangiogenesis suitable for gene therapy approaches include endostatin, angiostatin, thrombospondin-1, and uPA-fragment. Endostatin gene transfer in mouse models has been successful in suppression of endothelial cell proliferation and antitumor effects in several human solid tumors. Although much is yet to be learned about the delivery of angiogenesis inhibition, gene therapy could allow a continued delivery of drug rather than the more conventional peak and trough delivery of current drug therapies (Biagi et al. 2003; Rubanyi 2001; Wilson 2002).

13.2.5 Gene Marking

Gene marking of hematopoietic progenitor cells provides information that can be useful to improve therapeutic options using autologous stem cell transplantation. Additionally, gene marking has been used to investigate cancer biology and normal bone marrow reconstitution, evaluating ways to enhance immune reconstitution and determining the sources of relapse after stem cell (Biagi et al. 2003).

13.2.6 Cell Therapy

The immune response to a tumor can be modified by altering the specificity or effector function of immune system cells. Immunotherapy refers to any approach designed to enhance the immune system's ability to fight diseases. Adoptive immunotherapy, including vaccines and donor lymphocyte infusions, offer strategies for generating immune responses to inadequately presented tumor-associated antigens or for boosting the existing immune responses to eradicate malignant cells. Tumors are able to grow in part because the immune system fails to recognize them as abnormal. Two strategies that have been implemented are to insert genes into the tumor cells, acting like large neon signs that help the immune system "see" the tumor, and to introduce genes into the immune cells so that they are better able to detect the tumor. Tumor vaccine studies may enhance immune recognition of tumors with poor immunogenicity. Transduced tumor cells are being used in vaccines as adjuvant therapy to prevent relapse in patients with presumed minimal residual disease. Thus far, these vaccines have been evaluated in over 300 clinical trials with few side effects. Vaccine trials for neuroblastoma have used both autologous and allogeneic transduced cells. Autologous vaccine trials have demonstrated an increased frequency of tumor-specific cytotoxic T-lymphocytes (CTLs) and have provided a mixed response of disease stabilization in patients with advanced disease. Subsequent allogeneic vaccine studies for neuroblastoma demonstrated that the use of two stimulating agents at different phases of the immune response may be superior to a single agent approach. Combining two agents to act at different phases of T-cell activation is being evaluated in pediatric and adult high-risk acute leukemias (High and Brenner 2005).

Another example of adoptive transfer is the use of CTLs generated in the laboratory that are directed against viral or tumor antigens. Clinical studies have demonstrated the feasibility and safety of administering Epstein–Barr virus (EBV) CTLs to prevent and treat Epstein–Barr virus-lymphoproliferative disease (EBV-LPD) that can occur following allogeneic transplant or solid organ transplant. These CTLs also have been evaluated in pediatric patients with EBV-positive Hodgkin's disease and nasopharyngeal carcinoma (Gottschalk et al. 2006). To improve on this concept, clinical trials are currently evaluating CTLs that recognize multiple antigens expressed on the tumor cells, thereby improving the effectiveness of CTL therapy and minimizing tumor cell evasion.

13.3 Method of Delivery

Gene therapy is a multicomplex biological process. It begins with the introduction of an appropriate vector (carrier) for a single gene or genetic material into the body either locally by direct injection or into the blood circulation, which provides systemic delivery. Once the vector finds the target tissue, it enters the target cell, travels through the cytoplasm, and enters the cell nucleus. The therapeutic transgene is then transcribed into therapeutic proteins. These proteins act on receptors either on the cell that produced it, on neighboring cells, or at distant sites after entering the blood circulation. An appropriate biological effect can then occur after the proteins interact with receptors (Rubanyi 2001).

Several methods of delivering genes into cells have been developed, including transfer via viruses, plasmids, tumor cells, and immune system cells.

13.3.1 Viral Vectors

Viral vectors use the inherent ability of viruses to carry foreign genetic material into cells. Viruses that are used for gene transfer are first modified to remove the replication genes of that virus. Viral-based vectors are the most frequently used mode of delivery of genetic material into cells and this process is called viral transduction. Examples of viral vectors are the adenovirus (AV), the adeno-associated virus (AAV), and the herpes-simplex virus (HSV). In addition, other viral and nonviral vectors that can achieve similar functions are also being tested. Examples of nonviral vectors include liposomes and plasmid DNA (naked chunks of DNA). The use of these natural vectors, all of which demonstrate significant ability to infect human cells, requires specialized knowledge in terms of how to inactivate them from causing human disease before transducing them into patients (Rubanyi 2001; Wilson 2002).

The most widely used vector system in cancer gene therapy has been the replication-incompetent recombinant AV. AVs are respiratory tropic viruses with a double-strand DNA genome and a naked protein capsid coat. Recombinant vectors have been created by genomic deletion of viral gene functions involved in replication and provision of these functions by a packaging cell line (Zhang 1999). The deleted gene regions then can be replaced with expression cassettes containing the desired gene under the control of general or tumor-specific promoters. This vector system offers a number of advantages, including high-efficiency transduction in a wide range of target cells (including nondividing cells) and high expression levels of the delivered transgene (Yeh and Perricaudet 1997).

The most common viruses used as vectors in pediatric oncology gene therapy are AAV and HV.

13.3.2 Plasmid Vectors

Plasmid vectors are small particles of raw DNA. The advantage of using plasmids is that there is less chance of the patient becoming infected by a virus particle that regenerates the ability to become infectious. However, the use of plasmids are often limited to skin cancer, where they can be delivered directly and easily to the patient's cancer cells.

13.4 Potential Side Effects

Gene therapy continues to require consideration of the potential risks and benefits. Current vector systems may need to be modified, and additional efforts are required to better understand the biology of the diseases that are viable for therapeutic genetic intervention. This information will enable risk classifications for specific vectors and transgenes, as well as assessment of the risk factors that are unique to each clinical trial. With this approach, the therapeutic potential of somatic gene transfer may be realized through the application of appropriate prevention strategies (Williams and Baum 2003).

Some of the potential side effects of gene therapy include viruses infecting more than one type of cell, being inserted in the wrong location in the DNA (for example, in the middle of a critical gene), and possibly causing cancer or other cellular damage. Other concerns include the possibility that the transferred genes could be "over expressed," producing so much of the missing protein as to be harmful, resulting in inflammation or immune reaction as well as the slight chance of introducing the genetic material into the patient's reproductive cells (National Cancer Institute 2009). The development of T-cell leukemia has now been reported in 5 of 17 patients who were successfully cured of their primary immune disorder. Of these patients, four achieved remission after treatment with chemotherapy (Hacein-Bey-Abina et al. 2008; Howe et al. 2008; Fischer and Cavazzana-Calvo 2008).

The most frequently observed side effect associated with tumor vaccines is inflammation at the injection site. Vaccine trials in adults are combining specific tumor cells with IL-2 and side effects with these vaccines are similar to those observed in patients receiving biotherapy (e.g., chills, fever, flu-like symptoms) (National Cancer Institute 2009).

13.5 Special Considerations

Given the nature of this approach, many regulatory bodies oversee the design and conduct of gene therapy trials. In the UK, the Gene Therapy Advisory Committee (GTAC) has ethical oversight of gene therapy protocols. They work with other government agencies including the Medicines and Healthcare products Regulatory Agency (MHRA), the Health and Safety Executive (HSE), and the Human Tissue Authority (HTA). In the USA, gene therapy protocols must be approved by the U.S. Food and Drug Administration (FDA), which regulates all gene therapy products. In addition, trials that are funded by the National Institute of Health (NIH) must be registered with the NIH Recombinant DNA Advisory Committee (RAC) (National Cancer Institute 2009).

Nurses must be knowledgeable about the clinical trial, treatment schema, potential toxicities, and symptom management, as monitoring and documenting short- and long-term toxicities is essential. An understanding of genetics and its relationship to cancer and gene therapy are needed to enable explanation of the purpose, procedures, limitations, and risks associated with cell and gene therapy. Nurses should have an appreciation of the ethical, social, and cultural concerns associated with gene therapy and be aware of the specific implications these have for staff and patients participating in these clinical trials.

13.6 Future Perspectives

Gene therapy is a new approach to treating children with cancer, and despite some recent setbacks, it holds significant promise for the future. Scientists have made great progress in the last decade in understanding the molecular architecture of viruses used for gene therapy, and based on these advances, more sophisticated vectors have been designed. The progress is hopeful; however, there remains a need for continued advancement in this field.

In addition to identifying disease-specific risk factors, there are three ways to limit the possible deleterious side effects of genetic interventions: The first is to develop vectors with improved safety profiles, including a reduced propensity for insertional "genotoxicity." The second is to define "safe integration sites" in the genome and to design integration vectors that are targeted to these sites (Nienhuis 2008). The third is to reduce the number of vector-exposed cells (and thus vector integrations) that are infused into the patient; for example, by correcting a very small number of stem cells ex vivo and genetically characterizing them before they are infused back into the patient (Williams and Baum 2003).

Gene therapy is still in the early phases despite the fact that it has been an area of research and clinical trials since 1990. It is hoped that although barriers and challenges remain, gene therapy will be FDA-approved and offer successful cancer treatment and reduce the impact that the disease has on pediatric patients. Gene transfer is already being used successfully to complement conventional therapies for malignant disorders, and cancer vaccines are still in development and are being tested in clinical trials against various diseases. However, the benefits of these new technologies can only increase as current limitations are progressively, albeit slowly, surmounted (High and Brenner 2005).

References

Biagi E, Bollard C, Rousseau R, Brenner M (2003) Gene therapy for pediatric cancer: state of the art and future perspectives. Journal of Biomedicine and Biotechnology 1:13–24

Blaese RM (1993) Development of gene therapy for immunodeficiency: adenosine deaminase deficiency. Pediatric Research 33(1 Suppl):S49–S53

Fischer A and Cavazzana-Calvo M (2008) Gene therapy of inherited diseases. Lancet 371:2044–2047

Gottschalk S, Rooney C, Brenner M (2006) Cell and gene therapies. In: Pizzo P, Poplack D (eds) Principles and practice of pediatric oncology, 5th edn. Lippincott Williams & Wilkins, Philadelphia, pp 433–451

Hacein-Bey-Abina S, Garrigue A, Wang G, Soulier J, Lim A, Morillon E, Clappier E, Caccavelli L, Delabesse E, Beldjord K, Asnafi V, MacIntyre E, Dal Cortivo L, Radford I, Brousse N, Sigaux F, Moshous D, Hauer J, Borkhardt A, Belohradsky B, Wintergerst U, Velez M, Leiva L, Sorensen R, Wulffraat N, Blanche S, Bushman F, Fischer A, Cavazzana-Calvo M (2008) Insertional oncogenesis in 4 patients after retrovirus-mediated gene therapy of SCID-X1. Journal of Clinical Investigation 118:3132–3142

High K, Brenner M (2005) Gene transfer for hematologic disorders. In: Hoffman R, Benz E, Shattil S, Furie B, Cohen H, Silberstein L, McGlave P (eds) Hematology: basic principles and practice, 4th edn. Elsevier, Philadelphia, pp 1829–1841

Howe S, Mansour M, Schwarzwaelder K, Bartholomae C, Hubank M, Kempski H, Brugman M, Pike-Overzet K, Chatters S, de Ridder D, Gilmour K, Adams S, Thornhill S, Parsley K, Staal F, Gale R, Linch D, Bayford J, Brown L, Quaye M, Kinnon C, Ancliff P, Webb D, Schmidt M, von Kalle C, Gaspar H, Thrasher A (2008) Insertional mutagenesis combined with acquired somatic mutations causes leukemogenesis following gene therapy of SCID-X1 patients. Journal of Clinical Investigation 118:3143–3150

National Cancer Institute (2009) Gene therapy for cancer: questions and answers. http://www.cancer.gov/cancertopics/factsheet/Therapies/gen. Accessed 18 March 2009

Nienhuis AW (2008) Development of gene therapy for blood disorders. Blood 111(9):4431–4444

Rubanyi G (2001) The future of human gene therapy. Molecular Aspects of Medicine 22:113–142

Williams D, Baum C (2003) Gene therapy: new challenges ahead. Science 302:400–401

Wilson D (2002) Viral-mediated gene transfer for cancer treatment. Current Pharmaceutical Biotechnology 3:151–164

Yeh P, Perricaudet M (1997) Advances in adenoviral vectors: from genetic engineering to their biology. The FASEB Journal 11:615–623

Zhang WW (1999) Development and application of adenoviral vectors for gene therapy of cancer. Cancer Gene Therapy 6:113–138

Biological and Targeted Therapies

Lindsay Gainer

Contents

14.1 Introduction . . . 283
14.2 Principles of Treatment . . . 284
14.3 Description of Treatment . . . 285
14.3.1 Cytokines . . . 285
14.3.2 Interferons . . . 285
14.3.3 Interleukins . . . 286
14.3.4 Colony-stimulating Factors . . . 286
14.3.5 Fusion Proteins . . . 286
14.3.6 Monoclonal Antibodies . . . 287
14.4 Cancer Vaccines . . . 288
14.5 Other Immunomodulating Agents . . . 288
14.5.1 Nonspecific Immunomodulating Agents . . . 288
14.5.2 Retinoids . . . 289
14.5.3 Thalidomide . . . 289
14.6 Adoptive Immunotherapy . . . 289
14.7 Molecular Targeted Therapy . . . 289
14.8 Method of Delivery . . . 290
14.9 Potential Side Effects . . . 291
14.10 Future Perspectives . . . 292
References . . . 293

14.1 Introduction

Biotherapy and molecular targeted therapies are innovative methods of treatment for cancer and have recently become standard modalities for pediatric oncology, both alone and as adjuvants to other modalities such as surgery, radiation, and chemotherapy. Biotherapy uses the body's immune system, either directly or indirectly, to attack malignant cells or to minimize the side effects caused by traditional cancer treatments. Biotherapy is designed to repair, stimulate, or enhance the immune response.

Biotherapy is also called *biologic(al) therapy* or *immunotherapy* and the agents used are called *biological response modifiers* (BRMs). Targeted therapy involves the administration of biotherapeutic agents that selectively inhibit molecules associated with specific cell-signaling pathways involved in the development and progression of cancer. These agents stop tumor growth and progression by acting on growth factors and cell membrane receptors that control signaling pathways which regulate cell proliferation, apoptosis, angiogenesis, adhesion, and motility (Battiato and Wheeler 2005; National Cancer Institute 2006).

The pioneer of biotherapy was Coley, a bone surgeon in the early 1900s. Coley noted that postoperative infections in sarcoma patients seemed to reduce the incidence of tumor recurrence. Based on his observations, he used the bacterial toxins erysipelas and *Bacillus prodigious* to stimulate an immune response in patients with sarcoma. Patients who received the toxins with surgery or radiation had an improved outcome (Coley 1933).

In the past 25 years, there has been an increase in the understanding of immunology, cell-signaling pathways, and technologies to develop agents that mimic the body's defense and surveillance systems (Battiato and Wheeler 2005; Burks and McCune 2007; Fry and Lankester 2008). Scientific advances, such as the discovery and understanding of deoxyribonucleic acid (DNA), the discovery of interferon, the discovery of link between cancer and angiogenesis, and the development of hybridoma technology, opened the possibilities for the use of biotherapy and targeted therapies in cancer treatment (Battiato and Wheeler 2005; Burks and McCune 2007).

14.2 Principles of Treatment

The foundation of biotherapy is the immune response. To understand biotherapy, comprehension of innate and adaptive immunity is required:

- *Innate* immune response is mediated by myeloid cells (monocytes, macrophages, neutrophils, basophils, and eosinophils) and provides rapid, nonspecific protection.
- *Adaptive* immunity is mediated by lymphocytes and provides a slower immune response, but allows for antigen-specific recognition and memory.

Most biotherapy is focused on stimulating the *adaptive* immune response (Fry and Lankester 2008). The theory behind this focus is that adaptive immunity includes surveillance activity that can prevent the development of cancer or halt tumor growth (Rescigno et al. 2007).

The immune cells that are the most pertinent to biotherapy are B lymphocytes, T lymphocytes (cytotoxic and helper), natural killer (NK) cells, and dendritic cells (DCs). B cells mature into plasma cells that secrete antibodies, which recognize and attach to specific antigens. CD8+ cytotoxic T-cells release cytotoxins that directly attack infected, foreign, or cancerous cells and cause apoptosis. CD4+ helper T-cells regulate the immune response by releasing messenger proteins called cytokines to signal other immune cells to mount a response (National Cancer Institute 2006). NK cells are lymphocytes that have the potential to recognize and eliminate a wide range of tumors and virally infected cells. NK cells may have a dual function in the antitumor response as both direct effector cells and as initiators of the T-cell-mediated antitumor response (Fry and Lankester 2008). DCs are a crucial link between innate and adaptive immunity. DCs are antigen-presenting cells (APCs) and initiate the adaptive immune response (Fry and Lankester 2008). They respond to "danger signals," inflammatory substances produced by the innate immune response, by increasing their immune-inducing capacity. It also seems that DCs are able to sense and respond differently to the mode of cell death (Zwierzina 2008).

Molecular targeted therapies require an understanding of cell biology at the molecular level, and the differences between normal and malignant cells. These therapies are based on tumor biology and act on the cell-signaling pathways that control cancer cell growth and proliferation. Cell signaling is the communication of growth signals from outside of the cell to the nucleus of the cell. This complex system is made up of multiple cascades and chemical signals. The pathways are initiated by growth factors released by other cells that bind to cell surface receptors. This in turn activates those receptors, and this triggers multiple events eventually resulting in cell growth and division (Battiato and Wheeler 2005).

Tyrosine kinases (TKs), a class of these growth factor receptors, are key regulators of the cell-signaling process. Receptor TKs have a major role in cellular proliferation, migration, metabolism, differentiation, and survival. When alterations or mutations occur in receptor TKs, they become powerful oncoproteins (proteins associated with tumor cell growth). Abnormal activation of receptor TKs has been shown to be involved in many cancers. Altered TK activity both inhibits apoptosis and promotes tumor invasion, metastasis, and angiogenesis. One of the first receptor TKs to be discovered was the epidermal growth factor receptor (EGFR). EGFR was later found to be part of a family of receptors called the HER family, which are overexpressed or dysregulated in several types of solid tumors. Other TKs linked to cancers that have been discovered to date are BCR-ABL, platelet-derived growth factor receptor (PDGFR), and KIT (Battiato and Wheeler 2005).

Other targeted therapies are directed toward additional cell-signaling enzymes and growth factors, such as proteasomes and factors involved in angiogenesis. Proteasomes are involved in the cell cycle, angiogenesis, cell adhesion, cytokine production, and apoptosis. Basic fibroblast growth factor (bFGF), acidic fibroblast growth factor (aFGF), and vascular endothelial growth factor (VEGF) are growth factors that have been identified as crucial regulator in angiogenesis. Angiogenesis is the process of blood vessel formation. Judah Folkman was the first to hypothesize that tumor growth was dependent on angiogenesis in 1971 (Battiato and Wheeler 2005; Camp-Sorrell 2003).

In summary, biotherapy and targeted therapies manipulate the immune response and cell-signaling pathways in a variety of ways that are beneficial in cancer treatment. The mechanisms of action of biologic and molecular targeted therapies include:

- Stopping, controlling, or suppressing processes that permit cancer growth
- Making malignant cells more recognizable and more susceptible to destruction
- Enhancing the cytotoxic immune response of T-cells, NK-cells, and macrophages
- Altering the replication of cancer cells to promote behavior like that of healthy cells
- Blocking or reversing the process that changes a normal cell into a malignant cell
- Improving the ability to repair or replace cells damaged or destroyed by other forms of cancer treatment, such as chemotherapy or radiation
- Preventing metastases (National Cancer Institute 2006)

14.3 Description of Treatment

Biotherapy for oncology includes the use of cytokines (interferons (IFN), interleukins (IL), and colony-stimulating factors (CSFs)), monoclonal antibodies (MoAbs), cancer vaccines, other immunomodulating agents, and adoptive immunotherapy. Targeted therapies include TK inhibitors or MoAbs for receptor TKs, proteasome inhibitors, and angiogenesis inhibitors.

14.3.1 Cytokines

Cytokines are small signaling proteins that mediate and regulate immunity, inflammation, and hematopoiesis. They are secreted by cells to activate and recruit immune cells to increase the immune response. Cytokines act by binding to a specific cell-surface receptor. The receptor then signals the cell via second messengers, often TKs, to change the function of the cell by altering gene expression. Responses to cytokines include upregulation and/or downregulation of genes and their transcription factors, resulting in the production of other cytokines, and increasing or decreasing expression of membrane proteins, including cytokine receptors. Cytokines may act on the cells that secrete them (autocrine action), on nearby cells (paracrine action), or on distant cells (endocrine action) (Decker 2006).

Cytokines are used in biotherapy to enhance antitumor immune responses and regulate hematopoiesis. Cytokines are classed by family as IL, chemokines, tumor necrosis factors (TNF), IFN, and CSFs based on their function, cell of secretion, or target of action. Because T and B lymphocytes communicate with other immune cells by the secretion of cytokines and expression of surface molecules, administration of cytokines to patients can enhance their immune response. NK cell activation and cytolytic potential can also be increased with various cytokines, including IL and IFN (Fry and Lankester 2008). The most common cytokines used in the treatment of cancer are IFN, IL, and CSFs.

14.3.2 Interferons

IFN were the first cytokines produced for use in biotherapy (National Cancer Institute 2006). Three classes of IFN have been identified: α-IFN (derived from leukocytes), β-IFN (derived from fibroblasts), and γ-IFN (derived from T-lymphocytes) (Burks and McCune 2007). IFN produced using recombinant DNA technologies have been FDA approved for the treatment of several diseases including AIDS-related Kaposi's sarcoma, hairy cell leukemia, chronic myelogenous leukemia (CML), malignant melanoma, hepatitis B and C, genital warts, multiple sclerosis, chronic granulomatous disease, and osteopetrosis.

Studies have shown that interferon alpha may also be effective in treating other cancers such as renal cell carcinoma and non-Hodgkin's lymphoma (National Cancer Institute 2006).

14.3.3 Interleukins

IL function as messengers between cells of the immune system to assist in distinguishing and fighting cancer cells. Many IL have been identified, but IL-2 (Aldesleukin, Proleukin) has been the most widely studied in oncology. IL-2 stimulates the growth and activity of many lymphocytes, such as T-cells and NK cells that can destroy cancer cells. The FDA has approved IL-2 for the treatment of metastatic renal cell carcinoma and metastatic melanoma. Ongoing research is investigating the usefulness of IL to treat a number of other cancers, including leukemia, lymphoma, and brain, colorectal, ovarian, breast, and prostate cancers (National Cancer Institute 2006).

14.3.4 Colony-stimulating Factors

CSFs also called *hematopoietic growth factors*, are another type of cytokine used in cancer treatment. CSFs support hematopoiesis and are used for supportive care to expedite recovery from bone marrow suppression. The use of hematopoietic growth factors has improved cancer treatment because higher doses of chemotherapy and radiation can be administered without increasing the risk of infection or the need for transfusions. Examples of CSFs used in pediatric oncology include:

- Granulocyte-CSF (G-CSF) stimulates the bone marrow to produce neutrophils. The FDA approved a recombinant variant of G-CSF (filgrastim or Neupogen) in 1991 for controlling infections in patients receiving myelosuppressive therapy, in patients undergoing bone-marrow transplantation, and in patients with neutropenia. A long-acting version of G-CSF (pegfilgrastim or Neulasta) was approved in 2002 for use in adult patients.
- Granulocyte-macrophage CSF (GM-CSF) stimulates the bone marrow to produce neutrophils and macrophages. The FDA approved the recombinant equivalent of GM-CSF (sargramostim or Leukine) in 1991 for neutropenia after bone marrow transplant. Recently, GM-CSF has been studied for its ability to stimulate DCs, which play an important role in coordinating the immune tumor response. GM-CSF may have other antitumor properties such as enhancing monocytes, which have tumoricidal activity against some cancers; allowing DCs to enhance antibody-dependent cellular cytotoxicity (ADCC), and possibly inhibiting the angiogenic process of solid tumors (Buchsel and DeMeyer 2006).
- Erythropoietin (Epo) stimulates the bone marrow to increase red blood cell production. The first recombinant Epo (Procrit, Epogen) was FDA approved in 1989. A longer acting version of Epo that is administered weekly, darbepoetin alfa (Aranesp) was approved in 2002 for oncology patients with anemia secondary to chemotherapy and appears to be safe and effective in children in preventing and treating anemia.
- Oprelvekin (IL-11) stimulates the proliferation of hematopoietic stem cells and megakaryocyte progenitor cells and induces megakaryocyte maturation resulting in increased platelet production. Oprelvekin (Neumega) was approved by the FDA in 1997 for the prevention of severe thrombocytopenia and to decrease the need for platelet transfusions following myelosuppressive chemotherapy (Burks and McCune 2007; National Cancer Institute 2006; Mystakidou et al. 2007).

It should be noted that malignant tumors also produce cytokines that promote carcinogenesis. Cytokines such as IL-10, tumor growth factor (TGF)-β, prostaglandin (PG)-E2, and VEGF can assist tumors in escaping recognition by the immune system, and by promoting their growth and angiogenesis (Huber and Wölfel 2004; Rescigno et al. 2007).

14.3.5 Fusion Proteins

Fusion proteins are new therapeutic agents that employ cytokines. A fusion protein is made of a growth factor or cytokine linked to a toxin. Denileukin difitox (Ontak) was the first fusion protein to be FDA approved for cancer therapy in 1999. It consists of a diphtheria toxin fused to IL-2. The agent binds to cells with IL-2 receptors and initiates a series of reactions that inhibit protein synthesis, resulting in cell death. Denileukin difitox has shown promising results in non-Hodgkin's lymphoma and chronic lymphocytic leukemia (Battiato and Wheeler 2005).

14.3.6 Monoclonal Antibodies

MoAbs are agents that combine the concepts of biotherapy and molecular targeted therapy and are being used increasingly for diagnosis and targeted treatment of many types of cancer. Antibodies are proteins produced by B lymphocytes in response to antigens. After binding to a unique receptor on an antigen, antibodies induce cellular destruction by initiating an immune response to destroy harmful or non-self-substances. MoAbs are very specific antibodies created to be directed against one type of cell-signaling molecule, or against a specific antigen or receptor found on the surface of a cancer cell. Examples of targets for MoAbs include the CD20 antigen in the surface of a non-Hodgkin's lymphoma cell, the CD33 antigen on an acute myelogenous leukemia (AML) cell, the HER2 receptor on a breast cancer cell, or the VEGF molecule. After binding to their target, MoAbs activate the patient's immune system to destroy the tumor cell or to inhibit the growth factor or receptor (Battiato and Wheeler 2005; Burks and McCune 2007).

To create the original MoAbs, tumor-specific antigens were injected into mice. In response, the mouse's immune system made antibodies against these antigens. The mouse plasma cells that produced these antibodies were then removed and fused with laboratory-grown myeloma cells to create a "hybrid" cell line. These cells were called hybridomas. The hybridomas produced large quantities of MoAbs, which were then purified. When injected into humans, the mouse-derived product occasionally caused a human antimouse antibody (HAMA) response, which could negate the antitumor effect of the MoAb and prevent future treatment with the product. Newer molecular and genetic engineering techniques have refined the hybridoma process to produce chimeric (i.e., human and mouse origin) and humanized (i.e., human origin) MoAbs to prevent the HAMA response (Burks and McCune 2007; Gobel 2002).

The ability of MoAbs to bind to unique antigens and molecules allows for specifically targeted anticancer therapy. Because MoAbs are tumor-specific, they have a relatively low toxicity when compared to traditional cancer treatment such as chemotherapy and radiation. The mechanism of action of the MoAbs is different from these traditional therapies, which destroy all rapidly dividing cells. MoAbs affect only the cells that carry the specific target antigen on the cell surface or are influenced by the specific growth factor or receptor. Thus, many dose-limiting toxicities seen with traditional chemotherapy and radiation are not seen in treatment with MoAbs.

MoAbs are being used for cancer treatment in a number of ways. MoAbs that are targeted to specific tumor antigens can enhance a patient's immune response to the cancer. As well, MoAbs can be created to suppress cell growth factors, thus interfering with tumor replication. Newer generations of MoAbs are also being conjugated to radioisotopes, chemotherapy, or toxins. When these MoAbs bind to the antigens on the surface of cancer cells, they deliver the anticancer therapy directly into the malignant cells (Burks and McCune 2007; Fry and Lankester 2008). The clinical utility of MoAbs is not limited to antineoplastic therapy. Because of their ability to bind to specific antigens, MoAbs can also be attached to low-dose radioisotopes to image residual disease.

The majority of MoAbs have been developed for adult cancers, but they are increasingly being used in pediatric oncology. Rituximab (Rituxan) has been used successfully to treat children and adults with non-Hodgkin's lymphoma. It is targeted against the CD20 antigen on the surface of malignant B lymphocytes. Another promising MoAb being used to treat children with AML is gemtuzumab ozogamicin (Mylotarg). Mylotarg combines an antitumor antibiotic (calicheamicin) with an antibody targeted at the CD33 antigen found on leukemic cells. Two examples of radioimmunotherapeutic agents, MoAbs with a radioactive source attached, are ibritumomab tiuxetan (Zevalin) and iodine 131 tositumomab (Bexxar). Both are targeted at the CD20 antigen and used to treat non-Hodgkin's lymphoma. Other agents that are currently being studied in pediatric clinical trials include alemtuzumab (Campath) targeted at the CD52 antigen for acute lymphoblastic leukemia and lymphoma, CH 14.18 Chimeric MoAb AntiGD2 for neuroblastoma, epratuzumab targeted at CD22 for leukemia/lymphoma, trastuzumab (Herceptin) targeted at the HER2 receptor for osteosarcoma, and the bevacizumab (Avastin) targeted at VEGF, for solid tumors (Burks and McCune 2007).

14.4 Cancer Vaccines

Tumor vaccines are another form of biological therapy currently being studied in oncology. The goal for vaccine therapy is to enable the patient's immune system to recognize cancer cells. Cancer vaccines are designed to either treat existing cancers (therapeutic vaccines) or to prevent the development of cancer (prophylactic vaccines). Therapeutic vaccines are intended to activate the patient's immune system to induce a tumor-specific response. The advantage of a therapeutic vaccine is that, if successful, they can elicit long-lasting immunological memory that can protect against minimal residual disease and relapse (Rescigno et al. 2007). The types of therapeutic vaccines that have been developed and studied include those that use whole tumor cells, peptides derived from known tumor antigens, replication-deficient viruses expressing tumor antigens, and DCs loaded with tumor antigens (Fry and Lankester 2008). Currently, prophylactic cancer vaccines are designed to create immunity to viruses that can cause cancer. The human papillomavirus (HPV) vaccine (Gardasil) is an example of a prophylactic cancer vaccine, as it has been shown to prevent cervical cancer in some women.

The most promising therapeutic cancer vaccines to date are those based on the use of DCs as antigen presenters (Rescigno et al. 2007). DC-based vaccines are being investigated for a wide variety of malignancies (Buchsel and DeMeyer 2006). These vaccines can be made from general tumor antigens or from individualized antigens specific to the patient's tumor. Vaccines consisting of DCs that have been transduced with genes have shown an antigen-specific T-cell response. When these vaccines have been followed with chemotherapy, a higher clinical response has been demonstrated (Zwierzina 2008).

The future for prophylactic cancer vaccines may extend beyond immunization against cancer-causing viruses, and expand to include immunizations for patients who possess activated oncogenes or inactivated tumor-suppressor genes that predispose them to develop cancer. Research in animal models has shown evidence of potential for these vaccines to block the carcinogenic process driven by the overexpression of oncogenes and to prevent cancer (Rescigno et al. 2007).

The overall success with cancer vaccines has been limited (Rescigno et al. 2007). Further research, including randomized, controlled clinical trials are needed to fully understand the relationship between cancer vaccines and other cancer treatment modalities (Gabrilovich 2007). Thus far, the research with cancer vaccines in pediatric oncology is limited, but there have been promising clinical results in pediatric sarcoma (Fry and Lankester 2008).

14.5 Other Immunomodulating Agents

14.5.1 Nonspecific Immunomodulating Agents

Nonspecific immunomodulating agents are substances that stimulate or indirectly augment the immune system. Often, these agents target key immune system cells and cause secondary responses such as increased production of cytokines and cytotoxic cell activation (Battiato and Wheeler 2005). Coley's (1933) use of toxins in sarcoma patients was the first example of use of nonspecific immunomodulating agents in cancer patients. Nonspecific immunomodulating agents require that the patient is capable of mounting an immune response (Battiato and Wheeler 2005). Two nonspecific immunomodulating agents used in cancer treatment are bacillus Calmette-Guerin (BCG) and levamisole. BCG is an attenuated live strain of *mycobacterium bovis,* which causes tuberculosis, and has been used since the 1970s to treat bladder cancer. BCG is effective against the tumor because it leads to the infiltration of the epithelium with macrophages and

CD4+ T-lymphocytes. This causes the release of cytokines, including IFN γ, TNF, IL-2, IL-6, IL-8, and IL-10. This treatment is usually performed once a week for 6 weeks (Boyd 2003). Levamisole (Ergamisol), an antibiotic primarily used to control parasites in livestock, is another example of a nonspecific immunomodulator. It has been used as an adjuvant to chemotherapy in colon cancer, ovarian cancer, and breast cancer. Levamisole stimulates the immune response and may restore depressed immune function (National Cancer Institute 2006).

14.5.2 Retinoids

Retinoids are drugs that are relatives of vitamin A that were originally used to treat acne. Recently, they have been used in cancer treatment as immunomodulators. Retinoids have been successful in oncology because they induce cellular differentiation and suppress proliferation. The retinoids that have shown success in pediatric oncology are 13 cis-retinoic acid (Isotretinoin, Accutane) for high-risk neuroblastoma and all-trans retinoic acid (ATRA, Tretinoin, Vesanoid) for acute promyelocytic leukemia (Battiato and Wheeler 2005; Burk and McCune 2007).

14.5.3 Thalidomide

Thalidomide, a drug originally prescribed for morning sickness but taken off the market because it caused severe birth defects, has been found to be useful in cancer therapy. Thalidomide is classified as an immunomodulator with antiangiogenic activity. The immunomodulating effects of thalidomide include T-cell co-stimulatory activity and inhibition of TNF-α and other cytokines. Thalidomide has also been shown to inhibit bFGF, VEGF, and TNF, explaining its anti-angiogenic properties. Thalidomide has been studied in various cancers including multiple myeloma, AML, brain tumors, renal cell carcinoma, breast and prostate cancers, melanoma and myelofibrosis (Battiato and Wheeler 2005; Camp-Sorrell 2003). Structural analogs to thalidomide are being investigated for their immunomodulating effects and fewer side effects. These agents are known as immunomodulatory drugs (IMiDs) (Battiato and Wheeler 2005).

14.6 Adoptive Immunotherapy

Adoptive immunotherapy refers to the direct infusion of immune cells (T-lymphocytes, NK cells, DCs) to enhance the immune response in the patient. The concept of adoptive immunotherapy was first explored in the hematopoietic stem cell transplant (HSCT) setting. It was discovered that graft-versus-host disease (GvHD) in allogeneic HSCT recipients, which is mediated by T-cells, also caused a graft vs. leukemia effect, which led to a decreased incidence of relapse (Huber and Wölfel 2004). This led to the idea that selected T-cells could be infused into the patient to produce a desired immune response. The direct infusion of donor T-cells, called donor lymphocyte infusion (DLI), has been shown to induce remission in some patients who have relapsed after HSCT (Huber and Wölfel 2004; Fry and Lankester 2008). The withdrawal of immunosuppressive therapy after HSCT when a patient has relapsed has also been used to induce a graft vs. tumor response (Klingebiel et al. 2006). Newer adoptive immunotherapy protocols in HSCT are investigating the use of NK cells to contribute to an antitumor effect. Both autologous NK cells combined with IL-2 and allogeneic NK infusions have been researched (Huber and Wölfel 2004; Klingebiel et al. 2006).

Adoptive immunotherapy is being investigated in the oncology setting as well. Treatment of malignancies with adoptive immunotherapy involves the removal of lymphocytes from the patient, the stimulation of those lymphocytes to increase their immune capabilities, and the transfer of those cells back into the patient to fight the cancer. Antigen-specific cytotoxic T lymphocytes (CTLs) have been administered to patients for melanoma and Epstein Barr Virus (EBV) associated tumors with some success (Huber and Wölfel 2004; Klingebiel et al. 2006).

14.7 Molecular Targeted Therapy

Molecular targeted therapies for cancer are directed toward growth factors and receptors involved in cell-signaling pathways. Since different genes and proteins are involved in the growth and differentiation of different types of tumors, the best targets for therapy vary among cancers. Because receptor TKs have been found to be highly involved in cell growth and proliferation and seem to be overexpressed or mutated in many malignancies, they have become a promising target for cancer therapy. MoAbs for types of receptor TKs are discussed earlier. Other agents directed at TKs are tyrosine kinase inhibitors (TKIs). These agents act intracellularly to block the binding site of the TK enzyme. This blocks the ability of TK to function and limits cancerous growth and proliferation. Imatinib (Gleevec) was the first TKI to be approved by the US Food and Drug Administration for use in oncology in 2001. Imatinib inhibits BCR-ABL, which is the abnormal TK created by the Philadelphia chromosome mutation in CML (Battiato and Wheeler 2005).

The other category of promising targeted therapy in pediatric oncology is angiogenesis inhibitors. Angiogenesis is thought to be driven by many types of proangiogenic growth factors, including bFGF, aFGF, VEGF, TGF, TNF, several IL, and others (Camp-Sorrell 2003). Agents that inhibit angiogenesis may act by inferring with the stimulation of these growth factors, inhibiting endothelial cell proliferation or migration, or inhibiting microtubule formation for new capillaries. Both bevacizumab (Avastin), the MoAb targeted at VEGF, and thalidomide, which inhibits bFGF, VEGF, and TNF, are discussed here. Interferon alfa and IL-12 also seem to have some antiangiogenic properties (Camp-Sorrell 2003).

14.8 Method of Delivery

Biologic and targeted therapy agents can be administered to patients using a variety of methods. Some cytokines are delivered as continuous infusions in cycles, similar to traditional chemotherapy. IL-2 can be delivered as an intermittent intravenous (IV) infusion, a continuous IV infusion, or as a subcutaneous (SQ) injection. Interferon may be administered IV, SQ, or intramuscularly (IM) (Boyiadzis et al. 2007; Children's Oncology Group 2008). Most of the CSFs are given as SQ injections, and some can also be administered IV (Burks and McCune 2007). MoAbs are all given as intermittent IV infusions (Burks and McCune 2007; Children's Oncology Group 2008). The first dose of an MoAb is given slowly and the patient is monitored closely for an infusion reaction. If the first dose is tolerated, subsequent doses may be administered at a higher infusion rate (Children's Oncology Group 2008). Cancer vaccines can be administered by many different routes, including SQ, IM, IV, interdermal, intranodal, and intratumoral (Battiato and Wheeler 2005; Buchsel and DeMeyer 2006 Rescigno et al. 2007). To obtain optimal stimulation of the immune system, it appears that cancer vaccines need to be administered over several weeks to months. Ice and topical creams may affect DCs given in vaccine form, so these techniques should be avoided with these injections (Buchsel and DeMeyer 2006). BCG is given intravesically for the treatment of bladder cancer. It is instilled by gravity via a urethral catheter using aseptic technique, and retained in the bladder for 2 h if possible (Boyd 2003). Some nonspecific immunomodulators and targeted therapies, such as levamisole, cis-retinoic acid, ATRA, thalidomide, and imatinib (Gleevec) are available in oral preparations. This makes these agents convenient for long-term therapy at home. However, compliance may be an issue and nurses must educate patients on the negative effects of missed doses and dosing errors (Battiato and Wheeler 2005; Boyiadzis et al. 2007).

Until recently, exposure to most cytokines, MoAbs, and cell therapies was not considered to be hazardous (Battiato and Wheeler 2005; Conley 2007; Gobel 2002). Since most biotherapy agents act on the immune system and cell-signaling pathways rather than on DNA, they are not considered mutagenic. However, the National Institute for Occupational Safety and Health (NIOSH) does include multiple biotherapy and targeted therapy agents on their list of drugs that should be handled as hazardous. These include: aldesleukin, BCG, denileukin, imatinib, interferon alfa, several MoAbs, thalidomide, and tretinoin (National Institute for Occupational Safety and Health 2004). Nurses should use standard safe handling and disposal precautions when handling these biotherapy agents avoid unnecessary exposure, including using barriers such as gloves, gowns, and eye protection, avoiding contact with skin or mucous membranes and not generating aerosolization (Gobel 2002). As well, biotherapeutics that have been conjugated to chemotherapeutic drugs should be treated the same as chemotherapy, and safe administration and disposal guidelines should be followed. When working with biotherapy agents that have been conjugated to radioisotopes, radiation precautions must be maintained. The goal of radiation safety is to keep the exposure as low as reasonably possible using the principles of time, distance, and shielding (Gobel 2002). Nurses should collaborate with the radiation safety officer for compliance with this goal.

14.9 Potential Side Effects

As with other forms of cancer treatment, biological therapies can cause a number of side effects, which can vary widely by agent and individual patient. Some of the side effects can be very serious and potentially life-threatening. The side effects depend on the specific drug, dose, schedule, and combination of therapy. The stimulation of pro-inflammatory cytokines such as IL-6, interferon γ, GM-CSF, and TNF causes most of the frequent side effects of biotherapy (Newton et al. 2002). Some of the common side effects from biotherapy are flu-like symptoms, fever, arthralgia, myalgia, fatigue, rigors, nausea, vomiting, capillary leak syndrome, hypotension, and skin rashes (National Cancer Institute 2006; Newton et al. 2002).

BRMs can cause a local reaction with redness, swelling, pain, and itching at the site that they are injected (Buchsel and DeMeyer 2006). Cytokines such as IL-2 and interferon can cause a cutaneous skin reaction characterized by a dusky red rash, pruritis, flushing, and a sunburn sensation. Skin reactions from these agents typically begin a few days after therapy. The rash usually starts on the back and may spread to the arms, legs, and abdomen. The symptoms may last for 7–10 days after the last dose, and may also include skin peeling or sloughing (Burks and McCune 2007; Newton et al. 2002). For cutaneous reactions, the nurse should assess and document the rash and the patient's symptoms. The nurse should educate the patient to use alcohol- and perfume-free moisturizer on dry skin. Skin should be cleaned with gentle, non-drying soap, and patients should avoid hot showers and baths. Oatmeal baths and oral antihistamines may help with itching. Topical steroids should be avoided because of immunosuppression, which could negatively affect the antitumor effects of the biotherapy (Newton et al. 2002).

Other side effects vary with the type of treatment. In addition to skin reactions, IL-2 frequently causes flu-like symptoms and edema. IL-2 can also cause severe side effects such as hypotension, capillary leak syndrome, and pulmonary edema. Many of these side effects are dependent on the dose administered. Patients need to be closely monitored during treatment with high doses of IL-2. IFN can cause flu-like symptoms, abnormal liver function tests, and kidney damage. The side effects of CSFs include bone pain, fatigue, fever, and appetite loss. The side effects of MoAbs vary, and can include flu-like symptoms, diarrhea, electrolyte imbalances, and serious infusion reactions. Cancer vaccines can cause muscle aches, fever, chills, rash, sweats, general malaise, or allergic reaction. TKIs may cause edema, nausea, diarrhea, abdominal pain, musculoskeletal discomfort, an acne-like rash, fatigue, and headache. TKIs are also a local irritant, so patients should be educated to take them with food and a large glass of water (Battiato and Wheeler 2005; Burks and McCune 2007; National Cancer Institute 2006; Wilkes 2008).

The most serious side effects seen with biotherapeutic agents are liver toxicity, capillary leak syndrome, nerve toxicity, cognitive changes, and infusion reactions, a term that includes both hypersensitivity reactions and cytokine-release syndrome (Burks and McCune 2007; Wilkes 2008). Hypersensitivity or allergic reactions to biotherapy are mediated by IgE. In a hypersensitivity reaction, histamines, prostaglandins, leukotrienes, and cytokines are released by lysed mast cells. The symptoms seen in a hypersensitivity reaction range from flushing and rash, to fever, nausea and vomiting, to dyspnea and bronchospasm, to anaphylaxis with stridor, hypotension, and possibly respiratory and cardiac arrest. Because true hypersensitivity reactions are mediated by an antibody that forms in response to the initial exposure to the allergen, this type of reaction is rarely seen with the first dose of a new drug (Wilkes 2008). In contrast, cytokine release syndrome is common with MoAbs and therapeutic cytokines and develops soon after the beginning of the infusion. Cytokine release syndrome is due to elevated levels of cytokines and histamines as tumor antigen expressing cells are destroyed (Gobel 2007). Signs and symptoms of cytokine release syndrome include fever, flu-like symptoms, nausea, vomiting, pruritis, rash, rigors, chills, hyper or hypotension, tachycardia, and tumor pain (Wilkes 2008).

Infusion reactions can be seen with a variety of biotherapy agents, including IFN, IL-2, denileukin difitox, and most MoAbs (Gobel 2007). Despite the etiology of the infusion reaction or the causative agent, the nursing management is the same. If a patient develops symptoms of an infusion reaction, the infusion showed be stopped and the patient assessed. Airway, breathing, and circulation should be assessed initially and interventions should be made to address any issues found. Oxygen may be used if the patient is experiencing respiratory distress, and the patient may be placed supine or in the Trendelenburg position if hypotensive. Fluid boluses, antihistamines, and corticosteroids may be used to reverse the inflammatory response. If the reaction is severe, epinephrine, bronchodilators, and vasopressors may be needed (Gobel 2007; Wilkes 2008).

Premedications, such as antipyretics and antihistamines, can help manage infusion reactions and minimize the side effects of cancer vaccines (Buchsel and DeMeyer 2006; Burks and McCune 2007; Gobel 2007). For any type of administration, baseline vital signs are required and the patient should be monitored during the infusion. Slow titration of the rate of infusion and assessment for patient tolerance are helpful interventions when administering biotherapeutic agents that are known to have a high rate of infusion reaction. Nurses should identify patients at risk for severe reactions. Emergency drugs and equipment should be kept at the bedside (Gobel 2007; Wilkes 2008).

14.10 Future Perspectives

Although significant progress toward survival and quality of life has occurred in pediatric oncology, there is still a need for more effective and less toxic treatments for residual and refractory disease. Using biologic and targeted therapy to potentiate tumor-specific responses may hold the key to advancing pediatric oncology.

Advances in the understanding of immunology and cell biology have encouraged the development of targeted cancer therapies. As well, the success of the Human Genome Project now allows the description of the gene expression profile of many tumors in detail, which can be associated to the characteristics of the tumor to help select new targets for therapy (Argawal 2008). The Ludwig Institute for Cancer Research (LICR), an international non-profit institute, maintains the *Cancer Immunome Database*, a publicly available database that aims to document all immunogenic cancer antigens. Over 1,000 human tumor antigens have been identified to date (Huber and Wölfel 2004; Rescigno et al. 2007).

Newer concepts in cancer immunology are guiding the second generation of biotherapy. One of these is the theory of tumor escape mechanisms. Tumors evolve to avoid destruction by the immune system in a variety of ways. These include:

- Development of ways to escape recognition by the immune system
- Not sending "danger signals," to recruit and activate immune cells
- The release of immunomodulators (cytokines and chemokines) that alter immune cell function, favor angiogenesis, and encourage tumor growth (VEGF, prostaglandin (PG)-E2, IL-10, and TGF-β) (Rescigno et al. 2007)

These findings are driving the latest research in biotherapy. Future protocols will focus on both delivering tumor-specific targeted therapy and targeting the tumor's immune escape mechanisms. Combination therapies look the most promising for accomplishing these goals with the next generation of biotherapy (Rescigno et al. 2007).

A number of clinical trials combining chemotherapy and immunotherapy have shown promise. Studies have shown that some cytotoxic agents, such as cyclophosphamide, doxorubicin, gemcitabine, anthracylins, 5-fluorouracil, and taxanes stimulate antitumor immune responses. These responses occur through a variety of mechanisms, including cell death that signals the immune system, induction of cytokine production and the release of “danger signals,” increased macrophage activity, and the elimination of poorly functioning antitumor T-cells (Zwierzina 2008; Rescigno et al. 2007). In animal models, data suggest that a combination of immunotherapy and low doses of agents such as cyclophosphamide have the potential to eradicate resistant tumors. The combination of low-dose cyclophosphamide and immunotherapy is currently being studied in humans (Rescigno et al. 2007). Animal models have also shown that complete resection of a large tumor followed by a combination of gemcitabine and immunotherapy has a high cure rate, but cannot induce a long-term tumor-specific memory. However, if the tumor is only partially debulked, the data shows the same cure rate and a long-term immune memory response (Zwierzina 2008).

Cancer vaccines also hold promise for combination therapy. Studies have shown that there may be a synergistic effect between therapeutic cancer vaccines and cytokines, such as GM-CSF, IL-2, and interferon (Buchsel and DeMeyer 2006). As well, combination therapy with a DC-based prostate cancer vaccine and bevacizumab (Avastin), the MoAb against VEGF, showed a positive immunologic response in patients (Rini et al. 2006). Early studies have also created optimism around the use of vaccines for a synergistic effect between immunotherapy and chemotherapy in solid tumors. Several early phase clinical trials have suggested a positive correlation between immune response to vaccination and clinical response to chemotherapy. These studies have immunized patients with antigen-specific or dendritic cell vaccines before chemotherapy and have showed an improved tumor response to chemotherapy after the vaccine (Fry and Lankester 2008).

There have been successes in the field of biotherapy for cancer treatment, with the majority being in adult oncology patients and positive results have been inconsistent. Researchers continue to investigate the biology of cancer and immune response. As well, many questions remain about the scheduling, sequencing and dosing of biotherapy, and its use in combination with traditional cancer treatment (Zwierzina 2008). It will be very important to determine for each therapeutic approach the best combination of drugs and biologic agents, but also the optimal timing of administration to achieve the deletion of regulatory cells and the generation of a favorable environment before the activation of the immune response (Rescigno et al. 2007). Randomized, controlled clinical trials in translational research programs are needed to address these questions and optimize the use of biotherapy in cancer treatment (Zwierzina 2008). Adjuvant biotherapy and molecular targeted therapy hold promise for pediatric oncology, where remission can be easily induced with standard therapy for many patients, but preventing relapse is still a major challenge. Nurses play a critical role in the administration of agents, toxicity management, education, and advocacy for pediatric oncology patients receiving biologic and targeted therapy.

References

Argawal B (2008) Biological therapy for pediatric malignancy: current perspectives. Indian Journal of Pediatrics 75(8):839–844

Battiato LA, Wheeler VS (2005) Biologic and targeted therapy. In: Yarbro C, Goodman M, Frogge MH (eds) Cancer nursing: principles and practice, 6th edn. Jones and Bartlett, Sudbury, MA, pp 510–558

Boyiadzis MM, Lebowitz PF, Frame JN, Fojo T (2007) Hematology-oncology therapy. McGraw-Hill, New York

Boyd LA (2003) Intravesical bacillus Calmette-Guerin for treating bladder cancer. Urologic Nursing 23(3):189–199

Buchsel PC, DeMeyer ES (2006) Dendritic cells: emerging roles in tumor immunotherapy. Clinical Journal of Oncology Nursing 10(5):629–640

Burks C, McCune R (2007) Principles of biotherapy. In: Kline NE (ed) The pediatric chemotherapy and biotherapy curriculum, 3rd edn. APHON, Glenview, IL, pp 31–38

Camp-Sorrell D (2003) Antiangiogenesis: the fifth cancer treatment modality? Oncology Nursing Forum 30(6):934–941

Children's Oncology Group (2008) COG parenteral chemotherapy administration guidelines. https://members.childrensoncologygroup.org/_files/disc/Pharmacy/ChemoAdminGuidelinesmemo_TC.pdf. Retrieved 27 Mar 2009

Coley WB (1933) The treatment of sarcoma of the long bones. Annals of Surgery 97(3):434–460

Conley S (2007) Safe handling of chemotherapy and biotherapy agents. In: Kline NE (ed) The pediatric chemotherapy and biotherapy curriculum, 3rd edn. APHON, Glenview, IL, pp 31–38

Decker JM (2006) University of Arizona online tutorial: cytokines. http://microvet.arizona.edu/Courses/MIC419/Tutorials/cytokines.html. Retrieved 8 Nov 2008

Fry TJ, Lankester AC (2008) Cancer immunotherapy: will expanding knowledge lead to success in pediatric oncology? Pediatric Clinics of North America 55(1):147–167

Gabrilovich DI (2007) Combination of chemotherapy and immunotherapy for cancer: a paradigm revisited. The Lancet Oncology 8(1):2–3

Gobel BH (2007) Hypersensitivity reactions to biological drugs. Seminars in Oncology Nursing 23(3):191–200

Gobel BH (2002) Clinical Q&A: handling and disposal of monoclonal antibodies. Clinical Journal of Oncology Nursing 6(5):290–1

Huber CH, Wölfel T (2004) Immunotherapy of cancer: from vision to standard clinical practice. Journal of Cancer Research and Clinical Oncology 130(7):367–374

Klingebiel T, Bader P, Hollatz G, Koehl U, Lehrnbecher T, Meisel H, Dilloo D (2006) Immunotherapy in children: report from the Reisensburg – Symposium October 22–24, 2004 and recent advances. Klinische Pädiatrie 218(6):355–365

Mystakidou K, Potamianou A, Tsilika E (2007) Erythropoietic growth factors for children with cancer: a systematic review of the literature. Current Medical Research and Opinion 23(11):2841–2847

National Cancer Institute (2006) Biological therapies for cancer. http://www.cancer.gov/cancertopics/factsheet/Therapy/biological. Retrieved 27 Mar 2009

National Institute for Occupational Safety and Health (2004) Preventing occupational exposure to antineoplastic and other hazardous drugs in health care settings. Appendix A: drugs considered hazardous. http://www.cdc.gov/niosh/docs/2004-165/2004-165d.html. Retrieved 27 Mar 2009

Newton S, Jackowski C, Marrs J (2002) Biotherapy skin reaction. Clinical Journal of Oncology Nursing 6(3):181–182

Rescigno M, Avogadri F, Curigliano G (2007) Challenges and prospects of immunotherapy as cancer treatment. Biochimica et Biophysica Acta 1776(1):108–123

Rini BI, Weinberg V, Fong L, Conry S, Hershberg RM, Small EJ (2006) Combination immunotherapy with prostatic acid phosphatase pulsed with antigen-presenting cells (provenge) plus bevacizumab in patients with serologic progression of prostate cancer after definitive local therapy. Cancer 107(1):67–74

Wilkes G (2008) Managing drug infusion reactions: focus on cetuximab monoclonal antibody therapy. Clinical Journal of Oncology Nursing 12(3):530–532

Zwierzina H (2008) Combining immunotherapy with classical anticancer therapy. Annals of Oncology 19(Suppl. 7): vii252–vii255

Complementary and Alternative Medicine

Janice Post-White • Elena Ladas

Contents

15.1 Introduction . . . 295
15.2 CAM Modalities . . . 296
15.2.1 Acupuncture . . . 296
15.2.1.1 Indications . . . 297
15.2.1.2 Potential Risks/Side Effects/ Requirements . . . 297
15.2.1.3 Nursing Role . . . 297
15.2.2 Biological Therapies . . . 297
15.2.2.1 Indications . . . 297
15.2.2.2 Potential Risks/Side Effects . . . 298
15.2.2.3 Nursing Role . . . 299
15.2.3 Mind–Body Therapies . . . 299
15.2.3.1 Indications . . . 299
15.2.3.2 Resources . . . 300
15.2.3.3 Nursing Role . . . 300
15.2.4 Movement Therapies . . . 300
15.2.4.1 Indications . . . 300
15.2.4.2 Potential Risks/Side Effects . . . 300
15.2.4.3 Resources . . . 300
15.2.4.4 Nursing Role . . . 301
15.2.5 Aromatherapy . . . 301
15.2.5.1 Indications . . . 301
15.2.5.2 Potential Risks/Precautions/ Side Effects . . . 301
15.2.5.3 Nurse's Role . . . 301
15.2.6 Massage . . . 302
15.2.6.1 Indications . . . 302
15.2.6.2 Potential Risks/Side Effects . . . 302
15.2.6.3 Resources . . . 302
15.2.6.4 Nursing Role . . . 302
15.2.7 Energy Therapies . . . 303
15.2.7.1 Indications . . . 303
15.2.7.2 Potential Risks/Side Effects . . . 303
15.2.7.3 Resources for Nurses . . . 303
15.3 Future Perspectives . . . 303
References . . . 304

15.1 Introduction

Complementary and alternative medicine (CAM) encompasses practices and therapeutic modalities that fall outside of the mainstream of conventional medicine. The National Center for Complementary and Alternative Medicine of the National Institutes of Health (NCCAM, NIH) (2008) identifies four domains of CAM therapies, including mind–body, touch, energy, and biological therapies (www.nccam.nih.gov). Children with cancer use therapies from all domains; most often used are prayer and spiritual practices, mind–body-relaxation interventions, massage, and herbal therapies and supplements. In addition, NIH acknowledges whole medical systems that have philosophies and practices that are independent from conventional Western medicine and use a combination of therapies from the four domains, including traditional Chinese medicine, Ayurvedic medicine, Naturopathic medicine, and homeopathy. Most families use CAM therapies in combination with conventional medical therapy (complementary), as opposed to replacing mainstream treatment (alternative). Integrative pediatric oncology blends CAM with standard care to manage symptom distress and emphasize healing and wellness.

CAM use varies widely and is higher in children whose parents are more educated or use CAM for themselves (Nathanson et al. 2007). Children with cancer use CAM to reduce symptoms, promote comfort and relaxation, and help fight the disease (Sencer and Kelly 2006), while survivors of childhood cancer most often use CAM for specific symptoms related to previous diagnosis and treatment

(Mertens et al. 2007). Although there are few scientifically rigorous studies determining whether CAM therapies in children are effective, mind–body therapies, massage, aromatherapy, and acupuncture are considered safe and feasible in children with cancer and may help reduce symptoms (Ladas et al. 2006). No known published research exists on energy therapies or whole medical systems for children with cancer. A complete review of individual CAM therapies is beyond the scope of this chapter; more comprehensive reviews can be found elsewhere (Ladas and Post-White 2009a, b; Ladas et al. 2006).

The most important nursing role in CAM is to communicate a non-judgmental approach when assessing for CAM use and evaluating risks and benefits for the patient and family. The Oncology Nursing Society (2000) advises nurses to rely on credible sources and providers when giving information to patients; to evaluate CAM for safety, efficacy, cost, third-party payer coverage, ethics, and liability; and evaluate their own beliefs regarding CAM. It is especially important to ask patients and families what CAM they use; to document CAM use, including dosages, frequency, and reasons for use; and to evaluate how well the specific therapy is working for the patient and family (Table 15.1). Use of CAM and potential interactions with treatment should be assessed at diagnosis, during each hospitalization, and at every phase of medical treatment (e.g., before surgery, radiation, and chemotherapy). Parents should bring in bottles of vitamins or supplements used by their child.

Table 15.1. Assessing Use of CAM

Role of the Nurse
– Listen objectively to what therapies parents or adolescents are using or considering to use
– Document what is being used and why, including dosages and frequency
– Ascertain all known and suspected potential side effects and interactions with treatment
– Explore how the child, adolescent, or parent expects the therapy to help
– Offer supportive therapies that can be used at home at any time, such as acupressure, aromatherapy, massage by a parent or friend, music, relaxation, yoga, and meditation
– Provide a list of local resources, including practitioners who have pediatric experience
– Provide reliable resources for information on specific therapies, including where to obtain them
– Ask questions to ensure the family has considered the risks, benefits, and cost
– Discuss options for insurance reimbursement. Reimbursement typically requires a medical order and inpatient service; however, state laws and insurance policies vary
– Monitor the patient's response to any complementary and alternative medicine (CAM) therapies used. Ask at each transition in treatment if CAM therapies are still being used and whether they have been helpful
– Assess for negative responses, including allergic reactions, side effects, emotional distress, or financial hardship
– Periodically assist the family to evaluate the need and value of the therapy
Expected patient and family outcomes
– The family makes informed decisions regarding choice of CAM therapies for their child
– Families work with trained providers who have experience with pediatric patients
– Resources consulted by families are current, reputable, and reliable
– Families report to their providers their use of CAM, any side effects, and perceived benefits attributable to CAM therapies

Adapted from Post-White (2008)

15.2 CAM Modalities

15.2.1 Acupuncture

Acupuncture is the insertion of thin sterile single-use needles placed at points along meridians (invisible channels of energy flow) to balance energy (qi or chi) in the body to prevent or treat a condition. Disease results when chi is blocked. Acupuncture accesses the meridians through the specific points to help restore the flow of chi. Acupuncture is a component of Chinese Medicine that can be used in concert with other therapies, such as herbs and diet.

15.2.1.1 Indications

Acupuncture is effective for adult nausea and vomiting secondary to surgery and chemotherapy (NIH Consensus Conference 1998). It is currently being studied for effectiveness in delayed nausea and vomiting in children, and is commonly used for constipation, diarrhea, pain, anxiety, insomnia, xerostomia, asthma/reactive airway, and sinus inflammation. Because meridians access multiple organ systems, acupuncture is capable of treating multiple side-effects simultaneously. Patients typically benefit the most if acupuncture is given several times a week or weekly for 8–10 weeks, depending on the condition. A temporary condition may resolve with 1–3 treatments. Acupuncture can be provided inpatient and outpatient and can be administered to infants and toddlers, with an experienced acupuncturist alert to unexpected movement.

15.2.1.2 Potential Risks/Side Effects/ Requirements

Although some children may shun needles, acupuncture uses very fine gauge needles that rarely hurt on insertion, although the child may feel sensations during the session (tingling, heaviness, movement), indicating that the chi is present and moving. Acupuncture is feasible in children with thrombocytopenia and neutropenia (Reindl et al. 2006; Taromina et al. 2007). The acupuncturist should be licensed (designated L.Ac.), have experience treating children, and be approved for practice in your institution. The National Certification Commission for Acupuncture and Oriental Medicine (NCCAOM) certifies acupuncturists, requiring a national certification exam, and individual states license practitioners. NCCAOM certification is a requirement for licensure in most states (National Certification Commission for Acupuncture and Oriental Medicine 2008).

15.2.1.3 Nursing Role

Prior to acupuncture administration, discussion should be held with the child and approval for use obtained from the parents. For children with fear of needles, a topical anesthetic cream, such as EMLA®, can be used over the specific acupuncture points to lessen the anxiety. Acupuncture can be especially beneficial for conditions not resolved with pharmaceutical intervention. One teenage boy receiving 6 weeks of radiation therapy for a brain tumor experienced retractable retching and vomiting, resulting in non-compliance with treatment. With his and his parent's consent, acupuncture needles were inserted prior to each daily radiation therapy session, removed in the radiology suite for the short treatment, and replaced immediately after. He subsequently completed his treatments and today remains in remission.

15.2.2 Biological Therapies

Biological therapies entail the use of herbal or nutritional supplements to treat the cancer or manage or prevent therapy-related side-effects. Dietary supplements are provided in many forms, including tablets, capsules, powders, geltabs, extracts, and liquids. Many patients obtain information on biological therapies from family, friends, their local health food store, and the internet. Although much information is available to patients and practitioners, little is based on scientific studies. Vitamins and herbs are among the most frequently used CAM therapies in cancer; they also have the greatest potential to interact with conventional treatment.

15.2.2.1 Indications

Families turn to biological therapies when side effects are inadequately managed or they prefer non-pharmacological interventions. Parents report using biological agents more often than other therapies for the purpose of "treating the cancer" or "increasing immune function." Other indications for herbs and supplements include: neuropathy (glutamine, B vitamins), fatigue (corticeps, l-carnitine), anxiety (valerian, passion flower, chamomile), hepatotoxicity/detoxification (milk thistle, lemon juice), immunosuppression (combination of mushroom extracts, beta glucan), thrombocytopenia (beet juice), and insomnia (lavender, valerian, chamomile). Antioxidants (Vitamin C, cuercitin, pycnogenol, Vitamin

E) are often chosen by patients to decrease the risk of adverse events or side effects or increase efficacy of chemotherapy or radiation therapy. Subsequent reviews on the topic have not found any evidence supporting these uses and theoretically may pose a risk (Ladas and Kelly 2008).

15.2.2.2 Potential Risks/Side Effects

The primary risk of any biological agent is interaction (inhibitory or synergistic) with chemotherapy or radiation therapy. Use of any ingested agent should be given careful consideration for risks or benefits (NCI/PDQ, Table 15.2). The risk is greatest when

Table 15.2. Resources on CAM use in clinical practice

CAM – General	National center for complementary and alternative medicine, National institutes of health (NIH)	http://nccam.nih.gov/health/
	National cancer institute, NIH	http://www.cancer.gov/CAM/
Acupuncture	Licensing site/website to locate licensed acupuncturist in your state	http://www.nccaom.org/
Biological agents	Advising patients and families	NCI, PDQ: www.cancer.gov/cancertopics/pdq/cam
		U.S. Food and Drug Administration http://cfsan.fda.gov
	Resources to evaluate therapies and interactions	Office of dietary supplements http://ods.od.nih.gov
		Herb research foundation www.herbs.org/index.html
		Consumer lab www.consumerlab.com
	Experts in CAM oncology	www.childrensoncologygroup.org
	Reference books	Hendler and Rorvik (2001)
		Gruenwald et al. (2007)
		Blumenthal (2003)
		Cassileth and Lucarelli (2003)
Mind–body therapies	The American music therapy association	http://www.musictherapy.org/
	National association for holistic aromatherapy	http://www.aromahead.com/course/aromatherapy-certification-program
	The institute of spiritual healing and aromatherapy	http://www.ishaaromatherapy.com/
	Continuing education certification programs	http://chirocredit.com/pages/aromatherapy.php
	Matching essential oils to indication	Buckle (2003); Essential Oils Desk Reference (2007)
Massage	Identify licensed massage therapists; state requirements	http://www.amtamassage.org/
Energy therapies	Healing touch international	http://www.healingtouchprogram.com/
	Therapeutic touch	http://www.therapeutictouch.org/

supplementing for the entire treatment plan or ingesting multiple agents or single agents at high doses. Pharmacists can cross-reference drugs and supplements for interaction. Immunoenhancing agents (astragalus, echinacea, and mushroom extracts) should be avoided in patients with hematologic or lymphoproliferative tumors or those receiving allogeneic transplants, so as not to increase the risk of graft versus host disease (GvHD). Most adverse events are due to contamination and impurity of products. The FDA promotes good manufacturing practices (GMP) for herbal and nutrition products; however, impurities remain an issue, especially with imported products that are inconsistently tested (Food and Drug Administration 1995). Contamination is of particular concern for an immunosuppressed child.

15.2.2.3 Nursing Role

The most important nursing role is to assess and document what is being used and why, including dosages and frequency of use, and to observe for and report increased or unexpected toxicities. Consult with physicians, pharmacists, or CAM experts about concerns regarding patient use of biological agents. Patients with advanced disease or those on Phase I studies are more likely to turn to CAM therapies for treatment despite advice to avoid biological therapies while on clinical trials.

Patients are more likely to disclose their CAM use in an open and nonjudgmental environment. Open communication with patients will foster a discussion about the safe use of biological agents. For example, many parents are concerned about the late-effects associated with cancer treatment, which drives them to investigate biological remedies in hopes of preventing the development of a late effect. Anthracylines are a class of chemotherapeutic agents often used for the treatment of pediatric cancers and are associated with both acute and delayed cardiotoxic effects. Patients may present multiple biological agents to their nurse in hopes of preventing cardiotoxicity; however, some evidence for safety is available for nurses. Biological agents; such as, l-carnitine or coenzyme Q10 can be recommended and will discourage patients from approaching their local health food store or internet for consultation. Additionally, this will set precedence for future inquiries. Approaching clinical situations in this manner empowers families to feel a part of the medical plan while allowing the healthcare team to use evidence to safely guide patients on their choice of biological agents.

15.2.3 Mind–Body Therapies

Mind–body interventions use a variety of techniques designed to enhance the mind's capacity to affect bodily function and symptoms. Several mind–body techniques that were previously considered CAM have become mainstream, especially for children (e.g., guided imagery/relaxation and cognitive–behavioral therapy). Other mind–body techniques include meditation, prayer, and therapies that use creative outlets such as art, music, or drumming. Several forms of music tap into the child's creative and expressive nature, with the music striking a vibrational or auditory connection that stimulates the amygdala and hypothalamus, directly affecting mood and stress responses. Music also offers choices and some control over the child's environment, and is something fun to share with family and the therapist.

15.2.3.1 Indications

Relaxation, guided imagery, and biofeedback are used to decrease anxiety, fatigue, pain, blood pressure, pulse, and respiration, and to induce sleep. Meditation is primarily used for body awareness and stress reduction, with the focus on a particular object, sound, or image. Several studies have shown that meditation yields positive results, although children find it difficult to meditate in the same focused manner as adults. Imagery is more creative and free flowing for children, even allowing for physical movement. The use of imagery for procedural pain was pioneered in children with cancer. Art and music therapy are most often used for exploration of feelings and distraction from symptoms and the stress of hospitalization or procedures. Creating pictures and music can provide insight into feelings and thoughts and release of emotions often hidden from consciousness. Shamanic drumming emanates from Native American practices and is a powerful inducer of meditative states and spiritual healing. The beat of the drum is used to transport the drummer into shamanic states of consciousness, which closely approximates the base resonant frequency of the Earth and can be measured scientifically.

15.2.3.2 Resources

Certification programs for guided imagery and hypnosis abound. The American Society of Clinical Hypnosis has state chapters and is gaining national recognition as a standard for the practice of hypnosis (American Society of Clinical Hypnosis 2007). Keys to a successful experience include finding a clinical training program with a focus on health, working with an experienced mentor, and practicing techniques clinically. Music therapists have a college degree and internship in music therapy. The American Music Therapy Association (2004) sets the education and clinical training standards for music therapists and the Certification Board for Music Therapists certifies music therapists to practice music therapy nationally.

15.2.3.3 Nursing Role

Pediatric nurses often use imagery in daily practice, sometimes without realizing that their suggestions to "imagine you are up in hot air balloon" are therapeutic and facilitate the child's dissociation from his/her body experiencing unpleasant symptoms (back on the ground). Nurses use creative visualization with children to encourage them to take medications ("send this pill sliding down the slide at your favorite park"), to get them through scary procedures ("tell me what you see as you fly over the country"), and to help distract them from painful or unpleasant events associated with cancer and its treatment ("blow the bubbles hard so they beat the other team to the finish line"). The ability of the child to go along with an image that is meaningful to them is a powerful intervention that should always be considered part of nursing care. Nurses can be advocates for hiring or hosting visiting music therapists, art therapists, or other trained professionals who have experience in hypnosis, biofeedback, and other mind–body techniques.

15.2.4 Movement Therapies

Movement therapies take the form of yoga, pilates, karate, and other martial arts or exercise.

Yoga is the use of poses (asanas), breathwork (pranayama), and meditation (dyhana) with the goal of uniting mind, body, and spirit for health and self-awareness. Pilates focuses on core (abdominal) strengthening, posture, and alignment.

15.2.4.1 Indications

Movement therapies are recommended for fatigue, anxiety, depression, and insomnia, and for maintaining muscle tone. Yoga encourages mild movement and is of particular benefit for patients who are experiencing a decrease in muscle tone or athletes who have been required to decrease physical activity either due to the nature of the sport or inability to continue sports during treatment. Yoga and other movement therapies can maintain muscle strength, flexibility, and cardiovascular capacity during treatment thereby shortening rehabilitation after therapy. A review of studies of yoga in adults with cancer found no negative effects, and although results are inconclusive, high satisfaction rates and positive effects on mood and sleep were consistent across studies (Smith and Pukall 2008). Movement therapies do not have to be rigorous to help with posture, self-esteem, muscle tone, and overall sense of well-being. Selecting a particular movement is patient-driven.

15.2.4.2 Potential Risks/Side Effects

There are few, if any, negative effects of movement if the intervention is matched to the patient's ability and limitations. (Bench pressing and free weights are contraindicated.) Yoga positions require guidance by a trained yogi to ensure proper alignment. A review of studies of yoga in adults with cancer found no negative effects, and although results are inconclusive, high satisfaction rates and positive effects on mood and sleep were consistent across studies.

15.2.4.3 Resources

Yoga programs and instructional DVDs are available for children, but will need to be modified for the ill child.

15.2.4.4 Nursing Role

Nurses can identify patients interested in and needing movement therapies, and can recommend particular therapies based on patient interest and underlying motivation and conditioning. Movement therapies are particularly useful for patients who are experiencing prolonged stays in the hospital. For these cases, nurses can suggest books, DVDs, electronic games (Nintendo® Wii™) to provide guidance to patients who are unable to attend movement classes. On discharge, nurses can recommend local yoga studios or instructors to provide direction on the safe integration of movement therapies. Nurses may also consult hospital physical therapists or rehabilitation specialists for direction on local resources.

15.2.5 Aromatherapy

Aromatherapy is the therapeutic use of essential oils from flowers, herbs, or trees for improving physical, emotional, and spiritual well-being. Essential oils are extracted and distilled into the air via nebulization, air filtration, or simply smelling the vial of essential oil passed under the nose.

15.2.5.1 Indications

Aromatherapy is primarily used as an inhalant for supportive care indications among children with cancer; however, topical application of aromatic oils, such as diluted tea tree oil, may be used as a treatment of skin conditions (e.g., topical fungal infections, acne, athlete's foot). The inhaled form of aromatherapy for therapeutic or medical purposes is most often used for respiratory or sinus congestion (eucalyptus, rosemary). Aromatic oils are nontoxic, easy to transport, and can be used in both the inpatient and outpatient setting.

Patient preferences often dictate the choice of aromatic oil; however, many oils have been historically used for certain indications. Ginger (*Zingiber officinale*), spearmint (*Mentha spicata*), and peppermint (*Mentha piperita*) are recommended for their antiemetic and antispasmodic effects on the gastric lining and colon. Uplifting aromatic oils such as citrus scents (bergamot, citrus, lemon) may be used for fatigue, and eucalyptus (*Eucalyptus globulus*) for sinus congestion. Lavender (*Lavandula angustifolia*) is often used for insomnia; however, spike lavender (*Lavandula spica*) is therapeutic for topical burns and as an expectorant. An aromatherapist may often use specialized systems of aromatic treatments, such as Rain Drop therapy, which systematically combines the use of multiple aromatic oils dropped along the length of the spine.

15.2.5.2 Potential Risks/Precautions/Side Effects

Lavender and tea tree oils have been found to have some hormone-like effects that mimic estrogen, and, if used topically, should be used in moderation with boys who have not yet reached puberty or patients with hormone-sensitive cancers (e.g., breast cancer). Topical application of aromatic oils may cause local skin irritation. To avoid local irritation, practitioners should test a small amount of the oil prior to use. Very high concentrations of some oils with high potencies can cause headaches, dizziness, and overall discomfort and tend to be patient-specific. With the exception of direct topical application or ingestion, aromatherapy poses little risk for an adverse event to occur, and is a safe CAM therapy that may be used to treat a variety of symptoms. Careful consideration should be given when using aromatic oils around other patients undergoing treatment, as smells that may be appealing to one patient may be perceived as noxious to another. Note that essential oils are not chemical fragrances, which are more likely to cause respiratory distress or adverse reactions. The label should read "pure essential oil" and list no fragrances (many products can be labeled aromatherapy, but include fragrances and not essential oils).

15.2.5.3 Nurse's Role

Patients can safely self-administer essential oils and nurses should feel comfortable allowing patients to drive the oil of choice and form of application. Nurses can provide information and resources on which essential oils are best used for certain conditions.

The National Association for Holistic Aromatherapy (NAHA) has national educational standards for Aromatherapists and an approved program providing Aromatherapy Certification. To be certified through NAHA you must have 200 h of training. Other programs also offer certification (Table 15.2). Helpful resources that can assist practitioners and patients in choosing a therapeutic oil are Buckle's book (2003) and PDR for aromatic oils. Oils that adhere to GMP are preferred so as to decrease the risk of contamination (mold, bacteria). Application of aromatic oils may be through a diffuser or simply through applying a few drops of the oil on a tissue or cotton ball and then placed near the patient or under the pillow. Essential oils lose their potency after 6–9 months and should be discarded after that to avoid contamination.

15.2.6 Massage

Massage is the use of therapeutic touch for the purpose of reducing fatigue and pain and restoring structure and function of the musculoskeletal and nervous systems. Massage techniques vary, and involve manual soft tissue manipulation, including holding, causing movement, and/or applying pressure to the body.

15.2.6.1 Indications

Although massage was at one time contraindicated in cancer, several Cochrane databases and meta-analyses support the use of massage in adults and children with cancer for management of anxiety, pain, fatigue, and distress (Ezzo 2007). The effects are consistent across studies, but tend to be temporary, with improvements lasting hours to days. No studies have demonstrated long-term effects of massage.

15.2.6.2 Potential Risks/Side Effects

There are few contraindications to massage, but massage should be individualized to the client and adapted under some conditions (e.g., avoiding solid tumor, radiation, surgical, and intravenous/central line sites, consideration for positioning of the patient). Touch in some form or another is almost always possible (American Massage Therapy Association 2008). Children with thrombocytopenia can receive light massage; aggressive forms of massage (e.g., Rolfing) should be avoided until platelets are above 20,000 mm^3. Massage therapists should be trained in standard precautions for infection and pancytopenia.

15.2.6.3 Resources

Licensing for massage is under state legislation. Currently, 42 states, the District of Columbia, and 4 Canadian provinces offer some type of credential to professionals in the massage and bodywork field – usually licensure, certification, or registration (Massage Magazine 2009). Although 36 states require a license to practice massage (LMT), the requirements are inconsistent and not transferable among states. All states require education from an accredited massage therapy school, but exams and certification are not consistent requirements (American Massage Therapy Association 2008). American Massage Therapy Association (AMTA) maintains a list of licensed massage therapists. Commission for Massage Therapy Accreditation (COMTA) is the official accrediting agency for Canadian massage schools (Walsh 2005). Many massage therapy-related modalities have national, and in some instances, international certification and set their own standards of competence, continued competence, and professional conduct. Today, there is no regulation in England like those that exist in Ontario or British Columbia. However, there are individual associations that govern members graduating from schools recognized within each massage therapy profession (e.g., shiatsu, aromatherapy). The Scottish Massage Therapists' Organization (SMTO) is the best organized Massage Therapists' organization in Scotland (Stone Waters Massage Education 2009).

15.2.6.4 Nursing Role

Backrubs, practiced by nurses for generations, are a form of massage. Hand massage and foot massage (reflexology) are also practiced by nurses, although reflexology requires special training in the corresponding organ response. Because state laws vary for nurses and for massage therapists, it is best to determine what the nursing and massage boards in your state require. Receiving massage by a licensed massage therapist (if indicated in your state) can be arranged for inpatients and outpatients to facilitate relaxation, sleep, anxiety reduction, and management of some symptoms. As many hospitals may have massage therapists on staff, nurses can inquire with human resources and provide patients with therapists who adhere to their institution guidelines.

15.2.7 Energy Therapies

Commonly used energy therapies include Reiki, Qi gong, Healing touch, TT, and Intercessory prayer. Practitioners of energy medicine believe in a universal healing energy and that illness results from disturbances of energy fields, either within the body (biofields) or external to the body (electromagnetic fields). Flow of energy can be restored where blockages occur, resulting in healing and energy balance. Therapeutic or healing touch uses light, gentle touch over a clothed body to affect the energy system physically, mentally, emotionally, and spiritually. Reiki is more often practiced without skin contact. Energy therapies are among the most controversial of CAM practices because neither the external energy fields nor their therapeutic effects have been demonstrated convincingly by any biophysical means.

15.2.7.1 Indications

TT and healing touch have been used to accelerate wound healing, decrease pain and swelling of arthritis, control pain and migraine headaches, reduce anxiety and fatigue, and promote relaxation and well-being. In a meta-analysis of 11 controlled TT studies, 7 had positive outcomes, and 3 showed no effect (Winstead-Fry and Kijek 1999). Healing touch energy therapies have impressive anecdotal evidence, but there is limited evidence for efficacy and no scientific evidence for the mechanism of action.

15.2.7.2 Potential Risks/Side Effects

Energy therapies carry low risk. There have been no negative effects reported from the use of energy therapies other than a lack of effect and investment of time and money. Although there is no evidence for efficacy, many patients report "feeling better" or "more relaxed," with less fatigue. Weighing the risks with potential benefits suggests that energy therapies are not likely to cause harm and may possibly do some good for some patients. Choosing energy therapies should be an individual choice. There is no certification or licensing for energy therapists. Some perceive the ability to detect energy fields as an innate gift. It is advised to first talk with the practitioner to determine style, beliefs, and expectations for the energy session.

15.2.7.3 Resources for Nurses

Many TT practitioners are nurses. A 3-level training program is offered to obtain expertise in TT, starting with a basic level, 5-day mentor workshop, intermediate workshop, and another 5-day mentor workshop at the intermediate level. The 5-day advanced TT workshop is intended for practitioners having 3 years of practice (Pumpkin Hollow Foundation 2004). Healing Touch International (Healing Touch Program 2009) offers a nursing continuing education multi-level certification program in which practitioners take a series of 5 or 6 workshops to advance to attain a certificate of completion. The Certification Board does not license the practice of an individual nor assume any legal responsibility for her/his practice.

15.3 Future Perspectives

Despite the prevalent use of CAM in both adults and children with cancer, at this time there are few scientifically rigorous studies determining whether CAM therapies in children are safe and effective and whether they lead to improved quality of life and positive clinical outcomes. Some therapies have more evidence for effectiveness (e.g., hypnosis and acupuncture) than others (e.g., herbal therapies and energy therapies). And some therapies require more caution prior to evidence of safety and efficacy because of known or potential interactions or toxicities (biological therapies), while others carry less risk (massage therapy, energy therapies). It is part of the nurse's role to evaluate evidence for efficacy and to determine, observe for, and report potential side effects and interactions with treatment.

A screening assessment tool for use and interest in specific CAM therapies would be a valuable addition to ongoing patient assessment and evaluation. The nurse could use the assessment tool to further evaluate specific therapies for potential risks, interactions, access to experienced and licensed or credentialed providers, and evaluation of perceived benefit. A check-off list of CAM therapies is more likely to capture accurate responses than simply asking "Do you use any CAM therapies, vitamins, or supplements?" Most importantly, maintaining a positive and non-judgmental approach will yield greater confidence and disclosure and more accurate reporting. The goal of CAM is to offer supportive interventions that enhance well-being and help manage or prevent complications or adverse effects of treatment.

References

American Massage Therapy Association (2008) Massage Information Center. http://amtamassage.org/infocenter/home.html. Retrieved 29 Mar 2009

American Music Therapy Association (2004). Professional requirements for music therapists. www.musictherapy.org. Retrieved 29 Mar 2009

American Society of Clinical Hypnosis (2007) ASCH Certification. http://asch.net/certification.htm. Retrieved 29 Mar 2009

Blumenthal M (2003) The ABC clinical guide to herbs. American Botanical Council, Austin, TX

Buckle J (2003) Clinical aromatherapy: essential oils in practice, 2nd edn. Churchill Livingstone, Edinburgh

Cassileth BR, Lucarelli C (2003) Herb-drug interactions in oncology. BC Decker, Lewison, NY

Essential Oils Desk Reference (2007) 4th edn. Essential Science Publishing, Orem, UT www.essentialscience.net 800-336-6308

Ezzo J (2007) What can be learned from Cochrane systematic reviews of massage that can guide future research? Journal of Alternative and Complementary Medicine 13(2):291–295

Food and Drug Administration (1995) Dietary and supplement health and education act of 1994. http://www.cfsan.fda.gov/~dms/dietsupp.html. Retrieved 30 Mar 2009

Gruenwald J, Brendler T, Jaenicke C (eds) (2007) Physicians desk reference for nutritional supplements. Thomas Healthcare, Montvale, NJ

Healing Touch Program (2009) Healing touch program information. http://www.healingtouchprogram.com/program/index.shtml. Retrieved 29 Mar 2009

Hendler SS, Rorvik E (eds) (2001) Physicians desk reference for herbal products. Thomas Healthcare, Montvale, NJ

Ladas EJ, Kelly KM (2008) The antioxidant debate. In: Abrams DI, Weil A (eds). Integrative oncology (Chapter 9:195–214). Oxford University Press, New York, in press

Ladas EJ, Post-White J (2009a) Complementary and alternative medicine. In: Carroll B, Findlay J (eds) Cancer in children (Chapter 41). Jones & Bartlett, Sudbury, MA

Ladas EJ, Post-White J (2009b) Complementary and alternative treatments in children with cancer. In: Baggott C, Foley G, Fochtman D, Kelly K (eds) Nursing care of children and adolescents with cancer and blood disorders, 4th edn. W.B. Saunders, Philadelphia, PA

Ladas EJ, Post-White J, Hawks R, Taromina K (2006) Evidence for symptom management in the child with cancer. Journal of Pediatric Hematology/Oncology 28(9):601–615

Massage Magazine (2009) Massage laws and legislation for the United States and Canada. http://www.massagemag.com/Resources/massage-laws-legislation.php. Retrieved 29 Mar 2009

Mertens AC, Sencer S, Myers CD, Recklitis C, Kadan-Lottick N, Whitton J, Marina N, Robison L, Zeltzer L (2007) Complementary and alternative therapy use in adult survivors of childhood cancer: a report from the childhood cancer survivor study. Pediatric Blood and Cancer. US: http://dx.doi.org/10.1002/pbc.21177. doi: 0.1002/pbc.21177

Nathanson I, Sandler E, Ramirez-Garnica G, Wiltrout SA (2007) Factors influencing complementary and alternative medicine use in a multi-site pediatric oncology practice. Journal of Pediatric Hematology/Oncology 29(10):705–708

National Center for Complementary and Alternative Medicine, National Institutes of Health (2008) NCCAM Publication No. D347. CAM Basics: What is CAM. http://nccam.nih.gov/health/whatiscam/. Retrieved 18 Feb 2009

National Certification Commission for Acupuncture and Oriental Medicine (2008) http://www.nccaom.org. Retrieved 29 Mar 2009

NIH Consensus Conference (1998) Acupuncture. JAMA 280(17):1518–1524

Post-White J (2008) Complementary and alternative treatments. Essentials of pediatric hematology/oncology nursing: a core curriculum, 3rd edn. Association of Pediatric Hematology/Oncology Nurses

Pumpkin Hollow Foundation (2004) Becoming a TT practitioner. http://www.therapeutictouch.org/practitioner.html. Retrieved 29 Mar 2009

Reindl TK, Geilen W, Hartmann R, Wiebelitz KR, Kan G, Wilhelm I et al (2006) Acupuncture against chemotherapy-induced nausea and vomiting in pediatric oncology. Interim results of a multicenter cross-over study. Support Care Cancer 14(2):172–176

Sencer S, Kelly KM (2006) Bringing evidence to complementary and alternative medicine for children with cancer. Journal of Pediatric Hematology/Oncology 28:186–189

Smith KB, Pukall CF (2009) An evidence-based review of yoga as a complementary intervention for patients with cancer. Psycho-Oncology 18(5):465–475. doi: 10.1002/pon.1411 (epub ahead of print)

Society ON (2000) Oncology nursing society position on the use of complementary and alternative therapies in cancer care. Oncology Nursing Forum 27:749

Stone Waters Massage Education (2009) History of regulation. http://www.stone-waters.com/clinicalwork/regulations.html. Retrieved 29 Mar 2009

Taromina K, Ladas E, Rooney D, Hughes D, Meyer A, Kelly KM (2007) Acupuncture is feasible in children with low platelet counts. Society for integrative oncology, Annual meeting, 14–17 Nov 2007

Walsh K (2005) Canada laws and regulation update. Massage magazine. http://www.massagemag.com/Resources/USCan/canadaLaw.php. Retrieved 29 Mar 2009

Winstead-Fry P, Kijek J (1999) An integrative review and meta-analysis of therapeutic touch research. Alternative Therapies in Health and Medicine 5(6):58–67

Clinical Trials

Biljana Dzolganovski

Contents

16.1 The Role of Clinical Trials 307
16.1.1 The Need for Research. 307
16.1.2 Phases of Clinical Trials 308
16.1.3 Study Types 308
16.1.4 Research Ethics: Principles, Policies, and Guidelines 308
16.1.5 Legal and Ethical Issues Regarding Participation of Children in Research . . 310
16.1.6 Research in Pediatrics 312
16.2 Research Networks 312
16.2.1 Cooperative Group Research 312
16.2.1.1 History of COG 313
16.2.1.2 History of UKCCSG. 313
16.2.1.3 History of BFM 313
16.2.2 Importance of Participation in Clinical Trials 314
16.3 Progress Made Through Clinical Trials 315
16.3.1 Treatments and Therapy Delivery 315
16.3.2 Quality of Life Measures and Supportive Care 319
16.3.3 Complementary and Alternative Medicine 320
16.3.4 Late Effects. 321
16.3.5 Palliative Care 321
16.4 Perception of Clinical Trials. 322
16.5 Future of Clinical Trials. 324
16.6 The Role of the Clinical Research Associate 324
16.6.1 Introduction 324
16.6.2 Clinical Research Associate. 325
16.6.3 The Role of the CRA 326
16.6.4 The Role of the Clinical Research Nurse 328
References 329

16.1 The Role of Clinical Trials

"The basic desire for new knowledge and understanding is the driving force for research" (Health Canada 2003, p1). The role of a clinical trial is to answer specific biomedical or health-related questions. Carefully conducted clinical trials, with human volunteers, are the safest and fastest way to find treatments that work and ways to improve health (Food and Drug Administration 2009), translating into benefits for as many people as possible.
Clinical trials include:

- Prevention trials that look for methods to prevent a particular disease, or that prevent a disease from returning. These approaches may include medications, vitamins, vaccines, minerals, or lifestyle changes
- Screening trials that test the best way to detect certain diseases or health conditions
- Diagnostic trials that identify better tests or procedures for diagnosing a particular disease or condition
- Treatment trials that test experimental treatments, new combinations of drugs, or new approaches to surgery or radiation therapy
- Quality of life (QOL) trials or supportive care trials that explore ways to improve comfort and the QOL for individuals with a chronic illness (National Institutes of Health 2007)

16.1.1 The Need for Research

Research involving human participants is premised on a fundamental moral commitment to advancing human welfare, knowledge, and understanding.

Participants may directly benefit from improved treatments for illnesses, and clinical research will also benefit particular groups and society as a whole (Health Canada 2003).

16.1.2 Phases of Clinical Trials

A clinical trial is the culmination of a long and well-thought-out research process. The process begins with the synthesis and discovery of molecules. This is followed by research involving an animal model, and then the trial is conducted in humans. The clinical-trial research phase is divided into four phases:

- Phase I

Researchers test an experimental drug or treatment in a small group of human subjects (20–80), for the first time, to evaluate safety, determine the maximum tolerated dose (MTD), and to identify side effects.

- Phase II

The experimental study drug or treatment is given to a larger group of people (100–300), to determine if it is effective in treating a particular disease or diseases, and to further evaluate its safety.

- Phase III

The experimental study drug or treatment is given to large groups of people (1,000–3,000) to confirm its effectiveness, to monitor side effects, to compare it with the commonly used treatments, and to collect information that will allow the experimental drug or treatment to be used safely.

- Phase IV

After a treatment has been approved and is being marketed for a particular indication, the manufacturer may choose to study it further. The purpose of phase IV trials is to evaluate the side effects, risks, and benefits of a drug over a longer period of time and in a larger number of people than in phase III clinical trials. Phase IV trials are also used when the manufacturer is collecting data to test the drug for a different indication (National Institutes of Health 2007).

Clinical trials are designed to answer a specific research question. Therefore, conducting them in this progressive step-by-step manner allows the researchers to obtain valuable and reliable information. After a phase I or phase II trial is completed, the researchers look carefully at the data collected and decide whether to continue with the treatment to the next phase, or to stop testing the treatment because it is not safe or effective. When a clinical trial is completed, the investigators evaluate the data and decide if the results have medical importance. If so, the results are presented at national or international meetings and published in scientific journals (National Institutes of Health 2001b). Most medical and scientific journals have a process of peer review, in which experts critique the report before it is published, in an effort to ensure that the analysis and conclusions are sound (National Institutes of Health 2001b).

The randomized control trial (RCT) is the gold standard of clinical research trials. It is the most rigorous way of determining whether a cause and effect relationship exists between the dependent variable (treatment) and the independent variable (outcome) (Sibbald and Roland 1998). RCTs involve the random assignment of subjects to different interventions (treatments or conditions). If the sample size is adequate and random assignment is used, both known and unknown confounding factors are evenly distributed among the treatment groups. A treatment or intervention that is proven to be safe and effective in an RCT often becomes the new standard of care.

16.1.3 Study Types

Clinical trials include:

- Interventional studies in which the research subjects are assigned to a treatment or other intervention, and their outcomes are measured (e.g., measuring responses to a new drug).
- Descriptive or quasi-experimental (noninterventional) studies in which individuals are observed and their outcomes are measured (e.g., review of medical records) (National Institutes of Health 2007).

16.1.4 Research Ethics: Principles, Policies, and Guidelines

The protection of human subjects is of paramount concern in all clinical trials. Table 16.1. shows an

Table 16.1. Historical summary of research ethics

Nuremberg code	• First international instrument that addressed the ethics of medical research, published in 1949 • Created as a consequence of the Doctors' Trial, physicians who had conducted atrocious experiments on unconsenting prisoners and detainees during the second world war • Designed to protect the integrity of the research subject; it set out ten conditions that must be met for the ethical conduct of research involving human subjects, • emphasizing their *voluntary* consent to research (The Nuremberg Code 1949)
The declaration of Helsinki	• First issued by the world medical association in 1964 • Comprehensive international statement of ethical principles for medical research involving human subjects, including research on identifiable human material and data • Ethical guidelines for researchers engaged in both clinical and nonclinical biomedical research • The first to address research issues in patient populations considered to be legally incompetent such as children (The World Medical Association 2008)
Belmont report	• Published in 1979 • Summary of the basic ethical principles identified by the National Commission for the Protection of Human Subjects of Biomedical and Behavioral Research (United States of America) • Establishes three fundamental ethical principles that are relevant to all research involving human subjects: respect for persons, beneficence, and justice (The National Commission for the Protection of Human Subjects of Biomedical and Behavioral Research 1979)
Code of Federal Regulations *Title 45, Part 46 ^Title 21, Parts 50 and 56	• Code of Federal Regulations (CFR) issued in 1981 • *Title 45 (public welfare), Part 46 (protection of human subjects) • ^Title 21 (food and drugs), Parts 50 (protection of human subjects) and 56 (Institutional Review Boards) • Created by the department of health and human services (DHHS)* and the food and drug administration (FDA)^, United States of America • Based on the Belmont report adopted by most federal departments and agencies sponsoring human-subjects research • *(United States Department of Health and Human Services 2005) • ^(Food and Drug Administration 1988)
Proposed international ethical guidelines for biomedical research involving human subjects	• First issued by council for international organizations of medical sciences (CIOMS) in 1982 CIOMS is an international, nongovernmental, nonprofit organization established jointly by the World Health Organization (WHO) and the United Nations Educational, Scientific and Cultural Organization (UNESCO) in 1949 • Guidelines are designed to be of use to countries in defining national policies on the ethics of biomedical research involving human subjects (Council for International Organizations of Medical Sciences 2002)
Good clinical practice (E6) R1	• Developed by International Conference on Harmonization of Technical Requirements for Registration of Pharmaceuticals for Human Use (ICH), in 1996 • ICH was designed to ensure that data generated from clinical trials are mutually acceptable to the regulatory authorities in the European Union, Japan, and the United States of America, by creating multiple guidelines under four major categories: quality (Q), efficacy (E), safety (S), multidisciplinary (M) • This Good Clinical Practice (GCP) document describes the responsibilities and expectations of all participants in the conduct of clinical trials, including investigators, monitors, sponsors, and research ethics boards (The International Conference on Harmonization of Technical Requirements for the Registration of Pharmaceuticals for Human Use 1996)

Table 16.1. (Continued)

Tri-council policy statement on the ethical conduct of research involving human subjects (TCPS)	• In 1998, Canadian institute of health research (CIHR), (formerly the medical research council of Canada), natural sciences and engineering research council of Canada (NSERC), and the social sciences and humanities research council of Canada (SSHRC) jointly published the TCPS as a single Canadian standard to replace their previous respective guidelines • Influenced by international codes of ethics, as well as professional association codes of ethics • The agencies have committed to keeping it a living or "evolving" document to respond to new developments and identified gaps (Health Canada 2003)
European Union Directive 2001/20/EC	• Legislative act aimed at harmonizing the circumstances in which clinical trials on medicinal products are conducted within any of the 25 member states in Europe • Commonly referred to as the clinical trials directive • Enhance participant protection • Simply administrative provisions governing clinical trials • Ensures credibility of data (DIRECTIVE 2001/20/EC 2001)

overview of the history of standards and guidelines that were created regarding the conduct of research and the treatment of research participants.

16.1.5 Legal and Ethical Issues Regarding Participation of Children in Research

Children represent a vulnerable group of research participants. Parents or guardians protect their children's interests because they are assumed to act in the best interest of their children when making decisions regarding participation in the research. With the limited exceptions that will be described in the following paragraph, all research with children require parental permission to be obtained (Diekema 2006; Macrae 2009). When children are involved in research, the investigator cannot rely on the conventional concept of informed consent, which pertains to decisions about research participation made by those with the legal and intellectual capacity to make such choices in their own right (National Institutes of Health 2001a). It was once assumed that children lacked the ability to consent to participation in clinical research, and therefore parents or legal guardians gave permission on their behalf. This approach has changed and a respect for children's maturity and independence has led to the development of guidelines and regulations, whereby researchers, when appropriate, seek to involve children in discussions about research and obtain their permission to participate, be it consent or assent.

In the United States of America, the Code of Federal Regulations (CFR), Title 45, Part 46, Subpart D, states that children who have not attained the legal age cannot give consent to treatments or procedures involved in the research (United States Department of Health and Human Services 2005). There are exceptions such as emancipated minors; however, the pediatric participant, as a rule, cannot provide consent. In Canada and throughout the UK, children younger than 18 years of age, and in some Canadian provinces, 19 years of age, are not adults; however, it may not be legally and ethically necessary for parent(s) or guardian(s) to give permission for their child's participation in clinical trials. For medical treatment, many adolescents can consent without their parent's permission. Many Canadian provinces such as New Brunswick, Saskatchewan, Manitoba, Prince Edward Island, Newfoundland, and Labrador define the age of consent for treatment to be 16 years, whereas in the province of Quebec, it is 14 years (Canadian Pediatric Society 2008). In Ontario, the Health Care Consent Act has no statutory age of consent (Canadian Pediatric Society 2008). Most Canadian legislation relates to consent for treatment and not consent for research, only Quebec has legislated consent for research, allowing minors over 14 years of age to consent in the absence of serious risks to their health (Canadian Pediatric Society 2008) However, Canadian guidelines, for provinces under common law, allow all those who have the mental ability to understand and appreciate the nature and consequences of their acts to make their own choices about participation in research studies, regardless of their age (National Council on Ethics in Human Research 1996). The Tri-Council Policy Statement: Ethical Conduct for Research Involving Humans (TCPS) defines competence as "the ability of prospective subjects to give informed consent in accord with their own fundamental values. It involves the ability to understand the information presented, to appreciate the potential consequences of a decision, and to provide free and informed consent." acknowledging that not all adults have the capacity to make free and informed decisions and not all children lack this capacity (Health Canada 2003). Even though there is no defined chronological age at which children can consent to research studies, the default position appears to be that consent for research may be given at the same age as that required for consent to treatment (Lind et al. 2003). In England and Wales, according to the Family Law Reform Act (1969), a person ceases to be a minor at the age of 18, and 16 and 17-year-olds are given the statutory right to give consent to medical treatment (McTiernan 2003). However, this statutory right does not cover participation in research. Under common law in England and Wales, children under the age of 16 can legally give consent to treatment if they have sufficient understanding of what is proposed (McTiernan 2003), and 16- and 17-year-olds, if deemed competent, can give consent to participate in research (British Pediatric Association 1992).

For children unable to give informed consent, researchers aim to obtain assent, which is the child's affirmative agreement to participate in research (Food and Drug Administration 1988). The National Commission for Protection of Human Subjects of Biomedical and Behavioral Research established that 7 years of age was a reasonable minimum age for involving children in some kind of assent process. It is felt that most children at this age can understand information tailored for their knowledge and developmental level (National Council on Ethics in Human Research 1996).

However, what happens if a child or adolescent refuses medical treatment? It would be reasonable to assume that a person would consent to treatment that was in his or her best interest, but what happens, for example, when a child is afraid of a procedure or drug that could be lifesaving? In this instance, it would be reasonable to say that the child does not have the ability to appreciate the consequences of his or her decision, and parental rights would override those of the child and they would provide consent on the child's behalf (Macrae 2009; Tomlinson 2004). Assent may be waived in therapeutic research studies when the participation of the child in an investigational treatment may be of such benefit that the welfare of the child would be significantly jeopardized by failing to provide assent (Afshar et al. 2005). However, for nontherapeutic research, dissent of the child overrides parental consent (Health Canada 2003; United States Department of Health and Human Services 2005). For example, a child can understand that needle sticks are painful and if there is no direct benefit to them and they will be subjected to pain, they should be allowed to dissent and have that dissent respected (Diekema 2006). Unwillingness to participate by the child should be noted in the child's medical record and is usually respected (Macrae 2009).

These are all mechanisms to encourage children as young as 7 years of age as well as adolescents to participate in decision-making to the extent that they are able to understand the purpose of the research. Informed consent and assent should be thought of as a process rather than an event. Parents and children should be able to ask questions about the research and the investigator should be available and willing to answer questions throughout the duration of the research study (Diekema 2006). Every effort should be made to assure that parents and children are informed in language and terms that they understand. Consent and assent forms are not contracts, but are voluntary, and participants can withdraw at any time.

Kamps et al. (1987) conducted a survey of parents whose children were in remission, to elicit their views on experimental therapy in children with cancer. Parents felt that children who are 12 years and older should be a part of the discussion between the parents and the physician, and that they should be involved in making decisions. These parents reported that they would allow the child to make his or her own decision if he or she were 16 years or older. Ellis and Leventhal (1993) conducted surveys discussing information needs and decision-making preferences in 50 children with cancer (aged 8–17) and 60 accompanying parents. They found that 96% of children did not want to make their own decisions about therapy, while 63% of adolescents 13 years and older wanted to make their own decisions about palliative therapy, and many patients felt that they should be allowed to make decisions about participation in medical research at the age of 14.

Debate will continue regarding the ethics of parental permission and child consent and assent, particularly when adolescents are involved; however, much attention presently focuses on more practical questions concerning interpretation and implementation of these concepts, and honoring their underlying ethical principles in research practice (National Council on Ethics in Human Research 1996). The researcher must appreciate the feelings of the parents or legal guardians and children.

16.1.6 Research in Pediatrics

Children and adults suffer from many of the same illnesses and are often treated in the same way. However, the physiology and disease processes in adults may be different than that of children (Macrae 2009). Many commercially available drugs contain either no or limited information regarding doses for pediatric patients (Committee on Drugs American Academy of Pediatrics 1995; Gans-Brangs and Plourde 2006). As few as 20% of medications used in children are actually licensed for pediatric use (Macrae 2009).

In 1997, in response to the lack of pediatric data, the United States Congress began to enact legislation mandating studies in children (Gans-Brangs and Plourde 2006). In 2000, the International Conference on Harmonization Guidance on the Clinical Investigation of Medicinal Products in the Pediatric Population was adopted by ICH member countries including the United States, European Union, and Japan; its purpose was intended to encourage and facilitate timely pediatric clinical trials, detailed critical issues in pediatric drug development, and ways to ethically study the safety and efficacy of drugs in the unique and vulnerable pediatric population (The International Conference on Harmonization of Technical Requirements for the Registration of Pharmaceuticals for Human Use 2000).

Medical research involving children is widely recognized as essential, and treatment cannot always be safely adapted from proven therapy for adults (Macrae 2009). The child's growth and development should be considered, along with any long-term impacts. Clinical research trials have provided important information on appropriate dosing, rates and types of adverse reactions, and efficacy for the treatment of pediatric illnesses (Salazar 2003).

16.2 Research Networks

16.2.1 Cooperative Group Research

One of the most effective means of generating high quality, adequately powered clinical research in critical care is to establish research collaborations or networks (Macrae 2009). As a subspecialty, pediatric oncology is rooted in clinical research. Owing to the vast majority of children with cancer being treated at academic medical centers, most children are eligible for participation in clinical research at the time of initial diagnosis (Adamson 2008). Studies carried out with oncology patients are necessary to investigate and ensure that approaches to cancer prevention, diagnosis, treatment, and supportive care are safe and effective. Studies also help to understand and improve QOL and long-term effects of treatment.

Although childhood cancer is rare, it remains the most common disease-related cause of death in children and adolescents aged 1–19, and the second leading cause of all deaths among children aged 1–14, after trauma (Public Health Agency of Canada 2005). Over the last half of the twentieth century, childhood cancer has gone from an almost universally fatal disease, with survival rates lower than 10%, to one that is curable in most patients. Remarkable progress has been made in the past two decades; more than 75%

of children diagnosed with cancer today will be long-term survivors (Reaman 2005). This progress is largely the result of high participation rates in well-organized multicenter clinical trials (Bond and Pritchard 2006), carried out through cooperative groups such as the Children's Oncology Group (COG), The United Kingdom Children's Cancer Study Group (UKCCSG), and Berlin-Frankfurt-Münster study group (BFM). The need for collaboration was absolutely necessary, as no individual cancer program or children's hospital had the number of patients that could support clinical investigation by themselves (National Cancer Institute 2008). Collaboration and cooperation between clinical investigators as well as laboratory investigators resulted in significant advances in the understanding of basic biologic mechanisms critical to the development of childhood cancer and relevant to the current and future therapy of childhood cancer (Reaman 2004).

16.2.1.1 History of COG

COG is presently a National Cancer Institute (NCI)-funded international multicenter clinical trials organization, with its headquarters in the United States, with more than 230 sites in North America, Australia, the Netherlands, and Switzerland (Reaman 2005). It brings together specialized professionals to conduct focused clinical investigations in children with cancer (Devine et al. 2008). Throughout the 1950s and early 1960s, chemotherapy consisted of single agents given as part of phase I or II trials. As a result of the establishment of cooperative groups, Phase III studies with multiple drugs were begun. In 1955, Children's Cancer Study Group (CCSG) was formed. Two other pediatric cooperative groups were formed shortly after CCSG was established, and these were the Southwest Oncology Group (SWOG) and Cooperative Acute Leukemia Group B (CALGB), (which included adult oncologists) (Wolff 1991). These were followed by the Children's Cancer Group (CCG), the Pediatric Oncology Group (POG), the National Wilms Tumor Study Group, the Intergroup Rhabdomyosarcoma Study Group (IRSG), and in 2000, these four legacy pediatric groups merged, for greater efficiency and collaboration, forming the COG. The mission of COG, through scientific discovery and compassionate care, is to cure and prevent pediatric cancer (Reaman 2005).

To carry out its mission, COG:

1. Designs and conducts clinical trials to define the best treatments
2. Conducts laboratory research that translates into improved therapy
3. Identifies the causes of childhood cancer
4. Conducts research to improve QOL and long-term survival (Reaman 2005)

16.2.1.2 History of UKCCSG

UKCCSG began in 1977. Pediatricians who had been treating children with cancer joined together to form a group with the aims of improving the management of children with cancer and to advance the knowledge and study of childhood malignancy. Since then, the UKCCSG has steadily expanded and now has over 500 members, working in 22 Pediatric Oncology Centers throughout the British Isles, and including about 60 corresponding members from other countries around the world. The membership of the UKCCSG is multidisciplinary and includes clinicians, pathologists, epidemiologists, and basic scientists (Children's Cancer and Leukemia Group 2007).

16.2.1.3 History of BFM

The Society for Pediatric Oncology and Hematology (Gesellschaft für Pädiatrische Onkologie und Hämatologie – GPOH) is an interdisciplinary, international German-language scientific organization, dedicated to comprehensive research, diagnosis, treatment, and follow-up care of children and adolescents suffering from malignant diseases and blood diseases (Gesellschaft für Pädiatrische Onkologie und Hämatologie 2007). The GPOH was formed in 1991 by combining two professional societies, the German Working Group for Leukemia Research (Deutsche Arbeitsgemeinschaft für Leukämie-Forschung – DAL), which specialized in the treatment of pediatric leukemia and lymphoma, and the Society for Pediatric Oncology (Gesellschaft für Pädiatrische Onkolgie – GPO), which specialized in the treatment of pediatric solid tumors (Gesellschaft für Pädiatrische Onkologie und Hämatologie 2007). GPOH is the overarching umbrella under which multiple working groups are represented, the BFM group being the best known among these. From 1970 to 1976, Dr. Hansjörg Riehm conducted the "West Berliner Pilot Studie" (West Berlin Pilot Study), an intensive combination chemotherapy protocol for acute lymphoblastic leukemia (ALL) patients, which was found to have better results than previous treatment strategies applied to childhood leukemia (Creutzig and Klussmann 2004). The success of this initial study led to the creation of the BFM Study Group, named after the three initiating study centers. The BFM group, founded by Dr. Riehm in 1976, and the "West Berliner Pilote Studie" came to be known as the first of the series of BFM protocols that have gained international recognition due to its treatment concept and high cure rate in pediatric patients with ALL (Gesellschaft für Pädiatrische Onkologie und Hämatologie 2006). Today pediatric oncologists in more than 70 clinics throughout Germany, Austria, and Switzerland participate in BFM trials (Gesellschaft für Pädiatrische Onkologie und Hämatologie (2006)).

16.2.2 Importance of Participation in Clinical Trials

Over the past 30 years, treatment outcomes for pediatric cancer patients has improved dramatically due to the expertise of coordinated, multidisciplinary teams and national cooperative group clinical trials. Without the randomized Phase III clinical trials, progress would have been stalled and patients would have been locked into ineffectual and excessively morbid cancer treatments as the standard of care (Murphy 1995). There is no question about the value of clinical trials to the subsequent generations of patients and to the society in general (Ferrari et al. 2008). Figure 16.1 represents increased survival rates in pediatric patients, less than 15 years of age, over a 25-year period.

It is important for all children to participate in cooperative group clinical trials if they meet the eligibility criteria. Even if consent is not obtained for official registration, many will receive treatment with reference to published or even currently active protocols. Patients treated on cooperative group trials have a significant survival advantage compared with those who are not. This may probably be because of the inclusion effect, which may be a result of stricter protocol administration, enforcing adherence to

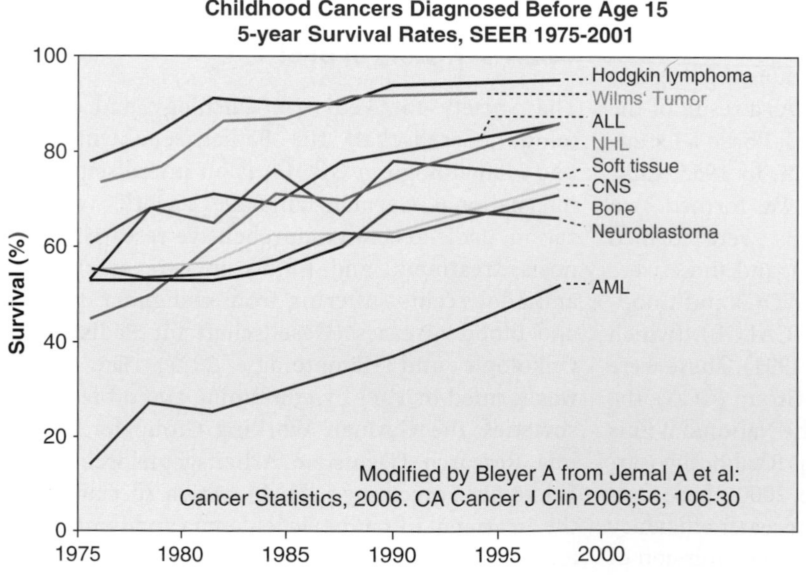

Figure 16.1 Survival rate trends from 1974 to 2001 (Bleyer, Personal communication, 2 March 2009)

chemotherapy dosage and schedule (Newburger et al. 2002). In addition, registration on a cooperative group trial provides immediate access to important protocol changes in response to ongoing data and safety monitoring, and patients have easier access to the expertise of national authorities in the field (Newburger et al. 2002). It could be argued that QOL is improved due to the expanded healthcare team, the extra attention paid to the clinical trial participants, a self-rewarding sense of altruism, and the indirect advantages of contributing to fellow and future patients (Ferrari et al. 2008).

Certain studies have shown a survival advantage for patients enrolled on clinical trials for children with ALL (Meadows et al. 1983), non-Hodgkin lymphoma (NHL) (Wagner et al. 1995), Wilms tumor (Lennox et al. 1979), and medulloblastoma (Duffner et al. 1982). In the United States and Canada, a comparison of 16–21-year-old patients with ALL or AML (acute myeloid leukemia) showed that the survival durations were superior in those treated on cooperative group trials than in those not treated on cooperative group trials (Nachman et al. 1993).

Even with these advancements in the treatment of pediatric cancer, adolescents have seen the least benefit in mortality reduction, mainly due to older adolescent patients not being consistently treated at institutions participating in cooperative group clinical trials (McTiernan 2003). The participation rate of 15–19-year-old patients in the United States on cancer treatment trials sponsored by the NCI during 1997–2003 was approximately half that of the corresponding rate of those less than 15 years of age (Bleyer et al. 2006). Data from the UKCCSG from 1992 to 1994 showed that 58% of 13–14-year-old patients were registered in the UKCCSG trials, compared with 73% of 10-year-old patients and 84% of children less than 9 years of age (Lewis 1996). The Clinical Studies Development Group in 2005 analyzed the inclusion of teenagers and young adults in phase III trials within the portfolios of the UK National Cancer Research Institute (NCRI) and the Children's Cancer and Leukemia Group (CCLG) for 2005–2007; they documented a substantial decline in the accrual beyond the age of 15 years. The most striking finding was that 56% of the patients aged 5 years entered into trials in England, Scotland, and Wales, but only 20% of 15–24-year-olds participated (Whelan and Fern 2008). Programs were not specifically developed for this age group and they fell within the gaps between adult and pediatric groups (McTiernan 2003).

In North America, France, Holland, Denmark, Italy, and the United Kingdom, older adolescents with ALL treated on pediatric clinical trials showed considerably better outcomes than those treated on adult leukemia treatment trials (Boissel et al. 2003; de Bont et al. 2004; Ramanujachar et al. 2007; Ramanujachar et al. 2006; Stock et al. 2008; Testi 2006). In Germany, older adolescents with Ewing sarcoma who were treated at pediatric cancer centers had better outcomes than those treated at other centers with the same protocol (Paulussen et al. 2003). In Italy, the outcome was better for older adolescents with rhabomyosarcoma if they were treated according to pediatric standards of therapy than if treated ad hoc or on an adult sarcoma regimen (Ferrari et al. 2003). Hence, there must be continued support of clinical trials research for pediatric cancer and there must be greater access for adolescents.

16.3 Progress Made Through Clinical Trials

16.3.1 Treatments and Therapy Delivery

Table 16.2. shows some examples of the progress that has been achieved through the establishment of cooperative group clinical trials. All these examples have led to the improvement in patient treatment, outcome, and QOL. The following section looks at some other key treatment and therapy delivery advances that have led to improvement in patient QOL.

Symptoms that the patient experiences during cancer treatment have been recognized to have a significant impact on QOL (Woodgate et al. 2003). Both the symptom and the distress associated with the symptom can have a significant impact on the overall well-being during treatment and ultimately on the outcome (Degner and Sloan 1995). Among the most frequently reported symptoms were lack of energy, pain, and drowsiness (Collins et al. 2000). Symptoms that patients experience during treatment can be related directly to the cancer itself, such as pain from

Table 16.2. Cooperative group clinical trial achievements

References	Summary
(Schrappe et al. 2000)	Results from four consecutive childhood acute lymphoblastic leukemia (ALL) clinical trials were completed between 1981 and 1995 by the Berlin-Frankfurt- Münster (BFM) study group • The probability for event free survival (EFS) at 8 years improved from 65.8% in the study by ALL-BFM to 81–75.9% in the study by ALL-BFM 90 • The cumulative incidence of recurrences with central nervous system (CNS) involvement was 10.1% in the ALL-BFM 81 study and 9.3% in the ALL-BFM 83 study, but was reduced to less than 5% in the ALL-BFM 90 study • For patients with adequate early response (90% of all), an 8-year probability of EFS of 80% was achieved in the ALL-BFM 90 trial • Four major findings were derived from this series of trials performed by 37–96 centers in Germany, Austria, and Switzerland – Reintensification is a crucial part of treatment, even in low-risk patients – Presymptomatic cranial radiotherapy can be safely reduced to 12 Gy, or even be eliminated if it is replaced by early intensive systemic and intrathecal methotrexate applied – Maintenance therapy given for a total of 24 months from diagnosis, provides a lower rate of systemic relapses than treatment for 18 months – Inadequate response to an initial 7-day prednisone window (combined with one intrathecal injection of methotrexate on day 1) defines about 10% of the patients with a very high risk of relapse
(Eden et al. 2000)	Results of three consecutive completed UK trials (1980–1997) for childhood ALL • The national accrual has progressively increased, so that over 90% of all the country's ALL cases were treated on the trial, UKALLXI • From 1980 to 1990, EFS and overall survival (OS) progressively improved, following adoption of an American therapy template and use of two postremission intensification modules • Since 1990, despite demonstration of the benefit of a third intensification module, the overall EFS has not improved further • Survival remains high due to a good retrieval rate especially for those relapsing post treatment after receipt of two intensification pulses • Cranial irradiation had been successfully replaced by a long course of intrathecal methotrexate injections for the majority of patients
(Gaynon et al. 2003)	• Survival rates for children with ALL are associated with successive series of randomized clinical trials spanning a 35-year period during which 10-year survival rates improved from less than 10 to 80% • Key components of successful therapy identified by this collaborative research included the use of – Empiric multiagent chemotherapy – Introduction of presymptomatic CNS-directed therapy – Use of post induction intensification therapy followed by antimetabolite-based maintenance therapy with periodic pulses of therapy Concept of risk-adjusted therapy

Table 16.2. (Continued)

References	Summary
(Ravindranath et al. 2005)	Results from four consecutive childhood acute myeloid leukemia (AML) trials conducted between 1981 and 2000. • Before 1981, patients were treated with regimens similar to those used to treat childhood ALL and the results of the AML treatment were poor • Clinical trials were conceived in which therapy consisting of anthracycline and cytarabine resulted in a rate of remission inductions and EFS estimates better than those from the treatment originally designed for ALL • The sequential pediatric oncology group (POG) studies demonstrated a stepwise increase in the long-term survival as therapy was intensified
(Cairo 2003)	Burkitt's and Burkitt's-like lymphoma • In four consecutive Children's Cancer Group (CCG) studies from 1977 through 1995, there has been a steady improvement in the 3-year disease-free survival (DFS) in children and adolescents with advanced Burkitt's and Burkitt's-like lymphoma. In the CCG study (CCG 5911 conducted from 1993 through 1995), in which participants received short but intensive chemotherapy (CHOP, ifosfamide + etoposide and DECAL or LMB-89 type therapy), the 3-year DFS improved considerably from 50 to 82% Anaplastic large cell lymphoma (ALCL) • In a report, children with localized (stage I/ II) ALCL achieved 100% EFS with 2 months of intensive combination chemotherapy (dexamethasone, ifosfamide, methotrexate, cytarabine, etoposide, and prophylactic intrathecal therapy). European Cooperative Group and POG studies have also shown promising results Lymphoblastic lymphoma • The prognosis for children with advanced lymphoblastic lymphoma has improved significantly over the past 25 years. The NHL-BFM-90 treatment regimen (high-dose methotrexate, dexamethasone, moderate doses of anthracyclines and cyclophosphamide with prophylactic cranial radiation, and treatment stratification based upon tumor response to induction therapy) has resulted in a 90% 3-year EFS
(Reaman 2005)	For the first time in 25 years, retinoblastoma is being evaluated in pediatric cooperative group studies. Three such clinical trials in retinoblastoma are now open. The studies are aimed at preserving vision in infants and young children who were previously managed with enucleation resulting in blindness and/or radiation therapy associated with a high risk of second cancers
(Abdullah et al. 2008)	• Medulloblastoma is the most common malignant CNS tumor in children • Major advances in the management of medulloblastoma have been achieved, since the first cooperative studies took place in the late 1970s • At that time, the standard treatment of medulloblastoma was based on surgery followed by craniospinal radiation • Pilot and randomized studies have contributed to refine the staging system, to identify risk groups, and to better tailor treatment according to risk factors • With the introduction of chemotherapy and improvement in surgical and radiotherapy techniques, 5-year survival rates in patients with average-risk medulloblastoma treated with craniospinal radiation and chemotherapy exceeded 80% • Improvements in survival have led to attempts to reduce the dose of craniospinal irradiation in average-risk patients, and the standard dose of craniospinal irradiation has dropped from 36 Gy in the 1980s and early 1990s to 23.4 Gy

Table 16.2. (Continued)

References	Summary
(Lukens 1994; Nesbit 1990)	• Solid tumors account for approximately 70% of malignant neoplasms in children younger than 15 years of age • The 5-year survival of children with solid tumors increased from 27 to 70% between 1960 and 1990 (Lukens 1994) *Wilms' tumor* • Survival rate has risen to 80% *Soft tissue sarcoma, brain tumors, and bone tumors* • Combination of preoperative chemotherapy, surgery, and radiotherapy followed by maintenance multiagent chemotherapy has resulted in a survival rate of 45–70% (Nesbit 1990) • The change in survival is a reflection of the nature of progress made through clinical trials Exploring novel strategies for the integration of different therapeutic modalities, clinical trials have identified indications for the use of – Presurgical chemotherapy – Preradiation chemotherapy – Second-look and delayed primary surgeries Refinements in the utilization of chemotherapy have been made possible by the evaluation of – New agents – The study of dose intensity – The use of the "window of opportunity" to identify active agents for tumors for which there is no effective treatment (Lukens 1994)

the presence of a tumor or may be a consequence of treatment such as nausea and vomiting (Linder 2005). In the early days of cancer treatment, antiemetics were ineffective and nausea and vomiting (N/V) was a source of much suffering for patients. Behavioral study of the problems of N/V was at the forefront of psycho-oncology research. After ondansetron was introduced in the early 1990s, for the first time, a highly effective, frontline antiemetic was available and N/V ceased to be a systemic problem requiring concentrated research efforts (Phipps 2005).

Pneumocystis carinii pneumonia (PCP) is a widely recognized opportunistic infection in immunocompromised pediatric oncology patients (Lindemulder and Albano 2007) that was associated with significant morbidity and mortality. Hughes et al. (1977) first demonstrated the efficacy of prophylactic daily administration of sulfamethoxazole-trimethorpim (SMX-TMP) in greatly reducing the incidence of PCP in pediatric oncology patients. Prophylactic SMX-TMP is now routinely used in pediatric oncology patients.

Invasive procedures such as bone marrow aspirations (BMAs) or lumbar punctures (LPs) are distressing for pediatric oncology patients, causing significant fear and anxiety (Holdsworth et al. 2003). At one time, they were perceived by parents and patients to be worse than the disease itself (Hilgard and LeBaron 1982). However, procedure-related distress decreased once the majority of BMAs and LPs were performed under conscious sedation, predominantly in the United States and Canada, or under general anesthetic, in the United Kingdom (Hain and Campbell 2001). This allowed the patient to be immobilized without restraint and provided a level of amnesia regarding the procedures.

Central venous catheters (CVC) today are essential for the care of pediatric oncology patients. CVCs ease the delivery of chemotherapy, blood products, and other supportive therapies by reducing the number of needle sticks that would be needed during the treatment Callahan C & De La Cruz H (2004). Some of the most distressing experiences for pediatric oncology patients are the pain from a needle stick and the associated phobia (Kettwich et al. 2007). CVCs decrease the need for the use of peripheral lines; frequently repeated peripheral cannulation can lead to destruction of the peripheral veins (McInally 2005). CVCs allow patients to conveniently receive certain treatment at home, such as cytosine arabinoside for ALL patients (Edwards and Breen 2002). CVCs have significantly improved pediatric oncology patient's experiences and QOL (Kettwich et al. 2007).

16.3.2 Quality of Life Measures and Supportive Care

QOL in pediatric oncology is multidimensional; it encompasses the cognitive, physical, and spiritual domains in addition to the emotional and social domains of the child and, when appropriate, their family (Bradlyn 2004; Rummans et al. 2006). It is influenced by individual experiences, beliefs, expectations, and perceptions (Sloan et al. 2002). Traditional endpoints such as disease-free survival (DFS), event-free survival (EFS), and overall survival (OS) reflect the effectiveness of the treatment, but these need to be supplemented to measure the impact of the treatment on the patients and sometimes their families (Bradlyn 2004).

McCaffrey (2006) conducted interviews with pediatric oncology patients, aged 5–15 years undergoing treatment and in remission, and their parents. The major stressors that they reported were treatment procedures, loss of control, the hospital environment, relapses, and fear of dying (McCaffrey 2006). Waters et al. (2003) conducted a health-related quality of life (HRQL) study in children, aged 5–18 years, with ALL. The results demonstrated that social and emotional health and well-being are significantly poorer in children with ALL than the health of their peers living without cancer (Waters et al. 2003). A study was carried out by Meeske et al. (2001) with 51 young adult survivors of childhood cancer 18–37 years of age. Eleven of the participants met the full criteria for posttraumatic stress disorder.

The QOL of the entire family is affected when a child is diagnosed with cancer. Family members have to adapt to physical absences of multiple family members due to inpatient hospitalizations and frequent medical appointments, interruptions to daily routines, new responsibilities, and financial strain (Robinson et al. 2007). Marital strain and divorce is a complication of childhood cancer (Weiner et al. 2005). For a family to adapt to a chronic pediatric condition, parental functioning and well-being are necessary (Goldbeck 2006). Parental distress has been linked to distress in their children (Robinson et al. 2007). Streisand et al. (2001) developed the Pediatric Inventory for Parents (PIP). A total of 126 parents of pediatric oncology patients, from birth to 21 years of age, at all stages of chemotherapy treatment and follow-up, completed the assessment. Younger parents, nonCaucasian parents, parents with younger children, and parents whose children had shorter illness duration reported more stress (Streisand et al. 2001). In a study comprising 122 parents, assessing the impact of the new diagnosis of a chronic pediatric condition on parental QOL, the parents described considerable restrictions on their emotional stability and general well-being. In addition, their physical/daily functioning was lower compared with that of parents of healthy children (Goldbeck 2006).

Nolbris et al. (2007) questioned the healthy siblings of cancer patients about their experiences of having a brother or sister with cancer. Healthy siblings reported that life had changed and would never be the same again. They reported feelings of anger and the difficulties in being loyal to a brother or sister with cancer when it conflicted with their own interests. They reported everyday life varied from periods of joy to worry and anxiety. Extra attention was thought to be given to the sibling with cancer, with their own emotional needs not being met. However, they also reported that it was good to have a sibling and how empty and lonely it would be without them. Zeltzer et al. (1996) conducted a seven-site study of 254 siblings (aged 5–18 years), of children with cancer, examining the overall health status, health-care utilization, somatization, and health-risk behaviors, and compared these factors with the matched controls or normative data. Siblings of pediatric cancer patients were found to be relatively healthy; most of them reported problems with sleeping and eating.

Health-risk behaviors were elicited from siblings aged 12 years and older. Among these 35% reported using alcohol more than once a month compared with the 3–33% from the normative data, and 26% reported using tobacco once a month compared with the 13–17.4% from the normative data. An important finding was that parents of these siblings were significantly less likely to seek medical help for a variety of conditions than were parents of control children (25% compared with over 50%). Another study assessed the HRQL of siblings of cancer patients attending the summer camp. The overall findings suggested that all the siblings, irrespective of whether or not their brother or sister had died, reported marked improvements in their HRQL, especially in the emotional and social domains. All the siblings described the camp as having a positive impact (Packman et al. 2005). These examples illustrate some of the QOL issues of the child with cancer and their family, and illustrate the larger scope of the problem.

A review of 70 pediatric oncology phase III clinical trials conducted from 1972 to 1991 demonstrated that less than 3% reported data on any HRQL dimension beyond toxicity (Bradlyn et al. 1995). Some patients may be too young or too incapacitated to report HRQL, in those cases the parent may act as a proxy (Russell et al. 2006); however, it is generally accepted that the patient is the best informant of their own HRQL (Bradlyn 2004). Vance et al. (2001) conducted a study on the relationship between child- and parent-reported QOL. Thirty-six parents and 32 children (8–12 years of age) completed the Pediatric Cancer Quality Life-32 (PCQL-32) scale. Based on the PCQL-32, parents rated their child's physical, cognitive, disease and treatment aspects of functioning as significantly poorer than their children rated themselves. Pediatric patients' self-report of HRQL is an important patient-based health outcome (Varni et al. 1999). Prior studies (Varni et al. 1987; Varni and Bernstein 1991) suggested that children as young as 5 years of age can self-report pain intensity using standardized Visual Analog Scales. The PedsQL is the first validated generic HRQL measure that was specifically designed for pediatric chronic health conditions (Varni et al. 1999). It is the first practical pediatric validated generic measure of HRQL that facilitates assessing risk, tracking health status, and measuring treatment outcomes.

Detmar et al. (2000) examined the extent to which adult palliative care patients and their physicians desired to discuss HRQL concerns and the impact on the routine communication of HRQL information upon clinical practice. They found a significant disparity between patients' and physicians' expectations with regard to the initiation of HRQL discussions, with each expecting the other to initiate the conversation. When HRQL information was routinely provided to physicians, more HRQL issues were discussed and more problems were identified; patients and physicians both rated this activity as beneficial. This study demonstrates the need for understanding the patient's HRQL issues and that there is a benefit to incorporating them into clinical studies. Even though there has been a dramatic increase in the development of pediatric HRQL measures over the last 20 years, there remain barriers to the inclusion of HRQL measures in pediatric oncology trials. These include a lack of acceptance and understanding of the available HRQL tools, a focus on the survival endpoints, and a lack of resource allocation (money and personnel) (Nathan et al. 2004). There is an increasing recognition that a thorough assessment of cancer treatment should include an evaluation of HRQL, in addition to the usual survival endpoints; HRQL measures offer an important and necessary tool in pediatric research.

16.3.3 Complementary and Alternative Medicine

Children with cancer use complementary and alternative medicine (CAM) to relieve symptoms, reduce side effects of treatment, and cope with the emotional aspects of having a life-threatening illness (Post-White et al. 2006). Surveys have shown that at least 31% of children with cancer use some form of CAM (Sencer and Kelly 2006). CAM can include exercise regimens, relaxation and massage therapy, hypnosis, diets, herbal remedies, individual or group counseling for the patients, family, and friends, art and music therapy, and spiritual guidance. However, some CAM therapies, particularly herbal remedies, may be unsafe. Unfortunately, very little research has been done to demonstrate the efficacy of such treatments or the potential interactions with cancer treatment. The State of Science Summit (SOS II) for pediatric oncology nursing, along with a working group meeting held in August 2003, titled "Moving the Research Agenda Forward for Children with Cancer," recommended a strategy for advancing this area of science by incorporating CAM studies into the ongoing COG clinical trials. Research in this area would allow researchers and practitioners to gain a better understanding of the alternative interventions and continue providing education on known interactions (Hare 2005). This would be a worthy endeavor as several studies have shown CAM to be popular among cancer patients (Nahleh and Tabbara 2003; Neuhouser et al. 2001; Saadat and Kain 2007; Swarup et al. 2006).

16.3.4 Late Effects

With the increasing number of pediatric cancer survivors, the intense effort to care for and cure a child with cancer does not end with survival. Continued surveillance and a variety of interventions may be needed to identify and care for either long-term or short-lived consequences of treatment which appear early on after therapy has ended, or decades later (Hewitt et al. 2003). More than two-thirds of the childhood cancer survivors experience late effects (Dickerman 2007). The emergence of late effects depends on many factors including age, exposures to chemotherapy and radiation during treatment (doses and parts of body exposed), and the severity of the disease. The most common late effects of childhood cancer include those that are neurocognitive and psychological, cardiopulmonary, endocrine, musculoskeletal, and those related to second malignancies.

Survivors may experience diminished cognitive functioning involving memory, quantitative skills, and abstract reasoning (Robison 2005). They may experience lower educational attainment (Robison 2005), have difficulty in gaining employment, and/or, if employed, have comparatively lower incomes (Apter et al. 2003).

Psychological and emotional problems can arise in adulthood related to issues such as marriage and fertility. Goodwin et al. (2007) surveyed health care providers about the issues surrounding cancer therapy and future fertility. Almost all providers agreed with the suggested recommendations to practice enhancement, including consulting with specialists ensuring that all patients at risk for infertility discuss preservation options, and that the need for additional training and information on the topic be available. The vast majority believed that children of any age should be included in discussions about fertility. Psychological issues also include the fear of a possible recurrence, a second malignancy, or some negative effect from treatment (Apter et al. 2003).

Families are essential for the care of the child with cancer (Kazak 2004); however, few studies have examined the caregiver's burden faced by parents of the childhood cancer survivors, and there is a paucity of studies that have examined family burden, related specifically to late effects. Family support and understanding of the needs of a child with neurodevelopmental late effects may limit the detrimental impact of these late effects (Peterson and Drotar 2006). A family systems approach to psychotherapy can possibly enhance the QOL of children and adolescent cancer survivors (Apter et al. 2003).

The issues of pediatric cancer survivorship differ from those of adults; there has been a huge movement in both North America and Europe to develop survivor programs to address these unique needs (Oeffinger et al. 2004; Taylor et al. 2004).

The AfterCare system in Ontario has so far been a remarkable success; it has been used as a model for the development of other survivor programs. As researchers and patients are becoming more aware of the risks associated with late effects, the number of patients currently found in the AfterCare system is expected to increase (Pediatric Oncology Group of Ontario 2005). This will provide the benefits of reaching a population-based cohort of survivors, and providing a unique opportunity for research in parallel with care delivery (Pediatric Oncology Group of Ontario 2005).

16.3.5 Palliative Care

Despite the successes in the treatment of childhood cancer, approximately a quarter of the patients may die as a result of their cancer or cancer treatment. The focus of pediatric oncology trials is curative. Few descriptive and even fewer intervention studies involving children at the end-of-life (EoL) have been published. Most palliative EoL studies are performed at single sites or limited number of institutions; thus, their finding are seldom generalizable. Larger, multi-institutional studies are required to decrease the suffering of children who are dying and to ease the suffering of bereaved survivors (Nuss et al. 2005).

Palliative research is conducted at a time when being a research participant may be extremely difficult. Researchers design studies keeping in mind the emotional and physical needs of the patient and family members (Hare 2005). The SOS II palliative and EoL consensus statements reflect the need to understand communication patterns to better understand suffering and grief, to respond to ethical dilemmas, and to design and implement interventions. Treatment decision- making takes on new challenges during relapse and EoL care. Differing expectations by family members and treatment providers may complicate the process of decision making (Kazak et al. 1997). Parents have identified EoL decisions as the most difficult treatment-related decisions that they face during their child's treatment (Hinds et al. 1997b).

A retrospective, descriptive study of parental perspectives of EoL, by the collaboration of researchers from three pediatric research centers – The Nebraska Medical Center, St. Jude's Children's Research Hospital, and Children's National Medical Center – found that when parents (12 mothers and 3 fathers) were asked open-ended questions about their child's death, the following themes/categories emerged from their analysis:

1. Abandonment
2. Acknowledging the child's wishes (giving all possible treatment or stopping treatment)
3. Anger (at God, at health-care professionals)
4. Communication (with health-care professionals, with family members, and friends)
5. Creating meaning (trying to find a purpose behind why the child has to die)
6. Experiencing the deceased (visualizing the child after death)
7. Visualizing specific phenomena, such as butterflies or rainbows
8. Faith (belief in God, spirituality)
9. Hope (that a miracle might occur)
10. Nursing actions (both positive and negative)
11. Regrets (wishing more had been done, wishing not to have agreed to a certain treatment)
12. Relationships (with health-care professionals, with family members, with friends)
13. Symptom management decreasing pain, easing dyspnea (difficulty breathing, shortness of breath) (Nuss et al. 2005)

The importance of EoL research regarding the experiences of dying children and their bereaved survivors is becoming more widely accepted. However, the gaps in research need to be addressed, particularly, related to interventions designed to prevent or minimize symptoms at the end of life; sadly, most parents reported the perception that their child suffered while dying (Nuss et al. 2005; Wolfe et al. 2000; Contro et al. 2002). The most promising of the intervention studies are those that include the perspectives, when possible, of the dying child or adolescent, the family members, and the health care providers (Nuss et al. 2005).

In single-site studies, interviews with bereaved parents indicated that approximately 25% suffer from substance abuse, marital dysfunction, or physical or mental illness, and that approximately one-third of surviving siblings experienced adaptation difficulties (Hongo et al. 2003; Rowa-Dewar 2002).

EoL research will directly benefit patients and their family members by easing their suffering, but it also has the promise of diminishing the suffering of health care providers by contributing to their sense of competence in providing EoL care (Nuss et al. 2005).

16.4 Perception of Clinical Trials

Current medical treatment practices center on evidence-based medicine (EBM). EBM is based on results obtained from RCTs or meta-analysis of RCTs (Anwar 2007). Before new therapies are approved, regulatory authorities require evidence from RCTs, to prove that a new therapy is as efficacious if not better than the current standard of care.

However, reasons why patients choose not to enroll in RCTs include the following:

- Random assignment of patients to treatment groups (Fallowfield et al. 1998).
- Patients should receive treatment and care based on their individual needs (Madsen et al. 2007).
- The patient would prefer to either make the decision themselves or have their doctor make the decision about which treatment they should receive (Slevin et al. 1995).
- Patients may perceive that one treatment option is better than another (Madsen et al. 2007).
- RCTs are viewed as experimentation, and patients do not want themselves to be used as "guinea pigs" (Ellis 2000).

Reasons why patients participate in a clinical research trial include:

- Benefiting others and advancing medical knowledge (Cassileth et al. 1982).
- Contributing to scientific knowledge (Slevin et al. 1995).
- Hope of receiving better care or treatment (Cassileth et al. 1980).
- Participation is the only way to the treatment (Madsen et al. 2007).
- Self interest (a more common reason for participating than altruism) (Edwards et al. 1998).

Madsen et al. (2007) carried out in-depth qualitative research interviews with female adult cancer patients who had either consented to participate or declined to participate in one of the three RCTs that included chemotherapy. Everyone, whether they chose to participate or not, in one of the three RCTs, expressed very positive attitudes towards clinical research, in general; they felt that clinical trials were pivotal for further development, and no patient saw trials as unnecessary. Most of the patients stated that the media was their major source for knowledge about clinical trials, and they judged the media to be untrustworthy, in general, and promoting disproportionately negative views of clinical trials.

Parents' perceptions are important to consider, as they are often the ones who decide if their child will participate in a research study. Rodriguez et al. (2006) conducted a study comprising 863 expectant parents, in which one of the objectives was to determine parent's willingness to allow children to participate in research. Seventy eight percent of the parents agreed with the statement that research in pediatrics is needed and 80% were willing to allow their child to become a research participant. However, half of the parents were unwilling to try a new treatment and the majority of parents would like the attending physician to evaluate the acceptable level of risk. Parents routinely seek their doctor's advice regarding clinical trial participation. Caldwell et al. (2003) conducted focus group discussions with 33 parents from a pediatric teaching hospital and a local school. All the parents who participated thought that those who had a child with a life-threatening condition would be more prepared to participate in the trials, in the hope of finding the "miracle cure" Parents whose child had cancer confirmed that they felt there was no choice about trial participation for their child's cancer treatment.

Deatrick et al. (2002) conducted a study on parents' views of their children's participation in phase I oncology trials. Some of the parent's expectations included: prolonging life, buying time for another therapy, and hope for a cure or a miracle. With regard to the decision about whether or not they should enroll their child on a phase I study, parents felt that they had limited choices or no choice at all in the decision-making process. It is a difficult decision for parents to decide between a phase I trial or stopping further active treatment for their child (Hinds et al. 1997a).

Estlin et al. (2000) surveyed oncologists' perceptions of phase I pediatric trials and cited the following potential benefits of participation to patients and their parents: medical benefit, palliation, maintaining hope, and altruism. Discussion between physicians and patients about clinical trials is an important factor in patients' decisions about whether to participate in a clinical trial. The results of another study showed a significant relationship between oncologists' recommendations and patients' decisions to participate in clinical trials (Eggly et al. 2008). This finding also supports previous studies demonstrating that physicians' behavior influences patients' decisions regarding the clinical trials (Nurgat et al. 2005; Albrecht et al. 1999; Daugherty et al. 1995).

Chang (2008) conducted an exploratory survey of nurses' perceptions of phase I pediatric oncology

Table 16.3. Nurses' opinions of phase I trials (Chang 2008)

Potential benefits	Negative impacts
Improving future treatments	Toxicities
Medical benefit	False hope
Improved quality of life (QOL) and hope	Decreased quality of life

trials. Overall, the perception of phase I trials was positive. The nurses felt that they were necessary or important. Nurses' opinions of phase 1 trials are highlighted in Table 16.3. Age, experience, and practice settings may influence the nurses' perceptions. On the whole, a positive view of clinical research trials has been observed, and some of the issues that can be addressed to improve the perception of clinical trials may begin with the informed consent process. Informed consent documents are necessary to provide patients with complete and comprehensible information.

16.5 Future of Clinical Trials

Although the majority of children with cancer will be cured, 20–30% will still die as a result of refractory disease or complications of treatment (Smith and Gloeckler 2002). There remains a need for new chemotherapy drugs to reduce morbidity and decrease mortality. Pediatric phase I trials are critical for the evaluation of promising new anticancer agents. They determine a safe and appropriate dose and schedule for new anticancer agents that can be subsequently used in phase II trials to test for activity against specific childhood cancers. Attention is also being focused on preventing psychosocial, biological, and behavioral consequences of cancer treatment (Reaman 2004).

Information from the clinical trial research allows laboratory research to further develop, leading to improved patient therapy. Molecular profiling of cancer cells as well as the evaluation of gene polymorphisms in children with cancer will likely drive future pediatric clinical cancer research. Table 16.4. illustrates some laboratory achievements and advancement in cancer therapy.

Table 16.4. Laboratory achievements and advancement in cancer therapy (Reaman 2004)

- Biological explanations for clinical observations
- Risk-adjusted therapies for specific pediatric cancers through biologically directed therapy
- Investigation of the human genome and the application of molecular genetics and cell biology
  - Uncovered causative effects related to specific genetic abnormalities in nearly every diagnostic subtype of childhood cancer
  - Contributed to understanding biological differences in natural history and response to therapy based on the presence or absence of specific genetic abnormalities
- Evaluating relationships between genetic abnormalities and environmental conditions to provide
  - Explanations for the causes of childhood cancer
  - Open new avenues for potential prevention strategies
- New methodologies to evaluate the variations in gene expression between cancer cells and normal cells, and between various clinically distinct and biological subclasses of specific cancers. This will have the potential to
  - Identify potential candidate genes, which might serve as specific therapeutic targets for a variety of pediatric malignancies
  - Expand existing risk-adjusted therapy using genetic profiling

Over the past decade, the investigation of human genetics and disease has shown that common genetic variation is a key component to understanding pediatric cancer and its outcome. Genetic variation has been shown to be associated with altered risk for cancer and its outcomes; it provides genetic markers for disease and insights into the biological pathways that are altered in cancer, and continued studies should unravel the interaction between genes and the environment (Chanock and Yeager 2007).

16.6 The Role of the Clinical Research Associate

16.6.1 Introduction

For as many different types of research studies, there are as many different types of clinical research professionals, either facilitating research by helping the research team to conduct the research or as a member of the frontline team that monitors the research to ensure that research is being conducted properly.

Clinical research professionals are known by a multitude of titles including clinical research managers, coordinators, assistants, and nurses. In this chapter, we will use the title of clinical research associate (CRA).

CRAs can be found in both the private and public sector, in industry and health-care settings. CRAs can be employed by pharmaceutical companies, be full-time employees of hospitals or community-based facilities, while others may be independent monitors who work for a clinical research organization (CRO). However, they are all guided by the International Conference on Harmonization principles of Good Clinical Practice.

Good Clinical Practices (GCP), Efficacy Topic E6, is an international ethical and scientific quality standard for designing, conducting, recording, and reporting trials that involve the participation of human subjects. Compliance with this standard provides public assurance that the rights, safety, and well-being of trial subjects are protected, consistent with the principles that have their origin in the Declaration of Helsinki, and that the clinical trial data are credible (The International Conference on Harmonization of Technical Requirements for the Registration of Pharmaceuticals for Human Use 1996).

16.6.2 Clinical Research Associate

McMaster University's definition of a certified CRA is an individual who functions as administrator, coordinator, consultant, educator, and/or researcher in the management of clinical trials. They are responsible for the administration and progress of a clinical trial, while understanding the ethical and legal ramifications for all participants. This covers protocol development, data collection, analysis, monitoring, recording, auditing, ethics and regulations, and liabilities and responsibilities of conducting research with human subjects (McMaster University 2007).

The CRA should be aware of the complete clinical trial process; from protocol development to relationships with investigators, nurses, and pharmacists (Hayes 2003).

Many CRAs learn on the job, with little experience or orientation. However, as the clinical trial industry becomes more regulated, more research training programs are available and required. Certification is required and, in some instances, is mandatory, to work in certain research areas, particularly in the industry.

Various societies have emerged catering to the certification, continued development, and education of CRAs, namely:

- Society of Clinical Research Associate (SoCRA), http://www.socra.org/
- Association of Clinical Research Professionals (ACRP), http://www.acrpnet.org/
- Regulatory Affairs Professional Society (RAPS), http://www.raps.org/personifyebusiness/

Clinical trials can be industry-sponsored, part of a cooperative group, such as COG, and/or investigator-initiated. CRAs can be involved in one of these types of clinical trials as members of research teams in hospitals, doctors and other medical offices, pharmaceutical companies, or CROs. While there are many diverse aspects of each position, they have many overlapping primary responsibilities. Table 16.5 lists the duties and responsibilities of a CRA.

Interpersonal skills such as diplomacy, negotiation, creative and effective problem solving, teamwork abilities, and above all, communication (Hayes 2003) are necessary to be successful; interaction is necessary with study participants and people throughout the organization and externally.

In research, time pressures compete against standards of quality (Hayes 2003). Efficient study set-up, successful patient recruitment, complete and accurate data, rapid data analysis, management of supplies and resources, budgets, and quality standards are essential in any research study. Serious problems can occur when there is a deviation from project expectations. A CRA may be a central link to all the resources vital to the smooth operation of the project, and he/she must be aware of the steps necessary to ensure the successful conduct of a research study (Fig. 16.2).

Table 16.5. Clinical research-associated responsibilities

Assists with protocol development
Case report form development
Informed consent/assent form development
Study management tool development
Site qualification visits by sponsor
Study site initiation meetings
Coordinating investigator and study meetings
Assists with grant writing
Standard operating procedure (SOP) development
Preparation of site agreements
Contracts management
Budget creation
Prepare protocol submission to appropriate boards (REB/IRB/SRB/section meetings, etc.) for scientific and ethical review
Screening
Patient recruitment
Review participants' eligibility criteria
Obtain informed consent (if feasible)
Data abstraction/collection
Case report form completion
Data entry
Specimen preparation
Specimen shipment
Make and respond to phone/fax/email queries
Update/correct data
(S)AE reporting
Implement amendment(s), update consent/assent forms
Manage protocol deviations and violations
Routine onsite monitoring
Schedule study visits
Management of investigative sites; regular communication to collect accurate and complete clinical data
Verify source documents
Attend meetings, i.e., protocol review meetings, inpatient hospital rounds, staff meetings
Audit (prepare, conduct)
Write journal articles
Assists with clinical study reports
Study site closeout
Closeout visits

16.6.3 The Role of the CRA

One of the key aspects essential for the successful operation of any clinical trial is for the CRAs to oversee the conduct of the trial. Although the researcher or the Principle Investigator (PI) retains the ultimate responsibility for the study, the CRA assumes the management of the study, assuring accountability for many regulatory aspects, such as compliance with the regulatory standards set forth by agencies such as the food and drug administration (FDA) or Health Canada, initial and continued review and approval of the protocol and consent forms by the institutional REB, timely notification of any (serious) adverse event, toxicity, or death of an enrolled patient, and accurate and complete recording of study data (Pelke and Easa 1997). CRAs play a key role in the implementation of oncology clinical trials that goes beyond data collection and/or administrative support, and contributes directly to gathering good a quality data (Rico-Villademoros et al. 2004; Vantongelen et al. 1989), which is essential for the success and future progress of clinical trials. One of the many challenges that cooperative groups such as COG face is adequately accruing the number of patients, particularly for their nontherapeutic studies. Six nontherapeutic studies between 1996 and 2006 were closed before their objectives were achieved owing to inadequate enrollment. Reeves et al. (2006) chose a nontherapeutic COG study and developed an elaborate plan to demonstrate that they could successfully achieve enrollment goals. The study CRA developed and implemented a set of electronic prompts that encouraged sites to open the study, enroll eligible patients, and collect study data at appropriate time points, and identified CRAs at eligible institutions to act as contacts and onsite facilitators. They concluded that the study CRA's leadership in developing this plan was key to the successful accrual of the projected sample.

Often patients are heavily influenced by the recommendation of their physician when weighing treatment options (Levinson et al. 2005). CRAs have clearly suggested that the physicians' communications skills are important to the success of recruitment, and having a vested interest in a particular trial increased their motivation to recruit patients

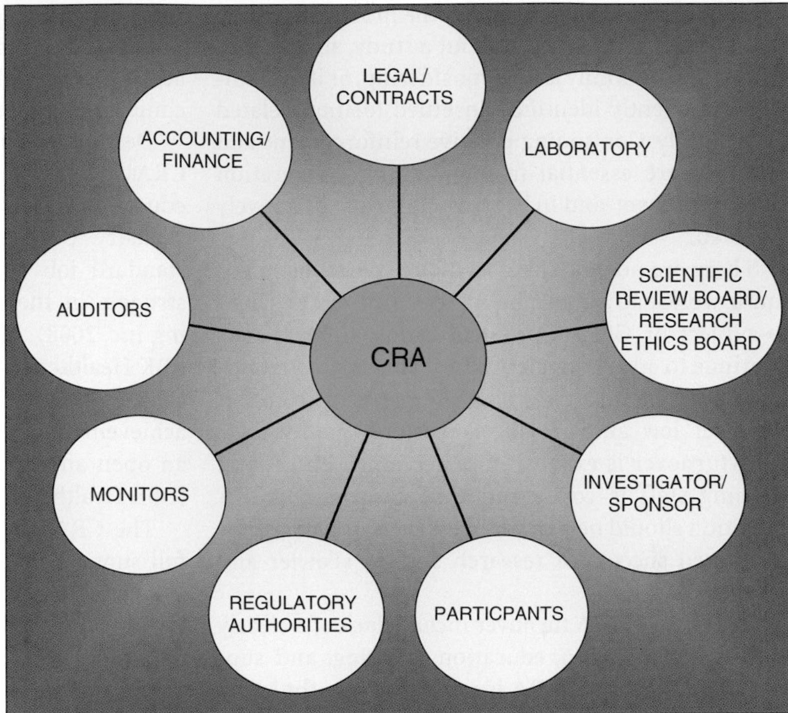

Figure 16.2
Representation of CRA as the central link to research resources

(Wright et al. 2002). They also conducted a descriptive study to explore the factors that influence the patients' decisions to enter RCTs. They suggested a potential for the CRA to influence patients' decisions that may be dependent on the level of involvement that the CRA has in the recruitment process (Wright et al. 2004). It would seem that the key to successful accrual is an interdependent consent process between the PI and CRA. Successful accrual indicates that study objectives can be realized, hypothesis can be examined, resources (e.g., time and money) can be saved, and that data gathered from the patients who participate are not merely discarded because the numbers are too few for analysis.

Collaboration between clinical care and research can be a challenge. For the research studies to be effectively implemented, it is important to involve those who are affected in any way as soon as possible (e.g., sponsor, PI, clinical staff). Inviting clinical staff to meetings to discuss the study allows the PI and the CRA to talk about the importance and relevance of the study and describe its potential benefits especially for enrolled patients (Pelke and Easa 1997). Sessions can clarify the roles of the research team, expectations of the clinic staff, and offer support to ensure the smooth operation of the study. This aims to engage the interest of clinic staff and alleviate any tension that may be caused because of disruption to their routine. In Ontario, provincial legislation requires that the initial contact for approaching a patient/family to participate in research is done by someone directly or following up that individual's care (Ministry of Health and Long Term Care 2004). Ellis et al. (2001) described a similar experience: if research is to take place in a setting where patient care occurs, the clinical staff needs to be made aware of the upcoming study activities. In-service training on general research methods and specific project expectations will help the nurses to understand the research process, and they frequently become a research team's best allies in finding and recruiting subjects (Ellis et al. 2001). For example, they can advise the researcher when it is the most convenient time to approach a family about a study, about other issues that the family is now considering, or if the family subsequently identifies unsettled feelings related to the study. Continuing positive reinforcement and feedback are essential in maintaining cooperation and enthusiasm, and in keeping clinical staff actively involved.

There are no guidelines to dictate what the maximum workload should be in terms of either CRA-to-subject or CRA-to-protocol ratios. Centers may continue to add or juggle studies. This is not an optimal management strategy if a site wants to keep staff turnover low and provide consistent quality data. CRA turnover is expensive for research centers and training staff is costly and time-consuming; CRA retention should be paramount if there is a desire for continued success of research studies (Fowler and Thomas 2003).

Reasons for CRA turnover include lack of a clearly defined job position, education, training, and support. The role of the CRA is not defined in the regulations or guidelines; neither US legislation nor ICH GCP guidelines include a definition of a CRA. Without proper training and education, CRAs may be unaware of the pertinent regulations, along with GCP guidelines. Table 16.6. lists some of the important agencies with regard to the good and ethical practice of clinical research. The CRAs can be held legally accountable for their actions during the conduct of a clinical research study (Wilson 2008).

Table 16.6. Agencies important to the good and ethical practice of research

European Union
FDA (Food and Drug Administration)
Health Canada
National Institutes of Health (NIH)
United States Department of Health and Human Services (DHHS)
Office for Human Research Protection (OHRP) (formerly OPRR)
World Health Organization (WHO)
Council for International Organizations and Medical Sciences (CIOMS)
International Conference on Harmonization of Technical Requirements for the Registration of Pharmaceuticals for Human Use (ICH)

Despite the importance to train and educate new CRAs, there remains a lack of standard training and education requirements within the clinical research industry. Until education and training becomes a standard job prerequisite, CRAs may continue to struggle in their roles (Clinical Research Consulting Inc. 2008). However, a survey carried out by the BBK Healthcare, Inc. revealed that 88% of CRAs had a strong sense of job satisfaction, 96% felt a sense of achievement, and that 91% reported that they enjoyed an open and responsive relationship with their PIs (BBK Healthcare Inc 2003).

The CRA cannot manage the study without the full support of the PI, and the PI cannot maintain adequate control of the study without the diligent attention of the CRA (Pelke and Easa 1997). Continued education, information, training, and support are essential for the successful development and retention of the CRA.

16.6.4 The Role of the Clinical Research Nurse

The role of the clinical research nurse (CRN) is unique, because they have the benefit of both the clinical and research knowledge of medical care. They can have a dual role in which they are both patient caregiver and clinical trial facilitator, sometimes having the role of the PI, CRA, or REB member. The CRN is responsible for safeguarding research participants, from the healthy to the acutely ill, and maintaining the integrity of the research study in settings ranging from ambulatory to inpatient (McCabe and Cahill Lawrence 2007). Discussion about the research study between the CRN and the research participant can pose an ethical dilemma, because they may have an undue influence on the participant. This is an area where the CRN must clearly delineate their role as care provider vs. researcher so that the research participant may make a truly informed consent decision. By clarifying the specific roles of healthcare personnel, therapeutic misconception can be avoided. Therapeutic misconception occurs when there is a blurred distinction between the goals of research and that of standard treatment in the view of the participant; they mistakenly attribute a therapeutic benefit to the research procedures when there may be none (Steinke 2004).

During the past 30 years, nursing research has had a positive impact on the specialty of pediatric oncology nursing. Nursing research has included work carried out by a single researcher at an institution to multidisciplinary research teams collaborating on the same study at numerous institutions. Research conducted by pediatric oncology nurse researchers has helped to optimize how childhood cancer is treated and how it is approached.

An example of a nursing research program that arose in response to an immediate need is the work of Dr. Ida Martinson (Schneider et al. 2001). Dr Martinson explored the dilemma of a physician having to admit a young boy with terminal cancer to the hospital to die. Out of a practical issue of improving the QOL for the child and his family, Dr. Martinson conducted a study in which she provided care for eight dying patients and their families in their homes (Martinson 1976). Because of her success with these initial eight cases, Dr. Martinson was awarded funding from the NCI to expand her work and eventually build a program of research designed to study the death of a child at home. The option for terminally ill children to go home to die is in large part because of Dr. Martinson's work (Schneider et al. 2001).

Research on cancer and treatment-related fatigue in children and adolescents with cancer has been led by nurse researchers (Davies et al. 2002; Hinds and Hockenberry-Eaton 2001; Hinds et al. 2007a, b; Hockenberry-Eaton and Hinds 2000; Hockenberry-Eaton et al. 1998; Ream et al. 2006). Fatigue is believed to contribute to the patient's overall morbidity (Davies et al. 2002). Fatigue during cancer treatment is more closely related to QOL than nausea, vomiting, or loss of appetite (Schumacher et al. 2002).

Historically, nursing has contributed significantly to the successful implementation of cooperative group clinical trials, by educating patients, families, and nurses about treatment protocols and clinical trials. In February 2000, the COG Nursing Discipline Committee took a more direct role, contributing to the COG scientific agenda, by creating the first-ever State of the Science Summit (SOS I) for Pediatric Oncology Nursing Research. The summit allowed nurses to put forward research questions of high priority to the nursing care of children and adolescents with cancer. Following the summit, four nursing research teams were created with the directive to contribute directly to the scientific mission of COG through their research efforts based on their own areas of defined expertise (Hinds and DeSwarte-Wallace 2000). The anticipated indicators of success for these nursing research teams included one or more of each of the following: productive committee placements within the COG committee structure, publications, concepts, research objectives nested within the therapeutic protocols, freestanding nurse-led protocols, research grants, and presentations (Hinds and DeSwarte-Wallace 2000). This past decade has witnessed nursing research thrive and expand with a strong foundation of committed individuals who share the same passion for quality of care. CRNs continue to provide practice changing contributions, improvements to the QOL of the pediatric patients and their families, along with continued contributions to their specialty and discipline.

References

Abdullah S, Qaddoumi I, Bouffet E (2008) Advances in the management of pediatric central nervous system tumors. Annals of the New York Academy of Sciences 1138:22–31

Adamson PC (2008) Advances in drug development: current challenges in pediatric drug development. Clinical Advances in Hematology and Oncology 6(12):883–884

Afshar K, Lodha A, Costei A, Vaneyke N (2005) Recruitment in pediatric clinical trials: an ethical perspective. Journal of Urology 174:835–840

Albrecht TL, Blanchard C, Ruckdeschel JC, Coovert M, Strongbow R (1999) Strategic physician communication and oncology clinical trials. Journal of Clinical Oncology 17: 3324–3332

Anwar S (2007) Evidence based medicine, systematic reviews and meta-analysis of literature: a powerful tool for the practising doctor. Journal of the College of Physicians and Surgeons – Pakistan 17:123–124

Apter A, Farbstein I, Yaniv I (2003) Psychiatric aspects of pediatric cancer. Child and Adolescent Psychiatric Clinics of North America 12:473–492

BBK Healthcare Inc (2003) Patient recruitment: a CRC perspective. available at: http://www.iptonline.com/articles/public/ICTTWO22NoPrint.pdf. Accessed

Bleyer A, Budd T, Montello M (2006) Adolescents and young adults with cancer: the scope of the problem and criticality of clinical trials. Cancer 107:1645–1655

Boissel N, Auclerc M-F, Lheritier V, Perel Y, Thomas X, Leblanc T, Rousselot P, Cayuela J-M, Gabert J, Fegueux N, Piguet C, Huguet-Rigal F, Berthou C, Boiron J-M, Pautas C, Michel G, Fiere D, Leverger G, Dombret H, Baruchel A (2003) Should adolescents with acute lymphoblastic leukemia be treated as old children or young adults? Comparison of the French FRALLE-93 and LALA-94 trials [comment]. Journal of Clinical Oncology 21:774–780

Bond M, Pritchard S (2006) Understanding Clinical Trials in Childhood Cancer. Pediatrics and Child Health 11:148–150

Bradlyn AS (2004) Health-related quality of life in pediatric oncology: current status and future challenges. Journal of Pediatric Oncology Nursing 21:137–140

Bradlyn AS, Harris CV, Spieth LE (1995) Quality of life assessment in pediatric oncology: a retrospective review of phase III reports. Social Science and Medicine 41:1463–1465

British Paediatric Association (1992) Guidelines for the Ethical Conduct of Medical Research Involving Children. Available (Accessed 25 Feb 2009)

Callahan C & De La Cruz H (2004): Central line placement for the pediatric oncology patient: a model of advanced practice nurse collaboration. Journal of Pediatric Oncology Nursing 21, 16–21

Caldwell PHy, Butow PN, Craig JC. Parents' attitudes to children's participation in randomized controlled trials.[see comment]. Journal of Pediatrics. 2003 May;142(5):554–9

Cairo M (2003) Advances in Non-Hodgkin's lymphoma treatments for children and adolescents available at: http://www.lymphoma.org/site/pp.aspx?c=chKOI6PEImE&b=1573485&printmode=1. Accessed 25 Feb 2009

Canadian Pediatric Society (2008) Advance care planning for pediatric patients. Canadian Paediatric Society 13:791–796

Cassileth BR, Lusk EJ, Miller DS, Hurwitz S (1982) Attitudes toward clinical trials among patients and the public. The Journal of the American Medical Association 248:968–970

Cassileth BR, Zupkis RV, Sutton-Smith K, March V (1980) Information and participation preferences among cancer patients. Annals of Internal Medicine 92:832–836

Chang A (2008) An exploratory survey of nurses' perceptions of phase I clinical trials in pediatric oncology. Journal of Pediatric Oncology Nursing 25:14–23

Chanock S, Yeager M (2007) The future of pediatric cancer and complex diseases: aren't they all? Pediatric Blood and Cancer 48:719–722

Children's Cancer and Leukaemia Group (2007) Background. Available at: http://www.cclg.org.uk/public/about_us/introduction/Background.html. Accessed 25 Feb 2009

Clinical Research Consulting Inc (2008) Clinical research coordinator: a career alternative for nurses available at: http://www.eclinicalresearchconsulting.com/career.php. Accessed

Collins JJ, Byrnes ME, Dunkel IJ, Lapin J, Nadel T, Thaler HT, Polyak T, Rapkin B, Portenoy RK (2000) The measurement of symptoms in children with cancer. Journal of Pain and Symptom Management 19:363–377

Committee on Drugs American Academy of Pediatrics (1995) Guidelines for the ethical conduct of studies to evaluate drugs in pediatric populations. Committee on drugs, American academy of pediatrics. Pediatrics 95:286–294

Contro N, Larson J, Scofield S, Sourkes B, Cohen H (2002) Family perspectives on the quality of pediatric palliative care [see comment]. Archives of Pediatrics and Adolescent Medicine 156:14–19

Council for International Organizations of Medical Sciences (2002) International ethical guidelines for biomedical research involving human subjects. Available at: http://www.cioms.ch/frame_guidelines_nov_2002.html.Accessed 25 Feb 2009

Creutzig U, Klussmann J-H (2004) Persönlichkeiten. In: Hildebrant B (ed) Chronik der Gesellschaft für Pädiatrische Onkologie und Hämatologie. Gesellschaft für Pädiatrische Onkologie und Hämatologie (GPOH), Hannover, p 37

Daugherty C, Ratain MJ, Grochowski E, Stocking C, Kodish E, Mick R, Siegler M (1995) Perceptions of cancer patients and their physicians involved in phase I trials [see comment] [erratum appears in J Clin Oncol 1995 Sep;13(9):2476]. Journal of Clinical Oncology 13:1062–1072

Davies B, Whitsett SF, Bruce A, McCarthy P (2002) A typology of fatigue in children with cancer. Journal of Pediatric Oncology Nursing 19:12–21

Deatrick JA, Angst DB, Moore C. Parents' views of their children's participation in phase I oncology clinical trials. Journal of Pediatric Oncology Nursing. 2002 Jul-Aug;19(4):114–21

de Bont JM, van der Holt B, Dekker AW, van der Does-van den Berg A, Sonneveld P, Pieters R (2004) Significant difference in outcome for adolescents with acute lymphoblastic leukemia treated on pediatric vs adult protocols in the Netherlands. Leukemia 18:2032–2035

Degner LF, Sloan JA (1995) Symptom distress in newly diagnosed ambulatory cancer patients and as a predictor of survival in lung cancer. Journal of Pain and Symptom Management 10:423–431

Detmar SB, Aaronson NK, Wever LD, Muller M, Schornagel JH (2000) How are you feeling? Who wants to know? Patients' and oncologists' preferences for discussing health-related quality-of-life issues. Journal of Clinical Oncology 18: 3295–3301

Devine S, Dagher RN, Weiss KD, Santana VM (2008) Good clinical practice and the conduct of clinical studies in pediatric oncology. Pediatric Clinics of North America 55:187–209

Dickerman JD (2007) The late effects of childhood cancer therapy.[erratum appears in Pediatrics. 2007 May;119(5):1045]. Pediatrics 119:554–568

Diekema DS (2006) Conducting ethical research in pediatrics: a brief historical overview and review of pediatric regulations. Journal of Pediatrics 149:S3–11

Directive 2001/20/EC (2001) Directive 2001/20/EC of the European Parliament and of the Council of 4 April 2001 on the approximation of the laws, regulations and administrative provisions of the Member States relating to the implementation of good clinical practice in the conduct of clinical trials on medicinal products for human use. Available at: http://europa.eu/eur-lex/pri/en/oj/dat/2001/l_121/l_12120010501en00340044.pdf. Accessed 25 Feb 2009

Duffner PK, Cohen ME, Flannery JT (1982) Referral patterns of childhood brain tumors in the state of Connecticut. Cancer 50:1636–1640

Estlin EJ, Cotterill S, Pratt CB, Pearson AD, Bernstein M. Phase I trials in pediatric oncology: perceptions of pediatricians from the United Kingdom Children's Cancer Study Group and the Pediatric Oncology Group. Journal of Clinical Oncology. 2000 May;18(9):1900–5

Eden OB, Harrison G, Richards S, Lilleyman JS, Bailey CC, Chessells JM, Hann IM, Hill FG, Gibson BE (2000) Long-term follow-up of the United Kingdom Medical Research Council protocols for childhood acute lymphoblastic leukaemia, 1980–1997. Medical Research Council Childhood Leukaemia Working Party. Leukemia 14:2307–2320

Edwards J, Breen M (2002) Intravenous chemotherapy for children at home. Cancer Nursing Practice 1:26–29

Edwards SJ, Lilford RJ, Hewison J (1998) The ethics of randomised controlled trials from the perspectives of patients, the public, and healthcare professionals. British Medical Journal 317:1209–1212

Eggly S, Albrecht TL, Harper FWK, Foster T, Franks MM, Ruckdeschel JC (2008) Oncologists' recommendations of clinical trial participation to patients. Patient Education and Counseling 70:143–148

Ellis E, Riegel B, Hamon M, Carlson B, Jimenez S, Parkington S (2001) The challenges of conducting clinical research: one research team's experiences [see comment]. Clinical Nurse Specialist 15:286–292; quiz 293–284

Ellis PM (2000) Attitudes towards and participation in randomised clinical trials in oncology: a review of the literature. Annals of Oncology 11:939–945

Ellis R, Leventhal B. Information needs and decision-making preferences of children with cancer. Psycho-Oncology. 1993 December;2 (4):229–301

Fallowfield LJ, Jenkins V, Brennan C, Sawtell M, Moynihan C, Souhami RL (1998) Attitudes of patients to randomised clinical trials of cancer therapy. European Journal of Cancer 34:1554–1559

Ferrari A, Dileo P, M C, Bertulli R, Meazza C, Gandola L, Navarria P, Collini P, Gronchi A, Olmi P, Fossati-Bellani F, Casali PG (2003) Rhabdomyosarcoma in adults. A retrospective analysis of 171 patients treated at a single institution. Cancer 98:571–580

Ferrari A, Montello M, Budd T, Bleyer A (2008) The challenges of clinical trials for adolescents and young adults with cancer. Pediatric Blood and Cancer 50:1101–1104

Food and Drug Administration (1988) 21 CFR Parts 50 and 56 Protection of Human Subjects; Informed Consent; Standards for Institutional Review Boards for Clinical Investigations. Available at: http://www.fda.gov/oc/gcp/preambles/53fr45678C.html. Accessed 25 Feb 2009

Food and Drug Administration (2009) Basic Questions and Answers about Clinical Trials. Available Food and Drug Administration (Accessed February 25, 2009)

Fowler DR, Thomas CJ (2003) Protocol acuity scoring as a rational approach to clinical research management. Research Practitioner 4:64–71

Gans-Brangs KR, Plourde PV (2006) The evolution of legislation to regulate pediatric clinical trials: present and continuing challenges. Advanced Drug Delivery Reviews 58:106–115

Gaynon PS, Angiolillo AL, Franklin JL, Reaman GH (2003) Childhood acute lymphoblastic leukemia. In: Kufe DW, Pollock RE, Weichselbaum RP, Bast RC, Gangler TS, Holland JR (eds) Cancer medicine. Decker, Hamilton, pp 2307–2316

Gesellschaft für Pädiatrische Onkologie und Hämatologie (GPOH) (2006) Therapy Optimising Trials. Available at: http://www.kinderkrebsinfo.de/e1664/e1676/e1758/index_eng.html. Accessed 25 Feb 2009

Gesellschaft für Pädiatrische Onkologie und Hämatologie (GPOH) (2007) GPOH: Who We Are. Available at: http://www.kinderkrebsinfo.de/e2260/e2298/index_eng.html. Accessed 25 Feb 2009

Goodwin T, Elizabeth Oosterhuis B, Kiernan M, Hudson MM, Dahl GV. Attitudes and practices of pediatric oncology providers regarding fertility issues.[see comment]. Pediatric Blood & Cancer. 2007 Jan;48(1):80–5

Goldbeck L (2006) The impact of newly diagnosed chronic paediatric conditions on parental quality of life. Quality of Life Research 15:1121–1131

Hain RD, Campbell C (2001) Invasive procedures carried out in conscious children: contrast between North American and European paediatric oncology centres. Archives of Disease in Childhood 85:12–15

Hare ML (2005) Comparing research priorities for pediatric oncology from two panels of experts. Seminars in Oncology Nursing 21:145–150

Hayes G (2003) The Clinical Research Associate. In: Stonier PD (ed) Careers with the Pharmaceutical Industry, 2nd edn. Wiley, New York, pp 67–78

Health Canada (2003) Tri-Council policy statement: ethical conduct for research involving humans. Available at: http://www.pre.ethics.gc.ca/english/policystatement/policystatement.cfm. Accessed 25 Feb 2009

Hewitt M, Weiner SL, Simone JV (2003) Late effects of childhood cancer. In: Council NR (ed) Childhood cancer survivorship: improving care and quality of life. The National Academies Press, Washington, pp 49–89

Hilgard J, LeBaron S (1982) Relief of anxiety and pain in children with cancer: quantitative measures and qualitative clinical observation in a flexible approach. The International Journal of Clinical and Experimental Hypnosis 30:417–424

Hinds PS, DeSwarte-Wallace J (2000) Positioning nursing research to contribute to the scientific mission of the Pediatric Oncology Cooperative Group. Seminars in Oncology Nursing 16:251–252

Hinds PS, Hockenberry-Eaton M (2001) Developing a research program on fatigue in children and adolescents diagnosed with cancer. Journal of Pediatric Oncology Nursing 18: 3–12

Hinds PS, Hockenberry M, Rai SN, Zhang L, Razzouk BI, McCarthy K, Cremer L, Rodriguez-Galindo C (2007a) Nocturnal awakenings, sleep environment interruptions, and fatigue in hospitalized children with cancer. Oncology Nursing Forum Online 34:393–402

Hinds PS, Hockenberry MJ, Gattuso JS, Srivastava DK, Tong X, Jones H, West N, McCarthy KS, Sadeh A, Ash M, Fernandez C, Pui C-H (2007b) Dexamethasone alters sleep and fatigue in pediatric patients with acute lymphoblastic leukemia. Cancer 110:2321–2330

Hinds PS, Oakes L, Furman W, Foppiano P, Olson MS, Quargnenti A, Gattuso J, Powell B, Srivastava DK, Jayawardene D, Sandlund JT, Strong C (1997a) Decision making by parents and healthcare professionals when considering continued care for pediatric patients with cancer. Oncology Nursing Forum 24:1523–1528

Hinds PS, Ruccione K, Kelly KP (1997b) Developing intergroup nursing research in pediatric oncology. Journal of Pediatric Oncology Nursing 14:135–136

Hockenberry-Eaton M and Hinds PS (2000) Fatigue in children and adolescents with cancer: evolution of a program of study. Seminars in Oncology Nursing 16:261–272; discussion 272–268

Hockenberry-Eaton M, Hinds PS, Alcoser P, O'Neill JB, Euell K, Howard V, Gattuso J, Taylor J (1998) Fatigue in children and adolescents with cancer. Journal of Pediatric Oncology Nursing 15:172–182

Holdsworth MT, Raisch DW, Winter SS, Frost JD, Moro MA, Doran NH, Phillips J, Pankey JM, Mathew P (2003) Pain and distress from bone marrow aspirations and lumbar punctures. Annals of Pharmacotherapy 37:17–22

Hongo T, Watanabe C, Okada S, Inoue N, Yajima S, Fujii Y, Ohzeki T (2003) Analysis of the circumstances at the end of life in children with cancer: symptoms, suffering and acceptance. Pediatrics International 45:60–64

Hughes WT, Kuhn S, Chaudhary S, Feldman S, Verzosa M, Aur RJ, Pratt C, George SL (1977) Successful chemoprophylaxis for Pneumocystis carinii pneumonitis. New England Journal of Medicine 297:1419–1426

Kazak AE (2004) Research priorities for family assessment and intervention in pediatric oncology. Journal of Pediatric Oncology Nursing 21:141–144

Kazak AE, Barakat LP, Meeske K, Christakis D, Meadows AT, Casey R, Penati B, Stuber ML (1997) Posttraumatic stress, family functioning, and social support in survivors of childhood leukemia and their mothers and fathers. Journal of Consulting and Clinical Psychology 65:120–129

Kamps WA, Akkerboom JC, Nitschke R, Kingma A, Holmes HB, Caldwell S, et al. Altruism and Informed Consent in Chemotherapy Trials in Childhood Cancer. Loss Grief & Care. 1987;1(3–4):93–110

Kettwich SC, Sibbitt WL Jr, Brandt JR, Johnson CR, Wong CS, Bankhurst AD (2007) Needle phobia and stress-reducing medical devices in pediatric and adult chemotherapy patients. Journal of Pediatric Oncology Nursing 24:20–28

Lennox EL, Stiller CA, Jones PH, Wilson LM (1979) Nephroblastoma: treatment during 1970–3 and the effect on survival of inclusion in the first MRC trial. British Medical Journal 2:567–569

Levinson W, Kao A, Kuby A, Thisted RA (2005) Not all patients want to participate in decision making. A national study of public preferences. Journal of General Internal Medicine 20:531–535

Lewis IJ (1996) Cancer in adolescence. British Medical Bulletin 52:887–897

Lind C, Anderson B, Oberle K (2003) Ethical issues in adolescent consent for research. Nursing Ethics 10:504–511

Lindemulder S, Albano E (2007) Successful intermittent prophylaxis with trimethoprim/sulfamethoxazole 2 days per week for Pneumocystis carinii (jiroveci) pneumonia in pediatric oncology patients. Pediatrics 120:e47–51

Linder LA (2005) Measuring physical symptoms in children and adolescents with cancer. Cancer Nursing 28:16–26

Lukens JN (1994) Progress resulting from clinical trials. Solid tumors in childhood cancer. Cancer 74:2710–2718

Macrae D (2009) Conducting clinical trials in pediatrics. Critical Care Medicine 37:S136–S139

Madsen SM, Holm S, Riis P (2007) Attitudes towards clinical research among cancer trial participants and non-participants: an interview study using a Grounded Theory approach. Journal of Medical Ethics 33:234–240

Martinson IM (1976) Why don't we let them die at home? RN 39:58–65

McCabe M, Cahill Lawrence CA (2007) The clinical research nurse. American Journal of Nursing 107:13

McCaffrey CN (2006) Major stressors and their effects on the well-being of children with cancer. Journal of Pediatric Nursing 21:59–66

McInally W (2005) Whose line is it anyway? Management of central venous catheters in children. Paediatric Nursing 17:14–18

McMaster University (2007) Certified Clinical Research Associate. Available at: http://www.mcmaster.ca/conted/programs/ccra/. Accessed 25 Feb 2009

McTiernan A (2003) Issues surrounding the participation of adolescents with cancer in clinical trials in the UK. European Journal of Cancer Care 12:233–239

Meadows AT, Kramer S, Hopson R, Lustbader E, Jarrett P, Evans AE (1983) Survival in childhood acute lymphocytic leukemia: effect of protocol and place of treatment. Cancer Investigation 1:49–55

Meeske KA, Ruccione K, Globe DR, Stuber ML (2001) Posttraumatic stress, quality of life, and psychological distress in young adult survivors of childhood cancer. Oncology Nursing Forum 28:481–489

Ministry of Health and Long Term Care (2004) Personal Health Information Protection Act, 2004. Ministry of Health and Long Term Care Available (Accessed February 25, 2009)

Murphy SB (1995) The national impact of clinical cooperative group trials for pediatric cancer [comment]. Medical and Pediatric Oncology 24:279–280

Nachman J, Sather HN, Buckley JD, Gaynon PS, Steinherz PG, Tubergen DG, Lampkin BC, Hammond GD (1993) Young adults 16–21 years of age at diagnosis entered on Childrens Cancer Group acute lymphoblastic leukemia and acute myeloblastic leukemia protocols. Results of treatment. Cancer 71:3377–3385

Nahleh Z, Tabbara IA (2003) Complementary and alternative medicine in breast cancer patients. Palliative and Supportive Care 1:267–273

Nathan PC, Furlong W, Barr RD (2004) Challenges to the measurement of health-related quality of life in children receiving cancer therapy. Pediatric Blood and Cancer 43: 215–223

National Cancer Institute (2008) Building on 50 years of cooperative cancer research. Available at: http://www.cancer.gov/ncicancerbulletin/NCI_Cancer_Bulletin_031808/page4. Accessed 25 Feb 2009

National Council on Ethics in Human Research (1996) Facilitating ethical research: promoting informed choice. Available at: http://www.ncehr-cnerh.org/english/consent/consente.html#s2. Accessed 25 Feb 2009

National Institutes of Health (2001a) Children's assent to clinical trial participation. Available at: http://www.cancer.gov/clinicaltrials/understanding/childrensassent0101. Accessed 25 Feb 2009

National Institutes of Health (2001b) How is a clinical trial planned and carried out? Available at: http://www.cancer.gov/clinicaltrials/learning/how-trials-are-done. Accessed 25 Feb 2009

National Institutes of Health (2007) Understanding clinical trials. Available at: http://clinicaltrials.gov/ct2/info/understand. Accessed 25 Feb 2009

Nesbit ME Jr (1990) Advances and management of solid tumors in children. Cancer 65:696–702

Neuhouser ML, Patterson RE, Schwartz SM, Hedderson MM, Bowen DJ, Standish LJ (2001) Use of alternative medicine by children with cancer in Washington state. Preventive Medicine 33:347–354

Newburger PE, Elfenbein DS, Boxer LA (2002) Adolescents with cancer: access to clinical trials and age-appropriate care. Current Opinion in Pediatrics 14:1–4

Nolbris M, Enskar K, Hellstrom A-L (2007) Experience of siblings of children treated for cancer. European Journal of Oncology Nursing 11:106–112; discussion 113–106

Nurgat ZA, Craig W, Campbell NC, Bissett JD, Cassidy J, Nicolson MC (2005) Patient motivations surrounding participation in phase I and phase II clinical trials of cancer chemotherapy. British Journal of Cancer 92:1001–1005

Nuss SL, Hinds PS, LaFond DA (2005) Collaborative clinical research on end-of-life care in pediatric oncology. Seminars in Oncology Nursing 21:125–134; discussion 134–144

Oeffinger KC, Mertens AC, Hudson MM, Gurney JG, Casillas J, Chen H, Whitton J, Yeazel M, Yasui Y, Robison LL (2004) Health care of young adult survivors of childhood cancer: a report from the Childhood Cancer Survivor Study. Annals of Family Medicine 2:61–70

Packman W, Greenhalgh J, Chesterman B, Shaffer T, Fine J, Van Zutphen K, Golan R, Amylon MD (2005) Siblings of pediatric cancer patients: the quantitative and qualitative nature of quality of life. Journal of Psychosocial Oncology 23:87–108

Paulussen S, Ahrens S, Juergens H (2003) Cure rates in Ewing tumor patients aged over 15 years are better in pediatric onology units. Proceedings of the American Society of Clinical Oncology 22:816a

Pediatric Oncology Group of Ontario (2005) Provincial Pediatric Oncology Plan (PPOP) 2005–2010. Available at: http://www.pogo.ca/_media/File/PPOP/PPOPFNL-WebVersion.pdf. Accessed 25 Feb 2009

Pelke S, Easa D (1997) The role of the clinical research coordinator in multicenter clinical trials. Journal of Obstetric, Gynecologic, and Neonatal Nursing 26:279–285

Peterson CC, Drotar D (2006) Family impact of neurodevelopmental late effects in survivors of pediatric cancer: review of research, clinical evidence, and future directions. Clinical Child Psychology and Psychiatry 11:349–366

Phipps S (2005) Commentary: contexts and challenges in pediatric psychosocial oncology research: chasing moving targets and embracing "good news" outcomes [comment]. Journal of Pediatric Psychology 30:41–45

Post-White J, Hawks R, O'Mara A, Ott MJ (2006) Future directions of CAM research in pediatric oncology. Journal of Pediatric Oncology Nursing 23:265–268

Public Health Agency of Canada (2005) The Canadian childhood cancer surveillance and control program (CCCSCP). Available at: http://www.phac-aspc.gc.ca/ccdpc-cpcmc/program/cccscp-pcslce/index-eng.php. Accessed 25 Feb 2009

Ramanujachar R, Richards S, Hann I, Goldstone A, Mitchell C, Vora A, Rowe J, Webb D (2007) Adolescents with acute lymphoblastic leukaemia: outcome on UK national paediatric (ALL97) and adult (UKALLXII/E2993) trials. Pediatric Blood and Cancer 48:254–261

Ramanujachar R, Richards S, Hann I, Webb D (2006) Adolescents with acute lymphoblastic leukaemia: emerging from the shadow of paediatric and adult treatment protocols. Pediatric Blood and Cancer 47:748–756

Ravindranath Y, Chang M, Steuber CP, Becton D, Dahl G, Civin C, Camitta B, Carroll A, Raimondi SC, Weinstein HJ, Pediatric Oncology G (2005) Pediatric Oncology Group (POG) studies of acute myeloid leukemia (AML): a review of four consecutive childhood AML trials conducted between 1981 and 2000. Leukemia 19:2101–2116

Reeves E, Keegan Wells D, Hinds PS, Kelly KP, Zhou T. The Study Clinical Research Associate (CRA) An Essential Co-Investigator to Facilitate Enrollment on Cooperative Group Protocols SOCRA Source. 2006(48):28–32

Ream E, Gibson F, Edwards J, Seption B, Mulhall A, Richardson A (2006) Experience of fatigue in adolescents living with cancer. Cancer Nursing 29:317–326

Reaman GH (2004) Pediatric cancer research from past successes through collaboration to future transdisciplinary research. Journal of Pediatric Oncology Nursing 21:123–127

Reaman GH (2005) Clinical advances in pediatric hematology and oncology: cooperative group research. Clinical Advances in Hematology and Oncology 3:133–135

Rico-Villademoros F, Hernando T, Sanz J-L, Lopez-Alonso A, Salamanca O, Camps C, Rosell R (2004) The role of the clinical research coordinator–data manager–in oncology clinical trials. BMC Medical Research Methodology 4:6

Rodriguez A, Tuvemo T, Hansson MG. Parents' perspectives on research involving children. Upsala Journal of Medical Sciences. 2006;111(1):73–86

Robinson KE, Gerhardt CA, Vannatta K, Noll RB (2007) Parent and family factors associated with child adjustment to pediatric cancer. Journal of Pediatric Psychology 32:400–410

Robison LL (2005) The Childhood Cancer Survivor Study: a resource for research of long-term outcomes among adult survivors of childhood cancer. Minnesota Medicine 88: 45–49

Rowa-Dewar N (2002) Do interventions make a difference to bereaved parents? A systematic review of controlled studies. International Journal of Palliative Nursing 8:452–457

Rummans TA, Clark MM, Sloan JA, Frost MH, Bostwick JM, Atherton PJ, Johnson ME, Gamble G, Richardson J, Brown P, Martensen J, Miller J, Piderman K, Huschka M, Girardi J, Hanson J (2006) Impacting quality of life for patients with advanced cancer with a structured multidisciplinary intervention: a randomized controlled trial. Journal of Clinical Oncology 24:635–642

Russell KMW, Hudson M, Long A, Phipps S (2006) Assessment of health-related quality of life in children with cancer: consistency and agreement between parent and child reports. Cancer 106:2267–2274

Saadat H, Kain ZN (2007) Hypnosis as a therapeutic tool in pediatrics [see comment]. Pediatrics 120:179–181

Salazar JC (2003) Pediatric clinical trial experience: government, child, parent and physician's perspective. Pediatric Infectious Disease Journal 22:1124–1127

Schneider SM, Hinds PS, Pritchard M (2001) From single site to societal belief: the impact of pediatric oncology nursing research. Journal of Pediatric Oncology Nursing 18: 164–170

Schrappe M, Reiter A, Ludwig WD, Harbott J, Zimmermann M, Hiddemann W, Niemeyer C, Henze G, Feldges A, Zintl F, Kornhuber B, Ritter J, Welte K, Gadner H, Riehm H (2000) Improved outcome in childhood acute lymphoblastic leukemia despite reduced use of anthracyclines and cranial radiotherapy: results of trial ALL-BFM 90. German-Austrian-Swiss ALL-BFM Study Group. Blood 95:3310–3322

Schumacher A, Wewers D, Heinecke A, Sauerland C, Koch OM, van de Loo J, Buchner T, Berdel WE (2002) Fatigue as an important aspect of quality of life in patients with acute myeloid leukemia. Leukemia Research 26:355–362

Sencer SF, Kelly KM (2006) Bringing evidence to complementary and alternative medicine for children with cancer. Journal of Pediatric Hematology/Oncology 28:186–189

Sibbald B, Roland M (1998) Understanding controlled trials. Why are randomised controlled trials important? British Medical Journal 316:201

Slevin M, Mossman J, Bowling A, Leonard R, Steward W, Harper P, McIllmurray M, Thatcher N (1995) Volunteers or victims: patients' views of randomised cancer clinical trials [see comment]. British Journal of Cancer 71:1270–1274

Sloan JA, Cella D, Frost M, Guyatt GH, Sprangers M, Symonds T, Clinical Significance Consensus Meeting G (2002) Assessing clinical significance in measuring oncology patient quality of life: introduction to the symposium, content overview, and definition of terms. Mayo Clinic Proceedings 77:367–370

Smith M, Gloeckler RL (2002) Childhood cancer: incidence, survival, and mortality. In: Pizzo P, Poplack D (eds) Principles and practice of pediatric oncology, 4th edn. Lippincott Williams and Wilkins, Philadelphia, pp 1–12

Steinke EE (2004) Research ethics, informed consent, and participant recruitment. Clinical Nurse Specialist 18:88–95; quiz 96–87

Stock W, La M, Sanford B, Bloomfield CD, Vardiman JW, Gaynon P, Larson RA, Nachman J, Children's Cancer G, Cancer and Leukemia Group B (2008) What determines the outcomes for adolescents and young adults with acute lymphoblastic leukemia treated on cooperative group protocols? A comparison of Children's Cancer Group and Cancer and Leukemia Group B studies. Blood 112:1646–1654

Streisand R, Braniecki S, Tercyak KP, Kazak AE (2001) Childhood illness-related parenting stress: the pediatric inventory for parents. Journal of Pediatric Psychology 26: 155–162

Swarup AB, Barrett W, Jazieh AR (2006) The use of complementary and alternative medicine by cancer patients undergoing radiation therapy. American Journal of Clinical Oncology 29:468–473

Taylor A, Hawkins M, Griffiths A, Davies H, Douglas C, Jenney M, Wallace WHB, Levitt G (2004) Long-term follow-up of survivors of childhood cancer in the UK. Pediatric Blood and Cancer 42:161–168

Testi A (2006) Differences in Outcome of Adolscents (14–17 Years) with Acute Lymphoblastic Leukemia Enrolled in Italian Pediatric (AIEOP) an Adult (GIMEMA) Treatment Protocols. Journal of Clinical Oncology Issue: 24 508S

The International Conference on Harmonisation of Technical Requirements for the Registration of Pharmaceuticals for Human Use (1996) Guidance for industry E6 good clinical practice: consolidated guidance. Available at: http://www.ich.org/LOB/media/MEDIA482.pdf. Accessed 25 Feb 2009

The International Conference on Harmonisation of Technical Requirements for the Registration of Pharmaceuticals for Human Use (2000) Guidance for industry E11 clinical investigation of medicinal products in the pediatric population. Available at: http://www.ich.org/LOB/media/MEDIA487.pdf. Accessed 25 Feb 2009

The National Commission for the Protection of Human Subjects of Biomedical and Behavioral Research (1979) The Belmont Report. Available at: http://ohsr.od.nih.gov/guidelines/belmont.html. Accessed 25 Feb 2009

The Nuremberg Code (1949) Trials of War Criminals before the Nuremberg Military Tribunals under Control Council Law No. 10. Government Printing Office, Washington DC, pp 181–182

The World Medical Association (2008) The Declaration of Helsinki. Available at: http://www.wma.net/e/policy/b3.html. Accessed 25 Feb 2009

Tomlinson D (2004) Physical restraint during procedures: issues and implications for practice. Journal of Pediatric Oncology Nursing 21:258–263

United States Department of Health and Human Services (2005) Title 45 Public Welfare; Department of Health and Human Services Part 46 Protection of Human Subjects. Available at: http://www.hhs.gov/ohrp/humansubjects/guidance/45cfr46.html. Accessed 25 Feb 2009

Vance YH, Morse RC, Jenney ME, Eiser C (2001) Issues in measuring quality of life in childhood cancer: measures, proxies, and parental mental health. Journal of Child Psychology and Psychiatry and Allied Disciplines 42:661–667

Vantongelen K, Rotmensz N, van der Schueren E (1989) Quality control of validity of data collected in clinical trials. EORTC Study Group on Data Management (SGDM). European Journal of Cancer and Clinical Oncology 25:1241–1247

Varni JW, Bernstein BH (1991) Evaluation and management of pain in children with rheumatic diseases. Rheumatic Diseases Clinics of North America 17:985–1000

Varni JW, Seid M, Rode CA (1999) The PedsQL: measurement model for the pediatric quality of life inventory. Medical Care 37:126–139

Varni JW, Thompson KL, Hanson V (1987) The Varni/Thompson Pediatric Pain Questionnaire. I. Chronic musculoskeletal pain in juvenile rheumatoid arthritis. Pain 28:27–38

Wagner HP, Dingeldein-Bettler I, Berchthold W, Luthy AR, Hirt A, Pluss HJ, Beck D, Wyss M, Signer E, Imbach P et al (1995) Childhood NHL in Switzerland: incidence and survival of 120 study and 42 non-study patients [see comment]. Medical and Pediatric Oncology 24:281–286

Waters EB, Wake MA, Hesketh KD, Ashley DM, Smibert E (2003) Health-related quality of life of children with acute lymphoblastic leukaemia: comparisons and correlations between parent and clinician reports. International Journal of Cancer 103:514–518

Weiner LS, Hersh S, Kazak A (2005) Psychiatric and Psychosocial Support for the Child and Family. In: Pizzo PA, Poplack DG (eds) Principles and Practices of Pediatric Oncology, 5th edn. Lippincott Williams and Wilkins, Philadelphia, pp 1414–1445

Whelan JS, Fern LA (2008) Poor accrual of teenagers and young adults into clinical trials in the UK. Lancet Oncology 9:306–307

Wilson S (2008) Role of Clinical Research Coordinator. Available at: http://www.wiziq.com/tutorial/11599-Role-Of-Clinical-Research-Coordinator. Accessed 25 Feb 2009

Wolfe J, Grier HE, Klar N, Levin SB, Ellenbogen JM, Salem-Schatz S, Emanuel EJ, Weeks JC (2000) Symptoms and suffering at the end of life in children with cancer [see comment]. New England Journal of Medicine 342:326–333

Wolff JA (1991) History of pediatric oncology. Pediatric Hematology and Oncology 8:89–91

Woodgate RL, Degner LF, Yanofsky R (2003) A different perspective to approaching cancer symptoms in children. Journal of Pain and Symptom Management 26: 800–817

Wright JR, Crooks D, Ellis PM, Mings D, Whelan TJ (2002) Factors that influence the recruitment of patients to phase III studies in oncology: the perspective of the clinical research associate [see comment]. Cancer 95:1584–1591

Wright JR, Whelan TJ, Schiff S, Dubois S, Crooks D, Haines PT, DeRosa D, Roberts RS, Gafni A, Pritchard K, Levine MN (2004) Why cancer patients enter randomized clinical trials: exploring the factors that influence their decision. Journal of Clinical Oncology 22:4312–4318

Zeltzer LK, Dolgin MJ, Sahler OJ, Roghmann K, Barbarin OA, Carpenter PJ, Copeland DR, Mulhern RK, Sargent JR (1996) Sibling adaptation to childhood cancer collaborative study: health outcomes of siblings of children with cancer. Medical and Pediatric Oncology 27:98–107

PART IV

Metabolic System

Deborah Tomlinson

Contents

17.1 Cancer Cachexia . . . 337
17.1.1 Incidence . . . 337
17.1.2 Etiology . . . 338
17.1.3 Treatment . . . 338
17.1.4 Prognosis . . . 339
17.2 Obesity . . . 339
17.2.1 Obesity in Survivors of Leukemia . . . 339
17.2.1.1 Incidence . . . 339
17.2.1.2 Etiology . . . 339
17.2.1.3 Treatment . . . 340
17.2.1.4 Prognosis . . . 340
17.3 Inferior Outcomes and Obesity . . . 340
17.3.1 Incidence . . . 340
17.3.2 Etiology . . . 341
17.4 Tumor Lysis Syndrome . . . 341
17.4.1 Incidence . . . 341
17.4.2 Etiology . . . 341
17.4.3 Treatment . . . 343
17.4.3.1 Patient Assessment . . . 344
17.4.3.2 Preventative Measures . . . 344
17.4.3.3 Management of Metabolic Abnormalities . . . 346
17.4.4 Prognosis . . . 347
17.5 Hypercalcemia . . . 347
17.5.1 Incidence . . . 347
17.5.2 Etiology . . . 347
17.5.3 Treatment . . . 347
17.5.4 Prognosis . . . 348
17.6 Impaired Glucose Tolerance . . . 348
17.6.1 Incidence . . . 348
17.6.2 Etiology . . . 348
17.6.3 Treatment . . . 349
17.6.4 Prognosis . . . 349
References . . . 349

17.1 Cancer Cachexia

17.1.1 Incidence

Cancer cachexia can be described as a syndrome characterized by weight loss, anorexia, muscle loss and atrophy, asthenia (general weakness including physical and mental fatigue), and anemia that occurs in cancer patients. A recent cachexia consensus conference agreed on a definition for cachexia: "Cachexia is a complex metabolic syndrome associated with underlying illness and characterised by loss of muscle with or without loss of fat mass" (Evans et al. 2008). Weight loss or the failure to gain weight are common adverse effects of cancer in children. Lange et al. (2005) found that 10.9% of 768 children with acute myelogenous leukemia (AML) were underweight at diagnosis, with the BMI ≤10th percentile. Picton et al. (1995) studied the nutritional status of 25 children with leukemia and 42 children with solid tumor malignancy. Nutritional status was assessed using weight-for-height index, triceps skinfold thickness, and mid-upper arm circumference. Table 17.1. shows the rates of cachexia seen in children in this study. Undernutrition has also been found to be significant (around 7%) in newly diagnosed children with acute lymphoblastic leukemia (ALL) (Reilly et al. 1999). In adults, a cachectic state at diagnosis is associated with a poor prognosis, but in children this association is debatable and may be of more importance in developing countries when associated with socioeconomic status and in social groups with relevant nutritional deficits (Rogers et al. 2005; Weir et al. 1998; Viana et al. 1994; Reilly et al. 1994). However, Lange et al. (2005) concluded that treatment-related

Table 17.1. Rates of cachexia seen in children with cancer (Picton et al. 1995)

	Cachexia at presentation (%)	Cachexia during treatment (%)
Solid tumors (*n*=42)	33	57
Leukemias (*n*=25)	12	28

complications significantly reduced survival rates in underweight (and overweight) children with AML (Lange et al. 2005). No significant differences were observed between underweight (or overweight) and children's gender, ethnicity, and race.

17.1.2 Etiology

Fundamentally, weight loss or growth failure is caused by a negative energy balance as a result of caloric/food intake that is inappropriate to meet energy expenditure. In growing children, energy balance should be positive to ensure adequate growth. Reduced intake commonly results from treatment-associated nausea and vomiting, gastrointestinal dysfunction, and/or taste disturbances. Reports have suggested that an increase in energy expenditure and/or altered metabolism may be another explanation for this energy balance. Anorexia of cancer may also be due to the disruption of the central nervous system appetite center by cancer metabolites. Other factors that contribute to cachexia in cancer patients include competition for nutrients between the tumor and the host and altered metabolism of nutrients.

Normally, a negative energy balance means that the body adapts to low nitrogen intake by reducing protein synthesis and breakdown, causing an overall reduced protein turnover. In children with cancer, the body does not adapt sufficiently, so protein turnover increases and muscle breakdown occurs. The increase in protein turnover in these children may be related to tumor, chemotherapy, or related conditions such as febrile neutropenia. Lipid metabolism is altered, with depletion of lipid stores, increased lipid in circulation, and increased free fatty acid turnover. Changes in carbohydrate metabolism include an increased whole body glucose turnover. Tumors appear to consume glucose, producing lactic acid that the liver must then metabolize and convert back to glucose. Energy is lost in this cycle. Carbohydrate metabolism may also be affected by chemotherapy. Endogenous mediators of cancer cachexia are undetermined but are thought to include tumor necrosis factor (TNF-a), also called cachectin, interleukin 1 (IL-1a), and interleukin 6 (IL-6). These cytokines are regarded as anorexigenic cytokines and have been reported to act on cells in the central nervous system and peripheral tissues in various conditions (Bayram et al. 2008; Saini et al. 2006).

Picton (1998) reported that some patients at high risk of developing cachexia could be identified at presentation by raised energy expenditure. However, a study that investigated the possibility of increased resting energy expenditure as a causative factor in the malnutrition frequently observed in children with stage IV neuroblastoma, concluded that this was not the case (Green et al. 2008). Malnutrition was thought to be due to decreased intake because of intra-abdominal mass and malignant malaise.

17.1.3 Treatment

Nutritional assessment is essential to identify nutritional status and anticipated problems. Aggressive nutritional intervention for these patients may help to prevent subsequent weight loss. This intervention may also be important for children on intensive chemotherapy regimes.

Symptom management of anorexia and cachexia should focus on

- Improving caloric intake
- Minimizing factors that create a negative energy balance

The oral intake of energy, protein, and carbohydrates for hospitalized children with cancer has been found to be below a recommended level (Skolin et al. 2001). When enteral, parenteral, and treatment-related glucose were taken into account, the level came close to that recommended for healthy children. However, children with malignant disease are likely to have increased energy and nutrient requirements. Supplementation with eicosapentenoic acid (EPA), an omega-3 fatty acid, has been shown to decrease cancer-induced weight loss in pediatric patients (Bayram et al. 2008). Cyproheptadine hydrochloride (Periactin) has also been shown to be a safe and effective supplement in the promotion of weight-gain in children with cancer or treatment-related cachexia (Couluris et al. 2008). Cyproheptadine hydrochloride is a serotonin and histamine antagonist that has produced unexplained weight gain when used as treatment for conditions that include allergic rhinitis and urticaria. Megestrol acetate (Megace) may similarly be effective in promoting weight gain in this population as it has been used effectively in adult populations. However, there have been reports of adrenal suppression with megestrol acetate supplementation in children (Azcona et al. 2000; Stockheim et al. 1999).

Chapter 29 will detail nutritional requirements, and the role of parenteral and enteral nutrition of the child and adolescent with cancer.

17.1.4 Prognosis

Weight loss is a serious complication of childhood cancer. Fortunately, developing strategies for providing enteral and parenteral nutrition can prevent major morbidity and mortality from this complication. Occasionally, nutritional strategies are insufficient to reverse a cachectic state. Metabolic changes can result in growth failure in pediatric cancer patients. Body tissue is then catabolized to meet the nutritional demands of the tumor, and nutritional death could be a possibility. Severe and prolonged undernutrition may result in atrophy of intestinal villi and can create lactose intolerance. Future treatment approaches may be able to combine different pharmacological approaches that target the cytokine factors involved. The resulting effects would be to reverse the metabolic derangements associated with the tumor and to ameliorate anorexia.

17.2 Obesity

Obesity, for study purposes, is often defined as a body mass index (BMI) of ≥95th percentile where BMI is calculated by weight (kg)/height $(m)^2$. In children with cancer, obesity presents as two issues:

1. Children and adolescents, partcularly girls younger than 5 years, treated with ≥20 Grays (Gy) of cranial radiation (CRT) have a tendency to gain excessive weight during and following treatment (Reilly et al. 2001a; Oeffinger et al. 2003; Rogers et al. 2005; Asner et al. 2008; Garmey et al. 2008; Oeffinger, 2008).
2. Potentially inferior outcomes for overweight children who received stem cell transplant or who were treated for leukemia (Lange et al. 2005; Rogers et al. 2005; Butturini et al. 2007; Bulley et al. 2008).

17.2.1 Obesity in Survivors of Leukemia

17.2.1.1 Incidence

Oeffinger and colleagues showed that females diagnosed with ALL between the ages of 0 and 4 years, and treated with CRT doses ≥20 Gy were almost 4 times as likely to be obese compared with healthy siblings (Oeffinger et al. 2003; Garmey et al. 2008).

However, Chow et al. (2007) reported that, despite reductions in the use of CRT, childhood survivors of ALL remain at an increased risk of obesity at least several years after the completion of treatment, with those exposed to higher doses of corticosteroids at greater risk.

17.2.1.2 Etiology

There may be several mechanisms by which CRT can cause obesity, including:

- Alterations in growth hormone production/secretion
- Leptin insensitivity
- Impact on physical function (Oeffinger 2008; Sklar et al. 2000)

Dalton et al. (2003) concluded that children treated for ALL had normal weight gain, but the loss of height caused by CNS treatment produced a higher BMI score that indicated obesity. Another study showed that the BMI catergory of the child at diagnosis was indicative of adult weight in long-term survivors of ALL and lymphoma (Razzouk et al. 2007).

The most significant abnormality in energy balance identified in the literature regarding ALL is reduced total energy expenditure as a result of reduced physical activity during and following therapy (Reilly et al. 2001a).

The effect of glucocorticoid therapy on energy balance and body weight control is accepted; however, there is little evidence of this effect, particularly in children with ALL. A study by Reilly and colleagues (2001a) was the first to show that energy intakes increased significantly when children were treated with glucocorticoids during the long-term maintenance phase of therapy. No significant difference was found between patients treated with prednisone and those treated with dexamethasone. This study concluded that glucocorticoid therapy substantially increases energy intake in patients with ALL and that this contributes to the development of obesity characteristic of these patients.

Another study carried out by Reilly et al. (2001b) found that adiposity rebound (AR) occurred much earlier in patients with ALL than in healthy children. AR occurs when BMI begins to increase after its nadir in childhood (usually between 5 and 7 years of age). This period is important for the regulation of energy balance and adult obesity risk, and early AR is associated with an increased risk of adult obesity.

Other effects on energy balance may include growth hormone status derangements (Van Dongen-Melman et al. 1995) and resting energy expenditure, although differences between patients treated for ALL and healthy controls have not been observed (Reilly et al. 1998). In patients who receive cranial irradiation as part of ALL therapy, the parameters of resting metabolic rate, physical activity, and growth hormone levels tend to be lower than normal, which would indicate causes for obesity in this group of patients. However, nonirradiated patients also have a tendency to obesity, which confounds the conclusions surrounding the etiology of obesity in this patient group (Mayer et al. 2000). It may be possible that obesity in childhood cancer survivors is related to familial background rather than treatment components (Asner et al. 2008).

17.2.1.3 Treatment

To reduce the incidence of obesity in this population, most children treated for ALL do not receive CRT, and if CRT is required for high-risk patients, then the dose is usually 18 Gy.

BMI (weight (kg)/height (m)^2), resting metabolic rate (measured by indirect calorimetry), caloric intake (24-h recall), and physical activity (questionnaire) are suggested parameters that can be used to identify and manage overweight and obesity (Mayer et al. 2000).

The main focus of treatment (and prevention) should concentrate on

- Achievable increases in habitual physical activity, working toward a more active lifestyle
- Modest restriction of dietary intake
- Monitoring of excess weight gain

Nutritional screening would identify patients who may require intervention and referral to specialist services.

17.2.1.4 Prognosis

Obesity can be an adverse effect for ALL survivors that may have considerable consequence because of their already higher risk for various health outcomes, including cardiovascular factors as well as general health, social, and emotional well-being (Oeffinger et al. 2004).

With the current emphasis on the quality of survival, it is vital that these patients and their families be educated about preventing later obesity. These efforts may take the form of encouraging a more active lifestyle.

17.3 Inferior Outcomes and Obesity

17.3.1 Incidence

The potential for outcome to be less favourable for overweight children compared with normal weight children treated for leukemia has been investigated more recently.

Inferior outcomes have been reported for overweight children with:

- ALL (Butturini et al. 2007), where obesity in children diagnosed with ALL after their tenth birthday were at greater risk of relapse..
- AML (Lange et al. 2005). This study reported that overweight and underweight children with AML are less likely to survive than patients with BMI in the 11th–94th percentiles. The inferior survival was attributed to early treatment-related mortality, which was mostly due to infection.
- Treatment of allogenic stem cell transplantation (SCT) (Bulley et al. 2008). Overweight children had inferior overall survival and increased treatment-related survival.

17.3.2 Etiology

Further research is required to determine the causes of poorer outcomes in obese children. Reasons may include, but are not limited to:

- Pharmacokinetics and pharmacodynamics: there are no pharmacological studies of bioavailability of chemotherapeutic agents in obese children. The opinion tends to be that obese adult patients receive too little rather than too much chemotherapy (Lange et al. 2005). However, it would probably be more favorable to have increased relapse if treatment-related mortality was decreased.
- Comorbidities. For example, persistent hyperglycemia and hypertension in overweight patients.
- Socioeconomic status.
- Growth factors and lymphokines can be directly secreted by adipocytes and may alter anticancer effects and chemotherapy toxicity (Butturini et al. 2007).
- The effect of obesity on cell growth as seen in a trend of higher initial white blood cell count in obese children (Butturini et al. 2007).

Standardized drug dose adjustment for overweight children may be an initial step that, at very least, would assist in investigations to the causal mechanisms. The use of an adjusted weight for drug calculation that is halfway between actual body weight and estimated body weight has been reported to be satisfactory (Rogers et al. 2005).

To proceed, retrospective reviews of completed studies could include analysis of survival and toxicities based on obesity and methods of dose calculation (Rogers et al. 2005).

17.4 Tumor Lysis Syndrome

Tumor lysis syndrome (TLS) is a potential life-threatening emergency that results from rapid spontaneous or treatment-related tumor cell death. The cell lysis releases large amounts of uric acid, potassium, phosphate, and other purine metabolites into the blood circulation. When these quantities of intracellular electrolytes exceed the excretory capacity of the renal system, TLS can occur.

17.4.1 Incidence

The incidence of TLS appears to be undefined, emphasizing identification of individual risk factors and preventative measures. Factors that influence the risk of TLS are shown in Table 17.2.. Large rapidly dividing tumors are most likely to be associated with TLS risk and in particular, Burkitt's lymphoma. Risk for renal failure may also be increased if there is kidney tumor infiltration or tumor compression on the ureters or renal veins. TLS typically occurs within 24–48 h after cytotoxic therapy begins, with rising serum potassium levels seen. It can then persist over 4–7 days as phosphate and urate levels rise. TLS normally occurs after commencement of the first treatment only.

17.4.2 Etiology

TLS is characterized by four metabolic abnormalitics (Fig. 17.1):

- Hyperuricemia
- Hyperphosphatemia
- Hypocalcemia
- Hyperkalemia

Table 17.2. Risk factors associated with tumor lysis syndrome (TLS) in children

Disease-related	Patient-related	Treatment-related
Bulky tumors (0.8–10 cm)	Increased uric acid level prior to treatment	Chemotherapy (main association)
High proliferative rate	Renal insufficiency leading to oliguria	Ionizing radiation therapy
Hematopoietic malignancies	Dehydration	Corticosteroids
Chemosensitive tumors	Male gender	Hormonal therapy
ALL (T-cell most commonly)	Immature tubular function (age <1 year) results in inefficient sodium and water regulation	Immunotherapy
Burkitt's lymphoma (and other nonHodgkin's lymphomas)	Children may have a decreased glomerular filtration rate	
AML with high WBC	Greater fluid needs per kilogram of body weight	
Neuroblastoma (on occasion)	Increased pretreatment lactic dehydrogenase	

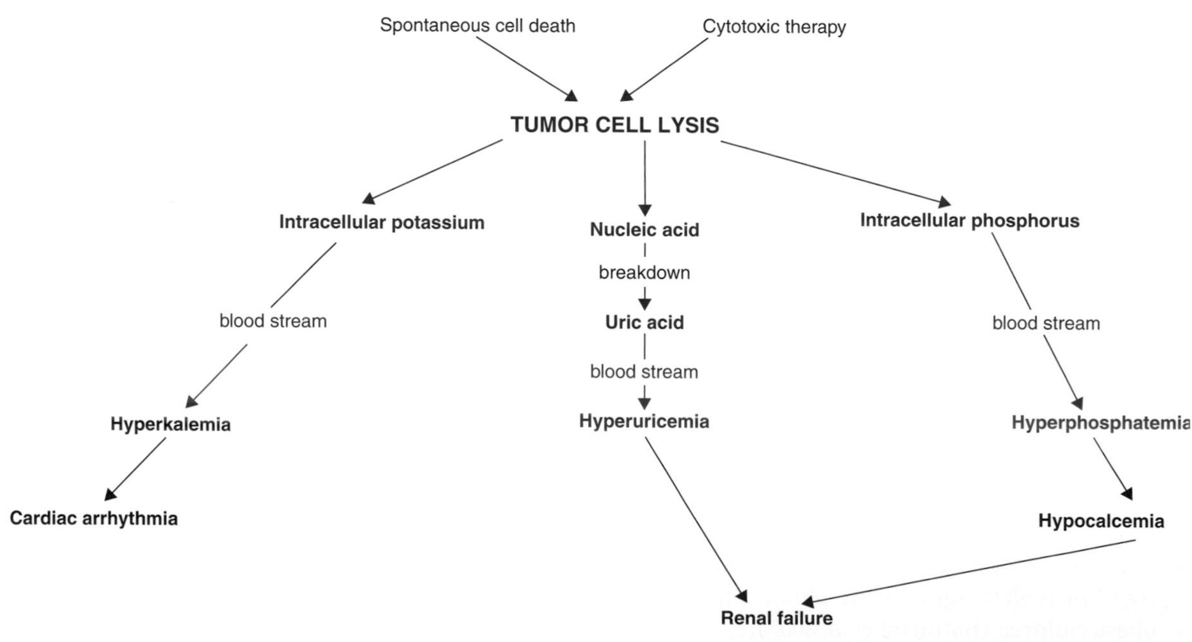

Figure 17.1
Metabolic consequences of tumor cell lysis

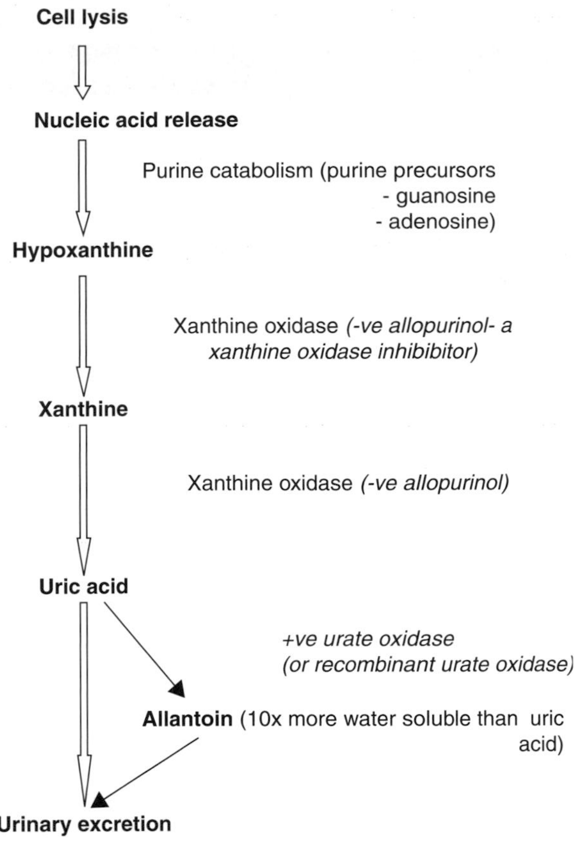

Figure 17.2

Uric acid metabolism (adapted from (Nicolin 2002))

These abnormalities may ultimately lead to seizures, acute renal failure, cardiac arrhythmias, and, in some cases, multiorgan failure and death.

Acute renal failure associated with TLS may be attributable to several factors. Uric acid, phosphorus, and potassium are primarily excreted by the kidneys. The release of intracellular purines from the nuclei of tumor cells increases the levels of uric acid in the blood. Uric acid crystals are formed when uric acid enters the acidic urine environment of the collecting ducts and ureters, causing precipitation of xanthine. (Xanthine is a by-product of nucleic acid destruction.) This can lead to a renal obstruction. Serum uric acid levels of 10–15 mg/dL can cause symptoms of lethargy, nausea, or vomiting, with renal failure usually seen as the level increases to 20 mg/dL (Allegretta et al. 1985). The drugs used to prevent TLS in these circumstances may also present a predisposition to renal failure. Allopurinol lowers the production of uric acid by inhibiting xanthine oxidase. Xanthine oxidase acts as a catalyst in the conversion of hypoxanthine to xanthine and xanthine to uric acid (see Fig. 17.2). Therefore, increased levels of xanthine and hypoxanthine are excreted in the urine. These products may then precipitate, especially in alkaline urine, and pose another contributing factor in acute renal failure.

Lymphoblasts are very rich in phosphorus compared with normal lymphocytes. Lysis causes increased serum phosphorus, which can lead to hypocalcemia or to calcium phosphate precipitation. Calcium phosphate precipitation may lead to tissue damage. Table 17.3. lists the clinical features associated with the metabolic abnormalities that occur in TLS.

Hyperkalemia is the most rapidly occurring, dangerous consequence of TLS. Potassium levels can rise because of its release during cell lysis and quickly reach life-threatening levels if there is associated acute renal failure. Serum potassium levels of 7.0 mEq/L (mmol/L) can show changes in electrocardiograph (ECG) readings with QRS widening and peaked T-waves. Ventricular arrhythmias and death can occur if there is no intervention to lower the serum potassium levels. However, the incidence of serum potassium reaching this level is particularly uncommon due to conventional hydration and acid–base management.

17.4.3 Treatment

The main treatment strategy for TLS concerns prevention. Nurses have a key role in the management of pediatric patients at risk of developing TLS. The main areas of focus are:

- Patient assessment prior to treatment administration
- Preventative measures
- Management of metabolic abnormalities

Table 17.3. Clinical features of tumor lysis syndrome

Hyperuricemia	Hypocalcemia	Hyperphosphatemia	Hyperkalemia	Acute renal failure
Gastrointestinal Nausea Vomiting Diarrhea *Renal* Anuria or oliguria Edema Hematuria Lethargy	*Neurological* Tetany, demonstrated by Trousseau or Chvostek's signs Irritability Tingling of extremities Carpopedal spasm Confusion Laryngospasm Convulsions Alterations in consciousness *Cardiovascular* Prolonged QT interval in the ECG Hypotension	*Renal* Oliguria or anuria Elevated blood urea and creatinine	*Gastrointestinal symptoms* *Neuromuscular* Weakness Paresthesias Paralysis *Cardiovascular* Widening QRS and peaked T-waves Blood pressure changes Ventricular arrhythmias	Oliguria or anuria Edema Hypertension

17.4.3.1 Patient Assessment

Identifying patients at risk should allow for prompt administration of prophylactic measures to avoid the complications associated with TLS. Patient assessment should include a patient history with respect to clinical features as described in Table 17.3.. Physical examination should assess blood pressure, heart rate and rhythm, neurological status, and respiratory status. Children should also be examined for lymphadenopathy, abdominal mass, ascites, edema, and weight changes. Radiological examinations including chest x-ray, renal ultrasound, or computerized tomography may be indicated. A renal scan may be indicated to anticipate renal infiltration that could add to the risk of TLS.

Baseline laboratory assessment should include a full/complete blood count, blood urea nitrogen, and electrolytes, including lactate dehydrogenase. If the serum potassium level is higher than 6.0 mEq/L, an ECG should be performed to rule out any cardiac abnormality. Blood urea nitrogen and electrolytes may need to be obtained every 6–8 h in the first few days of cytotoxic treatment.

17.4.3.2 Preventative Measures

Metabolic stability should ideally be achieved prior to administration of cytotoxic treatment as long as there is not too long a delay. The preventative measures are

1. Hydration
2. Alkalization
3. Uric acid reduction

Table 17.4. indicates the interventions that may be employed to achieve these three goals. However, the role of alkalization is controversial because of the risk of over alkalinization, which may result in life-threatening precipitation of calcium phosphate (see Table 17.4.). Recent consensus concludes that rasburicase (Elitek®, Fasturtec®) (recombinant urate oxidase) should be the drug of choice for TLS therapy and prophylaxis in high-risk patients, while allopurinol should be administered for prophylaxis in low-risk patients or when the use of Rasburicase is contraindicated (Tosi et al. 2008). In an attempt to define children with ALL with a low-risk of developing TLS, Truong et al. (2007) used the absence of the following four risk factors:

Table 17.4. Preventative measures in the management of TLS (Coiffier et al. 2008; Truini-Pittman and Rosseto, 2002; Nicolin 2002)

Preventative measure	Method
Hydration	IV fluids of 0.45% (or 0.225%) saline with 5% dextrose. No potassium added
	Generally, 2–4 times the usual maintenance requirements with approximately 3 L/m^2/day
	Maintain urine specific gravity at <1.010 and urinary output ≥3 mL/kg/h
	To avoid fluid overload, diuretics may be necessary: Furosemide/frusemide 1 mg/kg slow IV bolus q6h; mannitol 0.5 g/kg IV over 30 min q6h may also be required
	Avoid diuretics if hypovolemia present
Alkalization	Maintain urine pH at 7.0–7.5
	Sodium bicarbonate 50–100 mEq/L (mmol/L) added to IV maintenance fluids if advocated
	Note: Excess alkalization may be life-threatening as it may encourage precipitation of calcium phosphate and xanthine (phosphate precipitates at pH >7.5). Symptoms of hypocalcemia may also be aggravated by shifting ionized calcium to its nonionized form
	Reduce sodium bicarbonate if serum bicarbonate >30 mEq/L (mmol/L) or urine pH >7.5
Uric acid reduction	For low-risk to intermediate risk, allopurinol 50–100 mg/m^2 orally q8h (maximum 800 mg/day) or IV 200 mg/m^2/day in one to three divided doses (maximum 600 mg/day). IV allopurinol is compatible with dextrose and saline but not sodium bicarbonate. See Fig. 4.2. Uric acid production is blocked. Reduce dose of allopurinol in established renal failure. Allopurinol has a drug–drug interaction with 6-mercaptopurine and cyclophosphamide
	Alternatively, in high-risk or for treatment of TLS, urate oxidase 50–100 U/kg IV infusion over 30 min daily or recombinant urate oxidase (rasburicase) 0.15–0.2 mg/kg IV over 30 min 4 times daily for 5 days (Coiffier et al. 2008). This will convert uric acid to allantoin, which is 10 times more soluble than uric acid and promotes excretion by the kidneys. Use of urate oxidase targets a different step in uric acid metabolism that avoids build-up of xanthine and hypoxanthine. See Fig. 4.2. Do not administer urate oxidase as a bolus or through a filter. Infuse through a dedicated line
	Patients receiving either of these drugs should be monitored for hypersensitive-related adverse reactions (Brant 2002)

Pediatric daily maintenance fluids are determined as follows: 100 mL/kg for the first 10 kg of body weight, 50 mL/kg for the second 10 kg of body weight, 25 mL/kg for any remaining kg of body weight over 20 kg, Divide the sum of these three numbers by 24 to establish the hourly rate for maintenance fluids

- Age ≥10 years
- Splenomegaly
- Mediastinal mass
- Initial white blood count (WBC) ≥20 × 10^9/L

In the absence of these four factors, there was a 97% probability that TLS would not occur (Truong et al. 2007).

Laboratory values should be monitored on a regular basis as the patient's condition requires and should include the following:

- Complete/full blood count
- Blood urea nitrogen
- Electrolytes
- Creatinine

Nurses are in a position to perform the necessary assessments and interventions. In the event of alkalinization, nurses must be aware of the potential of precipitation of calcium phosphate. Nursing intervention should also include communication regarding physical findings and overall patient status while ensuring support and education for the patients and their families.

17.4.3.3 Management of Metabolic Abnormalities

The early identification of electrolyte imbalance along with prompt and aggressive treatment are essential and will minimize the need for hemodialysis. Table 17.5. outlines approaches in managing electrolyte imbalances.

When these methods are ineffective in correcting imbalances and improving urinary flow, some patients may require dialysis. Indications for dialysis include

- Volume overload
- Anuria
- Symptomatic hypocalcemia with hyperphosphatemia
- Hyperkalemia (>6.0 mEq/L or mmol/L) with cardiac changes
- Hyperuricemia
- Elevated serum creatinine with low urinary output

It is recommended that a renal consultation be obtained immediately if urine output is low, or if there is persisitent or elevated phosphate levels or in the case of hypocalcemia (Coiffier et al. 2008).

Hemodialysis, peritoneal dialysis, and continuous hemofiltration with or without dialysis have all been used to treat acute renal failure associated with TLS. Conventional hemodialysis is most efficient at correcting imbalances, but the continuous hemofiltration may benefit patients who cannot tolerate the osmotic shift of hemodialysis (Bishof et al. 1990). Peritoneal dialysis is much less efficient at clearing uric acid and is ineffective for removing phosphates.

Table 17.5. Approaches in the management of electrolyte imbalances associated with TLS (Coiffier et al. 2008; Truini-Pittman and Rosseto, 2002; Nicolin 2002)

Electrolyte imbalance	Treatment
Moderate hyperkalemia	Stop the intake of potassium-containing food and fluids, e.g., bananas, chocolate
Serum potassium >5.0–6.0 mEq/mL (mmol/mL)	Ensure that potassium is removed from IV fluids including parenteral nutrition Potassium-binding resin: polystyrene sulfonate resin 1 g/kg orally mixed with 50% sorbitol (0.25 g/kg q6h)
Severe hyperkalemia Serum potassium >6.0 mEq/mL (mmol/mL) or ECG shows arrhythmia or significant widening of QRS complex	Same as above, plus: Calcium gluconate 10% 0.3–0.5 mL/kg or 100–200 mg/kg/dose slowIV bolus (monitor for bradycardia); this augments myocardial conduction and shifts potassium intracellularly . Consider IV furosemide/frusemide 1 mg/kg (loop diuretic) if appropriate. Rapid reduction of potassium levels may be achieved by IV 25% glucose 2 mL/kg with IV insulin 0.1 U/kg; this promotes intracellular flow of potassium Salbutamol 2.5–5 mL nebulized or 4 mg/kg as slow IV bolus (5 min) to promote intracellular potassium flow Sodium bicarbonate 1–2 mEq/L (mmol/L) IV (diluted); this induces hydrogen efflux, leading to potassium influx Consider dialysis
Hyperphosphatemia	Low-phosphate diet
Serum phosphate ≥6.5 mg/dL	Aluminum hydroxide 50 mg/kg q8h Maintain urine output ≥3 mL/kg/h
Symptomatic hypocalcemi	Hyperphosphatemia treated first
Calcium ≤8.0 mEq/L (mmol/L) or Ionized calcium ≤1.5 mEq/L (mmol/L)	Maintain serum bicarbonate ≤30 mEq/L (mmol/L) IV calcium gluconate 10% 0.3–0.5 mL/kg slow bolus-5–10 min. Monitor for bradycardia. *Only used for symptomatic patients due to risk of calcium phosphate precipitation* Consider dialysis

Peritoneal dialysis is also contraindicated in patients with abdominal tumors (Stapleton et al. 1988). Dialysis should continue until metabolic stability is achieved.

Note that other concomitant therapies may contribute to metabolic abnormalities in pediatric patients with TLS:

- Oral and intravenous (IV) electrolyte and/or dietary supplements
- Nephrotoxic agents, e.g., aminoglycosides
- Radiographic contrast media (Morris and Holland 2000)

17.4.4 Prognosis

Life-threatening metabolic abnormalities may be observed at presentation in children with leukemia and lymphoma. TLS has a high morbidity, and rare cases may lead to multiorgan failure and death. However, if children at risk are identified, properly assessed, and treated with correct prophylactic measures, TLS can be prevented and/or treated before it reaches the stage of life-threatening complications.

17.5 Hypercalcemia

17.5.1 Incidence

Hypercalcemia can be defined as a serum calcium concentration >3.24 mEq/L (mmol/L) or 13 mg/dL. The incidence of hypercalcemia of malignancy is cited as approximately 0.4–0.7% (McKay and Furman 1993; Inukai et al. 2007). It is observed most frequently in children with ALL or alveolar rhabdomyosarcoma but has been associated with other types of malignancy in children. The incidence of hypercalcemia varies for each type of malignancy and has been noted to be as high as 18% in children with renal rhabdoid tumors (Vujanic et al. 1996).

17.5.2 Etiology

The cause of hypercalcemia may be multifactorial:

- Release of calcium from sites of skeletal metastases from localized bone destruction from invasive cancer cells (Mittal 2007)
- Production of humoral factors from tumor, including ectopic production of parathyroid hormone-related peptide (PTHrP), prostaglandin E2, tumor necrosis factor, osteoclast-activating factor, interleukin 1, and growth factor alpha. Osteoclastic bone resorption and renal resorption of calcium increases with renal phosphate loss (Inukai et al. 2007).
- Hypercalcemia interferes with the mechanisms of urinary concentration, with subsequent dehydration and a reduction in glomerular filtration rate. This causes reduction in renal calcium excretion and further hypercalcemia (Kelly and Lange 1997; Ralston 1994).

Symptoms of hypercalcemia are listed in Table 17.6. These symptoms are not always recognized in children because they may be attributed to other problems (Mittal 2007).

17.5.3 Treatment

Treatment for hypercalcemia focuses on the following:

1. Increasing renal calcium clearance
2. Inhibiting osteoclastic bone resorption
3. Reducing or eliminating the tumor burden

Table 17.7. outlines the approaches that may be taken in the management of hypercalcemia. Should approaches fail to reduce serum calcium levels, dialysis may be necessary.

Table 17.6. Symptoms of hypercalcemia

Mild hypercalcemia	Severe hypercalcemia
Generalized weakness	Profound muscle weakness
Poor appetite	Severe nausea and vomiting
Nausea	Decreased levels of consciousness
Vomiting	Bradyarrhythmias
Constipation	
Abdominal or back pain	
Polyuria	
Drowsiness	

17.5.4 Prognosis

Hypercalcemia is rare; however, it is difficult to correct. Immediate attention and appropriate treatment are essential to prevent a life-threatening situation.

17.6 Impaired Glucose Tolerance

17.6.1 Incidence

Although there are few documented studies regarding insulin-related metabolism glucose intolerance posthematopoietic cell transplant (HCT), the reported incidence in surviving patients is significant at 6–8%, which is higher than the general population (Taskinen et al. 2000; Hoffmeister et al. 2004). Impaired glucose metabolism can also occur during treatment for ALL due to therapy; however, this impairment may persist after therapy has been completed (Mohn et al. 2004).

Diabetes mellitus (DM) has also been reported following abdominal irradiation for Wilms' tumour (Teinturier et al 1995). Risk factors include: a diagnosis of leukemia, non-Hispanic white ethnicity, family history of diabetes and asparginase toxicity (Hoffmeister et al 2004). Growth hormone therapy has also been reported as a potential risk factor for type-2 diabetes (Cutfield et al 2000).

Transfer of DM type-1 by bone marrow transplant (BMT) (from donor to recipient) has been observed (Beard et al. 2002; Lampeter et al. 1998).

17.6.2 Etiology

Type-2 DM is caused by a combination of genetic causes and acquired factors. This type of DM is more common in adults, many of whom are overweight. Observations

Table 17.7. Management of hypercalcemia (Nicolin 2002; Kelly and Lange 1997)

Treatment aim	Management	Comments
Increase renal calcium	Increase IV fluid intake (3–6 L/m²/day)	Associated vomiting and polyuria will have caused hypovolemia
	Increase output with IV furosemide/frusemide (1–3 mg/kg q6h)	Promotes excretion of calcium and blocks its renal reabsorption in the loop of Henle
	Monitor fluid balance and electrolytes	*Treatment will cause fluid shifts and loss of sodium,potassium, and magnesium*
Inhibit osteoclastic bone resorption	Administer bisphosphonates (pamidronate) 1 mg/kg as an IV infusion with a rate not exceeding 1 mg/min Correct hypophosphatemia with oral phosphate 10 mg/kg/ dose 2 or 3 times a day	Bind to hydroxyapatite crystals, induce osteoclastic activity, and induce deposition of calcium into bone Use may be limited by severe diarrhea *IV phosphate is not recommended due to risk of calcium phosphate deposition*
Reduce or eliminate the tumor burden	Glucocorticoids (prednisolone) 1.5–2.0 mg/kg/day	Interfere with tumor-induced osteoclast-stimulating factors (osteoclast-activating factor and prostaglandins) Reduction in serum calcium may not be seen for 2–10 days
	May be used in conjunction with calcitonin (4 U/kg subcutaneously q12h)	Acts within hours by blocking bone resorption and promoting calcium excretion; *resistance develops within a day.*
	Alternatively: mithramycin, an antitumor antibiotic, given IV 25 mg/kg in 5% dextrose 50 mL over 3 h	Inhibits osteoclastic activity. Significant toxicity, *including thrombocytopenia, azotemia, proteinuria*

by Traggiai and colleagues (2003) suggest that radiation may compromise pancreatic alpha-cell function without the presence of autoantibodies. Damage to pancreatic beta-cell function attributed to chemotherapy has also been associated with alterations in glucose tolerance in children with ALL (Mohn et al. 2004).

In insulin resistance, a normal amount of insulin produces a subnormal biological response in peripheral target tissues. The impaired biological response to insulin, often as a result of steroids and/or cyclosporine, means that the serum insulin level rises to sustain normal blood glucose concentrations (Taskinen et al. 2000). Eventually, abnormal responses lead to the exhaustion of the pancreatic islet cells and to type-2 diabetes.

Type-1 DM is thought to be transferable because the immune system of the recipient destroys the B-cells of the recipient due to the myeloablative therapy received prior to the BMT. However, the risk of contracting type-1 DM from BMT is small, and type-1 DM in an otherwise eligible donor is not thought to be reason for exclusion (Lampeter et al. 1998).

17.6.3 Treatment

Given that diabetes can be symptom-free, follow-up for HCT patients should include monitoring for glucose intolerance. Laboratory investigations should include

- Serum lipids
- Fasting blood glucose
- Serum insulin

A diagnosis of DM requires urgent referral to a pediatric endocrinologist, and treatment will include dietary advice and possibly insulin therapy.

17.6.4 Prognosis

A diagnosis of DM presents challenges along with the other potential late effects of cytotoxic therapy. Early recognition may lead to early therapy and prevention of death from resulting coronary heart disease.

References

Allegretta GJ, Weisman SJ, Altman AJ (1985) Oncologic emergencies 1: Metabolic and space occupying consequences of cancer and cancer treatment. Pediatric Clinics of North America 32(3):601–611

Asner S, Ammann RA, Ozsahin H, Beck-Popovic M, von der Weid NX (2008) Obesity in long-term survivors of childhood acute lymphoblastic leukemia. Pediatric Blood Cancer 51(1):118–122

Azcona C, Sierrasesumaga L (2000) Adrenal suppression in children with malignant solid tumors treated with megestrol acetate. Journal of Pediatrics 137(1):141–142

Bayram I, Erbey F, Celik N, Nelson JL, Tanyeli A (2008) The use of a protein and energy dense eicosapentanaenoic acid containing supplement for malignancy-related weight loss in children. Pediatric Blood Cancer 52(5):571–574

Beard ME, Willis JA, Scott RS, Nesbit JW (2002) Is type 1 diabetes transmissible by bone marrow allograft? Diabetes Care 25(4):799–800

Bishof NA, Welch TR, Strife CF, Ryckman FC (1990) Continuous hemofiltration in children. Pediatrics 85(5):819–823

Brant JM (2002) Rasburicase: an innovative new treatment for hyperuricemia associated with tumor lysis syndrome. Clinical Journal of Oncology Nursing 6(1):12–16

Bulley S, Gassas A, Dupuis LL, Aplenc R, Beyene J, Greenberg ML, Doyle JJ, Sung L (2008) Inferior outcomes for overweight children undergoing allogeneic stem cell transplantation. British Journal of Haematology 140(2):214–217

Butturini AM, Dorey FJ, Lange BJ, Henry DW, Gaynon PS, Fu C, Franklin J, Siegel SE, Seibel NL, Rogers PC, Sather H, Trigg M, Bleyer WA, Carroll WL (2007) Obesity and outcome in pediatric acute lymphoblastic leukemia. Journal of Clinical Oncology 25(15):2063–2069

Chow EJ, Friedman DL, Yasui Y, Whitton JA, Stovall M, Robison LL, Sklar CA (2007) Decreased adult height in survivors of childhood acute lymphoblastic leukemia: a report from the Childhood Cancer Survivor Study. The Journal of Pediatrics 150(4):370–375.el

Coiffier B, Altman A, Pui CH, Younes A, Cairo MS (2008) Guidelines for the management of pediatric and adult tumor lysis syndrome: an evidence-based review. Journal of Clinical Oncology 26(16):2767–2778

Couluris M, Mayer JLR, Freyer DR, Sandler E, Xu P, Krischer JP (2008) The effect of cyproheptadne hydrochloride (Periactin) and megestrol acetate (Megace) on weight in children with cancer/treatment-related cachexia. Journal of Pediatric Hematology/Oncology 30(11):791–797

Cutfield WS, Wilton P, Bennmarker H, Albertsson-Wikland K, Chatelain P, Ranke MB, Price DA (2000) Incidence of diabetes mellitus and impaired glucose tolerance in children and adolescents receiving growth-hormone treatment. Lancet 355:610–613

Dalton VK, Rue M, Silverman LB, Gelber RD, Asselin BL, Barr RD, Clavell LA, Hurwitz CA, Moghrabi A, Samson Y,

Schorin M, Tarbell NJ, Sallan SE, Cohen LE (2003) Height and weight in children treated for acute lymphoblastic leukemia: relationship to CNS treatment. Journal of Clinical Oncology 21(15):2953–2960

Evans WJ, Morley JE, Argilés J, Bales C, Baracos V, Guttridge D, Jatoi A, Kalantar-Zadeh K, Lochs H, Mantovani G, Marks D, Mitch WE, Muscaritoli M, Najand A, Ponikowski P, Rossi Fanelli F, Schambelan M, Schols A, Schuster M, Thomas D, Wolfe R, Anker SD (2008) Cachexia: a new definition. Clinical Nutrition 27(6):793–799

Garmey EG, Liu Q, Sklar CA, Meacham LR, Mertens AC, Stovall MA, Yasui Y, Robison LL, Oeffinger KC (2008) Longitudinal changes in obesity and body mass index among adult survivors of childhood acute lymphoblastic leukemia: a report from the Childhood Cancer Survivor Study. Journal of Clinical Oncology 26(28):4639–4645

Green GJ, Weitzman SS, Pencharz PB (2008) Resting energy expenditure in children newly diagnosed with stage IV neuroblastoma. Pediatric Research 63(3):332–336

Hoffmeister PA, Storer BE, Sanders JE (2004) Diabetes mellitus in long-term survivors of pediatric hematopoietic cell transplantation. Journal of Pediatric Hematology/Oncology 26(2):81–90

Inukai T, Hirose K, Inaba T, Kurosawa H, Hama A, Inada H, Chin M, Nagatoshi Y, Ohtsuka Y, Oda M, Goto H, Endo M, Morimoto A, Imaizumi M, Kawamura N, Miyajima Y, Ohtake M, Miyaji R, Saito M, Tawa A, Yanai F, Goi K, Nakazawa S, Sugita K (2007) Hypercalcemia in childhood acute lymphoblastic leukemia: frequent implication of parathyroid hormone-related peptide and E2A-HLF from translocation 17;19. Leukemia 21(2):288–296

Kelly KM, Lange B (1997) Pediatric oncology: oncologic emergencies. Pediatric Clinics of North America 44(4):809–830

Lampeter EF, McCann SR, Kolb H (1998) Transfer of insulin-dependent diabetes by bone marrow transplantation. Lancet 351:568–569

Lange BJ, Gerbing RB, Feusner J, Skolnik J, Sacks N, Smith FO, Alonzo TA (2005) Mortality in overweight and underweight children with acute myeloid leukemia. The Journal of the American Medical Association 293(2):203–211

Mayer EI, Reuter M, Dopfer RE, Ranke MB (2000) Energy expenditure, energy intake and prevalence of obesity after therapy for acute lymphoblastic leukemia during childhood. Hormone Research 53(4):193–199

McKay C, Furman WL (1993) Hypercalcemia complicating childhood malignancy. Cancer 72:256–260

Mittal MK (2007) Severe hypercalcaemia as a harbinger of acute lymphoblastic leukemia. Pediatric Emergency Care 23(6):397–400

Mohn A, Di Marzio A, Capanna R, Fioritoni G, Chiarelli F (2004) Persistence of impaired pancreatic beta-cell function in children treated for acute lymphoblastic leukaemia. Lancet 363(9403):127–128

Morris JC, Holland JF (2000) Oncologic emergencies. In: Bast RC Jr, Hellman S, Rosenberg SA (eds) Holland Frei Cancer Medicine, 5th edn. BC Decker, Hamilton, Ontario

Nicolin G (2002) Emergencies and their management. European Journal of Cancer 38(10):1365–1377

Oeffinger KC (2008) Are survivors of acute lymphoblastic leukemia (ALL) at increased risk of cardiovascular disease? Pediatric Blood Cancer 50(2 Suppl):462–467

Oeffinger KC, Mertens AC, Sklar CA, Yasui Y, Fears T, Stovall M, Vik TA, Inskip PD, Robison LL, Childhood Cancer Survivor Study (2003) Obesity in adult survivors of childhood acute lymphoblastic leukemia: a report from the Childhood Cancer Survivor Study. Journal of Clinical Oncology 21(7):1359–1365

Oeffinger KC, Mertens AC, Hudson MM, Gurney JG, Casillas J, Chen H, Whitton J, Yeazel M, Yasui Y, Robison LL (2004) Health care of young adult survivors of childhood cancer: a report from the Childhood Cancer Survivor Study. Annals of Family Medicine 2(1):61–70

Picton SV (1998) Aspects of altered metabolism in children with cancer. International Journal of Cancer Supplement 11:62–64

Picton SV, Eden OB, Rothwell NJ (1995) Metabolic rate, interleukin 6 and cachexia in children with malignancy. Medical Pediatric Oncology 5(249):abstract 0–63

Ralston SH (1994) Pathogenesis and management of cancer associated hypercalcaemia. Cancer Surveys 21:179–196

Razzouk BI, Rose SR, Hongeng S, Wallace D, Smeltzer MP, Zacher M, Pui CH, Hudson MM (2007) Obesity in survivors of childhood acute lymphoblastic leukemia and lymphoma. Journal of Clinical Oncology 25(10):1183–1189

Reilly JJ, Odame I, McColl JH, McAllister PJ, Gibson BE, Wharton BA (1994) Does weight for height have prognostic significance in children with acute lymphoblastic leukemia? American Journal of Pediatric Hematology and Oncology 16(3):225–230

Reilly JJ, Ventham JC, Ralston JM, Donaldson M, Gibson B (1998) Reduced energy expenditure in preobese children treated for acute lymphoblastic leukemia. Pediatric Research 44(4):557–562

Reilly JJ, Weir J, McColl JH, Gibson BE (1999) Prevalence of protein-energy malnutrition at diagnosis in children with acute lymphoblastic leukemia. Journal Pediatric Gastroenterology Nutrition 29(2):194–197

Reilly JJ, Brougham M, Montgomery C, Richardson F, Kelly A, Gibson BES (2001a) Effect of glucocorticoid therapy on energy intake in children treated for acute lymphoblastic leukemia. The Journal of Clinical Endocrinology and Metabolism 86(8):3742–3745

Reilly JJ, Kelly A, Ness P, Dorosty AR, Wallace WHB, Gibson BES, Emmett PM, Alspac Study Team (2001b) Premature adiposity rebound in children treated for acute lymphoblastic leukemia. The Journal of Clinical Endocrinology and Metabolism 86(6):2775–2778

Rogers PC, Meacham LR, Oeffinger KC, Henry DW, Lange BJ (2005) Obesity in pediatric oncology. Pediatr Blood Cancer 45(7):881–891

Saini A, Al-Shanti N, Stewart CE (2006) Waste management – cytokines, growth factors and cachexia. Cytokine and Growth Factor Reviews 17(6):475–486

Sklar CA, Mertens AC, Walter A, Mitchell D, Nesbit ME, O'Leary M, Hutchinson R, Meadows AT, Robison LL (2000) Changes in body mass index and prevalence of overweight in survivors of childhood acute lymphoblastic leukemia: role of cranial irradiation. Medical and Pediatric Oncology 35(2):91–95

Skolin I, Hernell O, Whalin YB (2001) Energy and nutrient intake and nutritional status of children with malignant disease during chemotherapy after the introduction of new mealtime routines. Scandinavian Journal of Caring Sciences 15(1):82–91

Stapleton FB, Strother DR, Roy S 3rd, Wyatt RJ, McKay CP, Murphy SB (1988) Acute renal failure at onset of therapy for advanced stage Burkitt lymphoma and B cell acute lymphoblastic lymphoma. Pediatrics 82(6):863–869

Stockheim JA, Daaboul JJ, Yogev R, Scully SP, Binns HJ, Chadwick EG (1999) Adrenal suppression in children with the human immunodeficiency virus treated with megestrol acetate. Journal of Pediatrics 134(3):368–370

Taskinen M, Saarinen-Pihkala UM, Hovi L, Lipsanen-Nyman M (2000) Impaired glucose tolerance and dyslipidaemia as late effects after bone-marrow transplantation in childhood. Lancet 356:993–997

Teinturier C, Tournade MF, Caillat-Zucman S, Boitard C, Amoura Z, Bougneres PF, Timsit J (1995) Diabetes mellitus after abdominal radiation therapy. Lancet 346:633–634

Tosi P, Barosi G, Lazzaro C, Liso V, Marchetti M, Morra E, Pession A, Rosti G, Santoro A, Zinzani PL, Tura S (2008) Consensus conference on the management of tumor lysis syndrome. Haematologica 93(12):1877–1885

Traggiai C, Stanhope R, Nussey S, Leiper AD (2003) Diabetes mellitus after bone marrow transplantation during childhood. Medical Pediatric Oncology 40(2):128–129

Truong TH, Beyene J, Hitzler J, Abla O, Maloney AM, Weitzman S, Sung L (2007) Features at presentation predict children with acute lymphoblastic leukemia at low risk for tumor lysis syndrome. Cancer 110(8):1832–1839

Truini-Pittman L, Rosseto C (2002) Pediatric considerations in tumor lysis syndrome. Seminars in Oncology Nursing 18(3):17–22

Van Dongen-Melman JEWM, Hoekken-Koelaga ACS, Hakler K, de Groot A, Tromp CG, Egeler RM (1995) Obesity after successful treatment of acute lymphoblastic leukemia in childhood. Pediatric Research 38(1):86–90

Viana MB, Murao RG, Oliveira HM, de Carvalho RI, de Bastos M, Colosimo EA, Silvestrini WS (1994) Malnutrition as a prognostic factor in lymphoblastic leukaemia: a multivariate analysis. Archives of Disease in Childhood 71(4):304–310

Vujanic GM, Sandstedt B, Harms D, Boccon-Gibod L, Delemarre JF (1996) Rhabdoid tumour of the kidney: a clinicopathological study of 22 patients from the International Society of Paediatric Oncology (SIOP) nephroblastoma file. Histopathology 28:333–340

Weir J, Reilly JJ, McColl JH, Gibson BE (1998) No evidence for an effect of nutritional status at diagnosis on prognosis in children with acute lymphoblastic leukemia. Journal of Pediatric Hematology/Oncology 20(6):534–538

Gastrointestinal Tract

Anne Marie Maloney

Contents

18.1 Mucositis . . . 354
18.1.1 Incidence . . . 354
18.1.2 Etiology . . . 354
18.1.2.1 Iatrogenic . . . 354
18.1.2.2 Bacterial . . . 356
18.1.2.3 Viral . . . 356
18.1.2.4 Fungal . . . 357
18.1.3 Prevention . . . 357
18.1.4 Treatment . . . 357
18.1.5 Prognosis . . . 358
18.2 Dental Caries . . . 358
18.2.1 Incidence . . . 358
18.2.2 Etiology . . . 358
18.2.2.1 Iatrogenic . . . 358
18.2.3 Prevention and Treatment . . . 359
18.2.4 Prognosis . . . 359
18.3 Nausea and Vomiting . . . 359
18.3.1 Incidence . . . 359
18.3.2 Etiology . . . 359
18.3.3 Prevention . . . 360
18.3.4 Treatment . . . 360
18.3.5 Delayed Nausea and Vomiting . . . 361
18.3.6 Anticipatory Nausea and Vomiting . . . 361
18.3.7 Radiation-Induced Nausea and Vomiting . . . 362
18.3.8 Other Causes of Nausea and Vomiting . . . 363
18.3.9 Nonpharmacological Management . . . 363
18.3.10 Prognosis . . . 364
18.4 Constipation . . . 364
18.4.1 Incidence . . . 364
18.4.2 Etiology . . . 364
18.4.2.1 Iatrogenic . . . 364
18.4.2.2 Primary Constipation . . . 364
18.4.2.3 Secondary Constipation . . . 364
18.4.3 Prevention . . . 365
18.4.4 Treatment . . . 365
18.4.5 Prognosis . . . 366
18.5 Diarrhea . . . 366
18.5.1 Incidence . . . 366
18.5.2 Etiology . . . 366
18.5.2.1 Iatrogenic . . . 366
18.5.2.1.1 Chemotherapy-Induced Diarrhea . . . 366
18.5.2.1.2 Radiation-Induced Diarrhea . . . 368
18.5.2.1.3 Other Iatrogenic Causes of Diarrhea . . . 368
18.5.2.2 Viral . . . 368
18.5.2.3 Bacterial . . . 368
18.5.2.4 Other Infectious Etiologies of Diarrhea . . . 368
18.5.3 Prevention . . . 368
18.5.4 Treatment . . . 368
18.5.5 Prognosis . . . 369
18.6 Typhylitis . . . 369
18.6.1 Incidence . . . 369
18.6.2 Etiology . . . 370
18.6.2.1 Iatrogenic . . . 370
18.6.2.2 Fungal . . . 370
18.6.2.3 Bacterial . . . 370
18.6.3 Prevention . . . 370
18.6.4 Treatment . . . 370
18.6.5 Prognosis . . . 371
18.7 Perirectal Cellulitis . . . 371
18.7.1 Incidence . . . 371
18.7.2 Etiology . . . 371
18.7.2.1 Iatrogenic . . . 371
18.7.2.2 Bacterial . . . 371
18.7.3 Prevention . . . 371
18.7.4 Treatment . . . 371
18.7.5 Prognosis . . . 372
18.8 Acute Gastrointestinal Graft Vs. Host Disease . . . 372
18.8.1 Incidence . . . 372
18.8.2 Prevention . . . 372
18.8.3 Treatment . . . 373
18.8.4 Prognosis . . . 374
18.9 Chemical Hepatitis . . . 374
18.9.1 Incidence . . . 374
18.9.2 Etiology . . . 374
18.9.3 Prevention . . . 374
18.9.4 Treatment . . . 374
18.9.5 Prognosis . . . 375

18.10 Pancreatitis 375
18.10.1 Incidence 375
18.10.2 Etiology 375
18.10.3 Prevention 375
18.10.4 Treatment 375
18.10.5 Prognosis 375
References 376

18.1 Mucositis

18.1.1 Incidence

The mucosal lining of the GI tract, including the oral mucosal, is a prime target for treatment-related toxicity by virtue of its rapid cell turnover rate. Mucositis is an inflammation of the oral mucosa. Breakdown of the mucosal barrier can predispose patients to potentially fatal systemic infection. The estimated rates of the incidence of oral mucositis from standard multicycle chemotherapy for solid tumors range from 25 to 33%, and rise to nearly 100% in hematopoietic stem cell transplant patients (Sonis 2007). Chemotherapeutic agents differ in their potential for causing mucositis. Mucositis can also vary in intensity of pain and discomfort. Several grading systems have been developed to rate this common toxicity to cancer therapy. The World Health Organization (WHO) Mucositis Scale (Table 18.1) is a commonly used objective scale and The Oral Mucositis Assessment Scale (OMAS) (Table 18.2) is a commonly used subjective scale.

18.1.2 Etiology

18.1.2.1 Iatrogenic

Sonis (2004, 2007) proposed a Five-Stage Model of the Pathobiology of Oral Mucositis (Fig. 18.1):

1. *Initiation*: Radiation and/or chemotherapy causes direct DNA damage, stimulating the generation of Reactive Oxygen Species (ROS) that damage the connective tissue and cell membranes, and stimulate macrophages, which lead to the trigger of a

Table 18.1. WHO mucositis scale (WHO 1997)

Grade 0	None
Grade 1	Soreness with or without erythema, no ulceration
Grade 2	Erythema, ulcers. Patients can swallow solid diet
Grade 3	Ulcers, extensive erythema. Patients cannot swallow solid diet
Grade 4	Oral mucositis to the extent that alimentation is not possible

Table 18.2. Oral mucositis assessment scale (OMAS) (Sonis et al. 1999)

Location	Ulceration	Erythemia
Lip		
Upper	0, 1, 2, or 3	0, 1, or 2
Lower	0, 1, 2, or 3	0, 1, or 2
Buccal mucosa		
Right	0, 1, 2, or 3	0, 1, or 2
Left	0, 1, 2, or 3	0, 1, or 2
Tongue ventrolateral		
Right	0, 1, 2, or 3	0, 1, or 2
Left	0, 1, 2, or 3	0, 1, or 2
Floor of mouth	0, 1, 2, or 3	0, 1, or 2
Palate		
Soft	0, 1, 2, or 3	0, 1, or 2
Hard	0, 1, 2, or 3	0, 1, or 2
	0 = none, 1 = <1 cm^2, 2 = 1–3 cm^2, 3 = ≥ cm^2	0 = none, 1 = not severe, 2 = severe

cascade of biological mechanisms and molecules of the ceramide pathway.

2. *Upregulation and message generation*: The ceramide pathway signals the cells to enter apoptosis, leading to a biologic process that results in mucosal injury. The upregulation of genes due to chemotherapy- and radiation therapy-induced transcription factor activation results in the production of proinflammatory cytokines; TNF-α, IL-1β, and IL-6. Increased levels of these proteins have been found in the mucosa and their presence is likely to stimulate early damage to the tissues of the oral mucosa.
3. *Signaling and amplification*: Cytokines that have been unregulated not only continue to damage the tissue, but also provide a positive feedback loop to amplify the primary damage imitated by chemotherapy or radiation therapy.
4. *Ulceration*: The loss of mucosal integrity results in painful lesions that are prone to superficial bacterial colonization. Infection of the mucosa activates infiltrating mononuclear cells to produce and release pro-inflammatory cytokines.
5. *Healing*: In most cases, mucositis is a self-resolving condition once cancer therapy ends. Signals from the submucosal extracellular matrix govern the rate of epithelial-cell migration.

Oral complications associated with cancer treatment result from the following:

- The direct toxicity of antineoplastic agents and radiation therapy on the oral mucosa

Figure 18.1

The five phases of oral mucositis. Used with permission from Dr. Stephen Sonis, Brigham and Women's Hospital, Boston

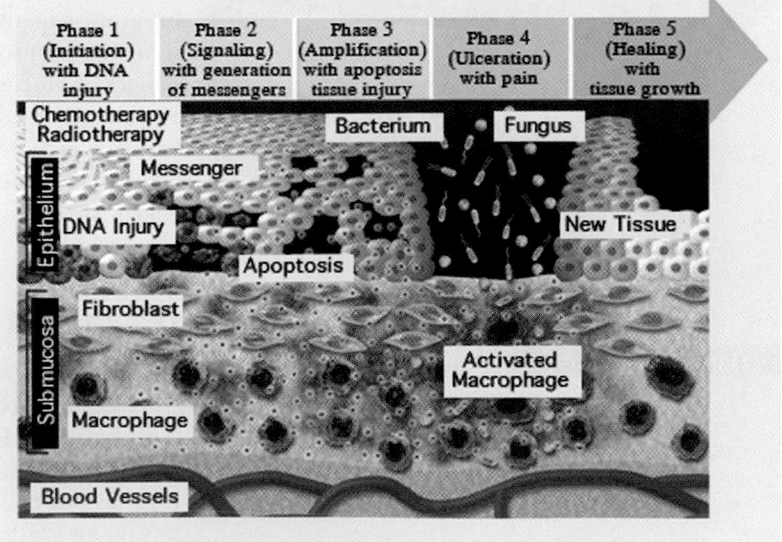

- The indirect effects of myelosuppression, consisting of hemorrhage and infection

The onset of oral mucositis, secondary to standard chemotherapy, is usually within three to seven days of therapy, with complete resolution observed fourteen days following the onset, which usually coincides with blood count recovery. Mucositis due to head and neck radiation therapy is the most troubling acute side effect experienced by patients (Otmani 2007). The combination of certain chemotherapeutic regimens along with radiation therapy can intensify mucositis. Figure 18.2 shows an example of ulcerative oral mucositis lesions. Chemotherapeutic agents that are commonly associated with mucositis are listed in Table 18.3.

Table 18.3. Chemotherapeutic agents commonly associated with mucositis

Alkylating agents	*Antitumor antibiotics*
Busulfan	Actinomycin D
Cyclophosphamide	Amsacrine
Ifosfamide	Bleomycin
Mellphalan	Mithramycin
Mechlorethamine	Mitomycin
Procarbazine	
Thiotepa	
Temozolamide	
Anthracyclines	*Taxanes*
Daunorubicin	Docetaxel
Doxorubicin	Paclitaxel
Epirubicin	
Idarubicin	
Antimetabolites	*Vinca alkaloids*
5-Fluorouracil	Vinblastine
Hydroxyurea	Vincristine
Methotrexate	Vinorelbine
Cytosine arabinoside	Etoposide
6-Mercaptopurine	
6-Thioguanine	

18.1.2.2 Bacterial

Oral mucositis is not an infectious process and oral decontamination regimens have been shown to be ineffective in reducing both the incidence and severity of mucositis (Treister and Sonis 2007). Mucositis, especially in the neutropenic patient, can predispose the patient to bacteraemia, septicemia, and fungaemia (Scully et al. 2006). The majority of bacterial infections are caused by opportunistic aerobic gram-negative bacilli that are seldom pathogenic in an immunocompetent host. Other bacterial etiologies of mucositis include Klebsiella, Enterobacter, Serratia, Proteus, and *Escherichia coli.* These lesions typically are creamy or yellow-white in color. They appear as moist glistening nonpurulent, smooth-edged surfaces seated on painful red superficial mucosal ulcers.

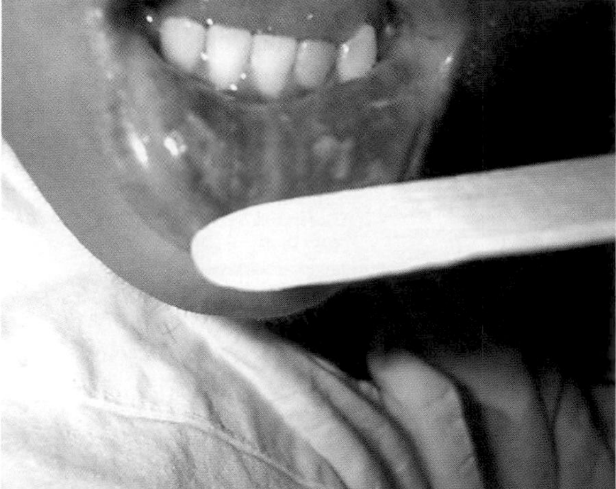

Figure 18.2

A case of ulcerative oral mucositis lesions of the labial mucosa. Reprinted with permission from: Cheng (2002). Oral care intervention to alleviate chemotherapy-induced oral mucositis in children with cancer. Unpublished PhD. Thesis, CUHK

18.1.2.3 Viral

Four different viral strains – herpes simplex virus (HSV) the most common, cytomegalovirus (CMV), varicella zoster, and Epstein–Barr virus (EBV) – commonly cause infection in the oral cavity. Perioral or intraoral HSV lesions usually appear as clear vesicles in clusters on an erythematous base. Intraoral lesions may appear as nondescript, and may be confused with mucositis associated with chemotherapy. Scraping of the lesion for viral cultures will confirm the etiology of the infection (Walsh et al. 2006).

18.1.2.4 Fungal

The most common oral mucosal superinfection is caused by *Candida albicans* (e.g., thrush), although other *Candida* species may be the causative agent. The incidence of oral candidiasis is variable and influenced by the underlying disease, immune status, intensity of cancer therapy, and salivary gland function (Lerman et al. 2008). Oral candidiasis presents as whitish plaques with slightly raised borders.

18.1.3 Prevention

Protocols and algorithms for the prevention and treatment of mucositis vary between institutions, and many preparations have been investigated in the prevention of chemotherapy-induced mucositis. In a Cochrane Database review, Clarkson et al. (2008) concluded that the only significant preventive measure for chemotherapy-induced mucositis is sucking on ice chips during 5-FU bolus dose administration. Certainly, this approach is not a viable option in younger children. To a lesser extent, this review concluded that Chinese medicine (various herbs given in combination), hydrolytic enzymes, and amifostine provided minimal benefit in the prevention of mucositis in patients with head and neck cancers and some solid tumors.

Palifermin, a recombinant keratinocyte growth factor, has recently been approved in the United States for the prevention of oral mucositis in patients undergoing stem cell transplant (Treister and Sonis 2007). A cooperative group phase III study id currently underway to investigate the efficacy of Palifermin in stem cell transplant patients.

18.1.4 Treatment

It is generally agreed that meticulous oral care is an important adjunct to the management of oral mucositis. A standardized oral care protocol was shown to reduce the incidence and severity of oral mucositis (Cheng et al. 2001). This study did not include a randomized comparison of agents. Given that the literature does not support the superiority of any particular agent in oral care, a simplified approach to oral care may be the best course of action. The American Academy of Pediatric Dentistry (2008) recommends that children undergoing cancer therapy continue toothbrushing 2–3 times a day, with a soft bristle toothbrush and a fluoridated toothpaste for as long as their oral condition allows. Toothbrushing should continue regardless of blood counts. Dental flossing and ultrasonic toothbrushes may be allowed if the patient has been properly trained in their use. Kennedy et al. (2003) reported that toothbrushes may become colonized with pathogenic organism; therefore, frequent replacement of toothbrushes is recommended. The American Academy of Pediatric Dentistry (2008) recommends replacement of toothbrushes every 2–3 months and that they be air-dried between uses.

Saline or sodium bicarbonate mouthwashes are non-irritating solutions that provide mechanical rinsing (Rogers 2001). These solutions have the benefit of being very cost-effective. Children with mucositis who are unable to brush their teeth should be instructed to rinse their mouth at a minimum of four times a day with one of these solutions. Commercially available alcohol-based solutions should be avoided as they may cause discomfort and dehydrate the tissues in patients with mucositis. Young children may have their mouths cleaned with a saline-soaked sponge "toothette" or gauze. Lips may be lubricated with lanolin-based creams or ointments that are more effective in moisturizing and protecting against damage than petroleum-based products (American Academy of Pediatric Dentistry 2008).

If feasible, a dental consultation should be obtained prior to the initiation of intensive chemotherapy, head and neck radiation therapy, and stem cell transplant, and the patient should continue to be evaluated by a dentist every 6 months during therapy (Shaw et al. 2000). Orthodontic appliances should be removed as they have the potential to harbor bacteria. If elective dental work is required during chemotherapy, it should be scheduled for a period when the patient is not expected to be pancytopenic. In patients with an ANC of more than 1,000/mm^3, antibiotic prophylaxis is not recommended (American Academy of Pediatric Dentistry 2008). Neutropenic patients requiring urgent dental care may require antibiotic coverage. Predental-care infective endocarditis prophylaxis in patients with central lines remains a controversial issue. The most recent guidelines for infective endocarditis prophylaxis do not cite the presence of a central line as an indication for treatment (Wilson et al. 2008).

Frequent assessment of the oral cavity is essential. Chemotherapy-induced mucositis can become further infected with *Candida* or HSV. Oral thrush, caused by *C. albicans*, appears as whitish plaques with slightly raised indurated borders. Herpetic lesions usually appear as clear vesicles, frequently in clusters on an erythematous base, either periorally or intraorally. Scrapings of suspicious lesions should be sent for culture. Culture-proven infections are treated with appropriate antimicrobials.

Pain is initially managed with topical anesthetics, and opioid analgesics may be eventually required. The patient's nutritional status must be carefully assessed, as inability to maintain adequate oral intake can quickly evolve into dehydration and nutritional deficits. A soft diet with cool and bland foods may be best tolerated. Ice chips and popsicles can be soothing and help to maintain hydration. In severe cases, intravenous hydration or total parenteral nutrition may be required.

18.1.5 Prognosis

Mucositis typically resolves with the resolution of neutropenia. In severe cases of mucositis, future chemotherapy cycles may need to be dose-reduced.

18.2 Dental Caries

18.2.1 Incidence

Dental side effects of cancer therapy can be of concern in the acute treatment period and in long-term follow-up. Although chemotherapy has little permanent effect on oral health, there is evidence that chemotherapy may result in an increased incidence of long-term dental problems. Minnicucci et al. (2003) described dental abnormalities, most frequently dental hypoplasia, in childhood leukemia survivors treated with chemotherapy alone. Radiation to the oral cavity results in changes in the composition of salvia and increased amounts of cariogenic oral bacteria, which leads to rapid decalcification of dental enamel and results in extensive caries known as radiation caries (Otmani 2007).

18.2.2 Etiology

18.2.2.1 Iatrogenic

The late effects of radiation therapy to the oral cavity are well established. The nature and severity of the potential side effects of radiation on the developing tooth vary with:

- The child's age at diagnosis
- The stage of tooth development
- The doses and schedules of treatment
- The anatomic region treated

The principal dental abnormalities caused by radiation include destruction of the tooth germ or tooth bud with failure of tooth development, stunted growth of the whole tooth or root, and incomplete calcification (Minicucci et al. 2003). The most severe disturbances on odontogenesis are seen when exposure to irradiation occurs in the preformative and differentiation phases of tooth development, rather than after dental maturation is complete. These changes in primary teeth can cause significant malocclusion and may adversely impact facial development (Otmani 2007).

Radiation caries is a rapidly progressive and destructive disease that develops between 2 and 10 months following treatment when radiation is delivered to the head and neck. When the major salivary glands are irradiated, all teeth within the field of radiation, as well as some outside the radiation field of treatment, have an increased risk of developing rampant caries. Radiation to the head and neck commonly damage the salivary glands, resulting in decreased salivary flow, changes in salivary composition, and increased salivary viscosity. These changes to the saliva reduce its buffering capacity, altering its concentration of electrolytes and changing its nonimmune and immune antibacterial systems. Children with functional impairment of their salivary glands face increased susceptibility to dental caries and oral infection (Otmani 2007).

18.2.3 Prevention and Treatment

Nurses can play a vital role in the establishment of proper oral hygiene practices in pediatric cancer patients. During the acute treatment period, the development of mucositis can often preclude the practice of effective oral hygiene practices. Poor baseline oral hygiene can be a predisposing factor in the development of infections. Gingivitis and peridonititis may cause infection and microorganisms may spread systemically (Raber-Durlacher et al. 2002). This suggests that dental cleanings should optimally be scheduled prior to chemotherapy or during periods when blood counts are anticipated to be satisfactory. Ideally, all potential foci of dental infection and bleeding should be removed before the start of cancer therapy.

Xerostomia can lead to an increased susceptibility to dental caries and erosion of tooth structure (Shaw et al. 2000). Interventions directed at increasing oral moisture and avoidance of refined sugar can help to prevent tooth decay. The American Academy of Pediatric Dentistry (2008) advocates the use of fluoride in toothpaste, supplement rinses, or topical applications to prevent the development of caries in children undergoing cancer therapy. Patients and families should be instructed regarding the increased risk of dental caries secondary to xerostomia. Strategies to achieve satisfactory oral hygiene during periods of painful mucositis should be addressed with the patient and family. Adequate pain control will help facilitate toothbrushing or at least oral cleansing with a toothette. Children should continue to have regularly scheduled dental examinations and cleanings during non-neutropenic periods, if possible.

18.2.4 Prognosis

Oral side effects from chemotherapy tend to be temporary. Increased susceptibility to dental caries can be a life-long problem following radiation therapy to the head and neck, or oral cavity and long-term abnormalities in dental enamel may occur after chemotherapy treatment. Preventive dental hygiene must be reinforced, and referral to a dentist familiar with the late effects of cancer therapy is indicated.

18.3 Nausea and Vomiting

18.3.1 Incidence

Nausea and vomiting are symptoms experienced by nearly all childhood cancer patients and are most commonly associated with chemotherapy and radiation therapy. However, the disease process, constipation, abdominal obstruction, infections, opioids for pain control, and other pharmacologic interventions can also contribute to nausea and vomiting in the pediatric oncology patient. Hockenberry (2004) reviewed the current literature on the symptom management of pediatric oncology patients and concluded that further research is needed to find measures to help alleviate nausea and vomiting in both acute and delayed phases of therapy. Unfortunately, research involving children experiencing cancer treatment-related nausea continues to be limited. Dupuis et al. (2006) developed the Pediatric Nausea Assessment Tool (PeNAT), an instrument to assess nausea in children receiving antineoplastic agents. The development of such instruments will facilitate research regarding the efficacy of interventions to manage nausea and vomiting in children. Advances in the understanding of the mechanisms of nausea and vomiting, the development of 5-hydroxytryptamine (5-HT_3) receptor antagonists, and the recent development of neurokinin-1 (NK1) receptor antagonists have greatly improved the outcomes in the antiemetic management of patients.

18.3.2 Etiology

The neurophysiologic mechanisms that control nausea and vomiting are mediated by the central nervous system by different mechanisms. Nausea is mediated through the autonomic nervous system. The vomiting center, located in the medullary lateral reticular formation, mediates vomiting. This center receives afferent input from five main sources:

1. Chemoreceptor trigger zone (CTZ)
2. Vagal and sympathetic afferents from the viscera
3. Midbrain receptors that detect changes in intracranial pressure
4. Labyrinthine apparatus that detects motions and position
5. Higher central nervous system structures (e.g., the limbic system)

The vomiting center in turn activates a series of efferent pathways, which include phrenic nerves to the diaphragm, spinal nerves to the abdominal musculature, and visceral nerves to the centrally mediated stimulation in the vomiting center, and act to induce actual vomiting (Berde et al. 2006).

The vomiting center contains neurotransmitter receptors of the serotonergic (especially 5-HT_3), dopaminergic (especially D2), histaminergic (especially H1), muscarinic cholinergic, endorphin cannabinoid, neurokinin (NK_1), and benzodiazepine types. The exact site and type of neurotransmitter involved in the pathogenesis of vomiting caused by each emetic stimulus is not known. The present understanding of pharmacologic control of emesis suggests that by blocking the effects of specific neurotransmitters for each stimulus, vomiting can be prevented or decreased. Acute emesis following chemotherapy is initiated by the release of neurotransmitters from cells that are susceptible to the presence of toxic substances in the blood or cerebrospinal fluid (CSF). Area postrema cells in the CTZ and enterochromaffin cells within the intestinal mucosa are implicated in the initiation and propagation of afferent stimuli that ultimately converge on the vomiting center. Delayed nausea and vomiting (DNV) is less well understood, and may involve an alternative pathway than those mediated through serotonin receptors (Billio et al. 2008).

Nausea and vomiting secondary to treatment experienced by pediatric oncology patients can be divided into three major categories:

1. Acute: nausea and vomiting experienced in the first 24 h following therapy
2. Delayed: nausea and vomiting that occurs 24 h following therapy
3. Anticipatory: nausea and vomiting that occurs prior to the start of subsequent cycles of chemotherapy.

Table 18.4 details the emetic risk of the commonly used chemotherapeutic drugs used in children with cancer.

18.3.3 Prevention

Prevention of nausea and vomiting is a cornerstone of good patient care. Good antiemetic control is best achieved by medicating with appropriate antiemetics prior to the initiation of therapy; it is very difficult to break the cycle of nausea and vomiting once it starts. Patient response to previous courses of chemotherapy should be assessed with each subsequent course of therapy, and an alteration to the antiemetic regimen is needed if a history of antiemetic failure is detected. Effective management of acute nausea and vomiting from the first exposure to treatment is important in the prevention of anticipatory nausea and vomiting (ANV).

18.3.4 Treatment

Successful management of chemotherapy associated nausea and vomiting requires an accurate assessment of the emetic potential of the chemotherapy regimen. The initial combination of antiemetics for a given chemotherapeutic regimen must be tailored to the emetogenic potential of that drug combination. Appropriate antiemetics must be initiated prior to the start of chemotherapy and given on a schedule, not on an "as needed" basis.

In pediatrics, commonly used antiemetic drugs include:

- 5-HT^3 antagonists such as ondansetron and granisetron
- Steroids such as dexamethasone

NB. However, the use of steroids may be contraindicated in some patients based on medical history or treatment protocol recommendations for supportive care.

Table 18.5 lists the antiemetics commonly used.

Table 18.4. Emetic risk of chemotherapeutic agents commonly used in pediatric oncology (Rolia 2006)

Emetic risk	Agents
High (>90%)	Cisplatin Mechlorethamine Streptozotocin Cyclophosph-amide > 1,500 mg/m^2 Carmustine Dacarbazine Cyclophosphamide plus antracycline Procarbazine
Moderate (30–90%)	Oxailiplatin Cytarabine >1 g/m^2 Carboplatin Ifosfamide Cyclophosphamide <1,500 mg/m^2 Doxorubicin Daunorubicin Epirubicin Idarubicin Irinotecan Etoposide P.O.
Low (10–30%)	Paclitaxel Docetaxel Mitoxantrone Topotecan Etoposide IV Pemetrexed Methotrexate Mitomycin Gemcitabine Cytarabine <100 mg/m^2 5-Fluorouracil Bortezomib Cetuximab Trastuzumab
Minimal (<10%)	Bleomycin Busulfan Fludarabine Vinblastine Vincrisitne Vinorelbine Bevacizumab

Reprinted with permission from Macmillan Publisher Ltd. (Jorn Herrstedt 2008)

The Multinational Association of Supportive Care in Cancer (MASCC) has set guidelines (Table 18.6) to determine the appropriate antiemetics to be prescribed based on the emetic risk of the chemotherapeutic agent (Herrstedt 2008).

There is limited evidence to suggest that if a patient fails one 5-HT$_3$ antagonist, switching to another drug in this class with subsequent chemotherapy cycles may be beneficial (de Wit et al. 2001). Thus, if the patient was initially treated with ondansetron and suffered an antiemetic failure, he would be switched to granisetron, tropisetron, or dolasetron for his next cycle of therapy. The management of acute nausea requires preventive around-the-clock dosing of antiemetics for 24 h, following the last dose of chemotherapy when the emetogenic potential is moderate or greater. Ideally, breakthrough antiemetics are ordered in case of antiemetic failure. Other antiemetics that may be used in pediatric oncology are listed in Table 18.7.

18.3.5 Delayed Nausea and Vomiting

DNV occurs 24 h or more after the last dose of chemotherapy, and may last up to 5 days or more following a cycle of chemotherapy. It is most often associated with cisplatin, carboplatin, and high-dose cyclophosphamide. Serotonin 5HT$_3$ antagonists have not been effective in the treatment of DNV; however, literature studies show that dexamethasone alone or in combination with metoclopramide is somewhat effective (Dupuis et al. 2001). Aprepitant, a NK-1 receptor antagonist, is a new antiemetic that has been recently introduced for the management of DNV in highly emetogenic chemotherapy protocols. Oral administration in combination with 5-HT$_5$ receptor antagonist and a corticosteroid has been shown to improve protection from both acute and DNV (Smith et al. 2005). The safety, efficacy, and dosing of aprepitant has not been established in children, and, therefore, its use may be limited to adolescents and young adults.

18.3.6 Anticipatory Nausea and Vomiting

ANV can occur anytime following the first cycle of chemotherapy. ANV can best be treated by the prevention of nausea and vomiting with the first

Table 18.5. Frontline antiemetics commonly used in pediatric oncology

Classification/ Drug	Dosing	Therapeutic considerations
5-HT_3 antagonist		
Ondansetron	5 mg/m^2 P.O./IV every 8–12 h Maximum dose = 8 mg P.O./IV	May cause headache, constipation with prolonged usage Expensive; oral form more cost-effective and equally efficacious. Oral disintegrating tablet (ODT) now available
Granisetron	20 µg/kg IV every 12 h	Adult oral dose = 2 mg P.O. daily. Currently, no pediatric oral dosing available. Some literature supports? up to 40 µg/kg/dose IV in pediatric patients; more research needed
Tropisetron	0.2 mg/kg P.O./IV every 24 h	Not available in North America
Dolasetron	1.8 mg/kg IV/P.O. every 24 h or 100 mg P.O. (adult dose)	Side effect: cardiac arrhythmias. Not approved in pediatrics
Palonosetron	0.25 mg and 0.75 mg IV single dose (adult dose)	No pediatric guidelines. Approved by FDA for acute and delayed nausea
Steroids		
Dexamethasone	8–12 mg/m^2 P.O./IV Maximum dose = 20 mg/dose	May be contraindicated in patients with brain tumors and patients on concurrent steroid therapy Risk of avascular necrosis
NK-1 receptor antagonist		
Aprepitant	125 mg P.O. prior to chemotherapy on day 1, and 80 mg P.O. on day 2 and 3	Pediatric dosing not established. Indicated only for use in highly emetogenic chemotherapy protocols. Potential interactions with medications metabolized via CYP3A4 enzyme in the liver

Table 18.6. MASCC guidelines to determine the appropriate prescribed antiemetics based on the emetic risk of a chemotherapeutic agent (Herrstedt 2008)

High emetic risk group: >90% risk
Acute: Serotonin antagonist plus dexamethasone plus aprepitant
Delayed: Aprepitant on days 2–3 plus dexamethasone on days 2–4
Moderate emetic risk group: 30–90% risk
Acute: Serotonin antagonist plus dexamethasone
Delayed: Dexamethasone on days 2–3 if corticosteroid contraindicated; may substitute serotonin antagonist
Low emetic risk group: 10–30% risk
Acute: Low-dose dexamethasone
Delayed: No routine prophylaxis
Minimal emetic risk group: <10% risk
Acute and delayed: No routine prophylaxis

administration of chemotherapy. Sights, sounds, or people associated with the administration of chemotherapy can precipitate ANV. Treatment of ANV can be pharmacologically managed with lorazepam or cannabinoids given the evening prior to chemotherapy. Assessment of the factors that trigger ANV can be helpful in developing nonpharmacologic approaches to treatment. Guided imagery, relaxation therapy, music therapy, and art therapy may be of benefit in the treatment of ANV.

18.3.7 Radiation-Induced Nausea and Vomiting

Total body, abdominal, cranial spinal, mantle, and hemi-body irradiation have been associated with radiation-induced emesis. 5-HT_3 antagonists have been effective when given prior to each radiation fraction and for 24 h following the treatment (Kris et al. 2006)

Table 18.7. Other antiemetics used in pediatric oncology

Classification/antiemetic	Indications
Benzodiazepine Lorazepam	Useful in the treatment of anticipatory and breakthrough nausea and vomiting. Route IV/P.O./SL dosing 0.025–0.05 mg/kg give 1 h prechemo and Q 6 h as needed maximum dose of 4 mg. Start with lower dose and increase as necessary. Monitor for excessive sedation
Oral cannabinoids Nabilone Marinol	Useful in the treatment of anticipatory nausea and break through nausea and vomiting. Some patients may not tolerate the euphoria associated with cannabinoids. Optimal dosing starts the night before chemotherapy
Phenothiazines Chlorpromazine Prochlorperazine Thiethylperazine Perphenazine	Major side effect is extra pyramidal reaction and agitation especially in younger children. Slow administration over 30–60 min and concurrent administration with antihistamines for 24 h after last phenothiazine dose will minimize these effects. Phenothiazines may be added to frontline antiemetic regimens with 5-HT$_3$ antagonist when these regimens fail
Procainamide derivative Metoclopramide	Major side effects are extra pyramidal reactions. Slow administration and concurrent antihistamine administration will minimize these reactions. Metoclopramide has both antiemetic and gastric emptying effect Dosing of 1 mg/kg every 2–4 h
Antihistamines Diphenhydramine Dimenhydrinate	Mild antiemetic properties. May be used in combination with other antiemetics. Sedating properties of antihistamines may be desirable for some patients

18.3.8 Other Causes of Nausea and Vomiting

In pediatric oncology, nausea and vomiting can be attributed to factors other than treatment-related causes. Metabolites of many tumors (especially in advanced disease), increased intracranial pressure (secondary to brain tumors), constipation, bowel obstruction, and opioid administration for pain control are some of the potential causes. Treatment is achieved with the control of the underlining cause of nausea and vomiting. If this is not feasible, control of symptoms may be achieved with standard antiemetic therapies. 5-HT$_3$ antagonists may be of benefit in opioids-induced nausea.

18.3.9 Nonpharmacological Management

Acupuncture, acupressure, and hypnosis have been used as complementary therapies in the management of chemotherapy-induced nausea and vomiting, and children are particularly sensitive to hypnosis as an intervention to manage both acute and delayed phase of nausea and vomiting (Ladas et al. 2006). Currently, a study is under way by the Children's Oncology Group to evaluate electroacupuncture, a type of acupuncture in which the needles are attached to low-voltage current to enhance the effect of the treatment of nausea and vomiting in pediatric oncology patients (Jindal et al. 2008). Relaxation or distraction therapy and self-hypnosis have also been described to decrease nausea and vomiting (Rheingans 2007). Nonpharmacologic approaches to the management of nausea and vomiting include controlling the patient's environment, including strong odors, bright lights, and noise. Patient education regarding strategies to manage nausea and vomiting are essential. Parents must be instructed to closely monitor their child for signs of dehydration. Small, frequent, bland meals maybe best tolerated. Giving the child the opportunity to request foods may also be successful. Uncontrolled nausea plays an important role in the development of food aversions; therefore, families should be counseled that children may develop this aversion to favorite foods after therapy, as taste alterations are common. Spicy foods may be appealing, as spices may mask alterations in taste (Skolin et al. 2006).

18.3.10 Prognosis

Nausea and vomiting are self-limiting sequelae to cancer therapy. These symptoms may also be the most debilitating symptoms associated with therapy. Effective antiemetic control is an essential component for the quality of life in a child with cancer.

18.4 Constipation

18.4.1 Incidence

Constipation is a common sequelae of childhood cancer treatment. Constipation can lead to complications such as nausea and vomiting, abdominal pain, anorexia, and subsequent delays in chemotherapy. In a recent study, Woolery et al. (2006) defined constipation as a change in the child's usual pattern of elimination including two or more of the following symptoms:

1. Decreased frequency from the child's normal pattern and/or less than three bowel movements per week
2. Difficulty passing stool
3. Painful passage of stool
4. Passage of hard stool and/or
5. Incomplete passage of stool

It is estimated that constipation accounts for 3% of the general population of pediatric outpatient visits and 25% of the visits to the pediatric gastroenterologist in the general pediatric population (Baker et al. 2006). In the pediatric oncology patients, constipation may be caused due to additional factor such as:

- Decreased gastric motility secondary to medications (especially vinca alkaloids and opioid analgesics)
- Tumor compression of the GI tract or spinal cord
- Hypokalemia
- Hypercalcemia
- Hypothyroidism
- Decreased mobility
- Anorexia
- Changes in toileting patterns

18.4.2 Etiology

The exact etiology of constipation in the child with cancer is often difficult to determine and is often multifocal. Constipation in the pediatric oncology patient can be categorized as primary, secondary, or iatrogenic.

18.4.2.1 Iatrogenic

The most common iatrogenic agents responsible for constipation in the pediatric oncology patient are opioid analgesics and vinca alkaloids. It is estimated that 50–95% of children receiving opioids and 30% of children receiving vincristine will experience constipation (Woolery et al. 2006). Opioids inhibit smooth intestinal muscle motility, resulting in decreased peristalsis and delayed stool transit time. Vinca alkaloids (e.g., vincristine and vinblastine) also decrease peristalsis. This results in increased transit time for the stool to pass, leading to increased absorption of water in the bowel and the formation of hard dry stools. Other iatrogenic causes of constipation include decreased peristaltic bowel activity following abdominal and pelvic surgery, and decreased oral intake due to chemotherapy-induced nausea and vomiting.

18.4.2.2 Primary Constipation

Primary constipation results from external factors such as:

- Dietary
- Decreased mobility
- Interruption in normal patterns of defecation

Children with cancer experience decreased oral intake and subsequent nutritional deficits, from nausea and vomiting, alterations in taste, or generalized malaise. A deficit in healthy food choices, especially in fiber intake, may also result. Hospitalized patients have their usual routine disrupted, and periods of privacy for toileting may predispose the patient to constipation.

18.4.2.3 Secondary Constipation

Secondary constipation in the child with cancer results from the pathology of the disease itself.

Abdominal tumors can cause partial or complete intestinal obstruction of the GI tract. Tumor growth along the spinal column can result in cord compression and decreased innervation of the bowel. Metabolic alterations, hypothyroidism, or metabolic conditions may lead to water depletion (i.e., renal acidosis, diabetes insipidus, and hyperkalemia may predispose the patient to constipation (Philichi 2007)).

18.4.3 Prevention

Prevention is crucial in the management of constipation. Families should receive anticipatory education regarding the potential for and treatment of constipation. Patients on opioid therapy should be empirically started on a bowel regimen. Careful assessment for constipation should be carried out in patients, prior to vincristine or vinblastine therapy. These patients may benefit from prophylactic stool softeners.

18.4.4 Treatment

A detailed physical examination and history, including dietary and defecation habits should be assessed in all patients. Children with constipation may present with:

- A decline in stool production
- Change in the characteristics of stool (hard, dry, and possibly blood-streaked)
- Hypoactive bowel sounds
- Distended or firm abdomen (a mass maybe noted in the left lower quadrant)
- Diffused abdominal tenderness
- Decreased appetite
- Feeling of satiety and nausea
- Straining with an attempt to have bowel movements
- Pain associated with defecation

The underlying causes of constipation should be identified and treated.

Dietary interventions include maximizing oral fluid intake; whole grains, fruits, and vegetables are recommended as part of a balanced diet. Supplemental fiber may actually worsen the symptoms in a severely constipated child (Philichi 2007). A dietary consult may be helpful in identifying foods that may predispose patients to constipation and those which may help to prevent this condition. Other non-pharmacologic interventions include encouraging physical activity, maintaining normal toileting routines, and providing privacy for defecation.

Pharmacologic interventions can be divided into two phases:

1. Disimpaction
2. Maintenance

In neutropenic patients, the rectal route of disimpaction must be avoided, owing to the risk of injury to the rectal mucosal and potential for perirectal infection. Disimpaction is necessary before initiation of maintenance therapy.

Disimpaction by the oral route, the rectal route, or a combination of the two has been found to be effective. In a medical position statement by the North American Society for Pediatric Gastroenterology, Hepatology, and Nutrition (Baker et al. 2006), the method of disimpaction is recommended to be determined after discussion with the child and family. The oral route may be less invasive, and the rectal route may be faster but more invasive. In pediatric oncology patients, the rectal route is reserved to children who are not neutropenic. High doses of mineral oil and/or polyethylene glycol–electrolyte solutions are highly effective agents for the oral route of disimpaction. The recommended dosage of mineral oil for disimpaction is 15–30 mL/year of age, up to 240 mL/day. Mineral oil can be associated with aspiration pneumonia and is not recommended in children under one year of age or those with impaired swallowing reflexes. Polyethylene glycol–electrolyte solution is recommended at a dosage of 25 mL/kg/h by nasogastric tube or oral route if tolerated, until clear up to a maximum dosage of 1,000 mL/h. However, it has been associated with nausea, bloating abdominal cramps, and anal irritation. High-dose magnesium hydroxide, magnesium citrate, lactulose, sorbitol, senna, or bisacodyl have all been successfully utilized to achieve disimpaction, although no clinical trials have been used to document their effectiveness. Once disimpaction of the fecal mass has been achieved, maintenance of a regular stooling must be achieved.

The pharmacological management of constipation includes a combination of laxatives and stool softeners to achieve a regular stooling pattern. Common medications used in the treatment of constipation are listed in Table 18.8. Stool softeners include mineral oil at a dose of 1–3 mL/kg/day or docusate sodium of 20–60 mg/day. Both these preparations can be given as a divided dose 1–4 times a day, titrated to maintain soft stools. The maintenance of soft stool ensures that the child does not have painful bowel movements which may lead to withholding of stool and result in stool impaction. Liquid docusate and mineral oil can be mixed with a variety of fluids and foods to aid in their palatability.

Magnesium hydroxide, lactulose, and sorbitol have been used in children experiencing constipation, showing good results. Long-term studies show that these therapies are safe and effective. As magnesium hydroxide, lactulose, and sorbitol seem to be equally efficacious, the choice of which laxative to use can be made on the basis of cost and patient preference. Stimulant laxatives, such as senna and bisacodyl are not recommended as daily therapy, and they should be reserved for intermittent therapy as a rescue to prevent recurrence of impaction (Baker et al. 2006).

18.4.5 Prognosis

Once a patient has experienced constipation, preventive regimens should be used to minimize recurrence. Constipation is rarely a long-term sequela of cancer or the associated therapy. Once the precipitating factors are removed, the patient usually returns to the previous bowel patterns.

18.5 Diarrhea

18.5.1 Incidence

Diarrhea is defined as an abnormal increase in the quantity, frequency, or liquidity of stool. This condition can predispose the patient to fluid and electrolyte imbalances, dehydration, renal failure, and impaired skin integrity. In the pediatric oncology patients, diarrhea can be a potentially serious sequela of the therapy or be caused by the disease process itself. Diarrhea may result in further hospitalization due to dehydration, and in severe cases, may result in delay of therapy. The most frequent cause of acute diarrhea is an infectious process. Other etiologies of diarrhea include drug reactions, dietary alterations, inflammatory bowel disease, intestinal ischemia, graft vs. host disease (GvHD) or overflow diarrhea secondary to fecal impaction. Chronic diarrhea can be complex and be caused by infections, inflammatory bowel diseases, irritable bowel syndrome, dietary alterations, surgeries, endocrine disorders, neoplasms, or radiation colitis (Cope 2001).

Chemotherapy-induced diarrhea (CID) can vary in intensity from mild and self-limiting to severe and requiring aggressive medical management. The exact incidence of CID is unknown; however, in the adult population, estimates suggest that 10% of patients with advanced cancer experience acute or chronic diarrhea sometime during their illness (Goldberg-Arnold et al. 2005). Chemotherapeutic regimens that contain fluoropyrimidines such as fluorouracil (5-FU) and irinotecan (CPT-11) have resulted in the incidence of diarrhea as high as 80% and incidence of grade 3–5 diarrhea of greater than 30% (Goldberg-Arnold et al. 2005).

18.5.2 Etiology

18.5.2.1 Iatrogenic

18.5.2.1.1 Chemotherapy-Induced Diarrhea

CID is a well-recognized side effect of a number of chemotherapeutic agents. Irinotecan (CPT-11) is one of the chemotherapy agents most commonly linked to CID. Wagner et al. (2008) described two distinct patterns of CID associated with Irinotecan. Early onset occurs within the first 4 h of administration, and is associated with cholinergic symptoms such as cramping, flushing, and diaphoresis. Table 18.9 lists the most common chemotherapeutic agents associated with diarrhea. Early onset diarrhea can be effectively prevented or treated with anticholinergic agents such as atropine. Late onset diarrhea develops in the second week of therapy and can be dose limiting. The mechanism of this toxicity are complicated and not completely understood. One factor seems to be the accumulation of the active metabolite of irinotecan, SN-38, in the gut, causing

Table 18.8. Common medications used in the treatment of constipation

Drug	Dose	Comments
Osmotic		
Lactulose	1–3 mL/kg/day in divided doses or 5–10 mL P.O. daily initially	Adult dose: 30 mL/day, increase dose daily until stool is produced. Well tolerated. Side effects include abdominal cramps
Magnesium citrate	<6 years, 1–3 mL/kg/day 6–12 years, 100–150 mL/day >12 years, 150–300 mL/day Maximum dose: 300 mL/day	Cathartic: Used for oral disimpaction. Monitor electrolytes
PEG 3350 MiraLax GlycoLax	10–30 kg, 8.5 g/day >30 kg, 17 g/day	Dissolve in 240 mL of water/juice
Sorbitol	2–11 years, 2 mL/kg Adults: 30–150 mL	Less expensive than lactulose. Side effects are nausea, vomiting, and diarrhea
Lavage		
Polyethylene Glycol–electrolyte solution	In severe impaction 25 mL/kg/h until clear Maximum = 1,000 mL	Most children will require NG tube as solution is not well tolerated. Side effects are nausea, vomiting, and cramps
Lubricant		
Mineral oil	Maintenance 1–3 mL/kg/day Disimpaction 15–30 mL/year up to 240 mL/day	Stool softener decreases water reabsorption; risk of lipoid pneumonia if aspirated; not to be used with children with neurological deficits or infants
Stimulants		
Senna	*Syrup*2–6 years, 3–5 mL/day 6–12 years, 5–10 mL/day *Granules* 2–5 years, 2.5 mL/day 6–12 years, 5 mL/day *Tablet* 6–12 years, 1–2 tablets/day	Stimulant laxatives should be used for short-term use only; not daily therapy
Bisacodyl	5 mg tablets, 1–3 tablets daily prn	Not for daily use Severe abdominal cramps

Data from (Baker et al. 2006; Philichi 2007)

Table 18.9. Chemotherapeutic agents associated with diarrhea

Cisplatin	Cyclophosphamide	Cytarabine
Daunorubicin	Doxorubicin	Fluorouracil
Hydroxyurea	Interferon	Interleukin-2
Irinotecan	Methotrexate	Thioguanine
Topotecan		

cytotoxicity, local inflammation, and secretory diarrhea. Within the bowel following biliary excretion, the inactive compound, SN-38 glucuronide, is converted back to active SN-38 by glucuronidases produced by enteric bacteria, which lead to further mucosal injury and diarrhea. Acute damage to the intestinal mucosa is caused by some chemotherapeutic agents such as irinotecan, leading to a loss of intestinal epithelium, inflammation, and superficial necrosis of the bowel. This inflammatory process and necrosis can stimulate secretion of fluids and electrolytes directly. Destruction of the terminal carbohydrate and protein digestive enzymes may also lead to increased secretion of fluid and electrolytes. Thus, the intestinal absorptive cells may not be able to manage the large volume of fluid and electrolytes that are produced, and consequently, diarrhea occurs (Cope 2001).

18.5.2.1.2 Radiation-Induced Diarrhea

Radiation therapy to the abdomen and pelvis is one of the major causes of chronic diarrhea in the child with cancer. Diarrhea associated with radiation therapy is a result of radiation colitis. Radiation colitis refers to radiation-induced changes in the colorectal mucosa, resulting in an ischemia of the gut wall. Acute colitis presents within a few days to up to 6 weeks following radiation therapy. The presenting symptoms of acute colitis are mucus discharge, diarrhea, and rectal urgency. The cumulative incidence of symptomatic radiation colitis is reported to be between 10 and 30% for grade 1 or 2 colitis, and between 2 and 3% for grade 3 or 4 colitis (Qadeer and Vargo 2008).

18.5.2.1.3 Other Iatrogenic Causes of Diarrhea

Medications used for the supportive care of children with cancer may also play a role in the development of diarrhea. Antibiotics may cause alterations in the normal flora of the GI tract resulting in diarrhea. Other supportive care medications, such as antacids, antihypertensive antiemetics, and especially electrolyte supplements, are associated with this condition. Frequent hospitalization places the pediatric oncology patient at risk for institution-acquired infectious diarrhea.

18.5.2.2 Viral

Rotavirus is the most important cause of viral gastroenteritis in infants and young children in the winter months, and accounts for 40–50% of admissions to pediatric hospitals for gastroenteritis (Rogers et al. 2000). Other common viral etiologies of diarrhea include adenoviruses and astroviruses.

18.5.2.3 Bacterial

Bacterial etiologies for diarrhea in the immunocompromised host include Salmonella, Campylobacter, Shigella, Yersinia, Aeromonas, and Plesiomonas. Children with a recent history of antibiotic therapy and prolonged hospitalization are at an increased risk of developing pseudomembranous colitis caused by the toxins produced by *Clostridium difficile*. This condition occurs in 0.2–10% of patients taking antibiotics (Sondheimer 2003).

18.5.2.4 Other Infectious Etiologies of Diarrhea

Diarrhea may also be secondary to a variety of parasitic infections, such as *Girardia* and *Entamoeba* and various tape worm species.

18.5.3 Prevention

In the hospital setting, strict adherence to infection control practices is the most important mechanism to prevent the spread of infectious diarrhea in immunocompromised patients. Patients experiencing diarrhea should be placed under enteric isolation precautions. Meticulous hand hygiene must be observed by all staff, families, and patients. Parent and patient education emphasizing on the strategies for preventing fecal–oral contamination is critical. Safe food-handling practices should be reviewed with the families, including food preparation and storage. Patients should avoid contact with others suffering from gastroenteritis.

Prevention of iatrogenic causes of diarrhea starts with patient education regarding the early detection of CID. In regimens associated with a high incidence of CID, families should be instructed to promptly treat diarrheic episodes with the prescribed antidiarrheal agent.

18.5.4 Treatment

The effective management of diarrhea is directly related to its etiology. Therefore, establishing the underlying cause is the first step in effective treatment. A detailed history including stooling patterns, volume and consistency of the stools, dietary practices, medication history, travel history, and exposures to potentially infectious persons should be completed by the nurse. Physical examination should focus on potential sequelae of diarrhea, including dehydration and skin breakdown. Infectious etiologies are determined by examining the stool for bacterial, viral, and *C. difficile* toxins. Stool should also be examined for ova and parasites if the patient history indicates.

C. difficile infections are common in the pediatric oncology patient due to the frequent use of antibiotic therapy. Once identified, *C. difficile* is treated with oral metronidazole or vancomycin. The use of vancomycin as a frontline therapy is discouraged because of the concerns of drug-resistant gram-positive bacteria. Unfortunately, there is a 10–20% rate of relapse, although most patients respond to a second course with the same or alternative therapy (Walsh et al. 2006).

The treatment of viral diarrhea is largely supportive care for the patients. Typically, viral diarrhea is a self-limiting process. *Medications directed at slowing bowel motility are contraindicated in infectious diarrhea, as they would slow the elimination of infectious pathogens.* Hospitalized patients with diarrhea must be assumed infectious until proven otherwise, and be placed under appropriate isolation practices.

CID is most frequently observed following the administration of irinotecan (CPT-11), a topoisomerase I inhibitor. Prompt management of acute diarrhea during administration of this drug is achieved with intravenous (IV) atropine. Late onset diarrhea is managed with loperamide. Wagner et al. (2008) described the use of cephalosporins as a safe and effective way to prevent CID in children receiving irinotecan. Cephalosporins selectively eradicate intestinal bacteria that produce glucuronidase that convert the inactivated metabolites of irinotecan to active metabolites within the gut. Irinotecan-induced diarrhea can have a sudden onset and result in life-threatening fluid and electrolyte imbalances. Patient education regarding loperamide administration and signs of dehydration is critical.

The management of patients with diarrhea focuses on prevention of dehydration and electrolyte imbalances. Frequent assessment of fluid and electrolyte status and the prompt correction of alterations are necessary. In severe cases, hospitalization and IV rehydration are required. Families should be taught to identify dehydration: decreased skin turgor, decreased urine output, dry mucus membranes, sunken fontanels, and alterations in activity. Careful assessment of the perianal area is indicated, as diarrhea can lead to skin breakdown and provide a portal for infection. Hygiene must be emphasized; sitz baths are effective to good hygienic practices and can be very soothing. Barrier creams to protect the perianal area are also indicated.

Nutritional support is addressed by increasing oral hydration to correct fluid losses in the stool. Oral rehydrating solutions can help replace lost salts. Families should be cautioned against diluting infant formula due to the risk of hyponatremia in young infants. Age-appropriate feedings (including breast feeding) should be continued and foods high in fat and simple sugars should be avoided.

18.5.5 Prognosis

Typically, diarrhea caused by *C. difficile* will resolve with the completion of an appropriate course of treatment. In viral etiologies of diarrhea, it is largely self-limiting. Iatrogenic causes of diarrhea usually resolve once sufficient time interval has passed to allow for healing of the GI tract. Unfortunately, chronic diarrhea associated with pelvic and abdominal radiation or with GvHD following stem cell transplant may have a lengthy recovery process.

18.6 Typhylitis

18.6.1 Incidence

Typhylitis or neutropenic enterocolitis (NE), or ileocecal syndrome is an inflammatory process of the terminal ileum and ascending colon (Hobson et al. 2005). This potentially life-threatening condition involves chemotherapy-induced damage to the intestinal mucosa and occurs in the face of neutropenia (van de Wetering et al. 2003). Typhylitis was historically seen in children with leukemia or aplastic anemia; however, with increasing intensity in therapy, it is now being diagnosed in the stem cell transplant and solid tumor populations (King 2002) (Alioglou et al. 2007). Children presenting with typhylitis usually have a history of neutropenia for more than 1 week, and the classic triad of fever, diffuse abdominal pain (or less frequently, right lower quadrant pain), and diarrhea (van de Wetering et al. 2003). In severe cases, patients with typhylitis may develop intestinal necrosis and perforation, eventually leading to septic shock. The incidence of clinical typhylitis varies with diagnosis, the chemotherapy regimen, and prophylactic antibiotics used. However, in an autopsy-based descriptive series, an incidence of up to 32% among children undergoing bone marrow transplant has been reported (Otaibi et al. 2002).

18.6.2 Etiology

18.6.2.1 Iatrogenic

The exact etiology of typhylitis remains uncertain, although several mechanisms have been proposed. The pathobiology of typhylitis is believed to be multifactorial and includes:

- Destruction of the normal mucosal structure due to chemotherapy, radiation therapy, or leukemic infiltrates
- Intramural hemorrhage due to thrombocytopenia
- Changes in the normal GI flora due to antimicrobial therapy and colonization by hospital flora (van de Wetering et al. 2003)

Steroids, common to many leukemia protocols and supportive care regimens, have long been associated with typhylitis. Neutropenia is a prerequisite for the development of typhylitis.

18.6.2.2 Fungal

There has been limited report on fungal typhylitis. Kamal et al. (1997) reported a case study of a child on antileukemia therapy who developed typhylitis associated with a *Candida* intraluminal mass. Other fungal isolates reported include *Candida* and *Aspergillus* in 53% of postmortem cases (Avigan et al. 1998).

18.6.2.3 Bacterial

A bacterial infectious etiology is most common in typhylitis. In one series, *Pseudomonas* was the most common isolated species; other common isolates include *E. coli*, *Staphylococcus aureus*, and *Klebsiella spp.* In addition, infections due to *C. difficile*, *Streptococcus viridans group*, and *Stenotrophomonas spp.* have also been reported (Alioglou et al. 2007).

18.6.3 Prevention

As typhylitis is associated with high-dose chemotherapy and resultant neutropenia, there is no specific preventive regiment. Management of typhylitis is directed at early detection and prompt treatment.

18.6.4 Treatment

The assessment of patients with suspected typhylitis should include a careful history and physical examination. Blood cultures, baseline CBC, and blood chemistries should be obtained. Frequent nursing assessments are vital in the prompt identification of life-threatening complications. Frequent vital signs and attention to fluid balance and urine output are also important for the early detection of shock. Assessment of the abdomen should include inspection, palpation, auscultation, and measurement of girth. Pain should be frequently assessed with a consistent age-appropriate tool. Changes in the intensity and quality of pain may be early indicators of deterioration in the patients' condition.

Abdominal X-rays are the least sensitive tool in diagnosing NE, but may be helpful in the exclusion of other bowel disorders such as intussusception. Perforation, obstruction, and pneumatosis intestinalis (interluminal air in the bowel wall) can easily be seen on plain film. Ultrasound is an easy and noninvasive technique to identify changes in the cecal mucosa, and can be used safely for frequent monitoring of the child with typhylitis, as radiation is not involved. CT scan is the most sensitive modality to assess cecal wall thickening (King 2002).

The management of patients with typhylitis is largely supportive in nature. Bowel rest, parenteral nutrition, broad spectrum antibiotics (including anaerobe coverage), titration of opioids to manage pain, and continuous patient assessment are included in the standard of care. Aggressive management of cytopenias and coagulopathies is essential. Granulocyte colony stimulating factor (GCSF) may be indicated to help decrease the period of neutropenia (Alioglou et al. 2007). Patients with typhylitis generally respond to medical management. However, consultation with a pediatric surgeon early in the clinical course may help facilitate identifying those rare patients for whom surgical intervention is required. It is generally agreed that surgical intervention is only required in the case of intestinal perforation or clinical deterioration despite appropriate medical management (Schlatter et al. 2002).

18.6.5 Prognosis

Typhylitis once had a very grim diagnosis in pediatric oncology patients. Fortunately, with the early detection of the condition and aggressive supportive treatment, majority of children survive this potentially life-threatening condition.

18.7 Perirectal Cellulitis

18.7.1 Incidence

Perirectal cellulitis involves inflammation and edema of the perineal and rectal area. Rectal tears or fissures can lead to perirectal cellulitis in the immunocompromised patients. Constipation and the traumatic passage of hard stools, rectal temperatures and enemas or suppositories, and perianal breakdown are the predisposing factors to perirectal cellulitis, and must be avoided. The incidence of anorectal infections has been reported to be as high as 5% in patients receiving myeloablative chemotherapy (Segal et al. 2001). The overall incidence of perianal cellulitis has decreased in the recent years, because of the early use of empiric antibiotics in febrile neutropenic patients. Nonetheless, the risk for perirectal cellulitis persists, especially for patients in the high-risk category, those with chronic (more than 7 days) and profound (less than 100 cells/mm^3) granulocytopenia (Walsh et al. 2006).

18.7.2 Etiology

18.7.2.1 Iatrogenic

Iatrogenic etiologies of perirectal cellulitis include neutropenia secondary to chemotherapy and tissue breakdown secondary to local radiation therapy. Rectal digital examination, rectal temperatures, or medications have been well-established predisposing factors to this condition. Constipation and passage of hard stools may predispose the patients to rectal tears and fistulas, which can become portals of infection.

18.7.2.2 Bacterial

The most common pathogens in perirectal cellulitis include aerobic gram-negative bacilli (e.g., *P. aeruginosa, K. pneumoniae, E. coli*), enterococci, and bowel anaerobes (Walsh et al. 2006).

18.7.3 Prevention

Prompt recognition of the signs of perirectal cellulitis and prompt initiation of appropriate therapy are critical in minimizing the potentially lethal sequelae of this infection. Measures to maintain the skin and tissue integrity of the perirectal area may minimize the risk of infection. These measures include meticulous hygiene, maintenance of soft daily bowel movements, and avoidance of rectal manipulation (e.g., rectal temperatures or suppositories, and enemas).

18.7.4 Treatment

Patients with perirectal cellulitis may present with fever, perianal pain, painful defecation, or constipation. On examination, the perianal area may be erythematous, irritated, and inflamed, and swelling and fissures may be present. In the neutropenic patients, localized reaction may be minimal or absent. In fact, the area may develop increasing inflammation and pain as neutrophil counts recover, with the occurrence of a localized granulocyte response. Daily assessment of the perianal area is mandatory in neutropenic patients. Radiological imaging of the retroperitonium using CT scan is required if abscess is suspected.

Treatment involves broad-spectrum antibiotics to control gram-negative organisms and anaerobes. GCSF may be indicated to help shorten the length of the neutropenia. Meticulous hygiene and frequent assessment of the area must be initiated. Sitz baths are often effective and soothing. Barrier creams should be applied to protect the affected area. Stool softeners must be started to help prevent constipation. Appropriate pain assessment and management is required. Patient controlled analgesia (PCA) may provide optimal pain control and facilitate the patient participation in ambulation and adherence to hygiene regimens. Digital rectal examination must be avoided due to the risk of trauma and infection. Surgical consultation may be required to have an abscess drained in severe cases that fail to resolve with medical management.

18.7.5 Prognosis

The outcome for children with perianal cellulitis is generally good with prompt diagnosis and appropriate medical management. Recovery from neutropenia is the most important prognostic indicator for a positive outcome (Segal et al. 2001).

18.8 Acute Gastrointestinal Graft Vs. Host Disease

18.8.1 Incidence

Acute graft vs. host disease (aGvHD), a sequela of allogeneic hematopoietic stem cell transplantation (HSCT), is an immune-mediated response that occurs within the first 100 days following stem cell transplant. Three organ systems are primarily affected: the skin, the GI tract, and the liver. Skin aGvHD is characterized by a maculopapular eruption that may range from a mild rash on the soles of the feet and palms of the hands (stage 1) to a generalized rash involving over 50% of the body with bullae formation and desquamation (stage 4) (Ball and Egeler 2008). Gastrointestinal aGvHD is characterized by copious diarrhea, abdominal cramping, and nausea and vomiting, and is staged by the volume of the stools passed each day. Liver aGvHD is characterized and staged by elevations in liver function studies. Staging and grading of gut and liver aGvHD are shown in Table 18.10. Diarrhea associated with aGvHD can vary from mild to copious, and may consist of several liters of bloody stool each day. Severe gut aGvHD is associated with anorexia, nausea, abdominal pain, GI bleeding, and may progress to ileus. The incidence of aGvHD following allogeneic bone marrow transplant varies with the specific disease entity being treated and the degree of genetic disparity between the donor and recipient. It has been estimated that 20–50% of all transplanted patients will experience grade 2 or greater aGvHD, despite immunosuppressive prophylaxis (Ball and Egeler 2008).

aGvHD is a clinical and pathologic syndrome of enteritis, hepatitis, and dermatitis which develops within 100 days of allogeneic HSCT. The effector cells are thought to be donor T-lymphocytes that recognize the antigenic disparities between the donor and the recipient. In addition, the altered host milieu promotes the activation and proliferation of inflammatory cells with resulting deregulated production of inflammatory cytokines. This cytokine network may be the final common pathway for the tissue damage associated with GvHD, and this entire cascade has been described as a "cytokine storm" (Guinan et al. 2002). GvHD is an iatrogenic etiology, resulting from HSCT. However, other causes of liver or gut dysfunction and infection are common, and must be ruled out in the acute transplant setting. A definitive diagnosis of GvHD can only be made with either liver or gut biopsy.

18.8.2 Prevention

The major risk factors for the development of aGvHD include:

- Histoincompatibility between the donor and the patient
- Older donor age
- Greater intensity of the transplant conditioning regimen
- Use of peripheral blood progenitor stem cells rather than marrow

In general, the patient's risk factors cannot be altered by the treating team. Nurses should be critical in the

Table 18.10. Organ staging of aGvHD

Stage	Skin	Liver	GI tract
0	No rash due to GvHD	Bilirubin <2 mg/100 mL or 35 µmol/L	None (<280 mL/m^2)
I	Maculopapular rash <25% of body surface area without associated symptoms	Bilirubin for 2 to <3 mg/100 mL or 35–50 µmol/L	Diarrhea >500–100 mL/day (280–555 mL/m^2); nausea and emesis
II	Maculopapular rash or erythema with pruritus or other associated symptoms >25% of body surface area or localized desquamation	Bilirubin from 3 to <6 mg/100 mL or 51–102 µmol/L	Diarrhea >1,000–1,500 mL/day (>833 mL/m^2); nausea and emesis
III	Generalized erythroderma; symptomatic macular, popular or vesicular eruption with bullous formation of desquamation covering >50% of body surface area	Bilirubin 6 to <15 mg/100 mL or 103–225 µmol/L	Diarrhea >1,500 mL/day (833 mL/m^2); nausea and emesis
IV	Generalized exfoliative dermatitis or bullous eruption	Bilirubin >15 mg/100 mL or 225 µmol/L	Diarrhea >1,500 mL/day (833 mL/m^2); nausea and emesis. Abdominal pain or ileus

Reprinted with permission from Macmillan Publisher Ltd. (Ball and Egeler 2008)

assessment and identification of the signs and symptoms of aGvHD (Deeg 2007).

The two major prophylactic regimens employed to prevent aGvHD include:

1. Immunosuppressive drugs such as cyclosporine, short-course methotrexate, or FK506
2. T-cell depletion of the donor bone marrow (Bollard et al. 2006)

18.8.3 Treatment

The medical management of aGvHD can be classified as either primary or secondary treatment. The mainstay of primary therapy is steroids, and a typical dosing regimen is methylprednisolone of 2 mg/kg/day for a 7–14 day course, followed by a gradual dose reduction if the patient responds. If the patient fails to respond to primary therapy, then second-line treatments are employed (Deeg 2007) (Table 18.11).

Ongoing assessment of the patient with gut GvHD is critical. Precise measurement of stool loss and fluid balance are required. Supportive care in the acute transplant period includes fluid and electrolyte replacement from diarrhea associated with GvHD. Patients with copious diarrhea often develop perianal skin breakdown. Frequent assessment of skin integrity and attention to good hygiene is essential in the nursing care of these patients. Transfusion of red blood cells is often required to replace gastric blood losses. These patients will require aggressive nutritional support and pain control.

Table 18.11. Second-line aGvHD therapies

Monoclonal antibodies Daclizumab Alemtuzumab Visilizumab
Pentostatin
Sirolimus (rapamycin)
ATG (antithymocyte globulin, ATGAM)
Infliximab (antitumor necrosis factor)
Extracorporeal photopheresis (ECP)

18.8.4 Prognosis

aGvHD remains a source of significant cause of morbidity and mortality in the stem cell transplant patients. Fifty percent of patients respond to first-line treatment (Messina et al. 2008). The prognosis for patients with aGvHD who do not respond to therapy is poor (Deeg 2007).

18.9 Chemical Hepatitis

18.9.1 Incidence

Chemical hepatitis or reactive hepatitis is a non-viral inflammation of the liver caused by exposure to chemical or other environmental toxins, such as chemotherapy, biotherapy, or radiation. Chemical hepatitis may range from asymptomatic elevations of liver transaminases and serum bilirubin levels to overt liver failure at the extreme end of the spectrum. Anti-inflammatory agents, antimicrobials, anticonvulsants, and other drugs metabolized by the liver and utilized in supportive care of children with cancer may contribute to drug-induced hepatitis (Table 18.12). The exact incidence of treatment-induced hepatotoxicity varies depending on the therapeutic and supportive care regimens utilized.

Typically, chemical hepatitis is identified in the routine prechemotherapy screening of liver function enzymes: alanine transaminase (ALT) and aspartate transaminase (AST). The patient may also exhibit clinical signs and symptoms of hepatitis including jaundice, prurtitis, pain, fever, diaphoresis, malaise, flu-like symptoms, nausea, vomiting, anorexia, and bruising or bleeding.

18.9.2 Etiology

Other potential disorders including infectious hepatitis and hepatic metastasis must be excluded to confirm the diagnosis of chemical hepatitis. Hepatocellular dysfunction usually is caused by a direct effect of either the parent drug or a metabolite, and is an acute event. Serum hepatic enzymes rise as cellular damage occurs. Fatty infiltration and cholestasis may occur as the toxic effect progresses (Weiss 2001). Patients with underlying infectious Hepatitis B and C are at increased risk for reactivation of dormant hepatitis viruses (Rodrigues-Frias and Lee 2007). There are no histological or biochemical features that are specific to drug-induced hepatotoxicity, and there is no simple and safe method for diagnosing this condition.

Table 18.12. Medications utilized in pediatric oncology associated with hepatotoxicity

Asparaginase
Methotrexate
Carmustine
Anticonvulsants
NSAIDS
Mercaptopurine
Lomustine
Vincristine
Dactinomycin
Antimicrobials
Thioguanine
Vinblastine
Doxorubicin
Idarubicin

18.9.3 Prevention

Prevention of this condition is limited to identification and avoidance, if possible, of hepatotoxic therapies. Most chemotherapy treatment protocols call for the routine monitoring of liver functions. Many of these protocols mandate dose adjustments of hepatotoxic agents based on the degree of elevation of liver transaminases or bilirubin.

18.9.4 Treatment

The treatment of chemical hepatitis is largely supportive. Removal of the causative factors of this condition is the initial step. Hepatotoxic chemotherapy and other drugs should be reduced or discontinued if possible. Total parenteral nutrition (TPN) should be avoided, if possible, secondary to the potential for liver damage. Careful monitoring of liver transaminases and coagulation studies is critical. Supportive care for the physical symptoms of hepatitis should be initiated and must include measures to minimize pruritus (e.g., cool baths and the application of moisturizing lotions). Daily weights and assessment for jaundice, ascites, or bleeding should be obtained, as these are common sequelae of hepatotoxicity. Dietary management includes a low fat and high carbohydrate diet.

18.9.5 Prognosis

Chemical hepatitis is usually self-limiting, with liver functions returning to normal parameters once the causative agent has been removed and the liver recovers. Unfortunately, chronic complications of chemical hepatitis can ensue and include chronic active hepatitis, cirrhosis, and a range of extrahepatic syndromes, including associated pulmonary injury and marrow compromise (Panzarella et al. 2002).

18.10 Pancreatitis

18.10.1 Incidence

Pancreatitis has been reported as a complication in 2–16% of patients undergoing L-asparaginase therapy for a variety of cancers (Top et al. 2005). It also has been associated, to a lesser extent, with mercaptopurine and steroid therapies.

18.10.2 Etiology

Pancreatitis is an acute inflammation of the pancreas. The clinical course of pancreatitis may range from very mild disease to multiorgan liver failure and sepsis. Veins and venules are often affected with granulocytic infiltration, thrombosis necrosis, and hemorrhage (Top et al. 2005). The adverse effects of L-asparaginase related to the development of pancreatitis are as a result of decreased protein synthesis, and include hypoinsulinemia, hypoproteinemia, and hypoalbuminemia (Alverez and Zimmerman 2000). Children with pancreatitis may present with acute abdominal pain, nausea, and vomiting. They may have elevations of serum amylase and lipase. However, the synthesis of amylase and lipase by L-asparaginase may result in normal levels of these markers, despite overt disease (Top et al. 2005). Abdominal ultrasound or CT scan may reveal the extent of inflammation of the pancreas and the presence of fluid collection.

18.10.3 Prevention

Chemotherapy-induced pancreatitis is an unavoidable complication of treatment for a small proportion of patients. There is no preventative treatment; therefore, early identification of symptoms and elevation of biochemical markers (lipase and amylase) and the prompt initiation of supportive therapy are imperative.

18.10.4 Treatment

The treatment of pancreatitis is largely supportive and includes bowel rest, fluid management, antiemetics, and antibiotics. Parental nutrition is indicated during periods of bowel rest. The role of nasogastric decompression has not been supported in the literature, but may provide symptomatic relief in the face of intractable vomiting. Analgesia is best achieved with meperidine, as morphine may cause constriction of the splinter of Oddi. Recent studies have indicated that octreotide may inhibit autodigestion of the pancreas and the resulting damage to the adjacent structures (Top et al. 2005; Reingold and Lange 2006). Surgical intervention may be required in severe cases to drain or debride an infected pancreas.

18.10.5 Prognosis

Majority of the patients with acute pancreatitis respond well to supportive measures. The development of pancreatitis may limit their ability to receive future doses of asparaginase therapy, the effect of which is unknown on the disease process. The reported mortality of patients with pancreatitis is between 2 and 5% (Alverez and Zimmerman 2000).

References

Alioglou B, Avci Z, Ozcay F, Arda S, Ozbek N (2007) Neutropenic enterocolitis in children with acute leukemia or aplastic anemia. International Journal of Hematology 86: 364–368

Alverez O, Zimmerman G (2000) Pegasparaginase-induced pancreatitis. Medical and Pediatric Oncology 34:200–205

American Academy of Pediatric Dentistry (2008) Guideline on the management of pediatric patients receiving chemotherapy, hematopoietic cell transplantation, and or radiation. http://www.aapd.org

Avigan D, Richardson P, Elias A, Demetri G, Shapriro M, Schnippper L, Wheller C (1998) Neutropenic enterocolitis as an complication of high dose chemotherapy with stemcell rescue in patients with solid tumors. Cancer 83:409–414

Baker S, DiLorenzo C, Liptak G, Ector W, Collettie R, Nurko S, Croffie J (2006) Clinical practice guideline Evaluation and treatment in infants and children: recommendations of the North American Society for Pediatric Gastroenterology Hepatology and Nutrition. Journal of Pediatric Gastroenterology and Nutrition 43:e 1–e 13

Ball L, Egeler R (2008) Acute GvHD: pathogenesis and classification. Bone Marrow Transplantation 41:S58–S64

Billio A, Clarke M, Morello E (2008) Comparison of clinical efficacy of serotonin receptor antagonist in highly emetogenic chemotherapy (protocol). Cochrane Database of Systematic Reviews Issue (4)

Berde C, Billett A, Collins J (2006) Symptom management in supportive care. In: Pizzo P, Poplack D (eds) Principles and practice of pediatric oncology, 5th edn. Lippincott Williams & Wilkins, Philadelphia, pp 1348–1373

Bollard C, Kranse R, Heslsop H (2006) Hematopoietic stem cell transplantation in pediatric oncology. In: Pizzo P, Poplack D (eds) Principles and practice of pediatric oncology, 5th edn. Lippincott Williams & Wilkins, Philadelphia, pp 476–500

Cheng KKF (2002) Oral care intervention to alleviate chemotherapy induced mucositis in children with cancer. Unpublished PhD Theses, Chinese University of Hong Kong, CUHK

Cheng K, Molassiotis A, Chang A, Wai W, Cheung S (2001) Evaluation of an oral care protocol intervention in the prevention of chemotherapy-induced oral mucositis in pediatric cancer patients. European Journal of Cancer 37(16): 2056–2063

Clarkson JE, Worthington HV, Eden OB (2008) Interventions for preventing oral mucositis for patients with cancer receiving treatment. Cochrane Database System Review (4)

Cope D (2001) Management of chemotherapy-induced diarrhea and constipation. Nursing Clinics of North America 36(4):695–708

Deeg HJ (2007) How I treat refractory acute GVHD. Blood 109:4119–4126

de Wit R, de Boer G, Linden G, Stoter G, Sparreboom A, Verweij J (2001) Effective cross-over to granisetron after failure to ondansetron, a randomized double blind study in patients failing ondansetron plus dexamethasone during the first 24 hours following highly emetogenic chemotherapy. British Journal of Cancer 85:1099–1101

Dupuis L, Lau R, Greenberg M (2001) Delayed nausea and vomiting in children receiving antineoplastics. Medical and Pediatric Oncology 37(1):115–121

Dupuis L, Taddio A, Kerr E, Kelly A, MacKeigan L (2006) Development anf validation of the pediatric nausea assessment tool for use in children receiving antineoplastics agents. Pharmacotherapy 26(9):1221–1231

Guinan E, Krance R, Lehmann L (2002) Stem cell transplantation in pediatric oncology. In: Pizza P, Pollack D (eds) Principles and practice of pediatric oncology, 4th edn. Lippincott Williams & Wilkins, Philadelphia, pp 429–452

Goldberg- Arnold RJ, Gabrail N, Raut M, Kim R, Sung JC, Zhou Y (2005) Clinical implications of chemotherapy-induced diarrhea in patients with cancer. Journal Supportive Oncology 3(3):227–232

Herrstedt J (2008) Antiemetics:an update and the MASCC guidelines applied in clinical practice. Nature Clinical Practice Oncology 5:32–43

Hockenberry M (2004) Symptom management research in children with cancer. Journal of Pediatric Oncology Nursing 21:132–136

Hobson M, Carney D, Molik K, Vik T, Scherer L, Rouse T, West K, Grosfeld J, Billmore D (2005) Appendicitis in childhood hematologic malignancies: analysis and comparison with typhilitis. Journal of Pediatric Surgery 40:214–220

Jindal V, Ge A, Mansky PJ (2008) Safety and efficacy of acupuncture in children; a review of the evidence. Journal of Pediatric Hematology and Oncology 30:431–442

Kamal M, Wilkinson A, Gibson B (1997) Radiological features of fungal typhylitis complicating acute lymphoblastic leukemia. Pediatric Radiology 27:18–19

Kennedy HF, Morrison D, Tomlinson D, Gibson BE, Bagg J, Gemmell C (2003) Gingivitis and toothbrushes: potential roles in viridans streptococcal bacteraemia. Journal of Infection 46(1):67–69

King N (2002) Nursing care of the child with neutropenic enterocolitis. Journal of Pediatric Oncology Nursing 19:198–204

Kris M, Hesketh P, Somerfeild M, Feyer P, Clark-Snow R, Koeller J, Morrow G, Chinnerry L, Chesney M, Gralla R, Grunberg S (2006) American society of clinical oncology guideline for antiemetics in oncology: update 2006. Journal of Clinical Oncology 24:2932–2947

Ladas E, Post-White J, Hawks R, Taromina K (2006) Evidence for symptom management in the child with cancer. Complementary and Alternative Medicine 28:601–615

Lerman M, Laudenbach J, Marty F, Baden L, Treister N (2008) Management of oral infections in cancer patients. The Dental Clinic of North America 52:129–153

Messina C, Faraci M, de Fazio V et al (2008) Prevention and treatment of acute GvHD. Bone Marrow Transplantation 41:S65–S70

Minicucci E, Lopez L, Crocci A (2003) Dental abnormalities in children after chemotherapy treatment for acute lymphoid leukemia. Leukemia Research 27:45–50

Otaibi A, Barker C, Anderson R, Sigalet D (2002) Neutropenic enterocolitis after pediatric bone marrow transplant. Journal of Pediatric Surgery 37:770–772

Otmani N (2007) Oral and maxillofacial side effects of radiation therapy on children. Journal of the Canadian Dental Association 73:257–261

Panzarella C, Rasco Baggott C, Cameau M, Duncan J, Groben V, Woods D, Stewart J (2002) Management of disease and treatment related complication. In: Rasco Baggott C, Patterson K, Fochtman D (eds) Nursing care of children and adolescents with cancer. Saunders, Philadelphia, pp 279–318

Philichi L (2007) When the going gets tough pediatric constipation and encopresis. Gastroenterology Nursing 31: 121–130

Qadeer M, Vargo J (2008) Approaches to the prevention and management of radiation colitis. Current Gastroenteology Reports 10(15):507–513

Raber-Durlacher J, Epstein J, Raber J, van Dissel J, van Winkelhoff A, Guiot H, vander Velden U (2002) Periodontal infection in cancer patients treated with high-dose chemotherapy. Supportive Care Cancer 10:466–473

Reingold S, Lange B (2006) Oncologic Energencies. In: Pizzo P, Poplack D (eds) Principles and Practice of Pediatric Oncology, 5th edn. Lippincott Williams & Wilkins, Philadelphia, pp 641–662

Rheingans J (2007) A systematic review of nonpharmacologic adjunctive therapies for symptom management in children with cancer. Journal of Pediatric Oncology Nursing 24:81–94

Rodrigues-Frias E, Lee W (2007) Cancer chemotherapy I: hepatocellular injury. Clinics in Liver Disease 11:641–662

Rogers B (2001) Mucositis in the oncology patient. Nursing Clinics of North America 36:745–760

Rogers M, Weinstock D, Eagan J, Kiehn T, Armstrong D, Sepkowitz K (2000) Rotavirus outbreak on a pediatric oncology floor: Possible association with toys. American Journal of Infection Control 28:378–380

Rolia F (2006) Prevention of chemotherapy and radiotherapy induced emesis: results of the 2004 Perugia international; antiemetic consensus conference. The antiemetic subcommittee of the multinational association of supportive care in cancer (MASCC). Annals of Oncology 17:22–28

Schlatter M, Synder K, Freyer D (2002) Successful management of typhylitis in pediatric oncology patients. Journal of Pediatric Surgery 37(8):1151–1155

Scully C, Sonis S, Diz P (2006) Oral mucositis. Oral Diseases 12:229–241

Segal B, Walsh T, Holland S (2001) Infection in the cancer patient. In: DeVita V, Hellman S, Rosenberg S (eds) Cancer principles and practice of oncology, 6th edn. Lippincott Williams & Wilkens, Philadelphia, pp 2815–2868

Shaw M, Kumar D, Duggal M, Fiske J, Kinsella T, Nisbet T (2000) Oral management of patients following oncology treatment: literature review. British Journal of Oral & Maxillofacial Surgery 38:591–524

Skolin I, Britt Wahlin Y, Broman D, Koivisto Hursti U, Vikstrom Larsson M, Hernell O (2006) Altered food intake and taste perception in children with cancer after start of chemotherapy: perspectives of children, parents and nurses. Supportive Care Cancer 14:369–378

Smith R, Repka T, Weigel B (2005) Aprepitant for the control of chemotherapy induced nausea and vomiting in adolescents. Pediatric Blood and Cancer 45:857–860

Sondheimer J (2003) Gastrointestinal tract. In: Hay W (ed) Current pediatric diagnosis and treatment, 16th edn. McGraw-Hill, New York

Sonis ST, Eilers JB, Epstein JB, LeVeque FG, Liggett WH Jr, Mulagha T et al (1999) Validation of a new scoring system for the assessment of clinical trial research of oral mucositis by radiation or chemotherapy. Mucositis Study Group. Cancer 85:2103–2113

Sonis S (2004) The pathobiology of mucositis. Nature Reviews 4:277–284

Sonis S (2007) Pathobiology of oral mucositis: novel insights and opportunities. The Journal of Supportive Oncology 5:3–11

Top P, Tissing W, Kuiper J, Pieters R, van Eijck C (2005) L-asparaginase induced severe necrotizing pancreatitis successfully treated with percutaneous drainage. Pediatric Blood and Cancer 44:95–97

Treister N, Sonis S (2007) Mucositis: biology and management. Current Opinion in Otolaryngology & Head and Neck Surgery 15:123–129

van de Wetering M, Kuijpers T, Taminiau J, ten Kate F, Caron H (2003) Pseudomembranous and neutrpenic enterocolitis in pediatric oncology patients. Supportive Care Cancer 11: 581–586

Wagner L, Crews K, Stewart C, Rodrigues-Galindo C, McNall-Knapp R, Albritton K, Pappo A, Furman W (2008) Reducing Irinotecan-associated diarrhea in children. Pediatric Blood and Cancer 50:201–207

Walsh T, Roilides E, Groll A, Gonzales C, Pizzo P (2006) Infectious complications in pediatric cancer patients. In: Pizzo P, Poplack D (eds) Principles and practice of pediatric oncology, 5th edn. Lippincott Williams & Wilkins, Philadelphia, pp 1270–1319

Weiss R (2001) Miscellaneous toxicities. In: DeVita V, Hellman S, Rosenberg S (eds) Cancer principles & practice of oncology, 6th edn. Lippincott Williams & Wilkens, Philadelphia, pp 2970–2971

Wilson W, Taubert n A, Gewitz M, Lockhart PB, Baddour LM, Levison M (2008) Prevention of infective endocarditis: Guidelines from the American Heart Association: A guideline from the American Heart Association Rheumatic Fever, Endocarditis and Kawasaki Disease Committee, Council on Cardiovascular Disease in the Young, and the Council on Clinical Cardiology, Council on Cardiovascular Surgery and Anesthesia, and the Quality of Care and Outcomes Research Interdisciplinary Working Group. Journal of the American Dental Association 139 Suppl:3S–24S

Woolery M, Carroll E, Feen E, Wieland H, Jarosinski P, Corey B, Wallen G (2006) A constipation assessment scale for use in pediatric oncology. Journal of Pediatric Oncology Nursing 23:65–74

World Health Organization (1997) Handbook for reporting results of cancer treatment. World Health Organization, Geneva, Switzerland, pp 15–22

Bone Marrow Function

Sandra Doyle

Contents

19.1 Introduction . . . 380
19.2 Anemia . . . 380
19.2.1 Incidence and Etiology . . . 380
19.2.2 Treatment . . . 380
19.2.2.1 Transfusion . . . 380
19.2.2.2 Use of Recombinant Human Erythropoietin . . . 381
19.3 Neutropenia . . . 381
19.3.1 Incidence and Etiology . . . 381
19.3.1.1 Fever (Pyrexia) and Neutropenia . . . 382
19.3.2 Treatment . . . 382
19.3.2.1 Antibiotic Management . . . 383
19.3.2.2 Special Consideration for the Management of Indwelling Intravenous Catheters . . . 385
19.3.2.3 Management of Candidiasis (Oropharyngeal Candidiasis and Candida Esophagitis) . . . 385
19.3.2.4 Infections Due to *Aspergillus* Species . . . 386
19.3.2.5 Management of Viral Infections . . . 386
19.3.2.6 Infections Due to *Pneumocystis jiroveci* (Formerly *Pneumocystis carinii*) . . . 386
19.3.2.7 Use of Colony Stimulating Factors in Children with Neutropenia . . . 388
19.3.2.8 Isolation . . . 389
19.4 Thrombocytopenia . . . 389
19.4.1 Incidence and Etiology . . . 389
19.4.2 Treatment . . . 389
19.5 Transfusion Issues . . . 390
19.5.1 Granulocyte Transfusions . . . 390
19.5.1.1 Transfusion-Related Acute Lung Injury . . . 390
19.5.2 Transfusion-Associated Graft vs. Host Disease . . . 391
19.5.3 Cytomegalovirus and Transfusions . . . 392
19.5.3.1 Treatment . . . 392
19.5.4 Platelet Refractoriness . . . 392
19.5.4.1 Treatment . . . 393
19.6 Disseminated Intravascular Coagulation . . . 393
19.6.1 Etiology and Manifestation . . . 393
19.6.1.1 Diagnosis . . . 394
19.6.2 Treatment . . . 394
19.7 Septic Shock . . . 395
19.7.1 Etiology . . . 395
19.7.2 Treatment . . . 395
19.7.3 Prognosis . . . 396
19.8 Immune Suppression . . . 396
19.8.1 Polymorphonuclear Leukocytes . . . 396
19.8.2 Lymphocytes . . . 397
19.8.3 Spleen and Reticuloendothelial System . . . 398
19.8.4 Other Factors Contributing to Immunocompromised States . . . 398
References . . . 398

19.1 Introduction

Bone marrow suppression may occur as a result of a child's disease or treatment of the disease process. Bone marrow suppression can result in a decrease in all the areas of hematopoiesis and is one of the most common dose-limiting toxicities of chemotherapy. There can be a decrease in red blood cells (RBCs), white blood cells (WBCs), and platelets. The time of most profound bone marrow suppression (nadir) occurs approximately 10–14 days after myelosuppressive treatment. Previous chemotherapy and radiation therapy can also prolong the recovery time and nadir. Table 19.1 summarizes the normal values and lifespans for hemoglobin, WBCs, and platelets.

Table 19.1. Normal blood values (data from Lodha 2003)

Component of blood	Lifespan	Age	Reference interval
White blood cell count ($\times 10^9$/L)	Hours to 300 days	6 days	9.0–30.0
		7–13 days	5.0–21.0
		14 days–2 months	5.0–20.0
		3–11 months	5.0–15.0
		1–4 years	5.0–12.0
		>5 years	4.0–10.0
Neutrophils ($\times 10^9$/L)	6–8 h	1 week	1.5–10.0
		2 weeks	1.0–9.5
		3 weeks–5 years	1.5–8.5
		6–10 years	1.5–8.0
		>10 years	2.0–7.5
Hemoglobin (g/L)	120 days	6 days	150–220
		7–30 days	140–200
		1 month	115–180
		2 months	90–135
		3–11 months	100–140
		1–4 years	110–140
		5–13 years	120–190
		Female, ≥14 years	120–153
		Male, ≥14 years	140–175
Platelet cell count ($\times 10^9$/L)	7–10 days	All ages	150–450

19.2 Anemia

19.2.1 Incidence and Etiology

Anemia is commonly encountered in pediatric oncology patients. This is usually due to chemotherapy-related myelosuppression, but can also be related to malignant infiltration of bone marrow, radiation, viral suppression, blood loss, and nonspecific processes (inhibitory effect of tumor necrosis factor, iron deficiency, or low endogenous erythropoietin) (Rizzo et al. 2002). Chemotherapy-associated anemia is characteristically an insidious and delayed complication of treatment.

19.2.2 Treatment

19.2.2.1 Transfusion

Transfusion was the traditional means of therapy in the 1990s. The usual recommended triggers for transfusion are a hemoglobin count of 60–70 g/L and no signs of imminent marrow recovery, or if hemoglobin >70 g/L and the child is symptomatic (i.e., decreased energy, fatigue, pallor, headache, tachypnea, tachycardia and/or gallop, and failure to take part in normal activities of daily living) (Steele 2003). Many radiotherapists request that transfusions be given to children receiving radiation therapy to maintain hemoglobin levels >100 g/L. This is to ensure well-oxygenated cells that can best respond to radiotherapy (Panzarella et al. 2002). Transfusions normally consist of 5–15 mL/kg of packed red blood cells (PRBC) that are leukocyte-filtered, irradiated, and cytomegalovirus (CMV)-negative if applicable (see Sect. 19.4) (Steele 2003). In an emergency, whatever blood is available can be used, with blood group

O rhesus (Rh)-negative being the universal donor. Nursing care includes the following:

- Being vigilant to the child's need for transfusion, assessing for increasing fatigue, headache, pallor, and a decrease in the normal activity level.
- Communicating with healthcare team members about pertinent laboratory values and the needs for transfusion.
- Vital signs should be recorded before, during, and after transfusions.
- Administration of transfusions through a sterile administration set with a standard pore size (170–260 μm) blood filter to remove clots or other debris.
- Adminsteration at a rate of no more than 2 mL/min during the first 15 min of transfusion; infusion rates of 2–5 mL/kg/h are the norm for paediatric patients (Chambers et al. 2007).
- Monitoring the child for transfusion reactions during blood administration.
- Educating the family members to recognize signs and symptoms of anemia.

19.2.2.2 Use of Recombinant Human Erythropoietin

Studies have explored the use of erythropoietin in a variety of oncology settings with small samples of predominantly adult patients (Rizzo et al. 2002). Before embarking on a trial of erythropoietin in children, it is important to correct other causes of anemia. Healthcare team members should obtain a thorough drug history, consider iron, folate, and B12 deficiency, and assess for occult blood losses (i.e., collection of stool specimens). The use of erythropoietin for children, particularly those with religious objections to blood transfusions, is a treatment option for patients with chemotherapy-associated anemia and a hemoglobin concentration <100 g/L (Rizzo et al. 2002). The recommended starting dose is 150 U/kg subcutaneously three times a week, or 40,000 U subcutaneously per week for a minimum of 4 weeks. If this does not improve the hemoglobin values, the dose is usually escalated to 300 U/kg subcutaneously three times a week, or 60,00 U subcutaneously per week for an additional 4–8 weeks (Rizzo et al. 2008). Injections once a week have been shown to increase the convience and compliance with treatment plans in adult patients. A rise of hemoglobin of at least 1–2 g/L/week has been seen with this dosing regimen. There is no benefit in extending the treatment regimen beyond 6–8 weeks after dose intensification, if there has been no response to more intensive dosing. Once hemoglobin levels rise above 120 g/L, dosing is withheld until hemoglobin levels drift down to bellow 100 g/L (Rizzo et al. 2008).

Darbopoetin at a dose of 2.25 μg/kg weekly or 500 μg every 3 weeks has also been employed in children. Because of the association between darbopoetin and thromboembolic events, the current recommendations are for use in children with chemotherapy-associated anemia and low-risk myelodysplasia. Risk factors such as previous history of thrombosis, surgery, prolonged periods of immobility, or limited activity, all preclude the use of darbopoetin in these patient groups (Rizzo et al. 2008).

Nurses will need to assess the family's learning needs with regard to acquiring the skills necessary to administer subcutaneous injections. Involvement of community nurses is often necessary to support families as they develop these new skills.

19.3 Neutropenia

19.3.1 Incidence and Etiology

Leukopenia is a decrease in the absolute number of WBCs, whereas neutropenia is a decrease in the number of neutrophils that fight infection. Neutropenia is a feature of hematological and malignant diseases and arises secondary to immunological disorders, infectious diseases, and drugs. Neutrophil levels are lower in some ethnic groups including Africans, African-Americans, and Yemenite Jews (Dale 2003). The relative risk of infection is determined by the absolute neutrophil count (ANC), calculated as total WBC count × neutrophils (% polys + % bands). Children with severe neutropenia, ANC $<0.5 \times 10^9$/L, are at risk for life-threatening infections that may be bacterial, fungal, or viral (Panzarella et al. 2002).

Although bacteria account for most infections in immunocompromised children, prophylactic strategies to combat all types of infections are important.

Measures such as careful handwashing before and after patient contact, vigilance in detecting potentially transmissible diseases (respiratory viruses, varicella zoster), and knowledge about the specific susceptibilities of the immunocompromised host are all important when caring for neutropenic children (Koh and Pizzo 2003).

19.3.1.1 Fever (Pyrexia) and Neutropenia

Fever in the neutropenic child must always be treated as an emergency, and therapy must be initiated promptly. Fever is regularly defined as temperature >38°C orally. There is a risk of morbidity with febrile neutropenia, and 10–20% of febrile neutropenic children have bacteremia on presentation. Patients who have received a bone marrow transplant within the previous 12 months should be considered neutropenic, regardless of full/complete blood count (FBC/CBC) result (Steele 2003). Some commonly associated infectious problems are listed in Table 19.2 (Koh and Pizzo 2003; Walsh et al. 2006).

19.3.2 Treatment

The management of a patient with fever and neutropenia should include the following guidelines:

- Instruct parents to monitor temperature and have a thermometer at home.
- Teach parents to understand their child's ANC and be aware of current ANC levels.
- Instruct families not to give antipyretics for fever unless instructed by the treating team.
- Instruct families to seek medical attention in the event of fever.
- Maintain ABCs if cardiorespiratory instability is present.
- Take a thorough history and carry out a physical examination with special attention to
  - Mucosa and perioral areas
  - Skin and indwelling catheters
  - Lungs
  - Perirectal areas
  - Any subtle sign of inflammation on the body
- Draw CBC and differential.

Table 19.2. Studies identifying "high- and low-risk" patients with febrile neutropenia

Reference	Type of study	Finding
Talcott et al. 1988	Retrospective review evaluating risk factors for serious medical complications/death during episodes of fever and neutropenia (F and N) in adults	"High risk" group were defined as those who were inpatients at time of diagnosis with F and N, and those as outpatients who had either co-morbid issues or uncontrolled cancer "Low risk" group were those outpatients without either comorbidities or uncontrolled cancers
Klastersky et al. 2000	Multinational Association for Supportive Care in Cancer developed a validated scoring system for identification of febrile neutropenic patients who were at low risk for infectious complications	Predictive factors for low risk of infectious complications included: absence of symptoms or mild/moderate symptoms, absence of hypotension, absence of chronic obstructive pulmonary disease, presence of solid tumor, absence of previous fungal infections, absence of dehydration, and age <60
Rackoff et al. 1996	Retrospective review focusing on the risk of bacteremias in pediatric oncology patients	Risk of bacteremia was associated with fever >39°C and an absolute monocyte count of less than 0.1×10^9/L at presentation of fever
Klassen et al. 2000	Prospective pediatric oncology patients	Children with presenting monocyte count of $>0.1 \times 10^9$/L and who had no comorbidity or an abnormal chest X-ray, were at low risk for significant bacterial infections
Freifeld et al. 1999	Prospective, double-blind study	In hospital therapy with either IV or oral antibiotic regimen, patients with low risk F and N demonstrated that the oral regimen was safe and effective

- Draw blood cultures from periphery, and culture any indwelling catheter from each lumen of the catheter. If the child has an Ommaya reservoir and fever, obtain cerebrospinal fluid for cultures.
- If ANC >500, treat with appropriate antibiotics if any infectious source is identified from history and physical examination.
- If ANC <500, promptly start broad-spectrum antibiotics. If the child has an indwelling catheter, rotate the administration of antibiotics through each lumen.
- Monitor the child closely for secondary infections requiring modification of initial therapy; obtain cultures daily as long as the child is febrile and if newly febrile. If the child has a positive blood culture, cultures should be repeated daily until results are negative.
- Avoid rectal temperatures, enemas, and suppositories while the patient is profoundly neutropenic (Steele 2003; Kline 2002; Koh and Pizzo 2003; Panzarella et al. 2002; Walsh et al. 2006).

19.3.2.1 Antibiotic Management

The standard approach to managing febrile neutropenia has been a combination antibiotic regimen. Practitioners should be aware of local bacterial sceptibilities and their institution's guidelines regarding appropriate drug coverage, toxicities of therapies, and cost differences. The first regimens with acceptable efficacy included aminoglycoside/alpha-lactam combinations. However, the advent of broad-spectrum alpha-lactam antibiotics with a wide spectrum of bactericidal activity have made monotherapies another option for treating febrile neutropenic children. Third-generation cephalosporins (ceftazidime) and carbapenems (imipenem) have excellent activity against *Pneumocystis aeruginosa,* and are also effective for the initial management of febrile children (Hughes et al. 2002). An example of an antibiotic regimen for febrile neutropenic children is as follows:

- Broad-spectrum coverage: piperacillin/tazobactam 80 mg/kg/dose intravenously (IV) every 8 h (maximum 4-g single dose) and gentamicin 2.5 mg/kg/dose IV every 8 h (maximum 20 mg/dose before serum monitoring).
- Children with piperacillin allergy have a limited choice of antibiotics for treatment of fever, and may require consultation with a specialist in infectious diseases.
  - As there is an incidence of cross-reactivity between penicillins and cephalosporins, one treatment regimen comprises ciprofloxacin 10 mg/kg/dose IV every 12 h (maximum 400 mg/dose) and tobramycin and clindamycin 8 mg/kg/dose every 8 h (maximum 600 mg/dose).
- Antibiotics specifically directed toward identified organisms should be added to broad-spectrum coverage, but broad-spectrum coverage should not be replaced by specific antibiotics alone in neutropenic patients.
- Antibiotic therapeutic drug-level monitoring should be done as appropriate, especially if the child is receiving other concurrent nephrotoxic drugs (amphotericin, acyclovir); follow renal function closely.
- Children who deteriorate clinically should be switched to meropenem 20 mg/kg/dose IV (maximum 1 g/dose) and tobramycin and vancomycin 15 mg/kg/dose IV every 6 h (maximum 1 g/dose).
- Persistent fever or recurrent fever without other signs of clinical deterioration is not a reason to change the initial broad-spectrum therapy.
- Consider adding amphotericin after 5–7 days of persistent fever after a fungal work-up has been initiated (sinus, chest, and abdominal CT scan).
- Duration of therapy:
  - Afebrile, ANC >500, cultures negative at 48 h: discontinue antibiotics
  - Afebrile, ANC <500, cultures negative at 48 h, IV antibiotics >48 h: consider discontinuing antibiotics
  - Afebrile, ANC >500, cultures positive: consider discontinuing broad-spectrum antibiotics but continue with specific therapy
- Discharge management:
  - No antibiotic therapy is recommended on discharge for those who meet the following criteria:
    1. Negative blood cultures
    2. Afebrile for a minimum of 24 h
    3. Fever no longer than 96 h
    4. Clinically well
    5. Evidence of marrow recovery with increasing monocytes, neutrophils, or platelet count

- Avoid routine use of oral antibiotics when discharging children, unless there is a localized site of infection that may require specific therapy
- Those who should remain in the hospital for IV therapy include:
  1. Children on induction therapy for malignancy known to significantly involve the bone marrow.
  2. Those with known or suspected noncompliance.
  3. Those with clinical sepsis at presentation.
- Encourage families to strictly adhere to follow-up.
- Recurrence of fever should be approached as a new fever in neutropenic hosts, and requires immediate reevaluation (Steele 2003).

Traditionally, febrile neutropenia in pediatric oncology patients has been managed aggressively with hospitalization and IV antibiotics. More recent literature suggests that less intensive, outpatient interventions may be effective for selected groups of children considered "low risk" of developing infectious complications during febrile neutropenia. Table 19.3 includes a sample of recent sudies with relevant clinical findings. Before embarking on an institutional policy switch in care of febrile neutropenic children, each institution must identify and validate criteria for the "low risk" child (Walsh et al. 2006). Nurses can play a vital role in providing some of the necessary supportive care infrastructure to implement an oral outpatient regimen for "low risk" children. Nurses often are the first link in the telephone triage network established for families to report febrile illnesses. They are also often the consistent healthcare

Table 19.3. Commonent problems associated with fever and neutropenia

Source of the problem	Common infectious problem	Predominant organisms
Central venous devices	Bacteremia	Gram-positive (coagulase-negative staphylococci) and enteric bacteria. *Corynebacterium jelkelum* Gram-negative
	Candidemia	*C. albicans*, most common, followed by *Candida glabrata* and *Candida tropicalis*
	Localized infections including exit sites, pocket space abscesses, pocket space cellulites, and tunnel infections	Gram-positive cocci and gram-negative bacilli including *Pseudomonas* spp., and *Mycobacterium* spp.
CNS shunts, Ommaya reservoirs	Pathogens colonized from adjacent skin	Coagulase-negative and coagulase-positive staphylococci, *Corynebacterium* spp., and *Propionibacterium acnes*
Skin or mucosa	Localized skin infections	Bacteremias associated with *P. aeruginosa*, *S. maltophilia*, *Aeromonas hydrophilia*, and *Bacillus* spp.; fungemia associated with *Aspergillus* spp., *Candida* spp., *Trichosporon* spp., and *C. neoformans*; or viremia such as HSV, VZV, and CMV
	Mucositis, esophagitis	Bacterial, viral, and fungal pathogens
	Bacteremia	α-hemolytic streptococci, gram-positive and gram-negative bacteria
	Enterocolitis	*Clostridium difficile*
Neutropenia	Bacteremia, sepsis	Coagulase-negative staphylococci, *Staph. aureus*, α-hemolytic streptococci, enterococci, *Bacillus* spp., *Escherichia coli*, *Klebsiella* spp., *Pseudomonas* spp., *Enterobacter* spp., *Citrobacter*, *Serratia*, *Acinetobacter* spp., *Clostridium* spp.
	Localized fungal infections	*C. albicans*, *Aspergillus* spp., Mucor
	Fungemia	*Candida* spp.

team member who reviews compliance with oral antibiotic therapies and provides education to families with regard to transportation and emergency access of the medical system.

19.3.2.2 Special Consideration for the Management of Indwelling Intravenous Catheters

With the increased usage of indwelling venous devises, there has been a rise in catheter-associated bacteremic episodes. It is often hard to distinguish catherter-related vs. non-catheter-related bacteremias. Positive line cultures drawn from a central venous catheter can arise from one of three sources: infection from the line from external sources (skin or cathether hub), seeding of the catheter from internal sources via the blood stream, and contaminated infusions running through the line (platelets or blood contaminated with bacteria). In the past, clinicians have utilized comparisons between peripheral and central blood cultures in an attempt to differentiate the source of infection. As pheripheral blood cultures are painful, are often associated with contamination from normal skin flora, and often do not contribute to increased diagnositic yield of bacteremias, many centres have abandoned their use (Walsh et al. 2006). Nurses need to be aware of institutional policies with regard to timing and blood volume draws when obtaining blood cultures from central venous catheters. The volume of blood drawn is of vital importance for the recovery of bacteria from bloodstream infections and some institutions have suggested volumes based on the weight of the child (i.e., >30 kg child, draw total of 20 mL of blood from all sites) (Walsh et al. 2006).

Gram-positive bacterial infections, especially staphylococci, are the most frequent cause of catheter-related infection (Koh and Pizzo 2003). It is important to culture all lumina of an intravascular device and to administer antibiotic therapy through all lumina as well. Most simple catheter-related bacteremia and exit-site infections can be cleared by appropriate antibiotic therapy and do not require removal of the device. However, should bacteremia persist after 48 h of appropriate therapy or if the child shows signs of a tunnel infection, consideration should be given to removing the device. Failure of therapy is most common when infections are due to organisms such as *Candida albicans* and *Bacillus* species (Koh and Pizzo 2003).

19.3.2.3 Management of Candidiasis (Oropharyngeal Candidiasis and Candida Esophagitis)

Canadida albicans is present on the skin, mouth, intestinal tract, and vagina of immunocompetent children. Invasive diseases can occur in immunocompromised children and arise from endogenous colonizated sites. Neutropenic children, children on treatment with corticosteroids or cytotoxic chemotherapy are at increased risk for the development of invasive infections. The incubation period of these infections is unknown (American Academy of Pediatrics 2006). These children are particulariy prone to developing oropharyngeal or esophageal candidiasis, or thrush (Koh and Pizzo 2003). Thorough mouth care can be a challenge in the pediatric population; hence, use of soft toothbrushes and frequent mouth rinses are encouraged, along with inspection of the oral cavity for signs of infection. Creamy white patches on the mucosal surfaces, which may be friable and bleed easily when scratched, are typical for thrush. It can be hard to distinguish between mucositis caused by chemotherapy and *C. albicans. C. albicans* causes most of the infections (50–60%) (American Academy of Pediatrics 2006).

Antifungal agents for the treatment of oropharyngeal or esophageal candidiasis include oral nonabsorbent agents such as nystatin or clotrimazole; oral systemic absorbable agents such as ketoconazole, itraconazole, and fluconazole; and IV fluconazole or amphotericin B (Koh and Pizzo 2003). Data on the use of IV capofungin, microfungin, and anidulafungin in children is limitted at this time. IV agents are often used when the neutropenic child is unable to swallow. Amphotericin B is administered for a minimum of 5 days in the neutropenic child, and preferably until neutropenia is resolved. Prophylaxis is not recommended routinely for immunocompromised children; however, there is emerging data on the use of fluconazole prophylaxis for children undergoing allogenic strem cell transplantation, which show significant decrease in the number of candida infections (American Academy of Pediatrics 2006).

19.3.2.4 Infections Due to *Aspergillus* Species

Invasive aspergillosis occurs almost exclusively in immunocompromised children with prolonged neutropenia induced by cytotoxic chemotherapy. These infections usually involve pulmonary, sinus, cerebral, or cutaneous sites. The hallmark of invasive aspergillosis is angioinvasion with resulting thrombosis, dissemination to other organs, and occasionally, erosion of the blood vessel wall with hemorrhage (American Academy of Pediatrics 2006). *Aspergillus* species are ubiquitous molds that grow on decaying vegetation and in the soil. The principle route of transmission is by inhalation of the conidia spores, and nosocomial outbreaks can occur in susceptible hosts where exposure to a probable source of fungus has occurred, such as a nearby construction site or faulty ventilation. The incubation period is unknown. *Aspergillus* is diagnosed from biopsy specimens of a variety of body tissues and is rarely diagnosed from the blood (American Academy of Pediatrics 2006).

The treatment of choice for invasive infections is IV voriconazole or amphotericin B in high doses (1.0–1.5 mg/kg/day). Therapy is continued for 4–12 weeks or longer. Lipid formulations of amphotericin B should be considered in children who cannot tolerate conventional amphotericin B due to renal toxicities or severe reaction. Voriconazole is metabolized in a linear fashion in children, and hence, the recommended adult dosing may be too low. Optimal pediatric dosing is not yet known. Caspofungin has also been shown to have a good response for invasive aspergillosis. The pharmokinetics of dosing is different in chldren and is now being dosed on a body-surface area dosing scheme. Itraconazole by mouth has many drug interactions and is more poorly absorbed. Currently, the safety and efficacy of voriconazole, itraconozole, and caspofungin in children is being studied (American Academy of Pediatrics 2006).

19.3.2.5 Management of Viral Infections

Herpes simplex, varicella-zoster, and CMV are the most commonly occurring viral infections in immunocompromised children. Table 19.4 outlines the clinical manifestations, etiology, diagnostic tests, and treatments for these viral diseases.

19.3.2.6 Infections Due to *Pneumocystis jiroveci* (Formerly *Pneumocystis carinii*)

Pulmonary infections with *Pneumocystis jiroveci* have in the past been a major problem in children with malignancies (Koh and Pizzo 2003). Infants and children develop a characteristic diffuse pneumonitis with dyspnea at rest, tachypnea, oxygen desaturation, nonproductive cough, and fever. Intensity of symptoms may vary, and in some immunocompromised children, the onset can be acute and fulminant. Chest X-rays often show bilateral diffuse interstitial or alveolar disease. The mortality rate in immunocompromised children ranges from 5 to 40% if treated, and approaches 100% if untreated (American Academy of Pediatrics 2006). Diagnostic tests in children include bronchoscopy with broncheoalveolar lavage, sputum samples in older children, intubation with deep endotracheal aspiration, and open lung or transbronchial biopsies. A definitive diagnosis of PCP is made by positive findings in tissues or secretions. Polymerase chain reaction (PCR) assays for detection of *P. jiroveci* are currently experimental. The incubation period is unknown, but is thought to be 4–8 weeks from exposure to clinical symptoms.

The drug of choice for treatment is IV trimethoprim-sulfamethoxazole (trimethoprim 15–20 mg/kg/day and sulfamethoxazole 75–100 mg/kg/daily every 6 h). IV pentamidine (4 mg/kg/day once daily) is an alternative for children who cannot tolerate or do not respond to trimethoprim–sulfamethoxazole. Atovaquone, clindamycin with primaquine, dapsone with trimethoprim, and trimetrexate with leukovorin have also been administered orally in adults with mild infections. However, experience on their usages in children is limited (American Academy of Pediatrics 2006).

Prophylaxis for *Pneumocystis* in children with significant immunocompromise includes:

Table 19.4. Typical viral infections and suggested management (data from American Academy of Pediatrics 2006; Walsh et al. 2006)

Viral infection	Clinical manifestations	Etiology	Diagnostic tests	Treatments
Herpes simplex (HSV)	Severe local lesions, disseminated HSV infection with generalized vesicular skin lesions and visceral involvement; incubation period 2 days to 2 weeks	Double-stranded DNA virus, transmitted from people who are symptomatic or asymptomatic through direct contact with infected lesions or secretions;covering affected areas can prevent spread; HSV-1 usually involves face and skin above the waist; HSV-2 involves genitalia and skin below the waist	Readily grown in culture obtained from skin vesicles, mouth, or nasopharynx, eyes, urine, blood, or stool; PCR assays are also a sensitive method of detection, especially valuable in CSF specimens	IV acyclovir for treatment and prevention of mucocutaneous infections; topical acyclovir may also accelerate healing; contact precautions are advised; oral valacyclovir, famciclovir, and penciclovir have been used in adults following IV acyclovir, but usage has not yet been approved for children
Varicella-Zoster	Generalized, pruritic, vesicular rash with mild fever; progressive severe varicella with encephalitis, hepatitis; pneumonia can develop; incidence of pneumonitis is up to 30% with mortality in nearly1/3 of these children; incubation period is 10–21 days after contact; may be prolonged to 28 days after receipt of VZIG or IVIG	Member of herpes virus family; highly contagious and spread through contact with mucosa of the upper respiratory tract; person-to-person transmission by airborne spread from respiratory secretions	Vesicular scraping and fluid from lesions: readily detected by viral DNA and PCR assays	IV antiviral therapy with acyclovir within24 h or onset of rash (dose 80 mg/kg/day divided into four doses for 7 days); selected low-risk patients receiving high-dose oral acyclovir; utilize standard airborne and contact isolation precautions; post exposure immunization of VZIG within 96 h; dose 125 U/10 kg body wt to a maximum of 625 units IM
Cytomegalovirus (CMV)	Interstitial pneumonitis, gastrointestinal infections such as mouth sores, esophagitis, colitis, and retinitis; incubation period is unknown	Transmitted by person-to-person contact with secretions and via transfusions of blood, platelets, and WBCs from previously infected people; virus persists in latent form after primary infection and reactivates particularly under conditions of immunosuppression	Development of serum immunoglobulin IgM CMV-specific antibody; virus can also be isolated in cell cultures from areas of CMV infection (urine, pharnyx, peripheral blood, and other tissues); detection by vora, DNA and PCR assays	Ganciclovir and CMV-immune globulin IV has been used to treat retinitis caused by CMV infections; foscarnet is more toxic but may be used in ganciclovir-resistant infections; oral valganciclovir has replaced oral ganciclovir in usage in children; cidofovir has been used in adults but not yet been fully studied in children; good hand hygiene for prevention of spread – CMV antibody-negative donor blood and platelets, removal of buffy coat or filtration to remove WBCs

- Trimethoprim–sulfamethoxazole (trimethoprim 150 mg/m^2/day, sulfamethoxazole 750 mg/m^2/day) administered orally in divided doses twice a day, 3 times a week on consecutive days
- Alternatives include the following:
  - Trimethoprim 150 mg/m^2/day, sulfamethoxazole 750 mg/m^2/day orally as a single daily dose, 3 times a week on consecutive days
  - Trimethoprim 150 mg/m^2/day, sulfamethoxazole 750 mg/m^2/day orally in divided doses, 7 days a week
- Alternative regimens if trimethoprim–sulfamethoxazole is not tolerated include:
  - Dapsone (children ≥1 month of age) 2 mg/kg orally once a day or 4 mg/kg (maximum 200 mg) orally every week
  - Aerosolized pentamidine (children ≥5 years of age, who are capable of following instructions and utilizing a nebulizer) 300 mg administered via inhaler monthly
  - Atovaquone (children 1–3 months and >24 months of age) 30 mg/kg orally, once a day; and 45 mg/kg orally (children 4–24 months of age), once a day (American Academy of Pediatrics 2006)

19.3.2.7 Use of Colony Stimulating Factors in Children with Neutropenia

Most children treated for cancer are treated on clinical research protocols. Chemotherapy for pediatric patients tends to be more intensive, and myelosuppression is more frequent and severe in the pediatric population. Infants receiving chemotherapy are at a particular risk for neutropenic morbidity because of the immaturity of their hematopoietic and immune systems. These factors combine to increase the incidence of febrile neutropenia in children and the potential for life-threatening infections. The use of colony stimulating factors (CSFs) in the pediatric population is largely determined by the requirements of research protocols (Ozer et al. 2000). A review of practices by the Pediatric Oncology Group (Parsons et al. 2000) revealed that:

- Primary prophylaxis with CSFs is common and guided by the anticipated duration of neutropenia (>7 days).
- Primary prophylaxis is not uniform across protocols or diseases.
- Practices are influenced by the physician's preference.
- Reduction in chemotherapy dosage is rarely selected as an alternative to the use of CSFs.
- The majority of pediatric oncologists use CSFs in children who have complicated illnesses with frequent febrile neutropenia; however, they do not use CSFs in uncomplicated fever and neutropenia.
- CSF doses are 5 µg/kg/day for G-CSF (filgrastim) and 250 µg/m^2 for GM-CSF (sargramostim) subcutaneously.

Several recent reviews have been completed to examine the utility of CSFs in the treatment of children receiving myleosuppresive chemotherapy. Sung et al. (2004) conducted a meta-analysis of randomized controlled trials in the prophylactic use of CSFs to decrease febrile neutropnia in children undergoing cancer chemotherapy treatments. The authors of this meta-anylsis concluded that CSFs were associated with a 20% reduction in the incidence of febrile neutopenia and in shorter duration of hospitalization. There was however, no reduction in infection-related mortality with CSF usage (Sung et al. 2004). In a Cochrane review of CSFs for the prevention of myelosuppressive threapy-induced febrile neutropenia in children with acute lymphoblastic leukemia (ALL), published in 2005, the authors concluded that children with ALL do benefit from shorter hospitalization and fewer infections if a regimen of CSF were utilized. There was, however, no evidence for a shortened duration of neutropenia episodes, fewer treatment delays, and no useful information with regard to changes in survival. This review concluded that the role of CSFs is still uncertain and further more rigorous studies are needed (Sasse et al. 2005). A meta-anaylysis of randomized controlled trials in children receiving prophylactic CSFs during myelosuppressive chemotherapy regimens by Wittman et al. (2006) concluded that prophylactic CSFs significantly decreased the incidence of febrile neutropenia and the duration of severe neutropenia, hospitalization, and antibiotic use in children, but did not significantly decrease the number of documented infections (Wittman et al. 2006). CSFs continue to be part of most pediatric cancer treatment protocols. Nurses play a pivotal role in coordinating care and teaching with regard to administration of CSFs, both within the hospital and in outpatient management of neutropenic children.

19.3.2.8 Isolation

Reverse isolation (i.e., placing the patient in a single room and requiring healthcare personnel to wear gowns, masks, and gloves) after the onset of neutropenia will not necessarily prevent infection. This is because most of the organisms that infect patients arise from the patient's endogenous flora. However, the use of total protective environments can reduce infection in the profoundly neutropenic child, such as one who has just received a bone marrow transplant (Koh and Pizzo 2003). These protective measures include the use of a high-efficiency particulate air (HEPA)-filtered laminar air flow room, an aggressive program of surface cleaning, use of sterile objects within the patient's room, and a bacterially reduced diet (no fresh fruits or vegetables, no fast foods or restaurant foods, and use of completely and thoroughly cooked foods).

The most efficacious and practical intervention that can be performed to decrease the aquisition of potential pathogens in pediatric cancer patients is adherence to strict handwashing rountines (Walsh et al. 2006). Nurses play a pivotal role in educating children and parents about the importance of handwashing both within the hospital environment and at home. Families should be taught and should practice the simple rule that no one should have contact with a child undergoing cancer treatment who does not first wash his or her hands.

19.4 Thrombocytopenia

19.4.1 Incidence and Etiology

Thrombocytopenia in children is usually due to myelosuppression from chemotherapy or malignancy. The risk of spontaneous hemorrhage increases when platelets fall below 10×10^9/L (Steele 2003).

19.4.2 Treatment

Prophylactic platelet transfusions are administered to children with thrombocytopenia resulting from impaired bone marrow function to reduce the risk of hemorrhage when platelets fall below a predefined level, such as 10×10^9/L. Several recent studies have demonstrated that the risk for spontaneous life-threatening hemorrage does not occur until the platelet count falls bellow 5×10^9/L (Sloan et al. 2009). The threshold for platelet transfusion can vary according to the child's diagnosis, clinical condition, and treatment modality. Platelets for transfusion can be prepared either by separation of units of platelet concentrations from whole blood, which is pooled before administration, or by aphaeresis from single donors. Studies have shown that the post transfusion increments, hemostatic benefits, and side effects are similar with either product. In most centers, pooled platelets are less expensive to obtain (Schiffer et al. 2003). Single-donor platelets from selected donors are reserved for histocompatible platelet transfusions (see Sect. 19.5.4). Transfusions may be necessary at higher levels in

- Newborns.
- Patients with signs of hemorrhage, high fever, hyperleukocytosis, rapid fall of platelet count, anticoagulant use, or coagulation abnormalities.
- Patients undergoing invasive procedures – ensure that the platelet count is greater than 50×10^9/L for minimally invasive procedures such as lumbar puncture and 80–100×10^9/L for surgery (Schiffer et al. 2003). A recent series of 956 consecutive paediatric patients newly diagnosed with ALL who underwent lumbar punctures, concluded that prophylactic platelets were unnecessary unless platelet counts fell bellow 10×10^9/L (Howard et al. 2000).

When platelet transfusion is necessary, 1 U/5–10 kg of pooled platelets to a maximum of 5–6 U is normally prescribed. Platelets are administered through a blood transfusion set with a standard blood filter. Infusions should be administered as rapidly as the child can tolerate, with the careful monitoring of vital sign before, during, and after transfusion. There is limitted evidence in the literature to determine the appropriate dose for platelet transfusions. Higher doses of platelets have been used historically; however, there is no evidence to suggest that these higher doses are more effective in the prevention or treatment of bleeding. Studies are needed to determine the optimum dosing of platelets by examining the effectiveness of dosing regimens with regard to total platelet utilization and donor exposure (Tinmouth 2007). A repeat platelet dose may be required in 1–3 days because of the short lifespan of transfused platelets of only 3–4 days (Chambers et al. 2007).

Patient safety should be ensured when platelets are low. Instruction should include avoiding activities that can cause injury when platelet counts fall below 50×10^9: cleaning teeth with a soft toothbrush, wearing protective equipment such as a bike helmet, and avoiding contact sports, diving, horseback riding, and other activities that could potentially lead to serious injury. Families should be educated about the proper method to stop nosebleeds or other profuse bleeding. Maintaining soft stools and avoiding rectal temperatures, enemas, or suppositories when platelet counts are low can prevent perirectal injury. Advice should include avoiding over-the-counter medications containing ibuprofen or aspirin, as well as Pepto-Bismol and Alka-Seltzer (Panzarella et al. 2002).

Nursing care during platelet transfusions includes the following:

- Being vigilant to the child's need for platelet infusion, assessing for increasing bruising and bleeding.
- Communicating with healthcare team members about pertinent laboratory values and the needs for infusion.
- Vital signs should be recorded before, during, and after infusions.
- Monitoring the child for infusion reactions and administering necessary premedications with subsequent infusions.

19.5 Transfusion Issues

19.5.1 Granulocyte Transfusions

In the 1970s and 1980s, several studies investigated the use of granulocyte transfusions in neutropenic patients. A comprehensive review by Strauss (1994) demonstrated that there is no benefit in the prophylactic administration of granulocyte transfusions. Interest in the use of granulocyte transfusions has decreased due to the following reasons:

- Granulocyte preparations are difficult to prepare and cannot be stored.
- Infusions have been associated with severe pulmonary reactions, especially in patients concurrently receiving amphotericin B.
- Survival from septic episodes is much improved with early introduction of antibiotic treatment and the availability of better antibiotics.
- Use of granulocyte stimulating factors (GSFs) to prevent prolonged periods of neutropenia (Hume 1999). Currently, granulocyte transfusions are reserved for patients with profound neutropenia, who are not expected to recover, in whom severe bacterial infection has been documented, and who are clinically deteriorating despite optimal antibiotic therapies (Strauss 1994).

A recent Cochrane review of eight parallel randomized control trials, which included 310 patient episodes revealed that there are many different policies and schedules for transfusion, methods of granulocyte procument, and processes for donor selection. Each study utilized different criteria for neutropenia and different definitions for the seriousness of the infection requiring treatment. The review found that granulocyte infusions of over one million cells may reduce deaths in patients; however, large-sized trials need to be undertaken to evaluate the effectivess and define the optimal patient selection and infusion schedules (Stanworth et al. 2005).

19.5.1.1 Transfusion-Related Acute Lung Injury

The etiology of transfusion-related acute lung injury (TRALI) is presently not fully defined. There are two postulated mechanisms that have been implicated:

- A passive transfer of human leukocyte antigen (HLA) or granulocyte antibodies from donor to blood-product recipient, or HLA or granulocyte

antibodies in the recipient (antibodies are detected in donor or recipient in 75% of the cases).
- Biologically active lipids in the transfused component.

Acute lung injury (ALI) is defined by acute onset, hypoxemia (as evidenced by oxygen saturation of less than 90% in the room), bilateral lung infiltrates on the chest X-ray, and no evidence of circulatory overload. In patients with no evidence of ALI prior to blood transfusion, TRALI is diagnosed if new ALI is present and this occurs during or within 6 h of the completion of a transfusion. The true incidence of this sydrome is unknown; however, it is estimated at 1 in 1,200–5,000 plasma-containing transfusions (Callum and Pinkerton 2007). TRALI is thought to be underdiagnosed and under reported.

TRALI presents with dyspnea, hypoxemia, fever, and hypotension. Chest X-ray reveals interstitial and alveolar infiltrates without elevated pulmonary pressures. It usually occurs with transfusion of RBCs, platelets, and plasma, but it can also, on rare occasions, occur with other bood products such as cryopercipitate and IVIG. It almost always occurs within the first 1–2 h after the start of a trasfusion and usually resolves within 24–72 h. Over 70% of reported cases of TRALI require mechanical ventilation, and death can occur in 5–10% of patients experiencing a TRALI reaction (TRALI is currently thought to be the most common cause of transfusion-associated fatality). Milder forms of TRALI are thought to exist and may present as transient hypoxia with or after transfusion (Callum and Pinkerton 2007).

The management for a child experiencing TRALI is supportive in nature, including diuretics, steriods, and mechanical ventilation. Accurate reporting to transfusion services is critical to identify implicated donors and prevent TRALI in other recipients. Nurses need to be aware of this newly emerging transfusion-related injury and report TRALI-type symptoms to team members and transfusion services according to institutional guidelines.

19.5.2 Transfusion-Associated Graft vs. Host Disease

Graft vs. host disease (GvHD), which results from the engraftment of immunocompetent donor T-lymphocytes into a recipient whose immune system is unable to reject them, is a recognized risk of blood transfusions. Donor lymphocytes engraft, proliferate, and mount an immunologic attack against recipient tissues. Almost all cellular blood components have been implicated in reported cases of transfusion-associated (TA)-GvHD. The threshold of the number of viable cells necessary to produce a GvHD reaction will vary depending upon the host's immune status as well as the antigenic similarity or disparity between donor and host histocompatibility antigens (Callum and Pinkerton 2007).

GvHD following blood transfusions generally manifests as an acute syndrome, the onset typically occurring within 4–30 days of transfusion. The initial clinical symptoms include a high fever occurring 8–10 days after the transfusion, appearance of a central maculopapular rash following the fever within 24–48 h, the rash's spread to the extremities, and in severe cases, the rash's progression to a generalized desquamation and pancytopenia 19 days post transfusion (Callum and Pinkerton 2007). Diagnosis of TA-GvHD is usually based on the clinical presentation and histological findings on skin biopsy, liver bilopsy, and bone marrow examination. TA-GvHD has been reported in children with hematological malignancies and solid tumors, who have received cytotoxic chemotherapy, radiation treatment, or both. Overwhelming infections are the most common cause of death and mortality in more than 90% if GvHD occurs (Callum and Pinkerton 2007).

As the treatment of TA-GvHD is almost always ineffective, efforts have focused on preventing and minimizing the risks by reducing or inactivating transfused donor lymphocytes. The methods available in blood banks to physically remove T-lymphocytes include washing or filtering blood products (Sloan et al. 2003). Current leukocyte reduction filters can achieve a three-log reduction in the leukocyte contents of blood components. This reduction is not sufficient to prevent TA-GvHD. Inactivation of transfused lymphocytes by alpha-irradiation of the blood components remains the most effective method for prevention of TA-GvHD. Irradiation decreases the number of viable lymphocytes in the blood product by direct damage to the nuclear DNA and/or by the generation of free radicals that cause cell damage.

The current dose of irradiation is 25 Gy, and the effects of this dose on platelet and other cell viability are not clinically significant (Sloan et al. 2003).

19.5.3 Cytomegalovirus and Transfusions

CMV belongs to the herpes family and is harbored in the lymphocytes. About 30–70% of the blood donors are CMV-seropositive, although there can be a great deal of regional differences due to donor demographics, such as age, sex, race, and socioeconomic status (Chambers et al. 2007). Primary infections occur in a seronegative recipient of blood products from a donor who is actively or latently infected. There is a wide clinical spectrum associated with post transfusion CMV. CMV infections may be asymptomatic and discovered by serologic tests, or they may produce significant morbidity and mortality (Sloan et al. 2003).

19.5.3.1 Treatment

The use of IgG-seronegative blood products is considered to be the gold standard. The availability of these products, however, is dependent upon the characteristics of the donor pool and may not be available in some areas. As the virus is carried in WBCs, manipulation that can reduce or attenuate leukocyte cell numbers should reduce the risk of transmission. These methods include washing, freezing followed by washing, and filtration with third-generation leukocyte-depletion filters (Tinmouth 2007). Recommendations based on the American Association of Blood Banks (1997, Bulletin 97–92) are included in Table 19.5.

19.5.4 Platelet Refractoriness

A major complication in the management of thrombocytopenia is platelet refractoriness. Refractoriness can be due to immune (presence in the recipient of HLA- or platelet-specific alloantibodies) or nonimmune causes (fever, infections, drugs including amphotericin B, vancomycin, or ciprofloxacillin, splenomegaly, disseminated intravascular coagulation, and bone marrow transplant) (Sloan et al. 2003). Alloimmune refractoriness can occur in up to 40% of patients receiving platelet transfusion. In Canada, this risk has been significantly reduced by the universal leukoreduction of all blood components (Tinmouth 2007).

In patients with poor response to platelet transfusions, measuring the post transfusion platelet count after a platelet transfusion may allow the determination of whether there is an immune or nonimmune cause.

The response to a platelet transfusion, known as the corrected platelet count increment (CCI), is determined by using the following formula.

$$\text{CCI} = \frac{\left[\left(\text{Post transfusion - pretransfusion}\right)\text{ platelet count} \times \text{body surface area}\right]}{\text{Number of platelets transfuse d}\left(\times 10^{11}\right)}$$

In general, a platelet transfusion is considered successful if the CCI is more than $7.5\times(10^9/\text{L})\text{m}^2$ within 10–60 min of a transfusion and more than

Table 19.5. CMV prophylaxis and transfusion therapy (data from Chalmers and Gibson 1999; Hambleton and George 2003)

Type of patient	Clinical circumstance	CMV-seronegative blood	Leukocyte-reduced (LR) blood; CMV unscreened
Patients who receive chemotherapy that produces severe immunosuppression	CMV-positive patient	Not indicated	LR blood to prevent viral reactivation
	CMV-negative patient	Either CMV-negative or LR blood	Either CMV-negative or LR blood
Patients receiving allogeneic or autologous progenitor cell transplants	CVM-positive recipient	Not indicated	LR blood to prevent viral reactivation
	CMV-negative recipient of a CVM-positive donor	Either CMV-negative or LR blood	Either CMV-negative or LR blood

5.0×10^9 if measured 18–24 h after transfusion (Tinmouth 2007). As most centers do not routinely obtain platelet counts of the infused product, a rough estimate of an absolute platelet increment is 3,500/m^2/U for children. Refractoriness to platelet transfusion is defined as a consistently inadequate response to platelet transfusion on two separate transfusions of adequate numbers of platelets.

19.5.4.1 Treatment

Management of a child who is refractory to random donor platelet transfusions includes, first, obtaining ABO-identical platelets for the child and, second, that the platelets should be as fresh as possible. When HLA alloimmunization is the cause of refractoriness, HLA-matched platelets should be used (Sloan et al. 2009).

It is important to note that some children may lose their antibodies over time and can again become responsive to random-donor platelet transfusions. The management of alloimmunized children who do not respond to interventions can be difficult. It is likely to be of no benefit to administer prophylactic platelets, and instead, one should administer platelets only in the presence of clinically significant bleeding (Tinmouth 2007). The administration of IV immunoglobulin may improve post transfusion platelet increments, but does not increase the platelet survival (Sloan et al. 2009).

19.6 Disseminated Intravascular Coagulation

Disseminated intravascular coagulation (DIC) is an acquired coagulopathy that is almost always acute in nature, and describes a disorder that is characterized by diffused fibrin deposition in the microvasculature, consumption of coagulation factors, and endogenous generation of thrombin and plasmin (Monagle and Andrews 2003). It results from disordered regulation of normal coagulation, and is characterized by excess thrombin generation with secondary activation of the fibrinolytic system.

19.6.1 Etiology and Manifestation

Infection is the most common cause of DIC in children. Bacterial infections predominate, but viruses, systemic fungal infections, malaria, and viral hemorrhagic fevers can trigger DIC. Many bacterial agents can trigger a consumptive coagulopathy; however, meningococcal meningitis remains one of the most frequent causes of severe DIC in children (Monagle and Andrews 2003). Table 19.6 outlines the common causes of DIC.

Any of these diverse diseases can lead to pathological activation of the coagulation system via the contact system, which follows endothelial injury, or via the tissue factor pathway following release of tissue factor. Figure 19.1 outlines a simplified pathway of blood coagulation.

Once the coagulation system has been activated and DIC is triggered, the pathophysiology basically remains the same regardless of the underlying etiology. Following activation, both thrombin and plasmin circulate systemically. Thrombin converts fibrinogen to fibrin, which then polymerizes. This is associated with the consumptions of procoagulant proteins and platelets. Fibrin deposits lead to microvascular and sometimes large vessel thrombosis, with impaired perfusion and subsequent organ damage. Coagulation

Table 19.6. Conditions associated with disseminated intravascular coagulation

Infections	Metabolic disorders	Tumors	Others
Bacteremia (meningococcus, streptococcus) Viremia (varicella, CMV) Fungemia	Hypotension Hypoxia Hyper/hypothermia	Tumor lysis syndrome Acute promyelocytic, myelomonocytic, or monocytic leukemias	Liver diseases Intravascular hemolysis (ABO incompatibility)

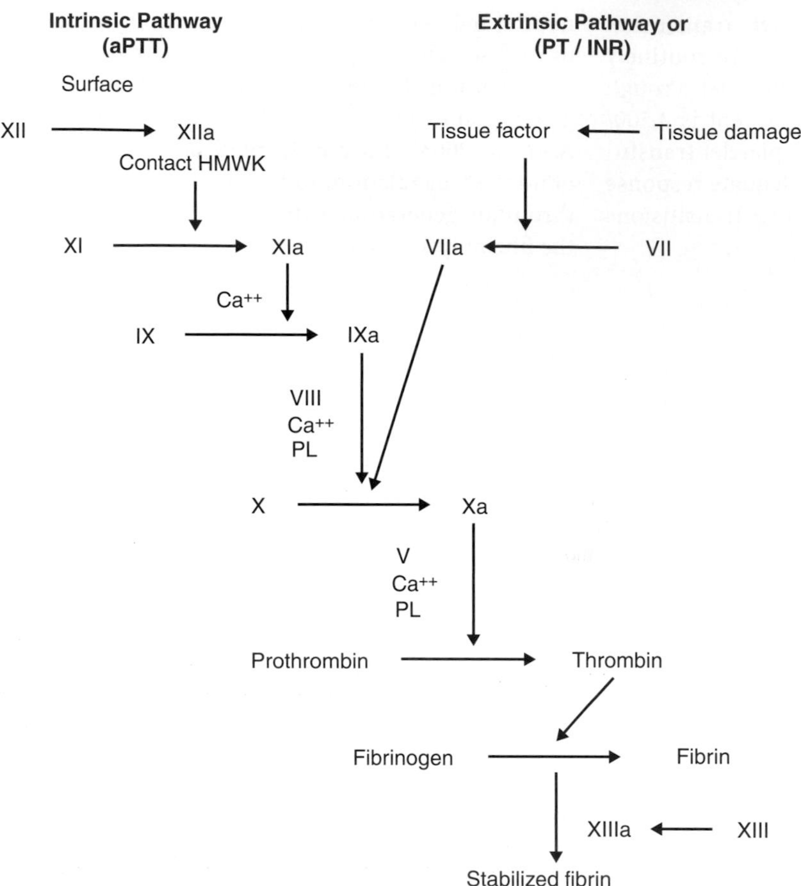

Figure 19.1

The pathway of blood coagulation (data from Shamsah 2003)

inhibitors also become depleted as thrombin continues to be generated. Circulating plasmin results in the generation of fibrin deregulation products, which interfere with fibrin polymerization and platelet function, leading to hemorrhagic problems (Monagle and Andrews 2003).

Hemorrhage is the most obvious manifestation of DIC, although spontaneous bruising, purpura, oozing from venipunctures, and bleeding from surgical wounds or trauma sites are common (Chalmers and Gibson 1999).

19.6.1.1 Diagnosis

The diagnosis of DIC is based on both procoagulant and fibrinolytic activation with concomitant inhibitor consumption (Monagle and Andrews 2003). Fulminant DIC is characterized by prolonged prothrombin time, activated partial thromboplastin time, and thrombin clotting time, combined with thrombocytopenia and increased fibrin regulatory products (Chalmers and Gibson 1999).

19.6.2 Treatment

As DIC is always a secondary phenomenon, the most important aspect of management is treating the underlying cause. Almost all the aspects of DIC management are controversial, and there has been no clear evidence supporting how to best manage this event (Chalmers and Gibson 1999). Blood product replacement is still a major component of most treatment

strategies. The choice of product – fresh frozen plasma (10–15 mg/kg body weight every 8 h), cryoprecipitate, platelets (1 U/5 kg body weight) or fibrinogen concentrate (1 bag/5 kg body weight), and PRBCs as required – the timing of administration, and the efficacy of treatment are still unclear (Shamsah 2003).
Nursing interventions include:

- Monitoring the patient for bleeding (observe skin for color and petechiae, monitoring potential sites of bleeding including mucosa, sclera, esophagus, joints, and intestine) and assessing tissue perfusion.
- Ensuring adequate circulation and oxygenation.
- Evaluating mental status to monitor for intracranial bleeding (Wilson 2002).
- Support the child and family by explaining interventions and providing open and honest answers to questions.

Prognosis has improved over the last 20 years because of advances in supportive care, including improved antibiotics, antifibrinolytic therapy, and platelet transfusions (Monagle and Andrews 2003).

19.7 Septic Shock

Septic shock is a systematic response to pathogenic microorganisms in the blood (Brown 1994). Children who have a compromised immune system from diseases such as human immunodeficiency virus (HIV), asplenia, or cancer chemotherapy have the greatest risk of developing septic shock. Fever is the first symptom of possible sepsis; however, the febrile neutropenic child will frequently not demonstrate clinical symptoms of sepsis until after the initiation of antibiotic therapy (Bruce and Grove 1992).

19.7.1 Etiology

As bacteria die, they release endotoxins into the bloodstream that interfere with the uptake and transportation of oxygen, leading to decreased tissue perfusion, cellular hypoxia, and cell death (Ackerman 1994). Sixty percent of all septic episodes in neutropenic cancer patients are from gram-positive organisms; however, the organisms involved in septic shock are usually gram-negative, and often arise from endogenous flora (Rheingold and Lange 2006). Septic shock can be defined as circulatory dysfunction (or a reduction of 40 mmHg from baseline systolic blood pressure) despite fluid resuscitation, leading to insufficient delivery of oxygen and nutrients to meet tissue needs. Compensated shock occurs when vital organ perfusion is maintained via endogenous compensatory mechanisms, whereas decompensated shock occurs when compensatory mechanisms have failed, and it results in hypotension and impaired tissue perfusion (Metha and MacPhee 2003). Risk factors include age (infants are at greater risk due to decreased production of T-lymphocytes), ANC less than 0.1×10^9/L, prolonged neutropenia, breaks in the integrity of the skin and mucous membranes, invasive devices such as central venous lines and Ommaya reservoirs, malnutrition, and asplenism (Ackerman et al. 1994).

19.7.2 Treatment

Treatment initially focuses on maintaining cardiovascular volume and blood pressure by administering hyperhydration, vasopressors, and blood and coagulation products. Interventions to support the respiratory system include keeping O_2 saturation at more than 90% or PaO_2 at more than 60 mmHg. Hemodynamic support interventions include:

- Isotonic crystalloid (0.9% saline or Ringer's lactate) 20 mL/kg bolus, then assess for response (heart and respiratory rate, capillary refill, sensorium, urine output); may repeat once or twice
- If not simple hypovolemia, consider early use of inotropes such as dopamine or epinephrine
- If hypovolemic and some response to fluids has occurred, consider isotonic colloid (5 or 25% albumin, dextran) or blood products
- Further boluses of 20 mL/kg as needed; central venous pressure monitoring
- May need to increase contractility and afterload, avoiding the use of large amounts of fluids in distributive or cardiogenic shock
  - Correct pH and other substrate abnormalities
  - $NaHCO_3$ (sodium bicarbonate) if pH still less than 7.2

- Glucose infusions; ensure that calcium and other electrolytes are normal (Metha and MacPhee 2003)

Investigations include full/complete blood count, platelets, coagulation screen, arterial blood gas (ABG), electrolytes, glucose, urea, creatinine, calcium, lactate, and liver functions. Blood cultures should be drawn followed by immediate administration of IV antibiotics, cross-match should be drawn if needed, and chest radiography and a septic work-up should be carried out if needed. Vital signs should be completed at least every 5–15 min, including blood pressures, pulse oximetry for O_2 saturation monitoring, and continuous cardiac monitoring. Bladder catheterization for urine output monitoring should be completed as well as an ABG if oximetry is unavailable (Metha and MacPhee 2003; Wilson 2002).
Nursing care of a child suspected of experiencing signs and symptoms of septic shock center around the following principles:

- Ensure reliable venous access.
- Observe the child's general condition.
- Administer all medications and supportive care measures promply.
- Provide support to the family and child, informing parents of any interventions; be open and honest concerning the child's condition.
- Educate the family and child regarding the importance of seeking help and guidance as soon as a fever is identified; educate the family to call for advise if lethargy is noted, or any changes in a child's skin color or respiratory rate (Selwood 2008).

19.7.3 Prognosis

Septic shock is one of the most common causes of treatment-related mortality in childhood cancer. Prognosis depends on the nature of the infectious organism, timely initiation of treatments, and the individual's response to the therapy. In the past two decades, the mortality due to infections of gram-negative organisms in the profoundly neutropenic child has dropped from 80 to 40%, with the prompt initiation of empiric antibiotics in the event of fever (Rheingold and Lange 2006).

19.8 Immune Suppression

The effector cells of the immune response include polymorphonuclear leukocytes (PMN), T-lymphocytes, B-lymphocytes, natural killer cells, peripheral blood monocytes, and fixed-tissue macrophages, including the cells of the spleen and reticuloendothelial system. Cancer or therapy-mediated immune dysfunction most severely affects PMNs, monocytes, and lymphocytes, whereas the cells of the reticuloendothelial system are relatively less sensitive to the effects of antineoplastic therapy (Alexander et al. 2002).

19.8.1 Polymorphonuclear Leukocytes

Susceptibility to infections in children receiving chemotherapy is related to the number of circulating neutrophils. The more profound and protracted the neutropenia, the greater is the likelihood of a serious infection. Persistent neutropenia lasting for more than 1 week is associated with increasing risk for recurrent or new infections (Bodey et al. 1966). Neutropenia can be secondary to a child's disease (acute leukemia or aplastic anemia), but is more commonly a consequence of cytotoxic chemotherapy or radiotherapy. Most bacteremias occur when the absolute neutrophil count is less than 0.1×10^9/L (Alexander et al. 2002).

Qualitative abnormalities of neutrophil function may occur as a result of underlying diseases (acute leukemias) or be secondary to antineoplastic therapy. Neutrophils from patients with leukemia have suboptimal chemo-attractant responsiveness, bactericidal activity, and superoxide production (Baehner et al. 1973). Radiation may cause myelosuppression if a large amount of bone marrow is radiated. Radiation to the pelvis, spine, and long bones can cause the development of neutropenia. Medications commonly used in treating children, such as opiates, corticosteroids, and antibiotics, may have a detrimental effect on neutrophil function (Dale and Peterdorf 1973). Patients with qualitative or quantitative defects in their PMPs are subject to bacterial infections from gram-positive or gram-negative bacteria and invasive fungi such as *Candida* and *Aspergillus* (Alexander et al. 2002, p 1241).

19.8.2 Lymphocytes

Cancer and the treatments involved in a child's care create abnormalities of lymphocytes that affect both the humoral (B-cell-mediated) and the cellular (T-cell-mediated) immune response. A significant alteration in the humoral immune response (alteration in the ability to generate antigen-specific neutralizing antibodies) occurs in persons with chronic lymphocytic leukemia. These patients are susceptible to infections by encapsulated bacteria, especially *Streptococcus pneumoniae*, *Haemophilus influenzae*, and *Neisseria meningitidis* (Hersh et al. 1976).

Children with Hodgkin's and non-Hodgkin's lymphoma have impaired cellular immune responses. Corticosteroids and radiotherapy can also contribute to lymphocyte dysfunction (Fisher et al. 1980). Children who receive T-cell-depleted bone marrow transplants are more susceptible to viral pathogens, especially CMV. CMV can also act to further suppress the host's defenses (Rouse and Horohov 1986). Children with deficiencies of cellular immunity are more prone to fungal, viral, and bacterial infection that replicates within the cells, such as *Listeria monocytogenes* and *Salmonella* species (Alexander et al. 2002).

Depletion of helper T-cells occurs as a result of cytotoxic chemotherapy. Studies have shown that lymphocyte numbers do not promptly recover after chemotherapy has ended. Lymphopenia may persist for many months, while neutrophil, monocyte, and platelet numbers recover to 50% of pretreatment values between the cycles of chemotherapy (Mackall et al. 1995). The capacity for T-cell regeneration after chemotherapy seems to decrease with age, so that younger children have a significantly greater recovery of T-cells, 6 months after chemotherapy, compared with young adults, who have persistent, markedly low levels of T-cells after completion of therapy. It is postulated that the thymus-dependent regeneration of T-cells plays a larger role in younger children, whereas in older children and adults the normal thymic involution that occurs with age results in dramatically less thymus-dependent generation (Mackall et al. 1995). Prolonged T-cell depletion contributes to the development of opportunistic infections such as herpes zoster or *Pneumocystis* pneumonia (Alexander et al. 2002).

Routine vaccination is an important part in the care of healthy children; however, vaccination schedules are often interrupted for children undergoing cancer treatment. There is no universally accepted recommendations for immunizing children undergoing therapies for cancer (Walsh et al. 2006). The following are guiding principles taken from recent publications:

- Information about the host's risk for infection needs to be balanced with safety and efficacy of each vaccine.
- Two main concerns to remember:
  - Will the host be able to mount/maintain an antibody response?
  - Could the vaccine itself cause the disease?
- Measles-mumps-rubella is a live attenuated virus vaccine that is contraindicated in children undergoing chemotherapy.
- Oral polio is a live virus vaccine that is also contraindicated in immunocompromised children and their household contacts; inactivated polio vaccine is safe to use.
- Varicella vaccine, which uses a live attenuated strain, is recommended for household contacts and healthcare workers who have no history of varicella and who are seronegative; there is still controversy surrounding the use of the varicella vaccine in immunocompromised children.
- Live viral vaccines are generally given 3–6 months post completion of chemotherapy treatments to allow the T-cells to repopulate.
- Inactivated bacterial vaccines (i.e., diptheria-pertusis-tetanus, pneumococcal polysaccharide vaccines) and inactivated viral vaccines (hemophilus influenzae type-B and annual influenza) are suggested as per mandated schedules, even while undergoing active chemotherapy regimens; an alternative approach is to immunize at the end of chemotherapy regimens to ensure greater immunogenicity in a "catch-up" schedule.
- Children undergoing hemoatopoeitic stem cell transplantation generally begin a revaccination schedule 12–24 months post transplantation with

the administration of live virus vaccines commencing 24 months post transplantation (American Academy of Pediatrics 2006; Walsh et al. 2006; Centers for Disease Control and Prevention 2009).

Nurses need to be aware of the local immunization schedules and practices, and should encourage families to have children and household contacts vaccinated following guidelines developed by their institutions.

19.8.3 Spleen and Reticuloendothelial System

The spleen and the fixed tissue cells of the reticuloendothelial system act as a mechanical filter and as an immune effector organ. The spleen is involved in the production of antibodies and acts as a filter to remove damaged cells and opsonin-coated organisms from the circulation (Rosse 1987). Children who have had a splenectomy are deficient in antibody production, especially to particulate type of antigens; have decreased levels of immunoglobulin M (IgM) and properdin (a component of the alternate complement pathway); and are deficient in the phagocytosis-promoting peptides (Spirer et al. 1977). Thus, these children are at increased risk for developing septicemias from encapsulated bacterial organisms, such as *Streptococcus pneumoniae*, *Haemophilus influenzae*, and *Neisseria meningitidis* (American Academy of Pediatrics 2006). It is important for nurses to educate the children and families about the immunization for encapsulated bacteria at least 2 weeks before splenectomy. If this is not possible, then immunization should occur as soon as is practical post surgery. Nurses also need to educate the families about the seriousness of any febrile episodes and the need to bring children in for assessment as soon as possible, after the identification of fever. Oral antimicrobial prophylaxis in the asplenic/splenectomized child is generally recommended for children younger than 5 years of age, for at least a year post splenectomy (oral penicillin V 125 mg twice a day for children younger than 5 years, and 250 mg twice a day for those older than 5 years) (American Academy of Pediatrics 2006).

19.8.4 Other Factors Contributing to Immunocompromised States

Several other factors can exacerbate the immunocompromised state of children with cancer. Malnutrition has a documented effect on immune function. Nutritional deficiencies in children affect B- and T-lymphocytes, polymorphonuclear leukocytes, mononuclear phagocytes, and the complement system functioning (Santos 1994). Chemotherapy and radiation therapy can cause decreased immunoglobulin concentration, deficient agglutination and lysis of bacteria, inadequate neutralization of bacterial toxins, and diminished opsonic activities, which inhibits phagocytosis of bacteria (Groll et al. 2001).

Tumor masses, either primary or metastatic, can promote infection by organisms that colonize sites of tumor mass, cause obstruction in the biliary tree, gastrointestinal or genitourinary tracts, or respiratory passages. Children with central nervous system tumors may be at increased risk of aspiration pneumonias related to a diminished or absent gag reflex or a decreased level of consciousness. Aspiration pneumonias and subsequent infections that develop can be exacerbated by decreased mucosal clearance mechanisms, damaged as a result of antineoplastic therapies (Alexander et al. 2002). Nurses need to assess at-risk children and look for signs of diminishing gag reflexes, and initiate referrals to occupational therapists and dieticians for suggestions regarding appropriate feeding/drinking suggestions. Nurses play an important role in counseling and teaching families regarding the need for initiation of nasogastric and gastric feeds.

References

Ackerman MH (1994) The systemic inflammatory response, sepsis, and multiple organ dysfunction: new definitions for an old problem. Critical Care Nursing Clinics of North America 6:243–250

Ackerman MH, Evans NJ, Ecklund MM (1994) Systemic inflammatory response syndrome, sepsis, and nutritional support. Critical Care Nursing Clinics of North America 6: 321–340

Alexander SA, Walsh TJ, Freifeld AG et al (2002) Infectious complications in pediatric cancer patients. In: Pizzo PA,

Poplack DG (eds) Principles and practices of pediatric oncology, 4th edn. Lippincott Williams & Wilkins, Philadelphia, pp 1239–1283

American Academy of Pediatrics (2006) Active and passive immunizations and summary of infectious diseases. In: Pickering LK, Baker CJ, Long SS, McMillan JA (eds) Red book: 2006 report of the committee on infectious diseases, 27th edn. American Academy of Pediatrics, Elk Grove Village, IL,pp 71–85, 200–734

American Association of Blood Banks (1997) Recommendations of AABB on use of CMV safe blood. Association Bulletin 97–92, April

Baehner RL, Neiberger RG, Johnson DG et al (1973) Transient bacterial defect of peripheral blood phagocytes form children with acute lymphoblastic leukemia receiving craniospinal irradiation. New England Journal of Medicine 289: 1209–1219

Brown KK (1994) Septic shock. American Journal of Nursing 94(10):21–22

Bruce JL, Grove SK (1992) Fever: pathology and treatment. Critical Care Nurse 12(1):40–49

Callum J, Pinkerton P (2007) Adverse Reactions. In: Stevens H (ed) Clinical guide to transfusion, 4th edn. Canadian Blood Services, Toronto, pp 82–111

Centres for Disease Control and Prevention (2009) Recommendations of the Advisory Committee on immunization Practices (ACIP). http://www.cdc.gov/nip/ACIP

Chalmers E, Gibson BE (1999) Acquired disorder of hemostasis during childhood. In: Lilleyman JS, Hann IM, Blanchette VS (eds) Pediatric hematology, 2nd edn. Churchill Livingstone, London, pp 629–649

Chambers K, Lentendre P, Whitman L (2007) Blood components. In: Stevens H (ed) Clinical guide to transfusion, 4th edn. Canadian Blood Services, Toronto, pp 14–32

Dale D (2003) Myeloid disorders. In: George JN, Williams ME (eds) ASH-SAP American society of hematology self assessment program. Blackwell, Massachusetts, pp 116–128

Dale DC, Peterdorf RG (1973) Corticosteroids and infectious disease. Medical Clinics of North America 57:1277–1290

Fisher RJ, DeVita VT, Bostick F (1980) Persistent immunological abnormalities in long term survivors of advanced Hodgkin's disease. Annals of Internal Medicine 92:595–598

Freifeld AG, Walsh TJ, Marshall D et al (1999) A double blind comparison of empiricao oral and intravenous antibiotic therapy for low risk febrile patients with neutropenia during cancer chemotherapy. New England Journal of Medicine 341:305–311

Groll AH, Irvin RS, Lee JW et al (2001) Management of specific infectious complications in children with leukemias and lymphomas. In: Patrick CC (ed) Clinical management of infections in immunocompromised infants and children. Lippincott Williams & Wilkins, Philadelphia, pp 111–143

Hambleton J, George J (2003) Hemostasis and thrombosis. In: George JN, Williams ME (eds) ASH-SAP American society of hematology self assessment program. Blackwell, Massachusetts, pp 249–288

Hersh E, Gutterman J, Mavligit GM (1976) Effect of haematologic malignancies and their treatment on host defense factors. Clinical Haematology 5:425–430

Howard SC, Gajjar A, Ribeiro RC, Rivera GK, Rubnitz JE, Sandlund JT, Harrison PL, de Armendi A, Dahl GV, Pui CH (2000) Safety of lumbar puncture for children with acute lymphoblastic leukemia and thrombocytopenia. Journal of the American Medical Association 284:2222–2224

Hughes WT, Armstrong D, Bodey GP, Bow EJ, Brown AE, Calandra T, Feld R, Pizzo PA, Rolston KV, Shenep JL, Young LS (2002) 2002 guidelines for the use of antimicrobial agents in neutropenic patients with cancer. Clinical Infectious Diseases 34(6):730–751

Hume HA (1999) Blood components: preparation, indications and administration. In: Lilleyman JS, Hann IM, Blanchette VS (eds) Pediatric hematology, 2nd edn. Churchill Livingstone, London, pp 629–649

Klastersky J, Paesmans M, Rubenstein E et al (2000) The Multinational Association for Supportive Care in Cancer risk index: A multinational scoring system for identifying low-risk febrile neutropenic cancer patients. Journal of Clinical Oncology 18:3038–3051

Klassen R, Goodman T, Pham B et al (2000) "Low risk" prediction rule for pediatric oncology patients presenting with fever and neutropenia. Journal of Clinical Oncology 18: 1012–1019

Kline NE (2002) Prevention and treatment of infections. In: Baggott CR, Kelly KP, Fochtman D, Foley GV (eds) Nursing care of children and adolescents with cancer, 3rd edn. W.B. Saunders, Philadelphia, pp 266–278

Koh AY, Pizzo PA (2003) Infectious complications in children with hematologic disorders. In: Nathan DG, Orkin SH, Ginsburg D, Look AT (eds) Nathan and Oski's hematology of infancy and childhood, 6th edn. W.B. Saunders, Philadephia, pp 1685–1708

Lodha A (2003) Laboratory reference values. In: Cheng A, Williams BA, Sivarajan VB (eds) The HSC handbook for pediatrics, 10th edn. Elsevier Canada, Toronto, pp 813–898

Mackall CL, Fleissher TA, Brown MR et al (1995) Age, thymopoiesis and CD4+ T-lymphocyte regeneration after intensive chemotherapy. New England Journal of Medicine 332: 143–149

Metha S, MacPhee S (2003) Emergencies. In: Cheng A, Williams BA, Sivarajan VB (eds) The HSC handbook for pediatrics, 10th edn. Elsevier Canada, Toronto, pp 1–38

Monagle P, Andrews M (2003) Acquired disorders of hemostasis. In: Nathan DG, Orkin SH, Ginsburg D, Look AT (eds) Nathan and Oski's hematology of infancy and childhood, 6th edn. W.B. Saunders, Philadephia, pp 1631–1669

Ozer H, Armitage JO, Bennett CL et al (2000) 2002 Update of recommendations for the use of hematopoietic colony-stimulation factors: evidence-based, clinical practice guideline. Journal of Clinical Oncology 18:3558–3585

Panzarella, C, Rasco Baggot, C, Comeau, M. et al. (2002). Management of disease and treatment-related complications.

In Baggot CR., Kelly KP, Fochman D, Foley GV (eds) Nursing care of children and adolescents with cancer, 3rd edn. W.B. Saunders, Philadephia, pp. 279–318

Parsons SK, Mayer DK, Alexander SW, Xu R, Land V, Laver J (2000) Growth factor practice patterns among pediatric oncologist; results of a 1998 Pediatric Oncology Group survey: Economic evaluation working group the Pediatric Oncology Group. Journal of Pediatric Hematology Oncology 22:227–241

Rackoff WR, Robinson C, Keissman SC et al (1996) Predicting the risk of bacteremia in children with fever and neutropenia. Journal of Clinical Oncology 14:919–924

Rheingold SR, Lange BL (2006) Oncologic emergencies. In: Pizzo PA, Poplack DG (eds) Principles and practices of pediatric oncology, 5th edn. Lippincott Williams & Wilkins, Philadephia, pp 1203–1230

Rizzo JD, Sommerfield MR, Hagerty KL et al (2008) Use of epoetin and darpoetin in patients with cancer: 2007 American Society of Hematology/American Society of Clinical Oncology Clinical Practice Guidelines Update. Blood 111(1): 23–41

Rizzo JD, Lichtin AL, Woolf SH et al (2002) Use of Epoetin in patients with cancer: evidence-based clinical practice guidelines of the American Society of Clinical Oncology and the American Society of Hematology. Journal of Clinical Oncology 20:4083–4107

Rosse WF (1987) The spleen as a filter. New England Journal of Medicine 317:705–706

Rouse BT, Horohov DH (1986) Immunosuppression in viral infections. Review of Infectious Disease 8:850–855

Santos JI (1994) Nutrition, infection and immunocompetence. Infectious Disease. Clinics of North America 8:243–250

Sasse EC, Sasse AD, Brandalise SR et al (2005) Coloncy stimulating factors for prevention of myelosupressive therapy induced febrile neutropenia in children with acute lymphoblastic leukemia. Cochrane Database of Systematic Reviews, Issue 3:CD004139. DOI: 10.1002/14651858.CD004139.pub2

Schiffer CA, Anderson KC, Bennett CL, Bernstein S, Elting LS, Goldsmith M, Goldstein M, Hume H, McCullough JJ, McIntyre RE, Powell BL, Rainey JM, Rowley SD, Rebulla P, Troner MB, Wagnon AH, American Society of Clinical Oncology (2003) Platelet transfusion for patients with cancer: clinical practice guidelines of the American Society of Clinical Oncology. Journal of Clinical Oncology 19:1519–1538

Selwood K (2008) Oncologic emergencies. In: Gibson F, Soanes L (eds) Cancer in children and young people. Wiley, London, pp 73–82

Shamsah A (2003) Hematology. In: Cheng A, Williams BA, Sivarajan VB (eds) The HSC handbook for pediatrics, 10th edn. Elsevier Canada, Toronto, pp 350–378

Sloan S, Benjamin RJ et al (2003) Transfusion medicine. In: Nathan DG, Orkin SH, Ginsburg D, Look AT (eds) Nathan and Oski's hematology of infancy and childhood, 6th edn. W.B. Saunders, Philadephia, pp 1709–1757

Sloan SR, Friedman DF et al (2009) Transfusion medicine. In: Orkin SH, Nathan DG, Ginsburg D, Look AT, Fisher DE (eds) Nathan and Oski's hematology of infancy and childhood, 7th edn. Saunders, Elsevier, Philadephia, pp 1624–1662

Spirer Z, Zakuth V, Diamant S et al (1977) Decreased tuftsin concentration in patients who have undergone splenectomy. British Medical Journal 2:1574–1576

Stanworth SM, Massey E, Hyde C, et al (2005) Granulocyte transfusions for treating infections in patients with neutropenia or neutrophil dysfunction. Cochrane Database of Systematic Reviews 2005, Issue 3: CD005339. DOI: 10.1002/14651858.CD005339

Steele M (2003) Oncology. In: Cheng A, Williams BA, Sivarajan VB (eds) The HSC handbook for pediatrics, 10th edn. Elsevier, Toronto, pp 609–639

Strauss, R.G. (1994). Granulocyte transfusion therapy. In: Mintz PD (ed) Transfusion medicine 1. Hematology Oncology Clinics of North America 8:1159–1166

Sung L, Nathan PC, Lange B et al (2004) Prophylactic granluocyte colony-stimulating factor and granulocytemacrophage colony-stimulating factor decrease febrile neutropenia after chemotherapy in children with cancer: a meta-analysis of randomized controlled trials. Journal of Clinical Oncology 22(16):3350–3356

Talcott JA, Finberg R, Mayer R et al (1988) The medical course of cancer patients with neutropenia. Clinical identification of low risk sub-group at presentation. Archives of Internal Medicine 148:2561–2568

Tinmouth A (2007) Platelet transfusion: alloimmunization and management of platelet refractoriness. In: Stevens H (ed) Clinical guide to transfusion, 4th edn. Canadian Blood Services, Toronto, pp 169–177

Walsh TJ, Roilides E, Groll AH et al (2006) Infectious complications in pediatric cancer patients. In: Pizzo PA, Poplack DG (eds) Principles and practices of pediatric oncology, 5th edn. Lippincott Williams & Wilkins, Philadephia, pp 1268–1329

Wilson KD (2002) Oncologic emergencies. In: Rasco Baggott C, Patterson Kelly K, Fochtman D, Foley GV (eds) Nursing care of children and adolescents with cancer, 3rd edn. W.B. Saunders, Philadelphia, pp 334–346

Wittman B, Horan J, Lyman GH (2006) Prophylactic colonystimulating factors in children receiving myelosuppressive chemotherapy: a meta-analysis of randomized controlled trials. Cancer Treatment Review 32(4):289–303

Respiratory System

Margaret Parr

Contents

20.1 Pneumocystis Pneumonia . . . 401
20.1.1 Incidence . . . 401
20.1.2 Etiology . . . 402
20.1.3 Treatment . . . 402
20.1.4 Prognosis . . . 404
20.2 Pneumonitis . . . 404
20.2.1 Incidence . . . 404
20.2.2 Etiology . . . 404
20.2.3 Prevention . . . 405
20.2.4 Treatment . . . 405
20.2.5 Prognosis . . . 405
20.3 Fibrosis . . . 406
20.3.1 Incidence . . . 406
20.3.2 Etiology . . . 406
20.3.3 Prevention . . . 406
20.3.4 Treatment . . . 406
20.3.5 Prognosis . . . 406
20.4 Compromised Airway . . . 407
20.4.1 Incidence . . . 407
20.4.2 Etiology . . . 407
20.4.3 Prevention . . . 407
20.4.4 Treatment . . . 408
20.4.5 Prognosis . . . 408
References . . . 408

20.1 Pneumocystis Pneumonia

The *Pneumocystis* infecting humans, once called *Pneumocystis carinii*, is now called *Pneumocystis jiroveci* (pronounced “yee-row-vetsee”). *P. carinii* now refers to *Pneumocystis* from other host species. It is now clear that *Pneumocystis* from humans and other animals are quite different and that there are multiple species in the genus. Analysis of protein sizes has shown that the organism tends to be host-specific (Stringer et al. 2002). Changing the name of the organism does not preclude using the acronym PCP (*Pneumocystis pneumonia*).

20.1.1 Incidence

P. jiroveci pneumonia (PCP) is caused by the pathogen *P. jiroveci*. PCP has been described in immunocompromised patients for many years (Stringer et al. 2002). This group would include patients who have undergone organ transplantation, bone marrow transplantation or chemotherapy treatment for a malignancy. It has also been described in people who are mildly immunocompromised, for example patients with chronic lung disease (Stringer et al. 2002). PCP incidence has reduced considerably in the child and adolescent cancer population since initiation of prophylaxis, sulfamethoxazole–trimethoprim (co-trimoxazole, Bactrim®) (Shanker and Nania 2007). Hematologic malignancies, brain tumors that necessitate prolonged corticosteroid therapy, hematopoietic stem cell transplantation, prolonged neutropenia, and lymphopenia are the most important risk factors in non-HIV patients (Shanker and

Nania 2007). The highest incidence of PCP is most often being observed in patients who have HIV infection (Wakefield 2002).

20.1.2 Etiology

PCP is caused by the pathogen *P. jiroveci*. Originally discovered in 1909, it was thought to be a protozoan until DNA analysis in the 1980s demonstrated that it was a fungus (Lee 2006; Wakefield 2002). It was thought that PCP in the immunocompromised child resulted from latent cysts being reactivated. Children who are not immunocompromised have been found to carry the antibody to *P. carinii* (*jiroveci*) (Freifield et al. 2002; Wakefield 2002). As the child becomes immunocompromised during treatment, the latent cysts reactivate and the pneumocystis infection occurs. However, there have been patients with recurrent PCP infections that have been found to have different Pneumocystis jiroveci genotypes each time, which would imply new infections rather than reactivation of latent cysts (Lee 2006). Patient-to-patient transmission has also been suggested. Clusters have been described in pediatric oncology and transplant patients (Wakefield 2002).
The children considered to be most at risk of developing PCP within the pediatric oncology population are:

- Children with lymphomas
- Children on maintenance chemotherapy for acute lymphoblastic leukemia; the prolonged immunosuppressive effect of 6-mercaptopurine is directly responsible for a predisposition to *P. carinii* (*jiroveci*) (Pinkerton et al. 1994)
- Children who have undergone a bone marrow transplant (BMT)

Children receiving chemotherapy for acute lymphoblastic leukemia (ALL), are given Sulfamethoxazole–trimethoprim (Co-trimoxazole) prophylactic treatment against *P. jiroveci*.

Sulfamethoxazole–trimethoprim has several side effects: fever, rash, pruritus, vomiting, headaches, and bone marrow suppression. If children are experiencing any of the side effects, it may not be advisable to use sulfamethoxazole–trimethoprim. Indeed, prolonged bone marrow suppression is the most common reason to discontinue the prophylactic dose of sulfamethoxazole–trimethoprim (Shanker and Nania 2007). If the child shows intolerance to the drug, pentamidine may be chosen as a substitute to maintain the prophylactic treatment with minimal disruption to the child. Alternatives to sulfamethoxazole–trimethoprim include oral dapsone and oral atovaquone. It is recognized that pentamidine has been linked to a number of toxicities, including metabolic and hematological abnormalities, pancreatitis, hypotension, and nausea and vomiting (Freifield et al. 2002). Walzer (1994 in Bastow 2000) reports minor adverse reactions in most patients when pentamidine is administered intravenously (IV) or intramuscularly (IM), with serious toxicity in 47% of patients. Administering pentamidine via the nebulized route seems to reduce the toxicity risk. It is important to note that the effect that nebulized pentamidine may have on the staff administering the drug is largely unknown; therefore, care must be taken. Although administration usually requires a visit to the hospital or clinic, nebulized pentamidine is administered monthly, and it can usually be planned to coincide with a routine clinic visit. It is recommended that the patients receive the treatment in a single patient room and, if possible, some method of extraction or ventilation should be used to enable removal of the airborne particles produced during the drug's nebulization. Access to the room should be limited during the administration.

Bronchospasm is a recognized side effect that may occur at the time of administration. Nebulized bronchodilators may be prescribed routinely to prevent this from occurring.

20.1.3 Treatment

A child presenting with a suspected diagnosis of PCP most commonly presents with pyrexia, cough, dyspnoea, tachypnoea, a characteristic X-ray, and possibly intercostal recession (Bastow 2000). The chest X-ray normally reveals a bilateral, diffuse interstitial infiltrate (Bastow 2000; Freifield et al. 2002), which may be described as a "ground glass pattern" (Shanker and Nania 2007). PCP in the pediatric oncology patient can be diagnosed by the monoclonal staining of induced sputum, a specimen that is recommended as the first approach to assist diagnosis (Freifield et al. 2002). However, obtaining sputum specimens from children can be difficult, particularly because a presenting feature of the disease is an unproductive cough. Induced sputum specimens involve administering nebulized hypertonic saline. This method enables the particles to penetrate smaller airways. The hyperosmolality of the saline causes fluid to be drawn into the lung interstitium which washes the cysts and debris into the larger airways from where they can be expectorated (Bastow 2000). The use of the physiotherapist and the play specialist to work with the child may reduce the difficulty and help to ease the distress of the procedure.

If obtaining a sputum specimen is not possible, or the result is negative, then bronchoalveolar lavage or open biopsy may need to be considered (Freifield et al. 2002). Not all centers treating oncology patients will have the facilities for these diagnostic tests, or the child's condition may render him or her too ill for the procedure. If this is the case, then the healthcare practitioner should proceed directly to treatment. The first-line treatment for a suspected or confirmed diagnosis of PCP is high-dose oral or IV sulfamethoxazole–trimethoprim (see Table 20.1), with IV being the primary route of choice. Although central venous catheters (CVC) are the most commonly used method of venous access in the pediatric cancer patient, some children may still receive treatment via peripheral veins. If the drug is administered through a peripheral vein, nurses should note that there is a risk of abscess formation and necrosis of the injection site. Staff should regularly observe the site for patency, flashback, pain, redness, or swelling. If patients show intolerance to sulfamethoxazole–trimethoprim or show no response in 5–7 days, then it is recommended that treatment be changed to pentamidine (Shanker and Nania 2007, BNF for Children 2008).

If the diagnosis has not been confirmed, erythromycin may be prescribed alongside the sulfame thoxazole–trimethoprim to include treatment for

Table 20.1. Common drugs used for prophylaxis and treatment of pneumocystis carinii pneumonia

Drug	Use	Route	Dose	Administration
Pentamidine	Prophylaxis	Inhalation	300 mg inhaled once per month	Continue monthly throughout duration of cancer treatment (Consult product literature for method of administration)
	Treatment	Intravenous	4 mg/kg/day	Infuse in glucose 5% or sodium chloride 0.9% for 14–21 days. Dilute (once dissolved in water for injection) in 50–250 mL. Infuse over at least 60 min
		Inhaled	600 mg/day	For 14–21 days
Sulfamethoxazole–trimethoprim-(co-trimoxazole)	Prophylaxis	Oral	Surface area (SA) 0.5–0.75 m^2 = 480 mg/day SA 0.76–1.0 m^2 = 720 mg/day SA >1.0 m^2 = 960 mg/day	Given in two divided doses on two or three days per week
	Treatment	Intravenous	120 mg/kg/day	2–4 divided doses for 14 days as infusion in glucose 5% or 10%; or sodium chloride 0.9% Dilute 5–125 mL (or to 75 mL if fluid restrictions apply) Infuse over 60–90 min

Mycoplasma, as PCP and *Mycoplasma* are the two most common pathogens to cause the diffuse pulmonary infiltrate (Pinkerton et al. 1994). The use of steroids in combination with sulfamethoxazole–trimethoprim has been found to improve outcomes of adult AIDS patients with moderate or severe PCP (Freifield et al. 2002). In response to this finding, some pediatricians are prescribing an adjuvant short course of steroids to patients diagnosed with PCP.

Nurses must also consider the supportive care required by a child with a suspected or confirmed diagnosis of PCP. Oxygen therapy is usually required to maintain oxygen saturation, and the child's condition may deteriorate to the stage where mechanical ventilation is necessary. The team managing the child with PCP must also consider maintenance of nutrition and fluid, electrolyte, and acid–base balance; the child may require enteral feedings or total parenteral nutrition. The child will require antipyretic medication for comfort and will also need psychological support, which will be particularly important if he or she is isolated due to the diagnosis.

Chemotherapy is most likely to be interrupted until the child's condition improves and neutropenia subsides.

20.1.4 Prognosis

PCP is now much less common in the pediatric oncology population, and although the condition is treatable, it must still be recognized as a potentially fatal condition. It is essential that parents be taught to recognize the signs and symptoms their child may present with if PCP develops: dyspnoea, tachypnoea, pyrexia, and a cough. The staff should emphasize to the parents the importance of administering prophylaxis and reassure them that they can contact the hospital or clinic if they have any concerns regarding their child's condition.

20.2 Pneumonitis

20.2.1 Incidence

Pneumonitis secondary to a diagnosis of childhood cancer is very rare, but nevertheless should be considered in children presenting with a cough, which may be non-productive to begin with (Marina et al. 2004), dyspnoea, chest pain/pleuritis and fever. Children most at risk of developing pneumonitis are those who have received radiotherapy to the thorax, mediastinum, mantle, spine or flank. Children who have received total body irradiation as conditioning for BMT may also be considered at risk.

Radiation to the thoracic area can cause esophagitis, indigestion, nausea, acute pneumonitis, restrictive obstructive lung disease, fibrosis and cancer (Dickerman 2007).

Several studies have shown a range of 0–18% incidence of pneumonitis in patients who receive full-dose radiation in the thoracic area (Marina et al. 2004) with asymptomatic X-ray abnormalities in 27–92% of all patients treated in those studies.

Acute pneumonitis can occur between 1 and 3 months after radiotherapy treatment (Marina et al. 2004). Radiotherapy in conjunction with chemotherapy (especially actinomycin or bleomycin) increases the risk of pneumonitis from 5% at 20 Gy to 50% at 24 Gy (Kun 1997). Pneumonitis may occur more quickly in patients treated with both.

20.2.2 Etiology

Radiation pneumonitis is thought to occur as the result of excess free radical generation following radiotherapy (Cottier et al. 1996). The pathophysiology of the condition is immediate injury to alveolar type II pneumocytes, endothelial cells, fibroblasts, and macrophages (Marina et al. 2004). Edema and sloughing of endothelial cells in smaller vessels allows the fluid to accumulate in the interstitial tissues. The cell linings of the alveoli are also affected, and the swelling and sloughing of these cells also causes excess exudate (Strohl 1992). Pneumonitis can occur with radiation doses higher than 7.5 Gy, even as a cumulative fractionated dose (Van Dyk et al. 1981). Pneumonitis can also be related to some chemotherapy agents (see Table 20.2); those known specifically to cause pneumonitis are carmustine (BCNU), lomustine (CCNU), busulfan, cyclophosphamide, and bleomycin (Dickerman 2007). They cause a decrease in type I pneumocytes and an increase and redistribution of type II pneumocytes into the

Table 20.2. Chemotherapy agents with the potential to cause pneumonitis

Drug	Cytotoxic classification	Route	Antitumour spectrum
Lomustine	Alkylating agent	Oral	Brain tumor, lymphoma, Hodgkin's disease
Carmustine	Alkylating agent	Intravenous	Brain tumor, lymphoma, Hodgkin's disease
Busulfan	Alkylating agent	Oral	CML, leukemias (BMT)
Bleomycin	Antitumor antibiotic	Intravenous Intramuscular Oral	Lymphoma, testicular and other germ cell tumors

Adapted from Balis et al. 2002

alveolar spaces, leading to pneumonitis (Selwood et al. 1999).

Chemotherapy is also thought to accentuate the effects of radiation on the lungs. Radiation pneumonitis can occur with much lower doses of radiation when combined with actinomycin D, bleomycin, cyclophosphamide, vincristine, or adriamycin (Dickerman 2007).

20.2.3 Prevention

The risk of radiation pneumonitis is directly linked to the dose of radiotherapy the child receives. The greater the total dose of radiotherapy and the larger the dose per fraction, the greater the risk of significant lung damage. Lowering the radiation doses to 15–25 Gy has virtually eliminated the problem.

Children who are receiving bleomycin as part of their treatment regime should not be exposed to unnecessary high levels of oxygen. Anesthetists should be made aware of the fact that these children received bleomycin as part of their cancer treatment. However, this should not preclude children receiving oxygen therapy when their condition requires it.

20.2.4 Treatment

A child with suspected pneumonitis will present with a cough, dyspnoea, fever and increased respiratory effort. The child may also complain of pleuritic pain. It is important that the parents be aware of the risk of pneumonitis following radiation therapy to the lungs or treatment with some chemotherapy agents and that they know the signs and symptoms to look for. It is also important that the child/young person is made aware of the risk of pnemonitis and that advice against smoking is given.

The signs that may lead parents or patient to consult a doctor and the doctor to consider pneumonitis are the cough and a reduced exercise tolerance. Parents should be given the confidence and support to contact the clinic or hospital if they become concerned that their child may be showing any indication of developing pneumonitis. The child may require hospitalization and, in some rare but severe cases, ventilation.

If the child is admitted, he or she will require rest, observation of respiratory effort oxygen therapy, oxygen saturation monitoring, possible treatment with corticosteroids and psychological support. Symptoms may resolve in 2–3 months.

20.2.5 Prognosis

Reduced respiratory function increases susceptibility to infection, which will increase the risk of serious complications.

All children and young people who have been treated for cancer will be followed up regularly and it is important that the patient's exercise tolerance be assessed at each clinic appointment. Lung function may also be assessed but usually only if the patient is displaying symptoms such as tachypnoea or a persistent cough.

20.3 Fibrosis

As pneumonitis is the acute interstitial complication of radiotherapy and chemotherapy, fibrosis is the chronic complication, and the former often leads on to the latter.

20.3.1 Incidence

Pulmonary fibrosis as a consequence of treatment for childhood cancer is very rare. Nevertheless, it should be recognized as a possible late effect of treatment, particularly of radiotherapy to the thoracic region. Chronic fibrosis can be seen many years after treatment but most commonly changes are present 1–2 years after treatment. The fibrotic changes may occur as early as 2–4 months after radiation (Marina et al. 2004).

The Childhood Cancer Survivor Study analyzed 12,390 survivors of childhood cancer and found that pulmonary complications can occur any time after treatment. The survivors were found to have a significantly higher incidence of lung fibrosis, emphysema, pneumonia, pleurisy and need for oxygen compared with sibling controls (Mertens et al. 2002).

20.3.2 Etiology

Rolla et al. (2000) suggest that injury to the lung from radiation does not occur just from direct damage to the cell membranes, proteins and DNA, but also from an inflammatory syndrome. A study by Rubin et al. (1995) was able to demonstrate that there is a continuous cascade of cytokines starting soon after radiation therapy begins and lasting until lung fibrosis develops. As the pneumonitis subsides and the regeneration of the cells begins fibrosis will occur. Fibrosis can also develop in tissue as a result of scarring from previous injury. Bleomycin may cause fibrosis and this effect may not occur for many years. Methotrexate, Cyclophosphamide and Vinblastine have also been associated with chronic pneumonitis and fibrosis (Galvin 1994; Chen et al. 2002). The fibrotic process will cause loss of volume, loss of compliance, and reduced diffusing capacity.

20.3.3 Prevention

Survivors of childhood cancer who are thought to be at risk of developing fibrosis of the lung will be followed up appropriately in the late-effects clinics. They will require assessment of lung function, particularly if they are starting to display symptoms of dyspnoea or a dry hacking cough. However, the length of time the patients would need to be followed up would be difficult to determine, as the time period for developing fibrosis is quite varied. The Childhood Cancer Survivors Study showed patients developing symptoms between 5 and 20 years more than 5 years after completion of cancer treatment (Boughton 2002).

20.3.4 Treatment

A patient presenting with fibrosis will have a dry hacking cough and dyspnoea requiring treatment with steroids and oxygen. On admission to hospital, the patient will require a chest X-ray and lung function tests to determine the extent of damage to the lung tissue. The patient should be observed for any signs of infection, which will exacerbate the condition. Oxygen saturation should be monitored. If the condition is severe, the patient may require mechanical ventilation. Once a patient has been ventilated for fibrosis, it may be difficult to wean him or her off the ventilator, and this may be a long process. Exercise tolerance may be a problem, and the patient will need a great deal of psychological support to cope with the impact of this new restriction on his or her life.

20.3.5 Prognosis

Reduced respiratory function increases susceptibility to infection, which will increase the risk of serious complications. If the patient with fibrosis goes on to require mechanical ventilation, then the prognosis is poorer than that of those patients who do not require ventilation. Late effects clinic is also an opportunity for the team to discuss lifestyle choices such as smoking again with the young person and to revisit the conversation about the risk of fibrosis. While it is recognized that smoking may not cause fibrosis will certainly further compromise lung function.

20.4 Compromised Airway

20.4.1 Incidence

The incidence of compromised airway in the child with cancer is very rare, but due to anatomical differences, can occur more easily in the pediatric patient than in the adult. Any tumor occurring within the thoracic area can give rise to a compromised airway. The pediatric airway is small and compliant, making it susceptible to collapse (Jenkins 2001). Although airway compromise is rare, when it occurs it can rapidly become an oncological emergency (Fig. 20.1).

20.4.2 Etiology

There are several possible causes of compromised airway in the child with cancer. Any tumor developing in the thorax could compromise the airway due to compression. 35%–55% of mediastinal masses occur in the anterior mediastinum, 15% in the middle mediastinum and 30%–40% in the posterior mediastinum (Lerman J 2007). Tumours commonly found in the anterior mediastinum are Thymoma, Teratoma, thyroid and lymphoma with lymphoma accounting for approximately 45%. Lymph node masses account for the majority of masses found in the middle mediastinum and more than 90% of masses in the posterior mediastinum are neurogenic in origin (Lerman J 2007). Ginsberg et al. (2002) reported that the data from 18 studies from Europe, the United States, and Japan over a 10-year period showed that 74% of peripheral PNETs occurred in the central axis and 60% occurred in the chest. Rhabdomyosarcoma, Ewing's sarcoma and PNET may also occur in the chest wall. Children with mediastinal masses may present with superior vena cava syndrome (SVCS) or superior mediastinal syndrome (SMS). SVCS is the term used when a child presents with symptoms of compression, obstruction or thrombosis of the superior vena cava; if the trachea, larger airways or pulmonary vessels are also compressed, then the term SMS is used (Nicholin 2002; Rheingold and Lange 2002). SVCS and SMS most commonly occur with non-Hodgkin's lymphoma, Hodgkin's disease and leukemia.

Other tumors, germ cell tumors, neuroblastoma, rhabdomyosarcoma and Ewing's sarcoma (Nicholin 2002), may also cause airway obstruction with rhabdomyosarcoma being the most common of the malignant laryngeal tumors (Ferlito et al. 1999).

Some tumors – for example, osteosarcoma and Wilms' tumor – commonly metastasize to the lungs and can increase the risk of compromised airway in that patient.

Mucositis in the immunocompromised patient has also been reported as a cause of compromised airway (Chaimberg and Cravero 2004), and thrombocytopenia will create a risk of bleeding into the airway.

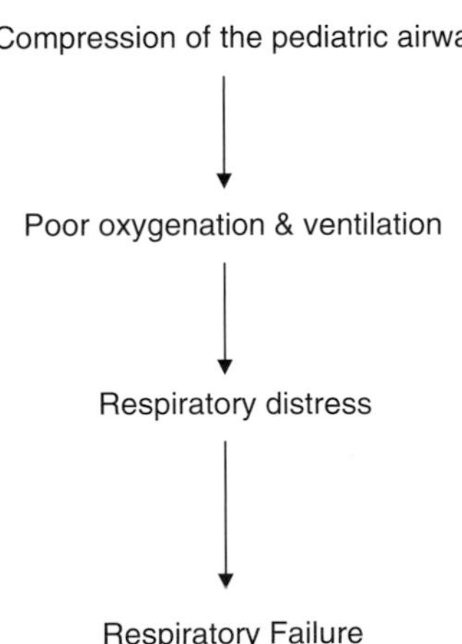

Figure 20.1
The pathway to oncological emergency

20.4.3 Prevention

It would be difficult to prevent a compromised airway from a tumor and therefore efforts should be concentrated on recognition rather than prevention. General practitioners and pediatricians should be educated to consider the possibility of a malignant diagnosis in children presenting to them with the signs and symptoms of airway compression and SVCS. This could then prevent wrong diagnoses, wrong treatment and deterioration in the child's condition.

20.4.4 Treatment

The signs and symptoms that the child may present with depend on the speed at which the condition arises. If the onset is slow and insidious, the child may present with cough, wheeze, tachypnoea, and possible stridor. If the onset is acute, then the child may present with fever, cough and mild shortness of breath, but may progress quickly to signs and symptoms of respiratory distress (Jenkins 2001). The child may also show signs of dyspnoea, orthopnoea, chest pain, jugular venous obstruction, and hoarseness. This condition can rapidly become an oncological emergency and must be managed promptly. If it is possible and time allows, then a biopsy for diagnosis would be the best option. However, several things must be taken into consideration: this group of patients is at high risk of respiratory or cardiac arrest if put in the supine position owing to impedance of venous return and airflow. Needle biopsy should only be considered if it can be undertaken under local anesthesia, as there is a high risk of arrest with either general anesthesia or sedation. A simple blood test could indicate whether leukemia is the underlying diagnosis. One could also take a blood sample for alpha-fetoprotein if a germ cell tumor is being considered, and a urine sample for catecholamines could be obtained if neuroblastoma were being considered.

This is one of the few occasions when medical staff may choose to start treatment without a definite diagnosis, and it would be advisable to nurse these patients within the intensive care unit until the acute phase has settled. To protect the child from obstruction, he or she may need ventilation until the tumor bulk has decreased. Neuromuscular blockade agents should be avoided during intubation because if the healthcare practitioner were unable to intubate past the obstruction, the child would be unable to breathe spontaneously (Jenkins 2001).

The team may choose to give chemotherapy and assess the situation; if the child's condition improves, they may then carry out the diagnostic tests. If the diagnosis is NHL, corticosteroids and possibly vincristine may be enough to improve the child's airway obstruction. It is important to note, however, that a child with mediastinal NHL or leukemia is at high risk of tumor lysis syndrome and the team should be advised to alert the renal team and the intensive care team.

If the chemotherapy does not improve the child's condition, the team may choose to give radiotherapy. There is a risk of the child deteriorating after radiotherapy, thought to be due to tracheal swelling post-radiotherapy (Rheingold and Lange 2002). There is also the chance that the child may suffer the risks of radiotherapy, i.e. pneumonitis, without seeing a benefit. NHL is both chemosensitive and radiosensitive, making biopsy and diagnosis difficult after treatment has already commenced. (With most of the other tumors, biopsy will still be possible.)

Compromised airway is a serious challenge for intensivists and oncologists and an aggressive approach is necessary to achieve best clinical result (Piastra et al. 2005). This will be a very frightening time for both the child and the family and they will require a great deal of psychological care and support.

20.4.5 Prognosis

The prognosis for recovering from compromised airway if due to tumor mass is very good. In their review of oncology patients requiring pediatric intensive care treatment, Keengwe et al. (1999) showed that four patients with tumor mass effect that resulted in respiratory compromise were admitted and ventilated and all four survived. A further study by Piastra et al. (2005) reported on seven children with mediastinal tumors all of whom required admission to intensive care, with two also requiring renal support. All seven children had successful discharge from intensive care.

References

Balis FM, Holcenberg JS, Blaney SM (2002) General principles of chemotherapy. In: Pizzo PA, Poplack DG (eds) Principles and practice of pediatric oncology, 4th edn. Lippincott Williams & Wilkins, Philadelphia, pp 237–308

Bastow V (2000) Identifying and treating PCP. Nursing Times 196(37):19

Boughton B (2002) Childhood cancer treatment causes complications later in life. Lancet Oncology 3(7):390

Chaimberg KH, Cravero JP (2004) Mucositis and airway obstruction in a pediatric patient. Anesthesia and Analgesia 99(1):59–61

Chen J, Wang PJ, Hsu YH, Chang PY, Fang JS (2002) Severe lung fibrosis after chemotherapy in a child with ataxia-telangectasia. Journal of Pediatric Hematology and Oncology 24(1):77–79

Cottier B, Cassapi L, Jack CIA, Jackson MJ, Fraser WD, Hind CRK (1996) Indicators of free radical activity in patients developing radiation pneumonitis. International Journal of Radiation Oncology, Biology and Physics 34(1):149–154

Dickerman JD (2007) The Late Effects of Childhood Cancer Therapy. Pediatrics 119:554–568

Ferlito A, Rinaldo A, Marioni G (1999) Laryngeal malignant neoplasms in children and adolescents. International Journal of Pediatric Otorhinolaryngology 49(1):1–14

Freifield AG, Walsh TJ, Alexander SW, Pizzo PA (2002) Infectious complications of in the pediatric cancer patient. In: Pizzo PA, Poplack DG (eds) Principles and practice of pediatric oncology, 4th edn. Lippincott Williams & Wilkins, Philadelphia

Galvin H (1994) The late effects of treatment of childhood cancer survivors. Journal of Cancer Care 3(2):128–133

Ginsberg JP, Woo SY, Johnson ME, Hicks MJ, Horowitz ME (2002) Ewing's sarcoma family of tumors: Ewing's sarcoma of bone and soft tissue and the peripheral primitive neuroectodermal tumours. In: Pizzo PA, Poplack DG (eds) Principles and practice of pediatric oncology, 4th edn. Lippincott Williams & Wilkins, Philadelphia, pp 973–1016

Jenkins TL (2001) Oncological critical care problems. In: Curley MAQ, Moloney-Harmon PA (eds) Critical care nursing of infants and children, 2nd edn. WB Saunders, Philadelphia, pp 853–874

Keengwe IN, Nelhans ND, Stansfield F, Eden OB, Dearlove OR, Sharples A (1999) Paediatric oncology and intensive care treatments: changing trends. Archives of Disease in Childhood 80(6):553–555

Kun LE (1997) General principles of radiotherapy. In: Pizzo PA, Poplack DG (eds) Principles and practices of pediatric oncology, 3rd edn. Lippincott Williams & Wilkins, Philadelphia

Lee SA (2006) A review of pneumocystis pneumonia. Journal of Pharmacy Practice 19:5

Lerman J (2007) Anterior mediastinal masses in children. Seminars in Anesthesia, Perioperative Medicine and Pain Pediatric anesthesia 26(3):133–140

Marina N, Sharis C, Tarbell N (2004) Respiratory complications. In: Wallace H, Green D (eds) Late effects of childhood cancer. Arnold, London

Mertens AC, Yutaki Y, Yan L, Stovali M, Hutchinson R, Ginsberg J, Sklar C, Robison L (2002) Pulmonary complications in survivors of childhood and adolescent cancer a report from the childhood cancer survivor. Study Cancer 95(11):2431–2441

Nicholin G (2002) Emergencies and their management. European Journal of Cancer 38:1365–1377

Paediatroc Formuary Committee. BNF for Children 2008. London BMJ publishing group; RPS Publishing and RCPCH Publications

Piastra M, Ruggiero A, Caresta E, Chiaretti A, Pulitano S, Polidori G, Riccardi R (2005) Life-threatening presentation of mediastinal neoplasms: report on 7 consecutive pediatric patients. American Journal of Emergency Medicine 23:76–82

Pinkerton CR, Cushing P, Sepion B (1994) Childhood cancer management: a practical handbook. Chapman & Hall, London

Rheingold SR, Lange BJ (2002) Oncologic emergencies. In: Pizzo PA, Poplack DG (eds) Principles and practice of pediatric oncology, 4th edn. Lippincott Williams & Wilkins, Philadelphia, pp 1177–1204

Rolla G, Ricardi U, Colagrande P, Nassisi D, Dutto L, Chiavassa G, Bucca C (2000) Changes in airway responsiveness following mantle radiotherapy for Hodgkin's disease. Chest 117(6):1590–1596

Rubin P, Johnston CJ, Williams JP, McDonald S, Finkelstein JN (1995) A perpetual cascade of cytokines postirradiation leads to pulmonary fibrosis. International Journal of Radiation, Biology and Physics 33(1):99–109

Selwood K, Gibson F, Evans M (1999) Side effects of chemotherapy. In: Gibson F, Evans M (eds) Paediatric oncology: acute nursing care. Whurr, London

Shanker SM, Nania JJ (2007) Management of Pneumocystis jiroveci pneumonia in children receiving chemotherapy. Pediatric Drugs 9(5):301–309

Stringer JR, Beard CB, Miller RF, Wakefield AE (2002) A new name (*Pneumocystis jiroveci*) for *Pneumocystis* from humans. Emerging Infectious Diseases 8(9):891–896

Strohl RA (1992) Ineffective breathing patterns. In: Hassey-Dow K, Hilderley L (eds) Nursing care in radiation oncology. WB Saunders, Philadelphia, pp 160–177

Van Dyk J, Keane TJ, Kan S, Rider WD, Fryer CJ (1981) Radiation pneumonitis following single dose irradiation: a re-evaluation based on absolute dose to lung. International Journal of Radiation Oncology, Biology and Physics 11(3): 461–467

Wakefield AE (2002) *Pneumocystis carinii* childhood respiratory diseases. British Medical Bulletin 61:175–188

Renal System

Fiona Reid

Contents

21.1 Nephrectomy . . . 412
21.1.1 Incidence . . . 412
21.1.2 Etiology . . . 412
21.1.2.1 Neoplasms . . . 412
21.1.2.2 Bacterial . . . 412
21.1.3 Treatment . . . 412
21.1.3.1 Preoperative Care . . . 412
21.1.3.2 Surgery . . . 414
21.1.3.3 Postoperative Care . . . 414
21.1.4 Prognosis . . . 416
21.2 Cytotoxic Drug Excretion . . . 417
21.2.1 Pharmacokinetics/Dynamics . . . 417
21.2.2 Metabolism . . . 418
21.2.3 Excretion . . . 418
21.2.4 Drug Interactions . . . 420
21.2.5 Dose Modification . . . 420
21.2.6 Safe Handling of Cytotoxic Excreta . . . 424
21.3 Nephrotoxicity . . . 425
21.3.1 Incidence . . . 425
21.3.2 Etiology . . . 426
21.3.2.1 Iatrogenic . . . 426
21.3.2.1.1 Radiation . . . 426
21.3.2.1.2 Chemicals . . . 426
21.3.2.2 Fungal . . . 427
21.3.2.3 Viral . . . 427
21.3.2.4 Bacterial . . . 427
21.3.3 Prevention . . . 427
21.3.4 Treatment . . . 430
21.3.4.1 Fluid Overload . . . 430
21.3.4.2 Metabolic Acidosis . . . 431
21.3.4.3 Electrolyte Imbalance . . . 431
21.3.5 Prognosis . . . 432
21.4 Hemorrhagic Cystitis . . . 432
21.4.1 Incidence . . . 432
21.4.2 Etiology . . . 433
21.4.2.1 Iatrogenic . . . 433
21.4.2.1.1 Radiation . . . 433
21.4.2.1.2 Chemical . . . 433
21.4.2.2 Fungal . . . 434
21.4.2.3 Viral . . . 434
21.4.2.4 Bacterial . . . 434
21.4.3 Prevention . . . 434
21.4.4 Treatment . . . 435
21.4.5 Prognosis . . . 437
References . . . 437

21.1 Nephrectomy

21.1.1 Incidence

In general, justifications for childhood nephrectomy include trauma, nephrolithiasis, or a nonfunctioning kidney, but within the field of oncology, surgery is performed predominantly for tumor control and occasionally for severe infections.

Nephrectomy of some kind is indicated in all cases of renal tumors, with certain cases needing bilateral nephrectomy. Wilms' tumor (nephroblastoma or WT) represents approximately 8% of all childhood malignancies and is the most common primary malignant renal tumor of childhood (90%), with an incidence of 7.8 per million children. Approximately 5% involve both kidneys, possibly displaying discordant histologies. Other renal neoplasms include renal cell carcinomas (0.1/million), clear cell carcinomas (2–4%), rhabdoid tumors (<2%), congenital mesoblastic nephroma (3%), and benign angiomyolipoma. It may be difficult to accurately diagnose these tumors as they could be confused with undifferentiated WTs, although they require different therapies.

In most cases of oncology patients requiring nephrectomy, there is enough time for appropriate radiography and assessment prior to surgery; however, primary emergency nephrectomy (3%) may occur in situations of massive bleeding due to tumor rupture, suspected "acute abdomen" or bowel occlusion.

21.1.2 Etiology

21.1.2.1 Neoplasms

Wilms' tumor has a peak incidence in children at 2–4 years of age. Few are seen after 7 years of age and rarely after 15 years of age; in bilateral cases the child tends to be younger. In most cases, WT is sporadic, but it is thought to have an inheritable link in 15–20% (see Chap. 3 on Solid Tumors).

There are also increased frequencies of associated congenital urological abnormalities (1%), in particular hypospadias, cryptorchidism, and renal function anomalies. These may be associated with the following:

- Beckwith–Wiedemann syndrome (BW) with a 25% increased risk of WT
- Hemihypertrophy
- WAGR complex (WT with aniridia, genitourinary malformations and retardation)
- Klippel–Trenaunay–Weber and Perlman syndromes
- Denys–Drash syndrome (DD), displaying pseudohermaphroditism, WT, and glomerulonephritis, or nephrotic syndrome leading to progressive renal failure

Many of the latter result in renal failure requiring dialysis and then renal transplantation following surgery for tumor removal (Ebb et al. 2001). Bilateral WTs are more commonly found associated with syndromes, with sporadic cases accounting for less than 4% (Ehrlich 2007).

21.1.2.2 Bacterial

Some renal infections leading to xanthogranulomatosis pyelonephritis are characterized by persistent chronic bacteruria and renal mass, which may be mistaken for WT, associated with renal pelvis calcification and destruction of renal parenchyma for which simple nephrectomy is the remaining option after failure to resolve with antibiotic treatment (Alp et al. 2002).

21.1.3 Treatment

21.1.3.1 Preoperative Care

The aims of preoperative evaluation are to:

1. Attempt to assess the function and renal vasculature of both kidneys
2. Locate tumor origin (WT is intrinsic to the kidney; neuroblastoma is adrenal in origin)
3. Exclude intracaval tumor extension (seen in 4–8% of WT patients)
4. Exclude ureteral invasion
5. Determine the relationship of the tumor to adjacent structures including lymph nodes
6. Assess renal vasculature (e.g., up to 30% may involve more than one renal artery)
7. Discover any metastases (usually pulmonary)
8. Exclude intrarenal neuroblastoma, as immediate surgery would not be appropriate and

catecholamine-secreting tumors can cause hypertension and pose particular anesthetic problems (Mitchell 2004)

Hypertension is present in 25–50% of WT patients because of raised renin levels as a result of renal artery compression. ACE inhibitors are a good option in normalizing blood pressure preoperatively (Maas et al. 2007) and in reducing operative morbidity. Hematuria is seen in 25%, but gross hematuria should lead to a suspicion of extension into the renal collecting system. Examination is needed to eliminate the associated syndromes (DD, BW, or congenital uro-anomalies). Laboratory investigations include complete/full blood count, blood urea nitrogen and electrolytes, serum creatinine, serum calcium, clotting studies, renal and liver function, and urinalysis. Acquired von Willebrand's disease has been found in a relatively high percentage of newly diagnosed WT patients (Will 2006), and serum calcium has been found elevated in rhabdoid tumors and congenital mesoblastic nephroma. Intravenous (IV) pyelograms have been superseded by ultrasound, which is particularly useful in differentiating solid and cystic lesions, venous tumor thrombosis, and extension into the renal pelvis. Computerized tomography (CT) scan, the spiral form of which is particularly valuable when partial nephrectomy and delineation for maximal parenchymal sparing needs evaluation, may be confusing because tumors thought to be invasive of adjacent structures on the scan may be found to be only compressive at the time of surgery.

Figure 21.1 shows a CT scan image using oral and IV contrast to demonstrate a large mass (WT) arising from the left kidney.

Preoperative imaging is necessary to establish the function of the contralateral kidney but there is controversy regarding the 100% accuray in the detection of synchronous bilateral tumors, with up to 7% of contralateral tumors missed by diagnostic imaging and found only at surgery in the NWTS-4 (Wiener et al. 1998). Chest radiographs are required to detect pulmonary metastases.

Preoperative chemotherapy has been shown to be useful in shifting toward a more advantageous stage distribution and therefore a reduction in therapy increases the possibility of laparoscopic removal, reduces the chances of tumor rupture and bleeding, small bowel occlusions (SBO) (Godzinski et al. 2001) and tumor embolism, and is useful in shrinking intracaval extensions and therefore reducing the requirement for cavotomy and cardiopulmonary bypass (Lall et al. 2006). However, there is an argument that preoperative chemotherapy has implications for altering tumor histology (through tumor necrosis or differentiation), and risking inappropriate treatment with increased relapse rate due to biopsies missing a definitive diagnosis of poor histology such as anaplasia, seen in up to 10% of cases (Hamilton et al. 2006). Cases of tumor seeding along the needle tract after percutaneous needle biopsy has also been reported (Aslam and Spicer 1996).

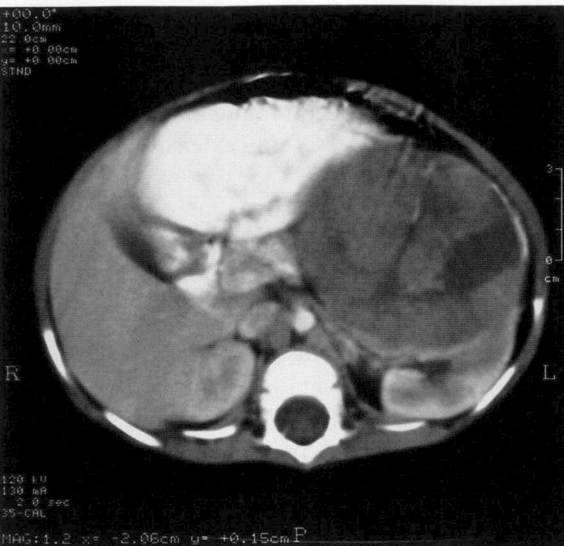

Figure 21.1

CT scan using oral and intravenous contrast demonstrating a large mass arising from the left kidney (Wilms' tumor). Image courtesy of Dr Sandra Butler, Consultant Radiologist, RHSC, Glasgow, Scotland

Presurgical chemotherapy treatment, with initial percutaneous needle biopsy, is generally accepted in the following situations:

- Solitary kidneys
- Bilateral renal tumors
- Tumors in a horseshoe kidney
- High inferior vena cava tumor extension
- Respiratory distress from extensive pulmonary metastases

Presurgical chemotherapy treatment could also be administered in cases where radical organ resection (which carries high morbidity and mortality rates) would otherwise be indicated.

Debate continues over the management of unilateral tumors in that Europe, through SIOP (International Society of Pediatric Oncology), prefers the option of biopsy and preoperative chemotherapy while North America, through the NWTSG (National Wilm Tumor Study Group), utilizes the primary nephrectomy and postoperative chemotherapy approach.

21.1.3.2 Surgery

Simple nephrectomy, involving the removal of the kidney from within Gerota's fascia, is usually performed for non-neoplastic disease states. In most renal tumors, radical nephrectomy (in which the entire contents of Gerota's fascia, including the kidney, perinephric fat, lymphatics, and ipsilateral adrenal gland, are removed to leave negative margins) is the ideal mode of choice, but only after a normal contralateral kidney has been established. Histopathology and tumor stage are the key determinants of prognosis and subsequent therapy in WT patients; therefore, surgical staging and careful technique are essential. In the past, a large transperitoneal, transabdominal, or thoracoabdominal approach has been recommended to enable full visualization of the contralateral kidney, with palpation for small bilateral tumors, assessment of other organs, lymph node involvement and biopsy, and careful manipulation and removal of tumor. Large necrotic, cystic, fluid-filled tumors, especially WT, are extremely friable and need to be removed en bloc. More recently, Duarte et al. (2006) have reported positive results using laparoscopic techniques for unilateral WT treated with careful imaging assessment and chemotherapy preoperatively. However, although postoperative recovery was uneventful and rapid, follow-up had only reached 23 months, and so relapse rates and late effects have yet to be established.

Partial or hemi-nephrectomy entails local tumor resection with least positive margins and leaving maximal normally functioning parenchyma. It has been reserved in the past, for situations of bilateral synchronous tumor or when radical nephrectomy would leave the patient either anephric or in renal failure, but more recently small favorable histology tumors have been removed in this way. Patients at high risk of developing second metachronous disease in the remaining kidney benefit from nephron sparing surgery. In these cases, prior chemotherapy is given to reduce tumor size and increase potential parenchymal sparing. It would appear that renal salvage procedures should aim to preserve 30% or more of renal volume to provide adequate renal function (Kubiak et al. 2004).

Figure 21.2 shows an image of the removal of a Wilms' tumor by radical nephrectomy.

Tumor spillage significantly increases local recurrence; therefore, its existence, local or diffuse, elevates staging and has repercussions for treatment intensification. The renal artery and vein are palpated to detect thrombus and intracaval extension and are ligated early, as close to the aorta as possible, and removed en bloc with the kidney to prevent tumor embolization and the risk of intracaval tumor dissection. The ureter is divided as low as possible, again after palpation, to rule out intraureteral extension. Any residual tumor may be marked with titanium clips to define areas needing future management. Renal vasculature anomalies are frequent and this should be borne in mind with rigorous preoperative assessment.

21.1.3.3 Postoperative Care

Complications of postnephrectomy may well be related to the type of excision, tumor histology and stage, place of incision, and intravascular tumor extension. High thoracoabdominal or flank incisions may result in pleural lacerations or pneumothorax requiring chest drain insertion. Pain related to the posture required during surgery and to the incision

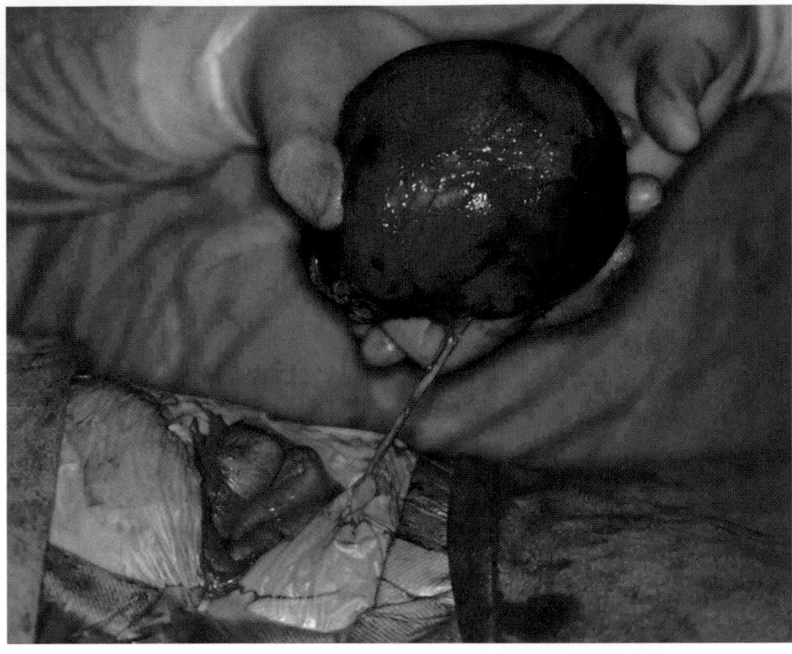

Figure 21.2
Image of removal of a Wilms' tumor by radical nephrectomy. Image courtesy of Mr. Gordon McKinlay, Consultant Pediatric Surgeon, RHSC, Edinburgh, Scotland

site predisposes to chest infections. Significant intraoperative hemorrhage is documented (6%) from tumor vessels (especially during partial nephrectomy) and adrenal glands and adjacent structures (particularly the liver and duodenum during right and the spleen during left radical nephrectomy). Distorted vascular anatomy increases the risks for iatrogenic injury to or incorrect ligation of the aortic arterial branches during surgery (Ritchey et al. 1992). Tumor rupture from friable Wilms' or highly vascular angiomyolipomas may lead to extensive hemorrhage. Bleeding may be exacerbated by preexisting coagulation disorders from neochemotherapy. SBO that can cause intestinal obstructions through adhesions or intussusception are the most common postoperative complication (7%) and may be exacerbated by edematous pressure necrosis of the bowel, which may lead to perforation and infection. Recognition of SBO may be difficult in the immediate postoperative period because of the relative frequency of paralytic ileus as a result of extensive bowel handling. This may be accentuated if vincristine has been part of the preoperative chemotherapy regime. Intravascular extension of the tumor and subsequent risks of embolization on mobilization can be reduced by early renal vessel ligation and palpation; however, this may risk tumor rupture and spillage. Hypercapnia can occur as a result of prolonged insufflation during laparoscopic procedures (Harrell and Snow 2005). Other problems that may arise following partial nephrectomy include the following:

- Blockage from postoperative bleeding into the ureter, with clot obstruction, perinephric hematoma or persistent urinary flank drainage that may suggest urinary fistula formation (Kubiak et al. 2004)
- Impaired wound healing and loss of host defense mechanisms as a result of chemotherapy and poor nutritional status, leading to increased risk of infection and delayed recovery
- Ureteral obstruction and varying degrees of renal insufficiency, which may require temporary dialysis

Table 21.1 summarizes the postoperative nursing management required following nephrectomy.

After the patient has recovered from surgery, both chemotherapy and occasionally radiation are often prescribed. Appropriate radiographic follow-up is

Table 21.1. Postoperative nephrectomy nursing management

Nursing action	Rationale	Potential problems detected
Vital signs, TPR, BP, SaO_2, air entry, abdominal distension	Signs of shock, infection, hypovolemia, respiratory depression, hypoxia, poor chest expansion	Hemorrhage, wound or chest infection, pneumothorax, thrombocytopenia, bowel obstruction, opiate-induced respiratory depression
Accurate fluid balance intake vs. urine and bowel output, care of urinary catheter	Assess renal function, urinary flow, vomiting, and bowel activity	Ureteral obstruction, renal insufficiency, edema, dehydration, bowel obstruction, paralytic ileus
Pain management, use of patient-controlled analgesia and pain tool, good postural support	Postural and procedural pain control aids mobility, well-being, and cooperation	Inadequate chest expansion leads to chest infections, delayed return of bowel activity due to immobility
Management of IV fluid and blood product replacement, introduction of oral fluids, diet, antiemetics	NPO for first 24 h or until bowel activity begins; nausea reduces oral intake; renal flow	Paralytic ileus, bowel obstruction, renal function reduced with dehydration, hypovolemia, anemia
Observation of wound site and any drainage systems	Ensure good healing, detect infection, assess bleeding/serous fluid loss. May be of poor nutritional status and immunocompromised	Wound infection, abscess formation, hematoma, urinary flank drainage, fistula formation
Laboratory investigations: urine and blood	Full/complete blood count, BUN, creatinine, electrolytes, osmolality, clotting, calcium, magnesium, renal and liver function, phosphate	Renal insufficiency, dehydration, fluid overload, electrolyte imbalance, infection, thrombocytopenia

required because clear cell carcinomas and renal cell carcinomas may metastasize to bone, rhabdoid tumors and clear cell carcinomas to the brain, and in particular WT to the lungs, with a potential for contralateral kidney tumor development.

21.1.4 Prognosis

Overall survival with multimodal therapy for WT of favorable histology is high at 90–95%. Follow-up for pulmonary metastatic recurrence and local recurrence is mandatory, alongside assessment of renal function and control of any presenting hypertension. Renal prognosis is also poorer with subsequent cytotoxic therapy. Appearance of a second WT in the remaining kidney is monitored, particularly in syndromes that have a predisposition to bilateral disease with ultrasounds 3–6-monthly up to the age of 10 years.

Renal hyperperfusion syndrome can follow unilateral nephrectomy, with focal glomerulonephritis and a deterioration in renal function leading to the need for dialysis and transplantation. Huang et al. (2006) found radical nephrectomy to be a significant risk factor in the development of chronic kidney disease arguing a case for partial nephrectomies for small cortical tumors.

Congenital mesoblastic nephroma presenting in neonates has survival figures nearing 100% cure after complete excision. However, 4-year survival for clear cell sarcoma and rhabdoid tumors is less encouraging, with high rates of cerebral metastatic disease.

Patients with bilateral disease responsive to chemotherapy may require unilateral nephrectomy with partial nephrectomy on the contralateral side that is least affected and/or with better histology with maximal parenchymal sparing (of more than 50%) and removal of positive margins. Dialysis may be needed to supplement renal function when the complexity of simultaneous chemotherapy temporarily reduces renal performance.

Survival rates for patients with bilateral nephrectomy and transplantation are dismal in the early stages due to sepsis or tumor reactivation from chemotherapy and immunosuppression (Ehrlich 2007). However, delaying the transplantation procedure with dialysis in the interim for approximately 2 years post completion of chemotherapy allows for recurrence of malignancy to be unlikely (Mitchell 2004).

Wilms' tumorigenesis is due to local rather than systemic factors, so recurrence in the transplanted kidney is unlikely (Mitchell 2004). Children with acquired solitary kidney are at risk of hypertension, proteinuria, Fanconi's syndrome, and renal insufficiency with compensatory renal hypertrophy.

After nephrectomy, patient education is of great importance regarding follow-up, hypertension management, any dietary restrictions, and awareness of the risk of urinary infections and trauma to the remaining kidney, and the patient should wear Medic Alert disks. Long-term renal follow-up investigations should include urinary protein, serum creatinine, and glomerular filtration rates (GFRs). Blood pressure monitoring is particularly warranted for those with an initial diagnosis of WT where up to 70% demonstrate hypertension or prehypertension as a late effect (Haddy et al. 2007).

21.2 Cytotoxic Drug Excretion

The mechanisms involved in effective drug administration are intricate on all occasions, but even more so when a variety of cytotoxic drugs is used whose primary aim of cell kill provides for multiorgan impact. Additionally, there is a high possibility of drug interactions.

Without careful control and intervention, a perpetuating cycle of increasing toxicity, organ failure, morbidity, and mortality may occur. Absorption, metabolism, and excretory patterns of antineoplastic agents are important determinants of therapeutic index (which is generally narrow), mechanisms of delivery, and drug dose modification. Recent advances in pharmacogenomics reveal that mutations in genes encoding drug-metabolizing enzymes, transporters, and target molecules may alter activity and affinity for drugs, so influencing pharmacokinetics/dynamics (Yamayoshi et al. 2005).

21.2.1 Pharmacokinetics/Dynamics

The bioavailability of a drug depends on absorption, distribution, biotransformation (metabolism), and excretion, and reflects total exposure of that drug, time vs. concentration, half-lives, and clearance, which are significant in predicting cytotoxicity and optimizing scheduling and methods of administration. Knowledge of half-lives can be important when estimating the lowest plasma cytotoxic activity for planning peripheral stem cell transfusion or granulocyte colony stimulating factor (GCSF) dosing. Third space fluid collections, such as ascites or pleural effusions, can substantially alter pharmacokinetics, with important ramifications for highly scheduled agents (e.g., methotrexate) and may require evacuation of these collections before therapy begins.

Pathways of drug clearance can be affected by:

- The patient's physiological state
- Genetic individuality
- The patient's prior exposure to the drug
- Drug interactions
- The patient's age
- The patient's sex
- Abdominal radiotherapy
- Graft vs. host disease (GvHD)

Pharmacodynamic variation between children and adults have led to different toxicities and altered outcomes of therapy. At times of major physiological change, such as infancy and puberty, pharmacokinetic variations also occur (see Fig. 21.3), making therapeutic drug monitoring and dose adjustment critical for safe, effective delivery in children. For example, methotrexate appears to have faster clearance in younger children (Borsi 1994a). Various physiological mechanisms mean that infants tolerate chemotherapy poorly:

- Body water content is higher at birth, reaching adult percentages after 1 year of age
- Plasma protein content changes over the first year
- Hepatic drug metabolizing enzymes acquire physiologic activity between 6 months and 1 year of age

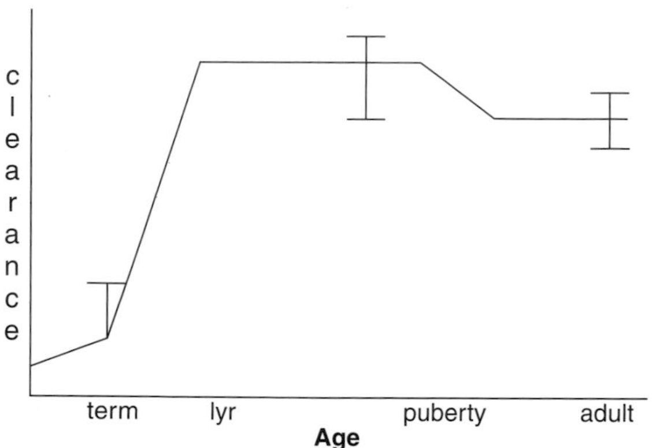

Figure 21.3

Representative developmental changes in drug clearance (Nies and Spielberg 1996) Copyright McGraw-Hill; reproduced with permission

- GFR attains comparable values to an adult at around 6 months of age (Vassal and Verschuur 2005)

There is a concept that drug clearance, and hence exposure, is based on body size. However, infants weighing <10 kg conventionally have their doses based on weight rather than surface area, with some protocols reducing doses further on the basis of tissue tolerance in infants being lower than in older children. Conversely, for some drugs, children may require a higher dose/kg than adults because of their relatively higher metabolic rate (BNF fo children 2007).

Dietary intake, nutritional status, gut motility, mucosal changes, and surgery may also affect oral absorption.

21.2.2 Metabolism

The metabolic activation and inactivation of drugs is carried out primarily by the liver, although enzymes are present in the small bowel that may be influenced by gut bacteria (and consequent antibiotic therapy) and deaminases in plasma and other normal tissues. Hepatic dysfunction through impaired blood flow, decreased biliary excretion, fatty changes, altered oral drug absorption from portal hypertension or decresed albumin production, malnutrition, viral hepatitis or genetic predisposition such as Gilbert's disease, may all affect metabolic capacity (Superfin et al. 2007). Evidence of liver failure will mean that some cytotoxics will require dose modification (Table 21.2). Mutations in enzymes involved in the metabolism of anticancer drugs can lead to slower metabolism and therefore increased toxicity. For example, deficiency of thiopurine methyltransferase in mercaptopurine use and dihydroprimidine dehydrogenase with fluoruaracil. In some instances, severe deficiency of a functional enzyme may preclude the use of that drug (Scurr et al. 2005).

Circadian timing of anticancer drugs (e.g., cisplatin) and biologic agents can result in altered metabolism, with improved toxicity profiles and enhanced tumor control (Wood and Hrushesky 1996).

21.2.3 Excretion

The kidneys are responsible for the majority of elimination of exogenously administered drugs, their active or inactive metabolites, and potentially dangerous endogenous compounds. Any significant decrease in renal function will be reflected by an increase in all body toxicities of anticancer drugs and their active or inactive metabolites dependant on this route, some of which are, themselves, nephrotoxic.

The main impediments to solute passage through glomerular capillary walls are particle size and charge (i.e., positive or negative). Serum proteins do not filtrate; therefore, drug protein binding affects the efficiency of excretion. Renal blood flow remains constant through a wide range of perfusion pressures, but autoregulation may be impaired by ischemic injury, furosemide use, or extracellular fluid depletion. Renal clearance of many acid/base drugs varies over the pH range. Alkalinization of tubular urine means that weak acids are excreted more rapidly. This is particularly relevant with methotrexate use, where coadministration of acids competing for excretion in the renal tubules or alkalinization with allopurinol can have potentially disastrous consequences (Tables 21.2–21.4).

Biliary excretion is secondary, but forms the primary elimination pathway for the vinca alkaloids. It involves a number of transport mechanisms that can

Table 21.2. Cytotoxic drug dose modification in organ failure (Tortorice 1997; Ignoffo et al. 1998; Neonatal and Pediatric Pharmaceutical Group 2001; Summerhayes and Daniels 2003; Superfin et al. 2007; BMJ 2008)

Drug	Organ dysfunction	Dose modification
Amsacrine	Hepatic – Bil >34 µmol/L Renal – GFR <10 mL/min	Reduce by 40% Reduce by 25–50%
Asparaginase		
Bleomycin	Renal – CrCl 40–50 mL/min CrCl 20–30 mL/min CrCl <20 mL/min	Reduce by 30% Reduce by 50% Reduce by 60%
Carboplatin	Specific formulas Renal – CrCl <20 mL/min	Avoid
Chlorambucil	Hepatic – gross dysfunction	Reduce
Cisplatin	Renal – CrCl >60 mL/min CrCl 40–50 mL/min CrCl <40 mL/min	100% dose Reduce by 50% Contraindicated
Cyclophosphamide	Renal – CrCl <10 mL/min Hepatic	Reduce by 50% Consider dose reduction
Cytarabine	Renal – CrCl <60 mL/min Hepatic – Bil >34 µmol/L	Reduce by 50% Reduce by 50%
Dacarbazine	Hepatic Renal – CrCl <10 mL/min	Consider dose reduction Avoid
Daunorubicin	Renal-Cr 100–260 µmol/L Cr >265 µmol/L Hepatic-Bil 20–50 µmol/L Bil >50 µmol/L	Reduce by 25% Reduce by 50% Reduce by 25% Reduce by 50%
Doxorubicin	Hepatic – Bil 1.2–3 mg/dL Bil 3–5 mg/dL Bil >5 mg/dL AST = 2–3 × ULN	Reduce by 50% Reduce by 75% Avoid Reduce by 25%
Epirubicin	Hepatic-Bil 24–50 µmol/L or AST 250–500 IU/L Bil >51 µmol/L or AST >500 IU/L	Reduce dose by 50% Reduce dose by 75%
Etoposide	Renal – CrCl >50 mL/min CrCl 10–50 mL/min CrCl <10 mL/min Hepatic – Bil 1.5–3 mg/dL or AST 60–180 U/L Bil >5 mg/dL or AST 180 IU/L+	100% dose Reduce by 25% Reduce by 50% Reduce dose by 50% Clinical decision
Idarubicin	Hepatic-Bil 21–34 µmol/L Bil >85 µmol/L Renal – CrCl <10 mL/min	Reduce by 50% Avoid Avoid
Ifosfamide	Renal – CrCl >50 mL/min CrCl 30–45 mL/min CrCl <10 mL/min Serum creatinine >120 µmol/L	100% dose Reduce by 25% Reduce by 50% Avoid

Table 21.2. (Continued)

Drug	Organ dysfunction	Dose modification
Mercaptopurine		Reduce dose with allopurinol administration
Methotrexate	Renal – CrCl 30–50 mL/min CrCl <30 mL/min Hepatic	Reduce by 50–75% Avoid Reduce especially with renal dysfunction
Mitoxantrone	Hepatic	Consider dose reduction
Procarbazine	Hepatic – Bil >85 μmol/L or AST >180 IU/L Renal – CrCl <10 mL/min	Avoid Avoid
Temozolamide	Hepatic	Consider dose reduction if severe
Thioguanine	Hepatic	Consider dose reduction
Thiotepa	Hepatic	Consider dose reduction
Vinblastine	Hepatic – Bil 1.2–3 mg/dL Bil >3 mg/dL Bil >51 μmol/L or AST >180 IU/L	Reduce by 50% Reduce by 75% Avoid
Vincristine	Hepatic – Bil 1.2–3 mg/dL Bil >3 mg/dL Bil >51 μmol/L or AST >180 IU/L	Reduce by 50% Reduce by 75% Avoid

CrCl creatinine clearance; *Cr* serum creatinine level; *GFR* must be adjusted for body surface area in pediatrics; *AST* serum aspartate aminotransaminase; *ULN* upper limit of normal

be inhibited by a variety of drugs and disease processes. After excretion, some may be broken down in the gut by bacterial enzymes and reabsorbed in the small bowel, leading to an enterohepatic circulation. The respiratory system and skin are lesser-documented pathways of excretion.

21.2.4 Drug Interactions

Given the complexity of most treatment regimens using multiple cytotoxics, analgesics, anticonvulsants, antiemetics, and steroids, relatively little specific data are available. Interactions may result in beneficial effect, improving therapeutic response or lessening toxicity. However, in most cases the reverse is true, with some drugs indirectly altering the eliminating function of end organs and so resulting in delayed clearance. Some patients may feel the need to complement treatment with homeopathic remedies that can enhance or decrease both effect and toxicity (see Table 21.4).

Selected drugs are known to enhance hepatic microsomal metabolism (cyclophosphamide, phenobarbital, phenytoin, rifampicin), whereas others inhibit (cimetide, alpha-interferon). Trimethoprim-sulfamethoxazole (co-trimoxazole, Bactrim®) can decrease protein binding of methotrexate and increase systemic exposure. Asparaginase may reduce hepatic clearance of vinca alkaloids.

Unfortunately, many of the drug interactions involve other medications commonly used in the oncology setting, and the potential for interaction increases with the number of drugs received.

21.2.5 Dose Modification

Understanding pharmacokinetics, pharmacodynamics, and drug interactions means that adaptive control

Table 21.3. Excretory pathways of cytotoxic drugs (Tortorice 1997; Ignoffo et al. 1998; Neonatal and Pediatric Pharmaceutical Group 2001; Summerhayes and Daniels 2003; Superfin et al. 2007; BNF 2008)

Drug	Use	Excretory pathway	Comments
All trans retinoic acid	APL	Renal	
Amsacrine	AML	Biliary	
Asparaginase	ALL, AML, CML	Biliary, minimal renal	May cause anaphylaxis
Bleomycin	Lymphoma, Hodgkins, germ cell tumors	50–60% Renal (40–60% as active drug)	Children <3 years have a faster clearance
Busulfan	BMT	Inactive metabolites renally	Requires hydration and allopurinol. May cause hepatotoxicity
Carboplatin	Solid tumors, BMT	70% Renal, extensive hepatic metabolism	Removed by hemodialysis in overdosage
Carmustine	Hodgkins, NHL, brain tumors	80% Renal, 10% as respiratory CO_2	
Chlorambucil		Mainly biliary, <1% renal	
Cisplatin	Solid tumors, germ cell, osteosarcoma, neuroblastoma	90% Renal, <10% hepatic	Magnesium wasting. May cause SIADH
Cyclophosphamide	ALL, AML, NHL, Ewing's, rhabdomyosarcoma neuroblastoma, BMT	Liver activated but exclusively renal elimination	May cause SIADH Use of MESNA to prevent hemorrhagic cystitis
Cytarabine	AML, ALL, lymphoma	90% Renal	Neurotoxicity may occur with high doses
Dacarbazine	Neuroblastoma, Hodgkins, sarcomas	50% Renal, some biliary	Hepatotoxic
Dactinomycin	Wilms', Ewings', NHL, Hodgkins, rhabdomyosarcoma	50% Biliary, 10% renal	Hepato-veno occlusive disease
Daunorubicin	AML, ALL	Mainly biliary, 20% renal	Turns urine red
Doxorubicin	ALL, Hodgkins, neuroblastoma, osteosarcoma	40–80% Biliary, 5–10% renal	Turns urine red
Epirubicin		27–40% Biliary	
Etoposide	ALL,AML,BMT, Ewings', soft tissue sarcomas, neuroblastoma	Mainly renal, some biliary	
Fludarabine		60% Renal in first 24 h	May cause pulmonary toxicity, hemorrhagic cystitis
Fluorouracil		Renal and hepatic	
Idarubicin		Mainly biliary, 10% renal	
Ifosfamide	Solid tumors	70–80% Renal	May cause tubular dysfunction or Fanconi syndrome. Use of MESNA to prevent hemorrhagic cystitis
Lomustine		Renal	
Melphalan	BMT	30% Renal, 30% fecal	Prior hydration required

Table 21.3. (Continued)

Drug	Use	Excretory pathway	Comments
Mercaptopurine	ALL	50% Renal (enormous individual variability in metabolism)	Allopurinol significantly reduces metabolic inactivation
Methotrexate	ALL, BMT, osteosarcoma	60–90% Unchanged renal excretion, 10% biliary (but increased with renal dysfunction)	Folinic acid rescue in high doses, urinary alkalinization, third space fluid collections slows clearance rate
Mitoxantrone		Mainly biliary, 5–10% renal	Transient blue–green urine discoloration
Procarbazine	Hodgkins	25–70% Renal as metabolites	
Temozolamide		Mainly renal	
Thioguanine	AML, ALL (pre-2003)	40–80% Renal	Can cause hepato-veno occlusive disease
Thiotepa	BMT	60% Renal as metabolites	
Vinblastine	Lymphoma, Hodgkins, histio-cytosis	35% Renal, mainly biliary	Can cause urinary retention
Vincristine	ALL, many cancers	10–20% Renal, 70% biliary	Can cause urinary retention

SIADH syndrome of inappropriate secretion of antidiuretic hormone

and, in some circumstances, individualization can be used to maximize the therapeutic effect within acceptable toxicity ranges. Dose modification due to impaired clearance or altered pharmacodynamics, use of modulating drugs (e.g., folinic acid given as calcium folinate/leucovorin) and careful monitoring of end-organ function form essential components of cancer chemotherapy management (see Table 21.2).

Methotrexate is an example where there is known faster clearance in younger children. Many acid-based drugs compete for tubular secretion, determining the need for accurate urinary pH regulation and good hydration/diuresis; consequently, creatinine clearance does not reflect methotrexate elimination. Folinic acid, a drug modulator, is used as "rescue" in high-dose regimens or in renal failure. Accurate measurement of plasma concentrations of methotrexate is available and should be implemented, particularly in high methotrexate dosages or when there is evidence of fluid collections. Such measurement can prevent the bone marrow, hepatic, nephrological, and, less commonly, neurological toxicities that can occur and can allow folinic acid treatment to be tailored appropriately.

Carboplatin clearance is closely correlated with GFR. If the dose is based on body surface area (BSA) and GFR is high, there is a risk of under-dosing, whereas a low GFR risks unacceptable toxicity. Hence, dosing formulas have been developed based on an individual's GFR and have been further adapted for pediatric use (Newell et al. 1993). It is important to remember that GFR is correlated with BSA, and smaller patients will appear to have poorer renal function unless the GFR is adjusted for the BSA (mL/min/m^2).

In view of enterohepatic circulation, serum bilirubin, although representative of hepatic function, may not reflect clearance of drugs that are primarily excreted through this route and should be complemented with a measurement of function, such as albumin or transaminase levels.

Table 21.4. Cytotoxic drug interactions (Tortorice 1997; Ignoffo et al. 1998; Neonatal and Pediatric Pharmaceutical Group 2001; Summerhayes and Daniels 2003; Nursing Drug Handbook 2004; Schellens 2005; Superfin et al. 2007; Wiffen et al. 2007; BNF 2008)

Drug	Interactions
Asparaginase	Increases vincristine associated peripheral neuropathy. Methotrexate reduces toxicity. May cause hyperglycemia with prednisone
Azathioprine	Increased leucopenia with ACE inhibitors and co-trimoxasole. May reduce cyclosporine levels. May decrease action of warfarin. Activation inhibited by allopurinol
Bleomycin	Half life increased with cisplatin increasing pulmonary toxicity. Decreases phenytoin and digoxin levels
Busulfan	Phenytoin increases clearance. Itraconazole decreases clearance. Plasma concentration increased with metranidazole. Hepatotoxicity increased with thioguanine
Carboplatin	Acute reduction in GFR when used with other cytotoxics. NSAIDs increase risk of bleeding. Nephrotoxicity enhanced with aminoglycosides and amphoterecin
Carmustine	Cimetidine may increase bone marrow toxicity. Reduces levels of phenytoin and digoxin
Chlorambucil	Anticoagulants may increase bleeding
Cisplatin	Toxicity increased by ifosfamide, aminoglycosides, vancomycin, furosemide, and amphoterecin. Enhances cytotoxicity of etoposide. Inactivated by MESNA. Decreases phenytoin levels. Increases bleomycin pulmonary toxicity
Cyclophosphamide	Allopurinol prolongs half life. Dexamethasone and chloramphenicol shortens half life. Barbiturates may enhance cytotoxicity. Reduces oral digoxin absorption. May reduce antimicrobial effect of ciprofloxacin. Prolongs neuromuscular blockade of succinylchloride (avoid)
Cytarabine	Inhibits methotrexate. Decreased activity of gentamicin against Klebsiella pneumoniae
Dacarbazine	Photosensitivity reactions in the sun
Dactinomycin	Reactivation of radiation reactions
Daunorubicin	Increased hepatotoxicity with other hepatotoxic drugs. Causes additive cardiotoxicity with doxorubicin
Doxorubicin	Neurotoxicity increased with cyclosporine. Decreases phenytoin and digoxin levels. Phenobarbitol increases doxorubicin clearance
Epirubicin	Increased risk of granulocytosis with clozapine. Levels increased by 50% with cimetidine (avoid)
Etoposide	Clearance enhanced by corticosteroids, cyclophosphamide, ifosfamide, phenobarbitol, phenytoin. Clearance decreased by erythromycin and clarithromycin. Cytotoxicity increased by cisplatin. Increases cyclosporine levels. Prolongs PT with warfarin
Ifosfamide	Activation decreased by erythromycin and clarithromycin. Metabolism increased by phenobarbitol. Prolongs warfarin PT. Increases cisplatin nephrotoxicity. May enhance anticoagulant effect of coumarins
Melphalan	Carmustine decreases threshold for pulmonary toxicity. Increased nephrotoxicity with cyclosporine and cisplatin. Cimetidine decreases melphalan concentrations. Nalidixic acid increases risks of severe necrotizing enterocolitis in children (avoid)
Mercaptopurine	Metabolic activity decreased by cotrimoxasole enhancing bone marrow toxicity. Shortens warfarin PT. Allopurinol reduces clearance. Antagonizes neuromuscular effect of non-depolarizing neuromuscular blockers.

Table 21.4. (Continued)

Drug	Interactions
Methotrexate	Competition for tubular secretion by salicylates, NSAIDs, aminoglycoside, penicillins, cisplatin, cephalosporins. Uptake inhibited by cytarabine. Increased toxicity with co-trimoxasole, cyclosporine, procarbazine, and phenytoin. May increase levels of thiopurines and theophylline. May decrease levels of phenytoin and digoxin. Increased pulmonary toxicity with cisplatin. Folic acid antagonizes methotrexate effect (may be used as rescue)
Procarbazine	Additive CN depression with narcotics, barbiturates, and phenothiazines. May decrease digoxin levels
Thioguanine	Can cause hepatic hyperplasia and portal hypertension with busulfan. Reduces digoxin absorption
Thiotepa	Increased apnea with pancuronium and succinylchloride (avoid)
Vinblastine	Increased clearance by corticosteroids cyclophosphamide, ifosfamide. Clarithromycin and erythromycin increase toxicity. Acute pulmonary reaction (bronchospasm) with mitomycin C. Decreases phenytoin blood levels
Vincristine	Increases asparaginase peripheral neuropathy. Erythromycin and clarithromycin increase toxicity. Decreases phenytoin and digoxin blood levels. Acute pulmonary reaction (bronchospasm) with mitomycin C. Potentiates hearing loss with other ototoxic drugs. Metabolism may be inhibited by itraconazole
Cyclosporine	Levels are reduced with phenytoin and barbiturates and increased with erythromycin, doxorubicin, and etoposide

GFR glomerular filtration rate; *NSAID* nonsteroidal anti-inflammatory drugs

Many herbal-drug interactions involve an effect on the efficacy of antiplatelet or anticoagulant drugs. Use herbal medication with caution in oncology, especially in the perioperative period

Herb	Drug Interaction	Consideration
Echinacea purpurea	Corticosteroids	Immune suppression can result from prolonged use of >14 days
St John's Wort	Cyclosporine, irinotecan	Loss or decrease in therapeutic effect

Useful agents should not be withheld because of potential toxicities, but preventative measures may reduce the risks. Preventative measures include

- Assessment of preexisting renal disease
- Use of ultrasound or isotope scans
- Dose modification
- Hydration, diuresis, and urinary pH adjustment
- Substitution with agents that have less similar/synergistic end-organ toxicity
- Monitoring of drug levels, creatinine clearance, uric acid, GFR, electrolytes, BUN (urea), full blood count, calcium, phosphate, magnesium, serum albumin, osmolality, liver function tests, and bilirubin
- Monitoring of urinary pH and urinary morphology, proteinuria, level of hydration, and volume of urinary output

Certain drugs are incompatible and may have their pharmacokinetic/dynamic properties altered if delivered concurrently or within the same infusion devices.

21.2.6 Safe Handling of Cytotoxic Excreta

Anticancer drugs are well documented as being irritative, carcinogenic, mutagenic, and teratogenic. They can also have many side effects, such as skin rashes, scarring, dizziness, and blurred vision. Safety measures regarding preparation, administration, and disposal of cytotoxically contaminated material are vital to protect healthcare professionals, patients, and their families. Pregnant women, whether they are medical personnel or, as is likely in the pediatric setting, mothers, in particular need education about the meticulous care required for both self and fetal protection. Avoidance of pregnancy is preferable but may be unrealistic. Contraceptive advice should be given.

Preparation and administration of cytotoxic agents is rapidly becoming more controlled as evidence becomes available about the potentially long-term damaging effects to all concerned. It is, however, understandable that many falsely view the less-invasive methods of administration (i.e., oral) to be less significant, and lapses in safeguards can occur. Suitability of protective clothing is a key factor in affecting permeation of cytotoxic agents (Allwood et al. 1997), with glove thickness and material (latex is better than vinyl) and completely absorbent disposable isolation gowns playing a role in preventing contamination. Awareness and staff attitude vary among different professional areas depending on the training they have received, regarding the significance of:

- Eye protection
- Inhalation from aerosolization
- Risks of skin contamination directly via drugs/excreta
- Contamination indirectly from contact during poor removal techniques of infected gloves, gowns, or aprons

It is for this reason that only individuals properly trained and regularly updated in safe handling of antineoplastics should be involved in their preparation or administration (Connor and McDiarmid 2006, Eisenberg 2009)

Healthcare workers should remember that all patient excreta should be considered potentially cytotoxic:

- Urine
- Skin
- Sweat
- Feces
- Blood
- Vomitus
- Breast milk
- Dressings/wounds/drains

Until recent years, the dangers of poor handling and disposal of cytotoxic drugs and excreta have been underestimated, and staff education in this area must be reinforced to protect all involved.

Certain measures effective in reducing risks of exposure to staff and families include wearing gloves whenever handling excreta and washing hands thoroughly after removing them. Males should be encouraged to sit to pass urine, and toilets should be double-flushed with lids closed to avoid aerosolization. Vomitus may contain high concentrations of chemotherapy for 2 h after oral administration. There is vast variation in clearance from urine and feces, but contact should generally be considered hazardous for up to 7 days after cytotoxic treatment.

21.3 Nephrotoxicity

21.3.1 Incidence

The kidneys form the elimination pathway for many drugs used in the oncological setting and are particularly vulnerable to toxicity because of their:

- Vascular supply
- Large endothelial surface area
- High metabolic activity
- Potential for accumulation/precipitation of drugs and their breakdown products within the glomerulus and tubular cells

The entire anatomical system, from glomerulus through distal tubule to ureter, is at risk. Renal failure can be caused by hypoperfusion, obstruction, or acute parenchymal failure. Nephrotoxicity is a dose-limiting side effect of some chemotherapeutic agents, and its presence will potentiate overall toxicities of many other drugs that depend on this excretory pathway (see Tables 21.2-21.4). Some drugs even cease to be effective when renal function is reduced. Acute renal failure with sudden loss of renal function will cause serious fluid and electrolyte imbalances and, without prompt action, result in severe short- and long-term morbidity and death. Nephrotoxicity leading to renal failure can be classified as prerenal, renal, or postrenal (see Table 21.5). Additional risk factors include the patient's nutritional status, hydration, radiation, unilateral or partial nephrectomy, duration of cancer therapy, large tumor bulk, preexisting renal disease, infection, and age.

Aminoglycoside antibiotics are thought to cause transient nonoliguric renal failure in 10–30% of patients and are one of the greatest causes of drug-induced acute nephrotoxicities. Renal toxicity from ifosfamide treatment ranges from 5 to 40%, with children under 5 years being at greatest risk. Some studies show the risk of dysfunction being as high as 9% for moderate and 9% for severe in the acute phase, leading to chronic tubular damage over a 5-year-period of 25–44% (Loebstein et al. 1999). This underlines the need to balance toxicity with efficacy.

Late-onset renal failure has occurred in up to 20% of bone marrow transplant (BMT) survivors, with total body irradiation (TBI) being a major factor, potentiated by chemotherapy (Cohen et al. 1995).

21.3.2 Etiology

21.3.2.1 Iatrogenic

21.3.2.1.1 Radiation

Fortunately, with the rise in neochemotherapy and surgery, the role of irradiation of renal structures has decreased; consequently, less radiation nephritis, is seen. Radiation nephropathy may result in chronic progressive renal dysfuncyion, glomerulosclerosis, and tubulointerstitial fibrosis. Acute radiation nephropathy can have an abrupt onset after a latent period of 6–12 months whereas chronic nephropathy may occur after an acute episode or be more indolent over 3–13 years, often associated with benign or malignant hypertension. In some cases, symptomless proteinuria may be the only sign of damage (Breitz 2004). Dosages of >2,300 cGy are a cause of damage to the epithelial lining in the acute phases and in chronic nephritis as a result of arterionephrosclerosis and vascular occlusion. Pediatric renal tolerance is lower than in adults; the National Wilms' Study Group (NWSG) showed a threshold of around 14 Gy (Cassady 1995). Conditioning regimens for BMT are near this dosage. In addition, nephrotoxic chemotherapy, aminoglycosides, antifungals, and immunosuppressants are prescribed; therefore, late chemoradiation marrow transplant renal dysfunction occurs. Thrombomicroangiopathy and hemolytic uremic syndrome (HUS) with hemoglobinuria can develop after BMT, resulting in renal insufficiency due to a combination of TBI, GvHD, and cyclosporine.

21.3.2.1.2 Chemicals

Treatment of large bulk, chemosensitive tumors in the initial phase leads to massive toxic breakdown of nucleic acid from tumor cells within 1–5 days, resulting in tumor lysis syndrome. Liberation of vast quantities of urate, phosphate, and potassium overwhelms the excretory capacity of the kidneys, causing hyperkalemia, hyperuricemia, and hyper-

Table 21.5. Classification and causes of oncological-related renal failure

Classification	Factors	Causes
Prerenal	Hypovolemia	Hemorrhage, hypoproteinemia
	Hypotension	Septicemia, hemorrhage, disseminated intravascular coagulation
Renal	Localized intravascular coagulation	Renal vein thrombosis, cortical necrosis, hemolytic uremic syndrome (HUS)
	Acute tubular necrosis	Chemicals, drugs, heavy metals, hemoglobin, shock, ischemia
	Acute interstitial nephritis	Infection, drugs
	Tumors	Renal parenchymal infiltration, uric acid nephropathy
Postrenal	Obstructive nephropathy	Tumor, *Aspergillus* spores, blood clots, calculi (uric acid)

phosphatemia (with secondary hypocalcemia). Precipitation of urate or calcium phosphate crystals in renal tubules or the development of calculi causes acute renal failure and worsening metabolic dysfunction, so even with prophylaxis, as many as 10% will experience some degree of renal deterioration.

Malignant infiltration of parenchymal tissue and ureters, or compression due to lymphoma or retroperitoneal masses, will only manifest loss of renal function if both kidneys are affected; however, surgical release can lead to brisk diuresis, hypovolemia, shock, and reduced renal perfusion. Bleeding may lead to blood clot and subsequent obstruction.

Nephrotoxic compounds may alter the kidneys either directly by reducing renal blood flow (causing obstruction during urine production) or through tubular necrosis, or indirectly through hypersensitivity reactions. Many chemotherapy agents are metabolized with the drug and/or metabolites being excreted by the kidneys (see Table 21.3), and notably cisplatin, carboplatin, ifosfamide, cyclophosphamide, and methotrexate are the instigators of most toxicities (see Table 21.6 for details of nephrotoxic drugs). Pediatric patients are particularly sensitive and can demonstrate subclinical glomerular dysfunction and tubular toxicity (Cachat and Guignard 1996). Fanconi's syndrome, caused by a number of medications, is demonstrated by renal phosphate and amino acid loss, which results in bone mineralization interference and renal rickets, growth failure, and decompensated renal tubular injury.

Hypotension can occur if drugs are given too rapidly (carmustine, etoposide) or as a result of anaphylaxis (asparaginase, cisplatin, amphotericin). Many of the supportive drugs used in oncology, such as salicylates, nonsteroidal anti-inflammatory medications, and medications used for immunosuppression and treatment of infection, are also nephrotoxic and additionally cause or potentiate damage to the already vulnerable renal system.

21.3.2.2 Fungal

The two most common opportunistic fungal infections seen in oncology patients are *Candida* and *Aspergillus*. Systemic invasion of these requires aggressive therapy in the immunocompromised patient. On rare occasions, *Aspergillus* spores have been known to invade renal vasculature, leading to medullary and cortical microabscesses and renal infarction, or spores may lodge in the filtration pathways and lead to an obstructive nephropathy that requires surgery. It is, however, the antifungal agents themselves, particularly conventional as opposed to lipid amphotericin B, that cause substantial nephrotoxicity, especially in conjunction with cyclosporine or aminoglycoside use.

21.3.2.3 Viral

Although a number of viruses are known to damage the epithelial lining of the bladder, little is documented with regard to kidney involvement. It should be noted, though, that renal manifestations of injury can be seen with acyclovir use (Bergstein 1996).

21.3.2.4 Bacterial

Renal infections, generalized septicemia or disseminated intravascular coagulation can result in dehydration, shock, hypovolemia, hypotension, and decreased renal perfusion, which will lead to a reduced GFR and acute renal failure. Aminoglycosides and vancomycin form the mainstay of gram-negative organism treatment but, unfortunately, are nephrotoxic, necessitating careful serum concentration measurement.

21.3.3 Prevention

Renal function is measured by the (GFR) through creatinine clearance (CrCl). The GFR changes in infancy becoming equal to the adult values by around 1 year of age and therefore formulas need to be adjusted for both age and surface area:

Neonate – CrCl = 30 × height (cm)/serum creatinine (μmol/L) measured in mL/min/1.73 m^2

Child over 1 year – CrCl = 40 × height (cm)/serum creatinine (μmol/L) measured in mL/min/1.73 m^2

- Normal values for 2–4 months of age is 60–80 mL/min/1.73 m^2

Table 21.6. Nephrotoxic drugs used in pediatric oncology (Tortorice 1997; Ignoffo et al. 1998; Neonatal and Pediatric Pharmaceutical Group 2001; Summerhayes and Daniels 2003; Nursing Drug Handbook 2004; Schellens 2005; Superfin et al. 2007; Wiffen et al. 2007; BNF 2008)

Drug	Mechanism of damage	Synergistic drugs	Risk factor	Other comments
BCNU/CCNU	Direct glomerular damage, tubular atrophy, interstitial nephritis		Cumulative dose of 1,200 mg/m^2	
Carboplatin	Interstitial nephritis, renal tubule damage, HUS (<cisplatin)	Prior use of nephrotoxics, aminoglycosides, amphoterecin	High doses for stem cell transplant	Transient, use pediatric GFR-based dose formula
Cisplatin	Platinum metal chelates in renal tubules, electrolyte imbalance, HUS; tubular nephritis, necrosis, atrophy	Ifosfamide Amphoterecin Aminoglycosides, vancomycin	Multidoses >50 mg/m^2 Damage dose-related and cumulative	Renal tubular injury salt-losing syndrome, SIADH, hypomagnesemia, hypokalemia, hypocalcemia, hypophosphatemia, hyperuricemia
Cyclophosphamide	Rarely, renal tubular necrosis	Cisplatin Vincristine	>50 mg/kg	Rarely SIADH
Ifosfamide	Glomerular and tubular toxicity, proteinuria, Fanconi's syndrome, diabetes insipidus	Prior use of nephrotoxics, Cisplatin, Radiotherapy	>119 g/m^2 very high risk >84 g/m^2 moderate risk Children <3 years high risk	Renal deterioration after cessation of treatment: toxicity cumulative
Methotrexate	Obstructive tubular precipitation of drug and metabolites, tubular necrosis	Other acids, NSAIDs, cephalosporins cisplatin, penicillins, co-trimoxasole salicylates, aminoglycosides	High dose >1 g/m^2 (plus leucovorin). Renal impairment accumulative	Azotemia
Mitomycin	Glomerular cell damage, deposition of platelets and fibrin, rise in creatinine	Vincristine	Risks increase with cumulative doses	Microangiopathic hemolytic anemia can develop later
Thioguanine (6TG)	Crystallization of 6-thiouric acid causes hematuria	Allopurinol	Massive intravenous doses of 6TG	Clears with drug cessation
Aminoglycosides	Proximal tubule necrosis, proteinuria, loss of protein concentration ability	Amphoterecin vancomycin, Piperacillin, Cephalosporin	Cumulative risk	Nonoliguric renal failure, hypomagnesemia, Fanconi's
Amphoterecin	Tubular transport defects and vasoconstriction, tubular acidosis	Aminoglycosides	Lipid form is less toxic	Salt-loading ameliorates toxicity, hypomagnesemia, hyponatremia

Table 21.6. (Continued)

Drug	Mechanism of damage	Synergistic drugs	Risk factor	Other comments
Cyclosporine	Increased renal vascular resistance, renal dysfunction (increased creatinine and urea), hypertension	Aminoglycosides Carboplatinum CisplatinAmphoterecin		Renal damage usually reversible, hypomagnesemia hyperkalemia, hyperuricemia
Others				
NSAIDs, penicillamines	Interstitial nephritis, nephrotic syndrome			
Pentamidine	Hypomagnesemia			
Salicylates	Interstitial nephritis, Fanconi's syndrome			
Sulfonamides	Interstitial nephritis, renal vasculitis			

- Normal values for 6–12 months of age is 80–110 mL/min/1.73 m^2
- Normal values for 12 months of age to adult is 85–110 mL/min/1.73 m^2 (Wiffen et al. 2007)

Mild renal failure (child/adult) CrCl 20–50 mL/min/1.73m^2 (approximate serum creatinine 150–300 μmol/L)

Moderate renal failure (child/adult) CrCl 10–20 mL/min/1.73m^2 (approximate serum creatinine 300–700 μmol/L)

Severe renal failure (child/adult) CrCl <10 mL/min/1.73m^2 (approximate serum creatinine >700 μmol/L) (BNF for children 2007)

Balancing the efficacy of chemotherapy and radiotherapy against possible side effects and short- and long-term morbidity makes for challenging sequencing of treatment. Risks should be reduced by:

- Substitution with nonnephrotoxic compounds
- Careful serum drug monitoring
- Serum biochemistry and antibiotic level monitoring
- Monitoring of fluid balance and hemodynamic parameters
- Dose modification/withdrawal (may be either a smaller dose at the same interval or the same dose at a longer dose interval depending on the type of drug)
- Avoidance of simultaneous and/or synergistic therapies

The main protective measure used in *all* cytotoxic drug administration emphasizes establishing hydration and good diuresis (in some cases forced with diuretics) prior to, during, and after their delivery.

- Prior hydration and allopurinol with urinary alkalinization when tumor lysis and urate production are anticipated
- Consideration of the elimination pathways and optimal conditions for excretion; e.g., alkalinization, avoidance of acid drugs, and leucovorin prophylaxis with methotrexate
- Awareness of cumulative dose effects

Prompt action in the event of febrile neutropenia should avoid septic shock. Increasingly, once-daily dosing with aminoglycosides given during the activity period of the day seems to reduce their nephrotoxicity (Beauchamp and Labrecque 2001). Liposomal amphotericin B for empirical antifungal therapy has been shown to be as effective as the conventional form but is associated with less nephrotoxicity and fewer breakthrough fungal infections (Walsh et al. 1999). Nephroprotective measures, including supplementation of potassium, sodium, and magnesium ions in conjunction with hydration to replace expected kidney losses, appear to meliorate amphotericin B nephrotoxicity (Doubek et al. 2002).

The use of selective renal shielding blocks provide evidence for reducing radiation-induced renal toxicity, especially with the implementation of TBI (Igaki et al. 2005).

21.3.4 Treatment

Signs of nephrotoxicity may initially be insidious and detectable only by blood analysis and monitoring of fluid balance. If the cause is prerenal with defective kidney perfusion and the underlying reason is anticipated and promptly corrected, then acute renal failure can be avoided.

In oliguric patients, there is a need to distinguish between hypoperfusion, in which urine is concentrated (urine osmolality >500 mOsm/kg and sodium content <20 mEq/L [mmol/L]), and impending tubular necrosis, in which urine is more dilute (osmolality is <350 mOsm/kg and sodium concentration >40 mEq/L [mmol/L]).

Acute renal failure develops when renal function is diminished functionally, resulting in decreases in GFR, tubular transport of substances, urine production, and renal clearance. Oliguria (urine volume <400 mL/m^2/day) is common, but nonoliguric renal failure may occur (e.g., aminoglycoside toxicity). Signs of acute renal failure include

- Anemia
- Diminished urine output
- Peripheral edema
- Vomiting
- Lethargy
- Hypertension
- Consequent complications of congestive cardiac failure
- Pulmonary and cerebral edema and seizures

Obstruction to the renal tract, which may be demonstrated by pain, dysuria, urinary retention, or renal dysfunction, may be excluded by radiography ± ultrasound. IV contrast agents should be avoided because of increased risks of tubular necrosis. Percutaneous nephrostomy may be required to reverse a blockage.

Hypovolemia and hypotension need correction with appropriate fluids (blood products/albumen bolus/saline infusions) depending on the cause, and possibly a dopamine infusion to raise blood pressure. If these conditions are associated with anaphylaxis, treatment will include hydrocortisone and adrenaline, or in the case of septicemia, treatment with antibiotics and/or antifungals will be required. A one-time dose of furosemide/frusemide or mannitol in the event of oliguria may be administered to attempt to effect a diuresis once hypovolemia and hypotension correction has been established. If there is no response, then fluid restriction and electrolyte balancing will need to commence. Figure 21.4 shows the algorithm for managing acute renal failure.

When known nephrotoxic agents have been employed, monitoring of drug serum levels, dose modification relative to creatinine clearance, or drug withdrawal might be required (see Table 21.2), and substitution with alternative nonnephrotoxic agents and avoidance of simultaneous nephrotoxics considered. In addition, certain drugs may have specific aids to reducing toxicity (see prevention) and treating a treatment overdose. For example,

Methotrexate overdose requires hemodialysis, charcoal hemofiltration, and cerebrospinal fluid exchange in the event of intrathecal overdose

Cisplatin overdose requires osmotic diuresis and plasmapheresis

Skill in accurate actual and anticipatory nursing management for acute renal failure heavily influences the ultimate outcome. Observation for fluid overload, metabolic disturbances, and electrolyte imbalance is essential.

21.3.4.1 Fluid Overload

- Weigh daily (or more often) at same time of day
- Strict fluid intake/output records
- Fluid intake restriction as per volemic status, ideally balanced throughout the 24 h; may need reassessed hourly if patient critically imbalanced
- Vital signs of temperature, pulse, respirations, and blood pressure
- Check for dependent edema: sacral, periorbital, pedal

Figure 21.4

Progressive algorithm for management of acute renal failure

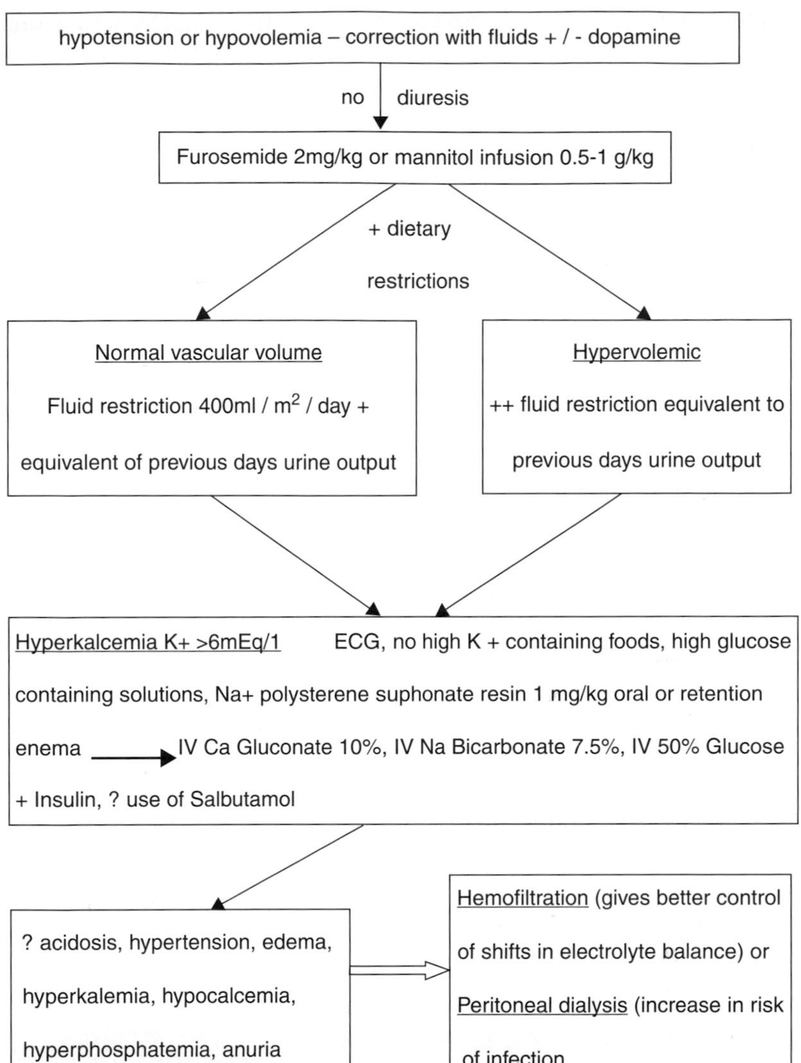

- Signs of respiratory edema or cardiac overload
- Urine specific gravity and urinalysis

21.3.4.2 Metabolic Acidosis

- Headache, nausea, vomiting
- Behavioral changes, lethargy, drowsiness
- Rapid, shallow respiration
- Restrict fat and protein intake to reduce acid end products
- Assist with bicarbonate dialysis if required

21.3.4.3 Electrolyte Imbalance

- Blood and urinary monitoring
- Strict dietary management

- Monitor for signs of electrolyte imbalance (see Table 21.7)
- Hemodialysis

21.3.5 Prognosis

The numbers of known adult survivors of childhood cancer have risen over the last 20 years but studies of long-term sequelae of treatment are restricted by the relatively recent development of intensive anti-tumoral therapy. Long-term outcomes are unknown, and careful monitoring for chronic toxicity is vital. The prognosis for recovery of renal function depends on its cause and the rapidity of response to diagnosis. Acute renal failure can be reversed if identified promptly before permanent damage occurs, which in its worst form may lead to a need for hemodialysis and transplantation. Renal tubulopathy effects are seen as metabolic acidosis, hypokalemia/magnesemia, proteinuria, Fanconi's syndrome, rickets, or a nephrogenic diabetes insipidus. Glomerular effects are demonstrated by a reduced GFR. Renal tubular dysfunction can persist for 2–4 years and may even be irreversible following cisplatin use, damage being accumulative (Skinner et al. 1998), and hypomagnesemia may be present in as many as 10% of patients. Ifosfamide-induced problems may or may not be reversible and may progress after cessation of treatment, eventually resulting in chronic failure necessitating dialysis (Loebstein et al. 1999). The tubular toxicity from aminoglycosides is generally reversible if the response to serum concentration levels is timely.

Radiation nephropathy is seen as a result of dose-related nephroarteriosclerosis or ureteral fibrosis, causing reduced GFR, obstruction, and hypertension. Late-onset renal failure can occur in up to 20% of BMT survivors. The BMT nephropathy, which is mainly attributed to TBI potentiated by prior chemotherapy, eventually stabilizes, and survival becomes dependent on control of hypertension (Cohen et al. 1995; Oyama et al. 1996). It is thought that the use of ACE inhibitors or angiotensin-converting enzyme inhibitors may mitigate the severity of radiation-induced injuries to the kidneys (Robbins and Diz 2006).

21.4 Hemorrhagic Cystitis

21.4.1 Incidence

The degree of vascularity and large surface area of the entire uroepithelium of the renal system mean that exposure to the causes of hemorrhagic cystitis (HC) can cause damage throughout the urological tract. The bladder is at particular risk because of the prolonged contact endured while storing urine that contains toxic elements, and its essential position making it susceptible during pelvic irradiation.

Table 21.7. Signs of electrolyte imbalance associated with nephrotoxicity

Electrolyte abnormality	Signs
Hypernatremia	Thirst, edema, weight gain, hypertension, tachycardia, dyspnea, CNS effects, seizures
Hyponatremia	CNS lethargy, coma, weakness, abdominal pain, muscle twitching, convulsions, nausea, vomiting, diarrhea
Hyperkalemia	Weakness, paralysis, paresthesias, nausea, diarrhea, abdominal pain, irregular pulse, muscle irritability, ECG changes, bradycardia, ventricular fibrillation, cardiac arrest
Hypokalemia	Weakness, paralysis, hypoventilation, polyuria, hypotension, paralytic ileus, nausea, vomiting, ECG changes
Hypocalcemia	Altered mental state, numbness/tingling of peripheries, muscle cramps, seizures, ECG changes, give high-calcium/low-phosphorus diet
Hypermagnesemia	Weakness, hypoventilation, hypotension, flushing, behavior changes
Hyperphosphatemia	Tetany, numbness of peripheries

HC can present:

1. Symptomatically
   - Bladder irritation
   - Suprapubic or flank pain
   - Dysuria/frequency/urgency, hematuria of differing degrees
2. With mucosal changes
   - Inflammation
   - Edema
   - Ulceration (epithelial loss)
   - Bleeding
   - Ischemia
   - Necrosis
3. With changes to renal/bladder function
   - Hydronephrosis/vesicoureteric reflux
   - Bladder tamponade
   - Smooth muscle fibrosis
   - Bladder perforation
   - Obstruction and renal failure

It is important to distinguish between red urinary discoloration caused by anthracyclines and true hematuria, which may range from minimal to life-threatening exsanguinating hemorrhage or renal failure. (See Table 21.8 for grading of HC.) Other causes such as bacterial infections, urinary calculi, or bladder neoplasms need to be excluded. The incidence of HC is broad-ranging, being related to cause, co-morbidity, and synergistic effects of treatment.

Onset may be:

- Acute: within hours of chemotherapy/weeks of radiation
- Chronic: months or years after BMT/radiation/chemotherapy

Table 21.8. Grading of hemorrhagic cystitis

Grade	Hematuria present
0	None
1	Microhematuria
2	Macrohematuria (gross), no clots
3	Macrohematuria (gross), with clots
4	Macroscopic hematuria with clots and elevated creatinine level secondary to obstruction. Severe bleeding/exsanguinating hemorrhage: transfusion required

An estimated 50–80% of patients receiving pelvic irradiation develop mild symptoms. As many as 50% have microhematuria and 15% have gross hematuria as a result of chemical cystitis (around 5–10% with cyclophosphamide and 20–40% with ifosfamide). Late-onset HC after BMT ranges from 7 to 25% and can be correlated with conditioning, viral activation, and degree of graft vs. host disease (GvHD) (Leung et al. 2002). The degree of myelosuppression heightens the risks and the severity as neutropenia allows for sepsis, and thrombocytopenia reduces clotting potential.

21.4.2 Etiology

21.4.2.1 Iatrogenic

Radiation and bladder-toxic chemotherapy (namely oxazophosphorine alkylating agents) are responsible for most HC cases; a minority can be attributed to coagulation disorders caused by myelosuppression, antifungals, antibiotics (penicillamines), and immunosuppressives (methotrexate and cyclosporine).

21.4.2.1.1 Radiation

Normal tissue tolerance of the bladder mucosa is 60–65 Gy (fractioned doses). Less radiosensitive tumors (e.g., rhabdomyosarcoma) may require 60–65 Gy to gain local control as a single form of treatment with huge morbidity; therefore, principles of management aim to reduce dosages to as low as 35 Gy using cytotoxic therapy and surgery prior to irradiation. The acute inflammatory response, seen within 4–6 weeks, can occur years after cessation of treatment, and the time between radiation and development of symptoms is proportional to the dose received. Simultaneous use of cyclophosphamide greatly increases the risks of radiation cystitis.

21.4.2.1.2 Chemical

HC is a major dose-limiting factor in the administration of cyclophosphamide and in particular ifosfamide. The drugs are metabolized through hydroxylation by microsomal hepatic enzymes to produce their inactive and active metabolites.

Figure 21.5 shows the sequence of events in the metabolism of these drugs.

Urinary excretion of acrolein, which binds to the bladder mucosa, is believed to be the source of urothelial damage. The degree of the problem is

- Cumulative
- Dose-related (especially intensive regimes)
- Experienced more with ifosfamide use than with cyclophosphamide
- Seen in children despite lower doses and with shorter duration of cyclophosphamide
- Increasingly affected by similarly timed or prior use of bleomycin, carboplatin, etoposide, vincristine, cisplatin, busulfan, pelvic irradiation, and GU cancers

BMT patients using TBI, cyclophosphamide and, in particular, high-dose busulfan in conditioning regimes are the most at risk of pre-engraftment HC, which tends to be transient and essentially self-limiting (Leung et al. 2005).

21.4.2.2 Fungal

Renal aspergillosis results in renal vascular invasion, leading to cortical and medullary microabscesses and renal infarction. Dissemination of infection through the system consequently evokes cystitis, hematuria, pyuria, and proteinuria. *Candida* can also be causative. Amphotericin may potentiate renal failure and should be used cautiously.

21.4.2.3 Viral

HC in BMT patients can be classed as pre-engraftment, when hematuria is brief and not more severe than grade 2, or as post-engraftment , when HC is more protracted and often of grade ≥3 and associated with GvHD. Immunosuppression therapy inclusive of cyclosporine risks new viruses or reactivation of dormant viruses such as adenovirus, cytomegalovirus (CMV), papovirus, or influenza A. Increasingly, human polyomavirus BK has been implicated in post-engraftment HC, associated with a raised BK viruria, which is a predictor for developing HC (Cesaro et al. 2008). It is thought that the uroepithelial cells damaged through conditioning therapy provides an environment for BKV replication, which together with the alloimmune response and acute GvHD results in the more severe form of HC. This explains why allogeneic recipients are at far greater risk than autologous patients (Leung et al. 2005).

21.4.2.4 Bacterial

Urosepsis is less commonly seen in children than adults and is usually associated with more intensive bone marrow suppressive schedules and episodes of urethral catheterization. Hematuria is usually mild, though exacerbated by concurrent use of other known HC causative agents. The use of penicillin including methicillin, piperacillin, and penicillin G has been implicated in 4–8% of patients with no other known cause (Relling and Schunk 1986).

21.4.3 Prevention

Prophylaxis is the primary management for HC. Preventative viral coverage post-BMT with acyclovir, ganciclovir, foscarnet and ensuring previous deliveries of CMV-negative and irradiated blood products

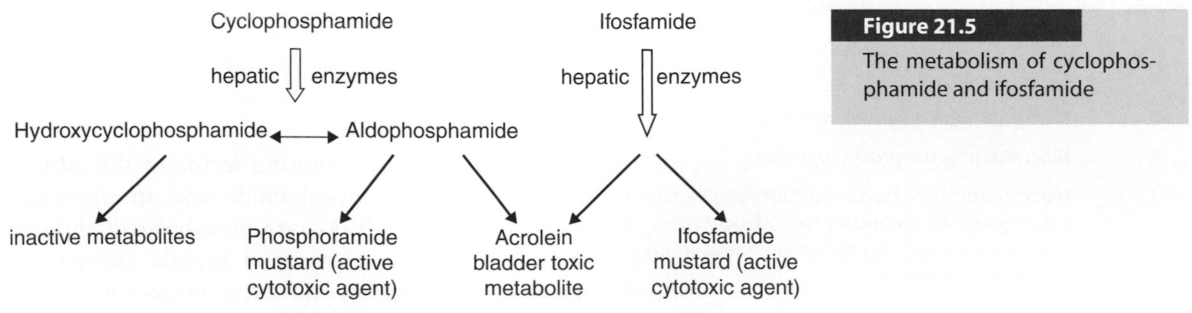

Figure 21.5 The metabolism of cyclophosphamide and ifosfamide

will lessen the risks. Prophylactic cidofovir to reduce BKV viral load is less preferable to the quinolone analog ciprofloxacin because it is myelotoxic and nephrotoxic (Leung et al. 2005). Neoadjuvant chemotherapy and surgery prior to irradiation can help reduce exposure fields in the pelvic region.

Anticipatory administration of mesna (mercaptoethane sodium sulfonate), an organ-specific uroprotective agent, has become a standard protocol with schedules involving cyclophosphamide or ifosfamide, but it only limits cystitis, not nephrotoxicity. Mesna does not compromise antitumor activity or BMT engraftment (Haselberger and Schwinghammer 1995); it reduces the incidence of oxazophosphorine-induced bladder cancers; and also inhibits the spontaneous breakdown of cyclophosphamide to acrolein in the urine. Cisplatin toxicity and side effects are also diminished with mesna, so it may be used as an antidote.

When absorbed, mesna undergoes oxidization to the dimerized form, dimesna. After glomerular filtration and tubular reabsorption, it is reduced back to its active form. The sulfhydryl group of mesna then complexes with acrolein to form a nontoxic thioether. Preexisting renal tubular damage leads to reduced mesna clearance and availability (Goren et al. 1987). Oral mesna tastes unpleasant, which, together with concomitant administration of emetogenic chemotherapy, makes for poor compliance. Early-morning chemotherapy allows for frequent daytime bladder emptying as opposed to nocturnal accumulation of toxic metabolites. The half life of mesna is 35 min, compared with 4 h for cyclophosphamide. Any timing error in delivery affords reduced uroprotection and crucially gambles the development of HC by up to 60%. To be effective, sufficient urine concentrations of mesna (10–20 mmol/mL) must be achieved during acrolein excretion (Borsi 1994b). A variety of protocols have been drawn up, but each adheres to these essential principles:

- Hyperhydration of 3 L/m^2/day ± furosemide/frusemide to attain adequate diuresis
- Close blood and urine monitoring; observation for signs of syndrome of inappropriate antidiuretic hormone (SIADH)
- Oral mesna dosage is twice cyclophosphamide dose, commences 2 h earlier, and is repeated after 2 and 6 h
- If the daily or total cyclophosphamide dose <300 mg/m^2 then hydrate only
- If the daily or total cyclophosphamide dose is equal to 300 mg/m^2, to1 g/m^2, then hydrate at 3 L/m^2/day, continuing for at least 6 h after cessation of chemotherapy
- If the daily or total cyclophosphamide dose >1 g/m^2 or any ifosfamide administration, then hydrate at 3 L/m^2/day plus mesna via either regime (a) or (b):
  a. IV loading dose of mesna 15 min precytotoxic delivery of 20–25% ifosfamide or 60–120% cyclophosphamide (mg:mg) dose and repeat every 4 h for three to five doses
  b. Continuous IV infusion of mesna beginning 3 h before chemotherapy and continuing for at least 12 h after completion, at 100–120% (mg:mg) of cyclophosphamide or ifosfamide dose

Hematuria appears to be greater in children who receive intermittent boluses, suggesting that 4 h is too long a gap and making continuous infusion the delivery mode of choice (Magrath et al. 1986). Continuous bladder irrigation together with MESNA and alkalization has been demonstrated to be beneficial in reducing both early and late-onset HC in adult BMT patients (Hadjibabaie et al. 2008).

21.4.4 Treatment

Prediction of risk and initiation of prophylactic measures is paramount in limiting oxazophosphorine-induced HC. Once severe bleeding has started, management becomes complex and morbidity high. Table 21.9 highlights the initial nursing interventions that are necessary.

Adherence to timely administration of mesna should prevent most cases of gross hematuria; those that do occur are often related to BMT in which conditioning included busulfan. Usually, escalation of hydration and mesna with or without forced diuresis and furosemide/frusemide are sufficient, but more invasive measures are occasionally required. Correction of thrombocytopenia, prothrombin time, and

Table 21.9. Nursing interventions in the management of hemorrhagic cystitis

Action	Rationale
Vital signs: temperature(*T*), pulse(*P*), respirations (R), blood pressure(BP)	*T* raised, *P* and BP up/down with infection, hypovolemia, or transfusion reaction
Monitor intake and output, check weight. Assess diuresis, need for furosemide	Signs of ifosfamide-induced renal tubular dysfunction (SIADH)
Maintain hydration (3 L/m^2/day)	Encourage diuresis, bladder voiding
Administer mesna as per protocol	Correct timing with antineoplastics influences amelioration of HC
Urinalysis q.i.d.	Degree of hematuria affects management
Encourage frequent voiding, maintain continuous bladder irrigation	Reduces clot production/retention and acrolein accumulation in urine
Administer anticipatory antiemetics, analgesics, and antispasmodics	Reduce discomfort, promote urinary voiding compliance and antispasmodics
Minimize constipation	Straining to eliminate exacerbates bleeding
Safe administration of blood products	Correct hypovolemia, thrombocytopenia, and PT time
Correct hypovolemia, thrombocytopenia, and PT time	Headache, nausea, diarrhea, and limb pain
Blood sampling: urea, electrolytes, creatinine, Hb, BUN, WCC, uric acid, HCT, serum albumen, serum bilirubin, ALT, AST[a]	Effects of hemodilution, hypovolemia, furosemide, obstructive nephropathy nephrotoxicity, toxic hepatitis, blood clotting disorders, SIADH

[a] AST (serum aspartate aminotransaminase) = SGPT (serum glutamic pyruvic transaminase)

hypovolemia using blood products, together with pain management using nonsalicylate analgesics and antispasmodics, antiemetics, and sedation are also needed. See Fig. 21.6 for the treatment pathway of HC.

Bladder irrigation via a 3-way Foley or suprapubic catheter to remove clots, helps prevent ureteral or urethral obstruction and improves efficiency of bladder emptying, so reducing the bladder mucosa's exposure to acrolein. Bladder instillation of chemical astringents using the least toxic materials, such as silver nitrate, a cauterizing agent, and alum, will stop bleeding but are not without risking long-term complications, especially in children, and monitoring for neurotoxicity with a view to discontinuing treatment is necessary.

The next stage is cystoscopy or suprapubic cystotomy to allow clot evacuation and electrofulguration of bleeding points and to treat bladder tamponade. Formalin 1% instillations are reserved for life-threatening HC refractory to more conservative measures, as the side effects of aluminum toxicity, bladder fibrosis, and contractions are severe. Prior ultrasound, cystogram, and removal of clots must be established to prevent ureteric reflux of caustic substances to the kidney. Instillation of formalin is painful and requires general anesthesia (Traxer et al. 2001).

If all of the above fail, then arterial ligation, selective vesical artery embolization (Palandri et al. 2005), or cystectomy with urinary diversion are a last resort to preserve life.

Prostaglandin instillation, which inactivates acrolein, causes severe bladder spasms requiring morphine and sedation and is of impractical use in pediatrics. Newer alternative treatments advocated include the use of 100% hyperbaric oxygen therapy (Bratsas et al. 2004), estrogen (Apozna ski et al. 2005), intravesical instillation of sodium hyaluronate, cidofovir or prostaglandins, and the use of fibrin sealants (Leung et al. 2005).

Because urosepsis is also causative of HC, exclusion of bacterial and, particularly post-BMT, viral

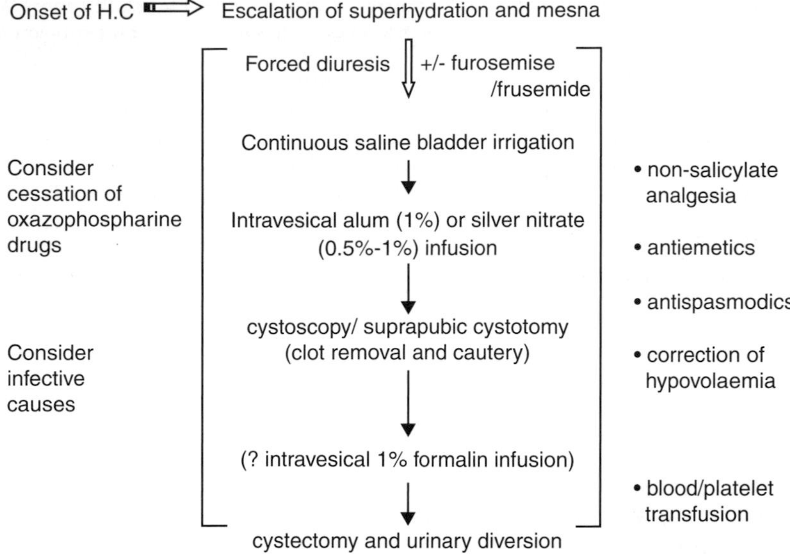

Figure 21.6
The treatment pathway for hemorrhagic cystitis

etiology should be taken into account. Vidarabine, cidofovir, and ganciclovir for viral infections have been deployed successfully, the latter being superior to foscarnet, which has been suggested to be bladder-toxic (Gonzalez-Fraile et al. 2001). Consideration of alternatives to penicillin-based antibacterials may be necessary if no other reasons are found.

21.4.5 Prognosis

The consequences of HC, including increased hospitalization and the effects on short- and long-term morbidity, cannot be underestimated and deaths have been known. Chronic mucosal changes may be seen as pale bladder mucosa, epithelial thinning, edema, small arterioles, and telangiectasia, and calcification and sclerosing endarteritis with radiation therapy. Patients receiving cyclophosphamide require thorough evaluation because of the increased danger of malignant lesions – commonly traditional cell carcinomas, although markedly abnormal cytologies seen during treatment may be confusing. Bladder biopsies should be performed with caution because the mucosa heals poorly.

Frequently seen effects, often developing as many as 23 years later, are chronic cystitis with or without hemorrhage or infection, bladder fibrosis/contraction, atrophy, prevention of bladder development in the young, loss of voluntary sphincter control, and ureteral/urethral strictures. The latter may lead to peri-urethral abscesses in boys as a result of high peri-urethral pressure causing extravasation of infected urine. Morbidity related to treatment for severe HC in the form of cystotomy, cystectomy with urinary diversion, exsanguinating hemorrhage, and bladder tamponade, and the effects of intravesical alum instillation leading to fibrosis, bladder rupture, and fistula can result in renal failure, mental changes, and encephalopathy (Murphy et al. 1992; Leung et al. 2005).

References

(2004) Nursing drug handbook, 24th edn. Lippincott Williams & Wilkins, Philadelphia

Allwood M, Stanley A, Wright P (1997) The cytotoxics handbook, 3rd edn. Radcliffe Medical, Oxford

Alp H, Orbak Z, Altinkaynak S, Gundogyu C, Ertekin V, Kilic A (2002) Xanthogranulomatosis pyelonephritis presenting as intra-abdominal tumor in a child. Pediatrics international 44(4):453–455

Apozna ski W, Sawicz-Birkowska K, Jaworski W, Szydelko T, Gorczy ska E (2005) Haemorrhagic cystitis as a complication after allogenic bone marrow transplantation. European Journal of Pediatric Surgery 15:44–47

Aslam AF, Spicer R (1996) Needle tract recurrence after biopsy of non-metastatic Wilms tumor. Pediatric Surgery International 11:416

Beauchamp D, Labrecque G (2001) Aminoglycoside nephrotoxicity: do time and frequency of administration matter? Current Opinion in Critical Care 7(6):401–408

Bergstein JM (1996) Toxic nephropathies: renal failure, pp 1513–1514. In: Nelson W, Behrman R, Kliegman R, Arvin A (eds) Textbook of pediatrics, 15th edn. W.B. Saunders, Philadelphia

Borsi JD (1994a) Clinical pharmacology of anticancer drugs in children I. Antimetabolites. In: Pochedly C (ed) Neoplastic diseases of childhood, vol 1. Harwood Academic, Switzerland, p p 186

Borsi JD (1994b) Principles of administration and monitoring chemotherapy in children. In: Pochedly C (ed) Neoplastic diseases of childhood, vol 1. Harwood Academic, Switzerland, pp 175–181

Bratsas KS, Stephanides AA, Spyropoulos E, Zachariades BP, Androulakakis PA (2004) Hyperbaric oxygen therapy for cyclophosphamide induced refractory hemorrhagic cystitis in a child. Journal of Urology 172(2):679

Breitz H (2004) Clinical aspects of radiation nephropathy. Cancer biotherapy & radiopharmaceuticals 19(3):359–362

British Medical Association, Royal Pharmaceutical Society of Great Britain (2008) British National Formulary (BNF) 55. BMJ, London

Cachat F, Guignard JP (1996) The kidney in children under chemotherapy. Review Medicale de la Suisse Romande 116:985–993

Cassady JR (1995) Clinical radiation nephropathy. International Journal of Radiation Oncology, Biology, Physics 31:1249–1256

Cesaro S, Facchin C, Tridello G, Messina C, Calore E, Biasolo MA, Pillon M, Varotto S, Brugiolo A, Mengoli C, Palù G (2008) A prospective study of BK-virus-associated haemorrhagic cystitis in paediatric patients undergoing allogeneic haematopoietic stem cell transplantation. Bone Marrow Transplantation 41:363–370

Cohen EP, Lawton CA, Moulder JE (1995) Bone marrow transplant nephropathy: radiation nephritis revisited. Nephron 70(2):217–222

Connor TH, McDiarmid MA (2006) Preventing occupational exposures to antineoplastics drugs in health care settings. CA: A Cancer Journal for Clinicians 56(6):354–365

Doubek M, Mayer J, Horky D (2002) Safety of long-term administration of conventional amphotericin B in oncology patients. Casopsis Lekaru Ceskych 141(5):156–159

Duarte RJ, Dénes FT, Cristofani LM, Odone-Filho V, Srougi M (2006) Further experience with laparoscopic nephrectomy for Wilms' tumour after chemotherapy. British Journal of Urology 98(1):155–159

Ebb D, Green D, Shamberger R, Tarbell N (2001) Solid tumors of childhood, chapter 44.2. In: DeVita (ed) Principles and practice of oncology, 6th edn. Lippincott Williams & Wilkins, Philadelphia

Ehrlich PF (2007) Wilms tumor: progress and considerations for the surgeon. Surgical Oncology 16(3):157–171

Eisenberg S (2009) Safe handling and administration of antineoplastic chemotherapy. Journal of Infusion Nursing 32(1):23–32

Godzinski J, Weirich A, Tournade M-F, Gauthier F, Buerger D, Moorman-Voestermans CGM, De Kraker J, Voute P, Ludwig R, Sawicz-Birkowska K, Vujanic G, Ducourtieux M (2001) Primary nephrectomy for emergency: a rare event in the international society of paediatric oncology nephroblastoma trial and study no.9. European Journal of Pediatric Surgery 11(1):36–39

Gonzalez-Fraile MI, Canizo C, Caballero D, Hernandez R, Vazquez L, Lopez C, Izarra A, Arroyo JL, de la Loma A, Otero MJ, San Miguel JF (2001) Cidofovir treatment of human polyomavirus-associated acute haemorrhagic cystitis. Transplant Infectious Disease 3(1):44–46

Goren MP, Wright RK, Horowitz ME, Pratt CB (1987) Ifosfamide-induced subclinical tubular nephrotoxicity despite mesna. Cancer Treatment Reports 71(2):127–130

Haddy TB, Mosher R, Revonda B, Reaman G (2007) Hypertension and prehypertension in long-term survivors of childhood and adolescent cancer. Pediatric Blood & Cancer 49(1):79–83

Hadjibabaie M, Alimoghaddam K, Shamshiri AR, Iravani M, Mousavi A, Jahani M, Khodabandeh A, Anvari Y, Gholami GA (2008) Continuous bladder irrigation prevents hemorrhagic cystitis in allogeneic hematopoietic cell transplantation. Urologic Oncology 26(1):43–46

Hamilton TE, Green DM, Perlman EJ, Argani P, Grundy P, Ritchey ML, Shamberger RC (2006) Bilateral Wilms' tumor with anaplasia: lessons from the National Wilms' Tumor Study. Jornal of Pediatric Surgery 41(10):1641–1644

Harrell WB, Snow BW (2005) Minimally invasive pediatric nephrectomy. Current Opinion in Urology 15(4):277–281

Haselberger MB, Schwinghammer TL (1995) Efficacy of mesna for prevention of hemorrhagic cystitis after high-dose cyclophosphamide therapy. Annals of Pharmacotherapy 29(9):918–921

Huang WC, Levey AS, Serio M, Snyder M, Vickers AJ, Raj GV, Scardino P, Russo P (2006) Chronic kidney disease after nephrectomy in patients with renal cortical tumours: a retrospective cohort study. The Lancet Oncology 7(9):735–740

Igaki H, Katsuyuki K, Sukamaki H, Saito H, Nakagawa K, Ohtomo K, Tanaka Y (2005) Renal dysfunction after total-body irradiation. Significance of selective renal-shielding blocks. Strahlentherapie und Onkologie 181(11):704–708

Ignoffo RJ, Viele CS, Dallon LE, Venook A (1998) Cancer chemotherapy pocket guide. Lippincott-Raven, Philadelphia

Kubiak R, Gundeti M, Duffy PG, Ransley PG, Wilcox DT (2004) Renal function and outcome following salvage surgery for bilateral Wilms' tumor. Journal of Pediatric Surgery 39(11):1667–1672

Lall A, Pritchard-Jones K, Walker J, Hutton C, Stevens S, Azmy A, Carachi R (2006) Wilms' tumor with intracaval thrombus in the UK Children's Cancer Study Group UKW3 trial. Journal of Pediatric Surgery 41(2):382–387

Leung AY, Mak R, Lie AK, Yuen KY, Cheng VC, Liang R, Kwong YL (2002) Clinicopathological features and risk factors of clinically overt haemorrhagic cystitis complicating bone marrow transplantation. Bone Marrow Transplantation 29(6):509–513

Leung AYH, Yuen K-Y, Kwong Y-L (2005) Polyoma BK virus and haemorrhagic cystitis in haematopoietic stem cell transplantation : a changing paradigm. Bone Marrow Transplantation 36:929–937

Loebstein R, Atanackovic G, Bishai R, Wolpin J, Khattak S, Hashemi G, Gobrial M, Baruchel S, Ito S, Koren G (1999) Risk factors for long-term outcome of ifosfamide-induced nephrotoxicity in children. Journal of Clinical Pharmacology 39(5):454–461

Maas MH, Cransberg K, van Grotel M, Pieters R, van den Heuvel-Elbrink MM (2007) Renin-induced hypertension in Wilms tumor patients. Pediatric Blood & Cancer 48(5):500–503

Magrath I, Sandlund J, Raynor A, Rosenberg S, Arasi V, Miser J (1986) A phase II study of ifosfamide in the treatment of recurrent sarcomas in young people. Cancer Chemotherapy and Pharmacology 18(Suppl 2):S25–S28

Mitchell CD (2004) Wilms' tumor. In: Pinkerton CR, Plowman PN, Pieters R (eds) Paediatric oncology, 3rd edn. Arnold, London

Murphy CP, Cox RL, Harden EA, Stevens DA, Heye MM, Herzig RH (1992) Encephalopathy and seizures induced by intravesical alum irrigations. Bone Marrow Transplantation 10(4):383–385

Neonatal and Paediatric Pharmaceutical Group (2001) Medicines for children. RCPCH, London

Newell DR, Pearson ADJ, Balmanno K, Price L, Wyllie RA, Keir M, Calvert AH, Lewis IJ, Pinkerton CR, Stevens MC (1993) Carboplatin pharmacokinetics in children: the development of a pediatric dosing formula. The United Kingdom Children's Cancer Study Group. Journal of Clinical Oncology 11(12):2314–2323

Nies A, Spielberg S (1996) Principles of Therapeutics. In: Hardman J, Limbird L, Molinoff P, Ruddon R, Goodman Gilman A (eds) The pharmacological basis of therapeutics, 9th edn. McGraw-Hill, New York, p 50

Oyama Y, Komatsuda A, Imai H, Ohtani H, Kamai K, Wakini H, Miura AB, Nakamoto Y (1996) Late onset bone marrow transplant nephropathy. Internal Medicine 35:489–493

Paediatric Formulary Committee (2007) British National Formulary for children. BMJ, London

Palandri F, Bonifazi F, Rossi C, Falcioni S, Arpinati M, Giannini MB, Ansaloni F, Bandini G, Baccarani M (2005) Successful treatment of severe hemorrhagic cystitis with selective vesical artery embolization. Bone Marrow Transplantation 35(5):529–530

Relling MV, Schunk JE (1986) Drug-induced hemorrhagic cystitis. Clinical Pharmacy 5:590

Ritchey ML, Lally KP, Haase GM, Shochat SJ, Kelalis PP (1992) Superior mesenteric artery injury during nephrectomy for Wilms' tumor. Journal of Pediatric Surgery 27(5):612–615

Robbins ME, Diz DL (2006) Pathogenic role of the rennin-angiotensin system in modulating radiation-induced late effects. International Journal of Radiation Oncology, Biology, Physics 64(1):6–12

Schellens J (2005) Clinical implications and mechanisms of variability in the response to anti-cancer agents. In: Shellens J, McLeod H, Newell D (eds) Cancer clinical pharmacology. Oxford University Press, New York

Scurr M, Judson I, Root T (2005) Combination chemotherapy and chemotherapy principles. In: Brighton D, Wood M (eds) The royal marsden hospital handbook of cancer chemotherapy. Churchill Livingstone, Philadelphia

Skinner R, Pearson ADJ, English MW, Price L, Wyllie RA, Coulthard MG, Craft AW (1998) Cisplatin dose rate as a factor for nephrotoxicity in children. British Journal of Cancer 77(10):1677–1682

Summerhayes M, Daniels S (2003) Practical chemotherapy-a multidisciplinary guide. Radcliffe Medical, Oxon

Superfin D, Iannucci A, Davies A (2007) Commentary: oncologic drugs in patients with organ dysfunction: a summary. The Oncologist 12(9):1070–1083

Tortorice PV (1997) Chemotherapy: principles of therapy, p. 299–301. In: Groenwald S, Hansen Frogge M, Goodman M, Henke Yarbro C (eds) Cancer nursing: principles and practice, 4th edn. Jones and Bartlett, Sudbury, MA

Traxer O, Desgrandchamps F, Sebe P, Haab F, Le Duc A, Gattegno B, Thibault P (2001) [Hemorrhagic cystitis: etiology and treatment]. Progres en Urologie 11(4):591–601

Vassal G, Verschuur A (2005) The principles of cancer chemotherapy in children. In: Voûte P, Barrett A, Stevens M, Caron H (eds) Cancer in children – clinical management. Oxford University Press, Oxford

Walsh TJ, Finberg RW, Arndt C, Hiemenz J, Schwartz C, Bodensteiner D, Pappas P, Seibel N, Greenberg RN, Dummer S, Schuster M, Holcenberg JS, Dismukes WE (1999) Liposomal amphoterecin B for empirical therapy in patients with persistent fever and neutropenia. The New England Journal of Medicine 340(10):764–771

Wiener J, Coppes M, Ritchey M (1998) Current concepts in the biology and management of Wilms Tumor. Journal of Urology 159(4):1316–1325

Wiffen P, Mitchell M, Snelling M, Stoner N (eds) (2007) Oxford handbook of clinical pharmacy. Oxford University Press, Oxford

Will A (2006) Paediatric acquired von Willebrand syndrome. Haemophilia 12(3):287–288

Wood PA, Hrushesky WJM (1996) Circadian rhythms and cancer chemotherapy. Critical Reviews in Eukaryotic Gene Expression 6(4):299–343

Yamayoshi Y, Iida E, Tanigawara Y (2005) Cancer pharmacogenomics: international trends. International Journal of Clinical Oncology 10:5–13

Cardiovascular System

Alison Hall

Contents

22.1 Cardiac Toxicity/Cardiomyopathy 441
22.1.1 Incidence 441
22.1.1.1 Recommendations During Treatment 442
22.1.1.2 Modification of Chemotherapy 442
22.1.2 Etiology 443
22.1.3 Treatment 445
22.1.4 Prevention 445
22.1.4.1 Limiting the Effects of Myocardial Concentrations of Anthracyclines and Their Metabolites 445
22.1.4.2 Concurrent Administration of Cardioprotective Agents . . 446
22.1.4.3 Developing Less Cardiac Toxic Therapies. 446
22.1.4.4 Lifestyle Advice. 446
22.1.4.5 Guidelines for Long-Term Follow-Up 446
22.1.5 Prognosis 447
22.2 Veno-Occlusive Disease 447
22.2.1 Hepatic Veno-Occlusive Disease 447
22.2.1.1 Incidence 447
22.2.1.2 Diagnosis 448
22.2.1.3 Etiology 448
22.2.1.4 Treatment 448
22.2.1.5 Prevention. 449
22.2.1.6 Prognosis 449
22.2.2 Pulmonary Veno-Occlusive Disease . . . 449
22.2.2.1 Incidence 449
22.2.2.2 Etiology 450
22.2.2.3 Treatment 450
22.2.2.4 Diagnosis 450
22.2.2.5 Prognosis 450
References 450

22.1 Cardiac Toxicity/Cardiomyopathy

More than half of all new pediatric patients with malignancies will receive therapy with cardiotoxic agents (van Dalen et al. 2007). As the number of survivors increases, the number of survivors developing cardiotoxicity also increases. Cardiac toxicity occurs primarily as a result of treatment with anthracyclines. Doxorubicin and daunorubicin are cited as having the greatest cardiotoxicity, though this may be because their effects have been studied more and the cardiac effects of mitozantrone, idarubicin, and amsacrine are less well documented. Prior to any anthracycline therapy, baseline cardiac function tests (normally an echocardiogram) should be performed.

Anthracycline-induced cardiotoxicity can generally be divided into three categories: (1) acute changes, (2) early-onset, chronic progressive cardiomyopathy, and (3) late-onset chronic progressive cardiomyopathy. Cardiotoxicity can manifest itself in patients as sub-clinical and clinical heart failure. Sub-clinical heart failure is defined as cardiac abnormalities detected in asymptomatic persons by various diagnostics (Wouters et al. 2005). Abnormalities in cardiac function increase over time and cardiac toxicity occurring early (within 1 year of completion of therapy) carries the highest risk for development of late/progressive cardiotoxicity (Wouters et al. 2005).

22.1.1 Incidence

The use of anthracyclines in childhood leukemia has resulted in improved long-term prognosis; however, these patients are subsequently at high risk of developing long-term cardiac damage, with studies 1suggesting that as many as 65% of survivors of childhood leukemia will develop cardiac abnormalities (Elliott 2006). The incidence of cardiomyopathy in hematology/oncology patients is related to the cumulative anthracycline dose. Actual incidence figures vary, due to differing methods of evaluation, baselines, and doses used in the studies reported. One literature review of 25 published studies reported frequencies between 0 and 57% (Kremer et al. 2002). Incidence also varies between groups of diseases and is more common in children with Down's syndrome and AML (O'Brien et al. 2008). There is increasing evidence of sub-clinical cardiac toxicity (even after low doses of anthracyclines, e.g. 90–200 mg/m^2 doxorubicin) in children who appear asymptomatic by echocardiogram (Guimaraes-Filho et al. 2007). New methods are being proposed as more sensitive screening tests for cardiac abnormalities, and include dobutamine stress echocardiography (Lanzarini et al. 2000), B-Type Natriuretic Peptide Markers (Aggarwal et al. 2007; Soker and Kervancioglu 2005), and Multigated Radionuclide Angiography (Corapçioglu et al. 2006). However, these tests are not routinely performed.

General incidence is summarized in Table 22.1.

Table 22.1. Incidence of cardiomyopathy related to anthracycline dosage (Lanzkowsky 1999)

Cumulative anthracycline dose (mg/m^2)	Percentage of patients affected
<400	11
400–599	23
600–799	47
800	100

Table 22.2. Diagnostic cardiac function tests

Test	Result if damage is present
ECG	Heart block, tachycardia, and may have wave changes
Echocardiogram (the most common test)	Fractional shortening (SF) <30%
Radionuclide cardiac cineangiocardiography (RNA or MUGA) (this is rarely used in the UK, but useful in patients in whom a good echocardiogram cannot be obtained)	A left ventricular ejection fraction (LVEF) of <55% indicates abnormal systolic function

Table 22.3. Criteria for progressive deterioration of cardiac function

Test	Result
ECG	SF <29% or decreased by absolute value of 10% from previous test
RNA/ LVEF	Value <55% or decreased by absolute value of 10% from previous test or absolute value decreased with stress

Children should have ongoing cardiac function tests during and post treatment (see Tables 22.2 and 22.3).

22.1.1.1 Recommendations During Treatment

Owing to lack of specific evidence, there is ongoing discussion as to the universal guidelines that should be in place for this monitoring. At present, individual guidelines for children during treatment are defined in the majority of pediatric protocols. As a general rule, if the child's cumulative anthracycline dose exceeds 200 mg/m^2, testing should be carried out (by either echo or MUGA) before, during, and after treatment. During treatment, testing schedules vary in frequency but often increase with higher anthracycline doses; some children receive cardiology review prior to every dose of anthracycline.

22.1.1.2 Modification of Chemotherapy

As with on-treatment testing, modification therapy may vary between protocols. An example of possible modifications is given in Table 22.4. However, any modifications depend on the grade of toxicity and are

Table 22.4. Modification of therapy associated with cardiotoxicity (Lanzkowsky 1999)

Investigation	Action
Abnormal SF & RNA LVEF	Anthracycline therapy should be stopped. Recommence only when both results normal in two consecutive tests, 1 month apart
Abnormal SF or RNA LVEF	Temporary discontinuation of anthracycline therapy. Repeat both tests at 1 month. If one still abnormal but no further deterioration resume therapy

Table 22.5. Cardiac toxicity after high-dose chemotherapy (Bearman et al. 1988)

Grade of cardiac toxicity	Presentation
Grade 1	Mild ECG abnormality, not requiring medical intervention; or noted heart enlargement on chest X-ray with no clinical symptoms
Grade 2	Moderate ECG abnormalities requiring and responding to medical intervention; or requiring continuous monitoring without treatment, or congestive heart failure responsive to digitalis or diuretics
Grade 3	Severe ECG abnormalities with no or only partial response to medical intervention; or heart failure with no or only minor response to medical intervention; or decrease in voltage by more than 50%

usually done in consultation with a cardiologist. Toxicity grading is included in many protocols, most using either the Bearman grading, or the Common Terminology Criteria for Adverse Events Version 3.0 (CTCAE) provided in Tables 22.5 and 22.6, respectively.

22.1.2 Etiology

Anthracyclines are unique in their requirements for limiting cumulative dose and it is thought that both the cumulative and peak dose of anthracyclines (doxorubicin, daunorubicin, and epirubicin) affects the child's risk of cardiac toxicity (Chang and Towbin 2006). Anthracycline-induced cardiac toxicity usually manifests as congestive heart failure. Permanent changes in the myocardium, most consistent with the contractile failure of cardiomyopathy occur (Iarussi et al. 2000; Ruggiero et al. 2008). Rarely, acute cardiotoxicity that is dose-dependent occurs. This manifests as transient tachycardia, non-specific ECG changes, and atrio-ventricular and bundle branch blocks (Langebrake et al. 2002).

More commonly, the cardiac toxicity is from free-radical-mediated myocyte death resulting in decreased thickness of the heart wall and interstitial fibrosis (Lipshultz et al. 2008). Cardiac cells are more susceptible to free radical damage because of their highly oxidative metabolism and relatively poor antioxidant defences. Additionally, anthracyclines have a very high affinity for cardiolipin, a phospholipid in the inner mitochondrial membrane. This affinity results in anthracyclines accumulating inside cardiac cells (Wouters et al. 2005).

The heart is unable to adequately compensate to meet the demands of growth, pregnancy, or cardiac stress, thus leading to late onset anthracycline-induced cardiac failure. This is mainly a progressive disorder that manifests itself with the symptoms highlighted in Table 22.7.

There is evidence, owing to long-term follow-up care, that cardiac damage may only become apparent over time as children with late decompensation are now becoming apparent (van Dalen et al. 2007). There may be an initial period during which SF may even almost return to normal as surviving myocytes compensate, via hypertrophic changes, for acute myocyte loss (Wouters et al. 2005). Therefore, the loss in cardiac function would become apparent

Table 22.6. Summary of common terminology criteria for adverse events (Version 3) grading of cardiac toxicity (formerly Common Toxicity Criteria (CTC), Cancer Therapy Evaluation Program 2003)

Grade of cardiac toxicity	Conduction abnormality/ atrio-ventricular heart block	Prolonged QTc interval	Ventricular arrhythmia	Cardiac ischemia/ infarction	Hypotension	Hypertension (remark: Use age and gender-appropriate normal values >95th percentile ULN for paediatric patients)
Grade 0	Asymptomatic, intervention not indicated	QTc >0.45–0.47 s	Asymptomatic, no intervention indicated	Asymptomatic arterial narrowing without ischemia	Changes, intervention not indicated	Pediatric: asymptomatic, transient (<24 h) BP increase >ULN; intervention not indicated
Grade 1	Non-urgent medical intervention indicated	QTc >0.47–0.50 s; >0.06 s above baseline	Non-urgent medical intervention indicated	Asymptomatic and testing suggesting ischemia; stable angina	Brief (<24 h) fluid replacement or other therapy; no physiologic consequences	Pediatric: recurrent or persistent (>24 h) BP >ULN; monotherapy may be indicated
Grade 2	Incompletely controlled medically or controlled with device (e.g. pacemaker)	QTc >0.50 s	Symptomatic and incompletely controlled medically or controlled with device (e.g. defibrillator)	Symptomatic and testing consistent with ischemia; unstable angina; intervention indicated	Sustained (>24 h) therapy, resolves without persisting physiologic consequences	Requiring more than one drug or more intensive therapy than previously
Grade 3	Life-threatening (e.g. arrhythmia associated with CHF, hypotension, syncope, shock)	QTc >0.50 s; life-threatening signs or symptoms (e.g. arrhythmia, CHF, hypotension, shock syncope)	Life-threatening (e.g. arrhythmia associated with CHF, hypotension, syncope, shock)	Acute myocardial infarction	Shock (e.g. acidemia; impairment of vital organ function)	Life-threatening consequences (e.g. hypertensive crisis)
Grade 4	Death	Death	Death	Death	Death	Death

Table 22.7. Signs and symptoms of cardiotoxicity

Signs & symptoms of cardiotoxicity	Cause
Dysnoea, tiredness, exercise intolerance	Incapability of heart to supply oxygen demands of the body
Peripheral edema Pulmonary rales Hepatomegaly	Diminished blood flow and accumulation of excess blood in tissues and organs as heart is unable to adequately circulate blood volume

only as the "overworked" myocytes fail and there is lack of further myocyte growth.

Certain factors also enhance the myocardial toxicity of anthracyclines:

- Exposure to other cytotoxic chemotherapy agents: cyclophosphamid[1–22], amsacrine, dactinomycin, mitomycin, darcarbazine, vincristine, bleomycin, and methotrexate
- Underlying cardiac abnormalities (tumor, uncontrolled hypertension)
- Mediastinal radiation[2–22]
- <5 years at exposure
- Female gender

Septic episodes affect cardiac function by decreasing left ventricular function, but this decrease is often subsequently recoverable. Progression of symptoms may also occur with anesthesia, pregnancy, use of illegal drugs (especially stimulants), and alcohol (Carver et al. 2007).

22.1.3 Treatment

Currently, the optimal treatment of cardiomyopathy remains unclear and cardiology consultation should be obtained. Although an angiotensin converting enzyme inhibitor such as captopril or enalapril may demonstrate symptomatic relief (i.e. lowering sodium and water retention and decreasing afterload), any long-term benefits are yet to be reported.

22.1.4 Prevention

Attempts to decrease the cardiac toxicity of anthracyclines fall into four categories:

1. Limiting the effects of myocardial concentrations of anthracyclines and their metabolites.
2. Concurrent administration of cardioprotective agents.
3. Developing less cardiac toxic therapies.
4. Lifestyle advice (Scully and Lipshultz 2007).

22.1.4.1 Limiting the Effects of Myocardial Concentrations of Anthracyclines and Their Metabolites

The principles of maximum dosing should be applied (see Table 22.8).

When the child will receive radiation involving the cardiac region, careful discussion with the radiation oncologist is required.

Because of the thought that a lower peak of serum anthracycline would help to limit cardiotoxicity, prolonged infusion times became the norm in the absence

Table 22.8. Maximum dosing guides for cardiotoxic chemotherapeutic agents

Drug	Maximum cumulative dose per m2 (mg)
Doxorubicin	<450
Daunorubicin	<450
Idarubicin[a]	125
Mitoxantrone[a]	160[b]

[a] Maximum doses of idarubicin and mitoxantrone are not definitively known

[b] Patients who have received a cumulative dose of 450 mg/m² of doxorubicin should not receive mitoxantrone. Recommended cumulative dose of mitozantrone for patients who have received doxorubicin is 120 mg/m²

[1] Cyclophosphamide: Cyclophosphamide-induced cardiac effects occur primarily with myeloblative BMT regimens and are not chronic effects. The drug causes intramyocardial edema and hemorrhage, often in association with serosanguineous pericardial effusion and fibrous pericarditis.

[2] Radiation: Cardiac radiation doses of up to 25 Gy are generally felt to be safe; evidence is stronger for cardiac effects in later life at doses of over 30–35 Gy.

of randomized trials. Since then, the results of some randomized trials investigating infusion length have cast doubt on this theory (Lipshultz et al. 2002, 2008). Controversy surrounding this issue remains (Langebrake et al. 2002) and administration times vary between bolus; 1; 6 h and continual infusion over 48 h. Research has indicated no benefit between 48-h infusions and <1 h in leukemic children (Lipshultz et al. 2002). In 2003, the British Medical Research Council (MRC) has recommended 1-h infusions.

22.1.4.2 Concurrent Administration of Cardioprotective Agents

The use of potentially cardioprotective agents has been evaluated; however, to date in preliminary studies only dexrazoxane (ICRF-187) has proven protective against acute cardiotoxicity without decreasing anti-tumor effect (Langebrake et al. 2002). Long-term benefits remain to be seen. Dexrazoxane is thought to act by binding to both bound and free iron, hence reducing the formation of anthracycline–iron complexes and the generation of free radicals that are toxic to cardiac tissues (Lipshultz et al. 2008). Following systematic review, Bryant et al. (2007) and van Dalen et al. (2007) offer a guarded opinion on the use of dexrazoxane in pediatrics until further research is done including cost-effectiveness and to ensure that it does not limit the anti-tumor efficacy of anthracyclines.

22.1.4.3 Developing Less Cardiac Toxic Therapies

Newer cytotoxic agents are potentially less cardiotoxic. Incorporating anthracyclines into liposomes, such as liposomal daunorubicin, appears to reduce cardiac toxicity (Langebrake et al. 2002). There is insufficient evidence to make recommendations as it is too soon to assess the longer-term chronic cardiotoxicity in children treated with this drug (Langebrake et al. 2002).

22.1.4.4 Lifestyle Advice

Lifestyle choices and non-smoking advice should also be emphasized. Healthy nutrition and regular exercise could reduce the risk of cardiovascular disease in later life (Scully and Lipshultz 2007; Wouters et al. 2005). Survivors of childhood ALL are at risk of hypertension, obesity and dyslipidemia, insulin resistance, and cardiovascular disease (Oeffinger et al. 2001).

Survivors who wish to take part in competitive sports and those considering pregnancy should be advised to have detailed cardiac assessment beforehand. Patients with cardiomyopathy are at risk of ventricle arrhythmias and should have 24 h ECG monitoring on a regular basis, adhering to institutional long-term follow-up guidelines.

22.1.4.5 Guidelines for Long-Term Follow-Up

The Children's Oncology Group have agreed and developed guidelines for long-term follow-up, similar to those available from the Scottish Intercollegate Guidelines Network (SIGN 2004; Landier et al. 2006; Shankar et al. 2008).

Key elements in cardiovascular care for survivors of childhood cancer include:

1. Assessment of individualized risk for cardiovascular disease by obtaining detailed treatment histories regarding cumulative dose and type of anthracyclines used, field and dose of radiation, and age at time of therapy
2. Assessment of additional cardiovascular risk factors, including dyslipidemia, hypertension, obesity, and family history of coronary artery disease
3. Obtaining detailed review of symptoms related to cardiovascular disease, such as effort intolerance, chest pain, palpitations, and dyspnea
4. Monitor cardiac function at baseline and periodically. The same method of testing for evaluation of systolic function should be used for follow-up evaluations for comparison with previous results
5. Counsel regarding weight management, regular physical activity, smoking abstinence, and heart-healthy diet
6. Monitor cardiac function with pregnancy and general anesthesia (Shankar et al. 2008)

22.1.5 Prognosis

Late onset anthracycline-induced cardiomyopathy portends a poor prognosis. Risk of death from cardiac-related events is eight times higher for long-term survivors than for the normal population (Wouters et al. 2005). Heart transplantation may be considered, as an earlier study of cancer survivor cardiomyopathy patients since 1970 treated with a heart transplant showed a favorable (74%) 5-year survival rate (Levitt et al. 1996).

There are many ongoing clinical trials and long-term follow-up studies to evaluate the various aspects of cardiotoxicity and preventative treatments described here.

22.2 Veno-Occlusive Disease

22.2.1 Hepatic Veno-Occlusive Disease

Hepatic veno-occlusive disease (HVOD) occurs as a result of liver damage by pre-transplant conditioning regimens (i.e. chemotherapy and radiation). It is also, though rare, recognized following some standard dose cytotoxic chemotherapy regimens (Cecen et al. 2007). HVOD has also more recently been named by the more descriptive term Sinusoidal Obstruction Syndrome (Chen et al. 2008). It is characterized by fibrous narrowing and sclerosis of the endothelial lining of both the sinusoids and terminal hepatic venules, leading to necrosis of the hepatocytes. As the hepatic veins become increasingly occluded with cellular debris and the blood flow obstructed, the protein-rich fluid content of the blood leaks out into the peritoneal cavity causing ascites.

Hepatic VOD is one of the most common life-threatening regimen-related toxicity in allogeneic SCT. The severity of the VOD is normally diagnosed retrospectively. It can be termed:

- Mild – when it is self-limiting and requires no treatment
- Moderate – when symptomatic and requires treatment
- Severe – when the child has multi-system failure, it lasts for over 100 days, and/or the child dies (Qureshi et al. 2008)

22.2.1.1 Incidence

VOD usually occurs within the first 30 days of transplant. Incidence is approximately 20% of allogeneic transplants and 10% of autologous transplants, though some literature reviews report an incidence of up to 60% (Gharib et al. 2006), reflecting differing diagnostic criteria. Though incidence does not appear to have changed over the last 10 years (indicating the need for more effective prophylaxis), there has been a recent unexpected rise in the rate of VOD. This may be due, in part, to the higher proportion of children with advanced disease (an identified risk factor) being transplanted. Patients with VOD have complex clinical pictures; so there may be other contributing factors that we are, as yet, unaware of (Gharib et al. 2006). There are case reports of children developing VOD following standard treatment, in particular Wilm's tumors treated with dactinomycin (Chen et al. 2008) and rhabdomyosarcoma (Cecen et al. 2007).

Clinical criteria vary, but those developed in Baltimore and Seattle are the most recognized (I-lun Chen et al. 2008) (see Table 22.9).

Other signs and symptoms include:

- Edema
- Jaundice
- Refractory thrombocytopenia
- Increase in almine-transferase (ALT)
- Hypoalbuminemia
- Clotting abnormalities (e.g. raised aPPT)
- Abnormal renal function

In severe cases, the child may require dialysis and ventilation; renal impairment expands the ascites, elevating the diaphragm and increasing respiratory impairment leading to decreased consciousness level. Late signs and symptoms include encephalopathy, often indicating terminal illness. All other causes of hepatic dysfunction, such as graft versus host disease (GVHD) of the liver, and infection and chemical hepatitis must be excluded before a diagnosis of VOD is made. Of these four, only VOD presents with fluid retention and unexplained weight gain. Early detection and treatment of VOD may help to limit the damage to the liver and is best attained with strict

Table 22.9. Baltimore and Seattle criteria for clinical criteria associated with venous occlusive disease

Baltimore criteria	Modified Seattle criteria
At least two of the following features within day +20	Hyperilirubinemia >34.2 μmol/L before day +21 and at least two of the following
Hyperbilirubinemia >34.2 μmol/L	Hepatomegaly and right upper quadrant pain
Hepatomegaly and upper right quadrant pain	Ascites
Ascities and/or unexplained weight gain >2%	Weight gain >5% from baseline

intake and output measurement in addition to twice daily weight and abdominal girth measurements so that the staff recognize any rapid changes.

22.2.1.2 Diagnosis

Doppler ultrasound may demonstrate a reversal in hepatic portal venous flow. This is the preferred radiological technique as it is non-invasive. A trans-venous liver biopsy or liver biopsy may be performed, though this is used infrequently as the child may have clotting abnormalities and is likely to be thrombocytopenic. Hepatic venous pressure gradient (HVPG) may be measured if bleeding risk is high (a balloon-tip catheter can be used).

22.2.1.3 Etiology

Though the actual cause of VOD is unknown, there are some risk factors:

- Conditioning agents, especially in high doses (e.g. Busulfan).
- 6-Thioguanine and myelotard have been implicated and may cause concomitant effects with the use of other hepatic-toxic drugs, particularly the "Azoles."
- Total body irradiation (TBI)
- Pre-existing hepatitis (one of the most predictive)
- Elevated liver function tests (LFT)
- Fever or infection invading the liver (immediately pre-transplant)
- Female gender
- Refractory leukemia
- >15 years old
- Underlying metastatic liver tumor
- Positive serological CMV status
- Mismatched or unrelated allogeneic transplants
- Second transplant

22.2.1.4 Treatment

The management of the child with VOD primarily provides supportive care. There is little consensus among clinicians about when to start specific treatments (Reiss et al. 2002). Symptomatic ascites is treated with diuretics (e.g. frusemide (ferosamide) and spironalactone); however, albumin may be required concurrently to maintain intravascular volume.

If the child has gross ascites that is not responding to treatment, it may be necessary to perform paracentesis with intravascular colloid replacement. This may improve the child's respiratory function and comfort.

In severe and deteriorating VOD, non-randomized studies have shown that in a number of cases, treatment with recombinant tissue plasminogen activator (rTPA) has been successful (Vogelsang and Dalal 2002). However, as rTPA can cause overwhelming bleeding, during such treatment the child requires careful observation and monitoring. Defibrotide is now increasingly being used with promising results, and its advantage is that, unlike rTPA, it causes no systemic anticoagulant effect (Qureshi et al. 2008; Bulley et al. 2007).

Adequate pain relief (s.c./i.v. morphine if necessary) is important. Observation should be made for petechiae, bleeding, and respiratory function. Platelets, albumin, and Fresh Frozen Plasma should be given as required and the platelet level should be kept above 20×10^9/L if possible.

Fluid volume and sodium content must be restricted and an accurate fluid balance chart is essential. Blood product infusions may or may not be included in the fluid intake depending on the institution; some centers restrict fluids to 75% of maintenance (using minimum drug dilutions and flushes) and maximize caloric intake (e.g. parenteral nutrition). Fluid balance should be calculated frequently (e.g. every 2 h). If in positive fluid balance, the child's weight, respirations, and blood pressure should be monitored and medical staff informed. Twice daily weights and abdominal girths should continue to be charted.

Blood pressure should be monitored every 4 h. Daily blood tests should include coagulation and LFT. Support and education for the child and family should be provided.

22.2.1.5 Prevention

Lower total doses of TBI or shielding of the liver during TBI[3–22] and the use of T-cell depleted marrow may all reduce VOD toxicity. Some studies have shown that heparin and low molecular weight heparin appears useful in preventing VOD but that this approach requires further study in the pediatric setting (Gharib et al. 2006). It is thought that the risk of VOD may also be reduced by dose adjusting the child's Busulfan regimen depending on their plasma Busulfan levels (Gharib et al. 2006). The most recent European Bone Marrow Transplant group (EBMT) trial is a prospective study looking into the incidence and outcomes of VOD with prophylactic use of defibrotide in the pediatric stem cell transplant setting.

Oral ursodeoxycholic acid (ursodiol) has been reported to reduce the incidence of non-fatal VOD in both randomized and historical control studies (Vogelsang et al. 2002). Many centers start ursodiol at a dose around 300 mg/m²/day in 2–3 divided doses, during conditioning and continuing until between day +28 and 80 depending on disease and regimen.

All compatible IV drugs should be administered with 5% dextrose (rather than 0.9% sodium chloride) to reduce the sodium load. Some centers test urinary sodium daily as an early warning sign. Scrupulous attention is required regarding intake and output; this, alongside twice-daily weight and abdominal girth charting, is a useful factor in early detection of the rapid weight gain and fluid retention indicative of VOD.

[3] In the setting of BMT for leukemia, this is difficult.

22.2.1.6 Prognosis

The outcome from VOD ranges from full recovery to hepatic failure and death. Differing classification of VOD has led to a great disparity in reported outcomes. In some studies, death rates of up to 47% have been reported (Reiss et al. 2002).

The severity of pathological change in the liver directly correlates with the severity of clinical symptoms the child presents. Classification of severity has sometimes been made retrospectively. Death before day +100 with ongoing VOD, or persistent VOD after day +100, is classed as severe and all other cases mild/moderate (McDonald et al., cited in Reiss et al. 2002).

Despite enhanced knowledge in the pathogenesis of VOD, overall incidence remains similar and the consequences severe. Research continues with regard to etiology, pathogenesis, prevention, and cure.

22.2.2 Pulmonary Veno-Occlusive Disease

Pulmonary veno-occlusive disease (PVOD) mainly affects children and young adults (Schwarz et al. 2005). PVOD causes pulmonary hypertension resembling the clinical picture of right-sided heart failure and pulmonary arterial hypertension. Fibrosis and thrombi narrow the pulmonary venules and veins leading to alveolar edema and hypertrophy of pulmonary arteries.

22.2.2.1 Incidence

PVOD is rare; literature reports it accounting for less than 10% of the 1–2 per million cases of primary pulmonary hypertension cases (Trobaugh-Lotrarion et al. 2003).

22.2.2.2 Etiology

Most cases are idiopathic. Several theories have been proposed, with viral infection being thought to be important (Schwarz et al. 2005); connective tissue disease, HIV, BMT, sarcoidosis, and pulmonary Langerhans cell granulomatosis are also cited (Montani et al. 2009). There remains paucity of literature on PVOD with 40 cases being reported in oncology patients between 1983 and 2003 (Trobaugh-Lotrarion et al. 2003).

22.2.2.3 Treatment

There is no definitive treatment for PVOD. Anticoagulation therapy, azathioprine, nifedipine, steroids, and treatment of infection have all been used with limited success. Lung transplantation may offer some hope, but patients do not tend to survive until a suitable donor would be available.

22.2.2.4 Diagnosis

It is difficult to diagnose PVOD antemortum. A chest X-ray commonly reveals signs of cardiac failure including cardiomegaly, dilated pulmonary arteries, pleural effusions, and Kerley B Lines (thin linear pulmonary opacities caused by fluid or cellular infiltration into the interstitium of the lungs). Dyspnea is a common symptom. PVOD can be diagnosed by lung biopsy. There are no conclusive blood tests for PVOD.

22.2.2.5 Prognosis

Most patients with PVOD die within 2 years of diagnosis. In the 40 reported cases in oncology patients, there were 4 survivors (Trobaugh-Lotrarion et al. 2003). Lung transplantation may be the treatment of choice (Montani et al. 2009).

References

Aggarwal S, Pettersen MD, Bhambhani K, Gurczynski J, Thomas R, L'Ecuyer T (2007) B-type natriuretic peptide as a marker for cardiac dysfunction in anthracycline-treated children. Pediatric Blood and Cancer 49(6):812–816

Bearman SI, Appelbaum FR, Buckner CD, Peterson FB, Fischer LD, Clift RA, Thomas ED (1988) Regimen-related toxicity in patients undergoing bone marrow transplantation. Journal of Clinical Oncology 6(10):1562–1568

Bryant J, Picot J, Baxter L, Levitt G, Sullivan I, Clegg A (2007) Clinical and cost-effectiveness of cardioprotection against the toxic effects of anthracyclines given to children with cancer: a systematic review. British Journal of Cancer 96(2):226–230

Bulley SR, Strahm B, Doyle J, Dupuis LL (2007) Defibrotide for the treatment of hepatic veno-occlusive disease in children. Pediatric Blood and Cancer 48(7):700–704

Cancer Therapy Evaluation Program (2003) Common terminology criteria for adverse events, version 3.0, DCTD, NCI, NIH, DHHS. http://ctep.cancer.gov. Accessed 10 June 2008

Carver JR, Shapiro CL, Ng A, ASCO Cancer Survivourship Expert Panel et al (2007) American Society of Clinical Oncology clinical evidence review on the ongoing care of adult cancer survivours: cardiac and pulmonary late effects. Journal of Clinical Oncology 25:3991–4008

Cecen E, Uysal KM, Ozguven A, Gunes D, Irken G, Olgun N (2007) Veno-occlusive disease in a child with rhabdomyosarcoma after conventional chemotherapy Pediatric Haematology and Oncology 24:615–621

Chang C, Towbin JA (2006) Heart failure in children and young adults. Saunders Elsevier, Philadelphia

Chen IL, Yang SN, Hsiao CC, Wu KS, Sheen JM (2008) Treatment with high-dose methylprednisolone for hepatic veno-occlusive disease in a child with rhabdomyosarcoma. Pediatric Neonatology 49(4):141–144

Corapçioglu F, Sarper N, Berk F, Sahin T, Zengin E, Demir H (2006) Evaluation of anthracycline-induced early left ventricular dysfunction in children with cancer: a comparative study with echocardiography and multigated radionuclide angiography. Pediatric Hematology and Oncology 23(1):71–80

Elliott P (2006) Pathogenesis of cardiotoxicity induced by anthracyclines. Seminars in Oncology 33(3 Suppl 8):S2–S7

Gharib MI, Bulley SR, Doyle JJ, Wynn RF (2006) Venous occlusive disease in children thrombosis Research 118:27–38

Guimaraes-Filho F, Tan D, Braga J, Rodrigues A, Waib P, Matsubara B (2007) Ventricular systolic reserve in asymptomatic children previously treated with low doses of anthracyclines. American Journal of Cardiology 100(8): 1303–1306

Iarussi D, Indolfi P, Galderisi M, Bossone E (2000) Cardiac toxicity after anthracycline chemotherapy in childhood. Herz 25(7):676–688

Kremer LC, van der Pal HJ, Offringa M, van Dalen EC, Voute PA (2002) Frequency and risk factors of subclinical cardiotoxicity after anthracycline therapy in children: a systemic review. Annals of Oncology 13(6):819–829

Landier W, Wallace WH, Hudson MM (2006) Long-term follow-up of pediatric cancer survivors: education, surveillance, and screening. Pediatric Blood and Cancer 46(2):149–158

Langebrake C, Reinhardt D, Ritter J (2002) Minimising the long-term adverse effects of childhood leukaemia therapy. Drug Safety 25(15):1057–1077

Lanzarini L, Bossi G, Laudisa ML, Klersy C, Arico M (2000) Lack of clinically significant cardiac dysfunction during intermediate dobutamine doses in long-term childhood cancer survivors exposed to anthracyclines. American Heart Journal 140(2):315–323

Lanzkowsky P (1999) Manual of pediatric hematology, 3rd edn. Academic Press, London

Levitt G, Bunch K, Rogers CA, Whitehead B (1996) Cardiac transplantation in childhood cancer survivors in Great Britain. European Journal of Cancer 32A(5):826–830

Lipshultz SE, Alvarez JA, Scully RE (2008) Anthracycline associated cardiotoxicity in survivors of childhood cancer. Heart 94:525–533

Lipshultz SE, Giantris AL, Lipshultz SR, Kimball Dalton V, Asselin BL, Barr RD et al (2002) Doxorubicin administration by continuous infusion is not cardioprotective: the Dana-Farber 91-01 Acute lymphoblastic leukemia protocol. Journal of Clinical Oncology 20(6):1677–1682

Montani D, Price LC, Dorfmuller P, Achouh L, Jais X, Sitbon O, Musset D, Simonneau G, Humbert M (2009) Pulmonary veno-occlusive disease. European Repiratory Journal 33: 189–200

O'Brien MM, Taub JW, Chang MN, Massey GV, Stine KC, Raimondi SC, Becton D, Ravindranath Y, Dahl GV, Children's Oncology Group Study POG 9421 (2008) Cardiomyopathy in children with Down syndrome treated for acute myeloid leukemia: a report from the Children's Oncology Group Study POG 9421. Journal of Clinical Oncology 26(3):414–20

Oeffinger KC, Buchanan GR, Eshelman DA, Denke MA, Andrews C, Germak JA, Tomlinson GE, Snell LE, Foster BM (2001) Cardiovascular risk factors in young adult survivors of childhood acute lymphoblastic leukemia Journal of Pediatric Hematology/Oncology 23(7):424–430

Qureshi A, Marshall L, Lancaster D (2008) Defibrotide in the prevention and treatment of veno-occlusive disease in autologous and allogenic stem cell transplantation in children. Pediatric Blood and Cancer 50:831–832

Reiss U, Cowan M, McMillan A, Horn B (2002) Hepatic venoocclusive disease in blood and bone marrow transplantation in children and young adults: incidence, risk factors and outcome in a Cohort of 241 Patients. Journal of Pediatric Hematology and Oncology 24(9):746–750

Ruggiero A, Ridola V, Puma N, Molinari F, Coccia P, De Rosa G, Riccardi R (2008) Anthracycline cardiotoxicity in childhood. Pediatric Hematology and Oncology 25(4):261–281

Schwarz MI, Collard HR, King TE (2005) Diffuse alveolar hemorrage and other rare infiltrative disorders. In: Mason RJ, Murray J, Broaddus VC, Nadel J (eds) Murray & Nadel's textbook of respiratory medicine, 4th edn. WB Saunders, Philadelphiam, chapter 56

Scully RE, Lipshultz SE (2007) Anthracycline cardiotoxicity in long-term survivors of childhood cancer. Cardiovascular Toxicology 7(2):122–128

Shankar SM, Marina N, Hudson MM, Hodgson DC, Adams MJ, Landier W, Bhatia S, Meeske K, Chen MH, Kinahan KE, Steinberger J, Rosenthal D, Cardiovascular Disease Task Force of the Children's Oncology Group (2008) Monitoring for cardiovascular disease in survivors of childhood cancer: report from the Cardiovascular Disease Task Force of the Children's Oncology Group. Pediatrics 121(2):e387–e396

Scottish Intercollegiate Guidelines Network (SIGN) (2004) Long term follow-up of survivors of childhood cancer: a national clinical guideline. http://www.sign.ac.uk/pdf/sign76.pdf Accessed March 2009

Soker M, Kervancioglu M (2005) Plasma concentrations of NT-pro-BNP and cardiac troponin-I in relation to doxorubicin-induced cardiomyopathy and cardiac function in childhood malignancy. Saudi Medical Journal 26(8):1197–1202

Trobaugh-Lotrarion A, Greffe B, Deterding R, Deutsch G, Quinones R (2003) Pulmonary veno-occlusive disease after autologous bone marrow transplant in a child with stage IV neuroblastoma: case report and literature review. Journal of Pediatric Hematology and Oncology 25(5): 405–409

van Dalen EC, Caron HN, Kremer LCM (2007) Prevention of anthracycline-induced cardiotoxicity in children: The evidence. European Journal of Cancer 43:1134–1140

Vogelsang GB, Dalal J (2002) Hepatic venoocclusive disease in blood and bone marrow transplantation in children: incidence risk factors and outcome. Journal of Pediatric Hematology and Oncology 24(9):706–709

Wouters KA, Kremer LC, Miller TL, Herman EH, Lipshultz SE (2005) Protecting against anthracycline-induced myocardial damage: a review of the most promising strategies. British Journal of Haematology 131(5):561–578

Central Nervous System

Jane Belmore • Deborah Tomlinson

Contents

23.1 **Spinal Cord Compression** 453
- 23.1.1 Incidence 453
- 23.1.2 Etiology 453
- 23.1.3 Treatment 454
- 23.1.4 Prognosis 454

23.2 **Fatigue** 454
- 23.2.1 Incidence 455
- 23.2.2 Etiology 455
- 23.2.3 Treatment 456
- 23.2.4 Prognosis 457

23.3 **Cognitive Deficits** 458
- 23.3.1 Incidence 458
- 23.3.2 Etiology 458
- 23.3.3 Prevention and Treatment 458
- 23.3.4 Prognosis 459

23.4 **Diabetes Insipidus** 459
- 23.4.1 Incidence 459
- 23.4.2 Etiology 460
- 23.4.3 Treatment 460
- 23.4.4 Prognosis 460

References 460

23.1 Spinal Cord Compression

23.1.1 Incidence

SCC is uncommon in children. Consequently, there is a paucity in the data concerning SCC in children; however, it has been reported to occur in 2.7–5% of children with cancer and in 4% of children at diagnosis of cancer (Kelly and Lange 1997).

SCC is most common in terminal stages of metastatic cancer, but 25–35% of cases occur as a presenting complaint, usually due to extension of a paravertebral neuroblastoma, Ewing's sarcoma, non-Hodgkin's lymphoma (NHL), or Hodgkin's disease through one or more intravertebral foramina – known as the "dumbbell tumor" (Nicolin 2002). SCC can also present as a manifestation of tumor recurrence that is most commonly seen in children with rhabdomyosarcoma or osteosarcoma.

23.1.2 Etiology

SCC occurs when the extension of a local or metastatic tumor invades the epidural space and compresses the cord along any part of the spine (Colen 2008). This causes compression of the vertebral venous plexus, leading to vasogenic edema, venous hemorrhage, demyelination, and ischemic cell death.

Presenting features of SCC include:

1. Back, neck, or leg pain
   - Localized: aching and dull, may be constant
   - Radicular: burning or shooting sensation caused by nerve root compression
2. Weakness or paralysis – limbs may feel weak or heavy

3. Localized spine tenderness
4. Sphincter disturbances – urinary retention or constipation or incontinence
5. Sensory disturbances – (difficult to ascertain in young children). May include numbness, tingling, inability to differentiate sharp and dull sensations
6. Gait disturbances – unsteady gait or ataxia (Nicolin 2002; Haut 2005; Marrs 2006; Colen 2008).

Back pain is unusual in children and should be investigated promptly. Pain may be aggravated by movement, neck flexion, or a recumbent position. Children with cancer and back pain should be considered to have SCC until proven otherwise. The more common cancers in children associated with SCC include non-Hodgkin lymphoma, sarcomas, and renal tumors. Local or radicular back pain occurs in 80% of children with cord compression. Pain can start weeks to months before diagnosis (Marrs 2006).

Any child who was previously ambulatory but is no longer ambulatory at the time of clinical presentation, independent of the duration of the dysfunction before evaluation, should undergo imaging immediately (Rheingold and Lange 2006).

Magnetic resonance imaging (MRI) is the preferred diagnostic imaging because radiographs are abnormal in only one-third of cases (Nicolin 2002; Marrs 2006). MRI gives high-quality images of the spinal cord, epidural space, and paravertebral areas.

If possible, lumbar puncture (LP) should not be performed until diagnostic imaging is completed when SCC is suspected due to the risk of impaction of the cord (spinal coning). If LP needs to be done urgently, close neurological monitoring is essential.

23.1.3 Treatment

The goal of emergency treatment of SCC is to restore neurological function and avoid irreversible neurologic damage. When SCC is confirmed, intravenous dexamethasone 1 mg/kg infused over 30 min should be administered. Further doses may be required over several days. Cases without neurological deficits may be given a lower dose of dexamethasone, 0.25–0.5 mg/kg orally every 6 h. Doses are empiric, and large doses of dexamethasone are not justified (Marrs 2006; Colen 2008).

Surgical debulking of the tumor may be necessary through laminectomy (removal of the posterior arch of the spinal canal) (Acquaviva et al. 2003). These procedures often lead to later problems, such as nerve damage, with further reconstructive spinal treatments required. Osteoplastic laminotomies, followed by orthopedic bracing for 6–8 weeks, are now the preference of some surgeons. Long-term incidence of deformities with this procedure has not yet been established.

If diagnosis has been confirmed, radiotherapy can be used in radiosensitive tumors (Nguyen et al. 2000). Low-dose radiotherapy is recommended because spinal radiation >2,000 cGy can cause late scoliosis and kyphosis, particularly in young children. Chemotherapy is also effective in relieving pressure on the spinal cord from chemosensitive tumors, such as neuroblastoma, NHL, Hodgkin's disease, and Ewing's sarcoma. Chemotherapy has the advantages of avoiding long-term deformities and gaining control of the cancer at the primary or metastatic sites.

23.1.4 Prognosis

The neurologic outcome for these children depends on the extent of cancer at diagnosis and the response to treatment.

Quality of life, however, depends on neurological recovery, which is related to the degree of disability at diagnosis. In turn, this is associated with the duration of symptoms and time to diagnosis. Patients who are ambulatory at diagnosis generally remain ambulatory, and about half of the children who are nonambulatory at diagnosis regain ability (Marrs 2006). Immediate treatment is essential.

23.2 Fatigue

A study carried out at two major cancer centers in the southern United States arrived at a definition for fatigue in children and adolescents with cancer after conducing focus group interviews with patients, parents, and healthcare providers. *Fatigue is a profound sense of being tired or having difficulty with movement, such as using arms and legs or opening eyes, and is influenced by environmental, personal/social, and treatment-related factors and can result in difficulties with play, concentration, and negative emotions, most typically anger and sadness* (Hockenberry-Eaton et al. 1999; Hockenberry et al. 2003). The profound sense of tiredness can be acute, episodic, or chronic, and is relieved by rest and distraction.

Seminal studies that investigate fatigue in adolescents are helping to influence healthcare professionals to acknowledge fatigue as a life-altering symptom that should be addressed in the planning of care for these children and adolescents (Hinds et al. 1999; Gibson et al. 2003; Davies et al. 2002; Hockenberry-Eaton et al. 1998; Langeveld et al. 2000).

23.2.1 Incidence

Healthy people seldom regard fatigue as a serious problem because it is usually a temporary phenomenon; however, for those with cancer, it is a chronic and frequently relentless symptom.

The actual incidence of fatigue in children or adolescents treated for cancer is unreported. It is acknowledged that fatigue is probably underrecognized and undertreated despite it being a prevalent problem in the pediatric population (White 2001). Data gained from a small-scale exploratory study conducted with cohorts of adolescents suggested that fatigue can be a considerable problem for adolescents during and after treatment, and it may not abate quickly (Ream et al. 2006). Fatigue is often reported as overwhelming by adolescents receiving treatment (Gibson et al. 2003); however, some individuals perceived that their quality of life remained compromised many years after treatment and it seemed that fatigue might play an important part in this (Gibson et al. 2003; Ream et al. 2006).

23.2.2 Etiology

The etiology of this type of fatigue is complex. There can be many contributing factors in the cause of this type of fatigue:

1. Physiological

Physiological causes include anemia, nutritional status, and biochemical changes secondary to disease and treatment. Fatigue may be attributed to bone marrow transplantation, surgery, radiation, or/and chemotherapy. Treatment for childhood cancer is aggressive, with every effort made to administer maximum doses of therapy when possible. Unlike adult regimens, dose-limiting parameters do not include fatigue as a side effect. A study by Hinds and colleagues (2007a) also indicated that dexamethasone treatment significantly altered sleep duration, nocturnal wakenings, and daily naps in children and adolescents with acute lymphoblastic leukemia (ALL). Therefore, dexamethasone was associated with behavioral responses of altered sleep and increased fatigue (Hinds et al. 2007a).

Young children may be unaware of changes in their physical stamina and activities of daily living, while parents and older children/adolescents may simply accept their fatigue and lack of energy as a consequence of having cancer.

2. Psychological

Anxiety and depression can lead to fatigue (Langeveld et al. 2000). These are complex issues because fatigue may be due to a depressed mood, or people may become depressed if they perceive that they are constantly fatigued (Langeveld et al. 2000). Additionally, depression and fatigue may co-occur in cancer patients, as they can both originate from the same pathology (Whitsett et al. 2008).

3. Situational

Sleep patterns are frequently changed, especially during hospital admission, which can be a contributing factor to fatigue. Some hospitalized patients experience 20 or more nocturnal awakenings (Hinds et al. 2007b).

The causes of fatigue and their contributing factors identified by children are listed in Table 23.1. Adolescents recognized the following as reasons for fatigue:

- Noise while hospitalized
- Inability to sleep
- Feeling upset

Table 23.1. Causes of fatigue identified by children (Hockenberry-Eaton et al. 1999)

Cause of fatigue	Contributing factors
Treatment	Chemotherapy, radiation, surgery Fatigue associated with being sick
Being active	Easily tired after play and activities
Pain	Being tired when experiencing discomfort such as pain
Hospital environment	Noises, frequent interruptions, location of bed. Trouble falling asleep
Sleep changes	Sleep patterns change making it hard to get to sleep or sleep all night
Low counts	Feeling tired when experiencing myelosuppression

- Fear
- Effects of treatment
- Boredom

(Hockenberry-Eaton et al. 1999)
Parents stated the following factors:

- Hospital sounds
- Interruptions
- Waiting
- Needing to interact with too many individuals

A study by Davies et al. (2002) found that children with cancer may experience three subjectively distinct types of tiredness: typical tiredness, treatment fatigue, and shutdown fatigue. Hospitalized children and adolescents with cancer who experience more nocturnal awakenings are more fatigued and sleep longer than they would at home (Hinds et al. 2007b).

23.2.3 Treatment

Because fatigue is commonly unrecognized in this patient population, interventions need to begin with an educational component that provides patients, parents, and staff with critical information about diagnosing fatigue and describing the type of fatigue experienced. It is only once the type of fatigue, i.e., physiological, psycological, and situational (see previous section), is identified that interventions can then be suggested. Precursors to fatigue identified in various studies have included physical, environmental, mental, and psychological causes that have implications for clinical care (Davies et al. 2002).

Cancer and cancer treatment can place an increasing demand on the child's energy. Fatigue may also be an issue related to mental health for pediatric oncology patients. Some of the common symptoms of fatigue may be misinterpreted as indications of depression. After careful nursing assessment for signs of fatigue vs. depression, the child/adolescent may need to be referred to the mental health team. This assessment may involve obtaining the views of parents/caregivers as it has been reported that children who identified themselves as depressed (in contrast to fatigued) were viewed by their parents as being more quiet/non-talkative compared with children who were highly fatigued (Whitsett et al. 2008). The relationship between nutrition and fatigue is also a concern because inadequate nutrition and anorexia can affect the child's energy levels. Efforts to optimize nutritional status, by concentrating on the pleasurable, rather than just nutritional, aspect of eating, can help support children through the potential for fatigue (Gibson et al. 2005).

An improved understanding of the contributing and alleviating factors associated with fatigue in this patient population will provide children with greater comfort during treatment. Within the plethora of information the families receive during treatment of their child's cancer, it is important for the nurse to discuss fatigue as a symptom both during and after treatment. Awareness of interventions that will decrease fatigue can also be discussed, both for the hospital and for the home. In the study by Hockenberry-Eaton et al. (1998), children and adolescents reported factors that may help overcome fatigue (see Table 23.2).

The realization that the hospital environment can be a major contributor to fatigue in children and adolescents is important. Awareness that fatigue during hospitalization occurs because of disrupted sleep due to noises, frequent interruptions, and even the location of the room can stimulate thoughts and ideas on how to make the hospital setting more conducive to rest and sleep.

Table 23.3 gives examples of nursing interventions that can relate to fatigue-alleviating factors (Hinds and Hockenberry-Eaton 2001).

Table 23.2. Children's and adolescents' description of what helps overcome fatigue (Hockenberry-Eaton et al. 1999)

Reported methods of help to overcome fatigue	Explanation
Naps/sleep	Resting during the day and night
Visitors	Someone coming to visit may help
Fun/activities	Going to the movies/listening to music/reading a book
Blood transfusion	Can re-energize
Protected rest time	Not getting interrupted during rest times
Going outside	Outside to enjoy the day and get some fresh air
Having fun	Doing something they like in hospital and at home

23.2.4 Prognosis

Any effort to define, measure, and decrease fatigue needs to take into consideration the major components of these children's and adolescents' treatment context. These components are multifactorial and can include hospitalization for treatment, which disturbs sleep patterns, and treatment with drugs such as dexamethasone. Fatigue is a problem for many long-term survivors of childhood cancer and may be multifactorial in nature. Fatigue may be associated with certain late effects of chemotherapy, including irreversible cardiac and pulmonary toxicities. Efforts should focus on educating survivors to avoid factors that may contribute to fatigue, such as lack of physical activity and lack of mental stimulation, disrupted sleep patterns (Gibson et al. 2005).

Most young children seem to recover their energy levels fairly quickly even between pulses of chemotherapy, whereas adolescents seem to take much longer to recover. Those who seem at risk of trying to fight off fatigue in the long term are those adolescents who have had some form of myeloblative therapy. Follow-up treatment for these patients can be lengthy, requiring many outpatient visits, which in turn can lead to psychological and physical distress that may manifest itself as increasing fatigue (Gibson et al. 2005).

As future work is carried out regarding fatigue in pediatric oncology patients, nurses should improve their understanding of the individuals' experiences and ultimately provide them with a greater sense of understanding and comfort during treatment for their cancer.

Table 23.3. Nursing interventions in the alleviation of fatigue (Hinds and Hockenberry-Eaton 2001)

Factor	Interventions
Hospital environment	Decrease unit noise levels Group nursing activities together Implement protected rest times Maintain quiet hours at the nurses' station
Personal/behavioral	Establish a routine/schedule in the hospital setting Offer choices in relation to care where possible Provide activities to prevent boredom in the hospital setting Encourage participation of care in a positive manner
Treatment-related	Assess the need for blood transfusion Consider physical exercise as part of the daily hospital schedule Support nutritional needs Manage other side effects that may enhance fatigue
Cultural/family/other	Educate families on the symptom of fatigue Inform parents that children/adolescents receive cues from their behavior Promote visits by family and friends Encourage quiet activities that expend minimal energy

23.3 Cognitive Deficits

23.3.1 Incidence

It is generally accepted that CNS treatments for childhood cancer can result in significant cognitive impairment, most commonly in the areas of attention and concentration. Neurocognitive problems are most frequently observed in survivors of ALL and brain tumors (Nathan et al. 2007).

Kingma et al. (2000) found that MRI of the brain revealed abnormalities, including cortical and subcortical white matter damage, in 63% of cases of children treated for ALL who received cranial irradiation and intrathecal methotrexate. However, there is no evidence to support the routine use of these imaging studies in survivors as it has no effect on management (Nathan et al. 2007). Resultant cognitive impairment is commonly manifested as lower intelligence (IQ) and memory capacity and poorer academic achievement and visual-motor functioning (Reimers et al. 2007). It would appear that there may be an ongoing decline in abilities over time, with plausible explanation including the disruption of aspects of attention, working memory, and learning that are necessary for the acquisition of new skills or the initiation of a process of neuronal damage by the cancer or its treatment that continues after the therapy is completed (Nathan et al. 2007).

The most important antecedent factors precipitating cognitive late effects in long-term survivors of childhood cancer are listed in Table 23.4.

23.3.2 Etiology

Damage to the CNS may result from the cancer (primary brain tumor, brain metastases, or CNS involvement of leukemia or lymphoma) or its treatment (cranial irradiation, cytotoxic drugs that penetrate the brain or cerebrospinal fluid, or surgery) (Nathan et al. 2007). The chemotherapy drugs most often associated with neurocognitive impairment are methotrexate, corticosteroids, and cytarabine (Nathan et al. 2007). There is evidence that children who have received cranial irradiation for treatment of ALL are likely to have resulting cognitive deficits (Moore et al. 2000; Precourt et al. 2002). Cranial irradiation of 18 Gy, in combination with methotrexate therapy, has been reported to show deficits in attention, concentration, and ability of sequencing and processing for survivors of ALL therapy (Langer et al. 2002).

Neuroradiological signs in ALL survivors include brain abnormalities such as calcification, white matter changes, and parenchymal atrophy. The underlying cerebral pathology includes necrotizing leucoencephalopathy and mineralizing microangiopathy.

23.3.3 Prevention and Treatment

CNS irradiation has been eliminated from most treatment protocols, particularly for infants and toddlers, and the avoidance of prophylactic CNS irradiation in low-risk patients is recommended (Langer et al. 2002). Although recent protocols for treatment of brain tumors have resumed cranial irradiation in young children to decrease the risk of disease recurrence, the field of irradiation is restricted to a smaller volume.

Patients with meningeal leukemia or those receiving bone marrow transplantation may be confronted with academic limitations following cranial radiation.

Table 23.4. Risk factors for cognitive effects following treatment for ALL (Nathan et al. 2007)

Precedent factor	Risk
Treatment modality	CNS radiation, TBI, intrathecal cytotoxics, high-dose systemic methotrexate
Age at time of initial CNS treatment	Increased risk if <3 years of age
Concomitant therapy	Combination of treatment modalities (CNS) irradiation and intravenous methotrexate
Dosage of irradiation	18 Gy or greater of whole brain irradiation for one or more treatments
Gender	Girls are more vulnerable than boys, particularly after ALL therapy

Initial studies have also shown that dexamethasone therapy (compared with prednisolone) may increase the risk for neurocognitive effects in children treated for ALL (Waber et al. 2000). Cognitive deficits will vary according to the level of skill development, because emerging, developing, and established skills are differentially vulnerable to the effects of childhood brain damage (Nathan et al. 2007).

School absenteeism may also be correlated with the degree of illness and medical complications, making periods of absence unavoidable. However, when children feel well enough to attend and are physically able, parents should be encouraged to send them to school as often as possible.

A study carried out in the United States found that cancer-surviving adolescents may require intervention to improve their decision-making skills that will assist their abstract and/or analytic abilities (Hollen et al. 1997). Poor-quality decision-making was also clearly linked to adolescents who exhibited more risk behaviors. Particular attention should be paid to the development of concentration, attention, short-term memory, and abstract reasoning ability in all children, with the development of verbal processing skills needing greater attention in girls.

Some work has been carried out to identify appropriate learning strategies for these survivors with neurocognitive deficits (Spencer 2006). Cognitive remediation principles were developed and applied to children who developed neurocognitive deficits as a result of cancer therapy (Butler et al. 2008). The model focuses on three disciplines:

1. Brain injury rehabilitation – the child focuses on a learning task for 15 min. The period of learning is alternated with more interesting activities such as games. This enables the child to maintain stamina over the 20 two-hour sessions that are involved in the cognitive remediation program. Children must obtain 50% correct: if less than 50%, then a more basic task is presented; if higher than 80%, the next level of difficulty is applied.
2. Special education/education psycology – instruction is focused on task preparedness (e.g., brief relaxation, prompts that the child has to do his/her very best work), on-task performance (e.g., talk to themselves to help self-monitoring, looking for shortcuts), and post-task strategies (e.g., check work, ask for feedback, reward yourself).
3. Clinical psychology - a cognitive behavioural approach that may include acknowledging weaknesses, reframing struggle into positive, learning strengths, internal dialogue, and becoming one's best friend (Butler et al. 2008).

Programs for at-risk children are vital for future academic achievement, social adjustment, and success. It is pertinent to inform patients and families of the possibility of cognitive delays and offer interventions and referrals to appropriate programs (Spencer 2006).

23.3.4 Prognosis

As the number of children surviving cancer for extended periods of time continues to increase, the phenomenon of symptoms that persist following completion of treatment is being recognized. Some children may benefit from special educational assistance to improve their educational outcomes. This is important for improving the quality of life of survivors and to help them achieve their maximum potential, initially at school and ultimately in the workforce. Some cognitive deficits are evident only at the point in development at which the requisite skills emerge and brain actively begins to contribute to the development of a new behavior or strategy for solving a problem, a point that may be several years removed from tumor diagnosis. For example, deficient executive and organizational skills after frontal lobe injury may be a latent deficit, a late-emerging impairment that becomes fully apparent only in adolescent or adult life (Walker et al. 2004).

23.4 Diabetes Insipidus

23.4.1 Incidence

Diabetes insipidus (DI) has been reported in 8–35% preoperatively and 70–96% postoperatively in patients with craniopharyngioma (Ghirardello et al. 2006; Smith et al. 2004). Although tumor-associated DI is uncommon in children under 5 years of age (Ghirardello et al. 2005), it is the most common clinical presentation of patients with CNS disease in Langerhans cell histiocytosis (LCH) where DI is present in 6% of patients at diagnosis (Grois et al. 2006). DI has also been reported as a permanent late sequalae of LCH 15–20% of children at 15 years from diagnosis (Mittheisz et al. 2007; Pollono et al. 2007; Bernstrand et al. 2005). DI may also be one of the presenting features in intracranial germ cell tumors (Crawford et al. 2007).

The clinical features of polyuria (>3,000 mL/m^2/24 h) and polydipsia, and on a flow of hypotonic urine (specific gravity <1,001–1,005) are usually dramatic (Grois et al. 2006). However, formal confirmation of the diagnosis by a water deprivation test is sometimes recommended. However, MRI may allow for identification of the posterior pituitary hyperintensity and of hypothalamic-pituitary abnormalities (Maghnie 2003).

23.4.2 Etiology

DI is associated with a disorder of antidiuretic hormone (ADH). There are two types:

1. Central or neurogenic DI: a defect in the synthesis or release of ADH
2. Nephrogenic DI: failure of the kidneys to respond to ADH

The diagnosis of DI is often based on the results of a water deprivation test to rule out primary polydipsia, where the water diuresis results from the suppression of arginine vasopressin (AVP) release by excessive fluid intake. Plasma sodium concentration and osmolality and urine osmolality are monitored. These results determine the progression of the test to enable the diagnosis of the type of DI.

23.4.3 Treatment

The aim of treatment is to treat the underlying disorder (germ cell tumor or LCH) and supply the body with pharmacologic preparations that contain the missing hormone. These preparations cannot be given orally because the gastrointestinal tract interferes with the action of the agent, so they must be administered parenterally or nasally. The preferred drug for treating chronic DI is 1-desamino-8-D arginine vasopressin (DDAVP). This can be given by intranasal spray and has a duration of action of 8–20 h. Despite appropriate management of patients with a fixed daily fluid intake and small, regular (2 or 3 times daily) doses of desmopressin, maintenance of fluid and osmotic balance often remains precarious (Hayward et al. 2004).

23.4.4 Prognosis

The most appropriate treatment for reversing DI-complicating LCH has yet to be determined (Grois et al. 2006). Most children with childhood craniopharyngioma developed DI postoperatively (Ghirardello et al. 2006; Smith et al. 2004). Patients with an initial diagnosis of idiopathic DI require vigilant medical follow-up including neuroimaging studies, particularly when there is evidence of evolving pituitary hormone deficiencies.

References

Acquaviva A, Marconcini S, Municchi G, Vallone I, Palma L (2003) Non-Hodgkin lymphoma in a child presenting with acute paraplegia: a case report. Pediatric Hematology and Oncology 20(3):245–251

Bernstrand C, Sandstedt B, Ahström L, Henter JI (2005) Long-term follow-up of Langerhans cell histiocytosis: 39 years' experience at a single centre. Acta Paediatrica 94(8):1073–1084

Butler RW, Copeland DR, Fairclough DL, Mulhern RK, Katz ER, Kazak AE, Noll RB, Patel SK, Sahler OJ (2008) A multicenter, randomized clinical trial of a cognitive remediation program for childhood survivors of a pediatric malignancy. Journal of Consulting and Clinical Psychology 76(3):367–378

Colen FN (2008) Oncologic emergencies: superior vena cava syndrome, tumor lysis syndrome, and spinal cord compression. Journal of Emergency Nursing 34(6):535–537

Crawford JR, Santi MR, Vezina G, Myseros JS, Keating RF, LaFond DA, Rood BR, MacDonald TJ, Packer RJ (2007) CNS germ cell tumor (CNSGCT) of childhood: presentation and delayed diagnosis. Neurology 68(20):1668–1673

Davies B, Whitsett SF, Bruce A, McCarthy P (2002) A typology of fatigue in children with cancer. Journal of Pediatric Oncology Nursing 1(1):12–21

Ghirardello S, Hopper N, Albanese A, Maghnie M (2006) Diabetes insipidus in craniopharyngioma: postoperative management of water and electrolyte disorders. Journal of Pediatric Endocrinology and Metabolism 19(Suppl 1): 413–421

Ghirardello S, Malattia C, Scagnelli P, Maghnie M (2005) Current perspective on the pathogenesis of central diabetes insipidus. Journal of Pediatric Endocrinology and Metabolism 18(7):631–645

Gibson F, Richardson A, Edwards J, Ream E, Sepion B (2003) A descriptive study to explore the impact of cancer and its treatment on adolescents: final report. Kings College London, University of London and Institute of Child Health, Great Ormond Street Hospital for Children, London

Gibson F, Mulhall AB, Richardson A, Edwards JL, Ream E, Sepion BJ (2005) A phenomenologic study of fatigue in adolescents receiving treatment for cancer. Oncology Nursing Forum 32(3):651–660

Grois N, Pötschger U, Prosch H, Minkov M, Arico M, Braier J, Henter JI, Janka-Schaub G, Ladisch S, Ritter J, Steiner M, Unger E, Gadner H, DALHX- and LCH I and II Study Committee (2006) Risk factors for diabetes insipidus in langerhans cell histiocytosis. Pediatric Blood Cancer 46(2):228–233

Haut C (2005) Oncological emergencies in the pediatric intensive care unit. AACN Clinical Issues 16(2):232–245

Hayward RD, Devile C, Brada M (2004) Craniophyrangioma. In: Walker DA, Perilopngo G, Punt JAG, Taylor RE (eds) Brain and spinal tumors of childhood. Arnold, London, pp 370–386

Hinds P, Hockenberry-Eaton M (2001) Developing a research program on fatigue in children and adolescents diagnosed with cancer. Journal of Paediatric Oncology Nursing 18(2):3–12

Hinds PS, Hockenberry-Eaton M, Quargnenti A, May M, Burleson C, Gilger E, Randall E, Brace-O'Neill J (1999) Fatigue in 7- to 12-year-old patients with cancer from the staff perspective: an exploratory study. Oncology Nursing Forum 26(1):37–45

Hinds PS, Hockenberry MJ, Gattuso JS, Srivastava DK, Tong X, Jones H, West N, McCarthy KS, Sadeh A, Ash M, Fernandez C, Pui CH (2007a) Dexamethasone alters sleep and fatigue in pediatric patients with acute lymphoblastic leukemia. Cancer 110(10):2321–2330

Hinds P, Hockenberry M, Rai S, Zhang L, Razzouk BI, McCarthy K, Cremer L, Rodriguex-Galindo C (2007b) Nocturnal awakenings, sleep environment interruptions and fatigue in hopitalized children with cancer. Oncology Nursing Forum 34(2):393–402

Hockenberry-Eaton M, Hinds P, O'Neill J, Alcoser P, Bottomley S, Kline N, Euell K, Howard V, Gattuso J (1999) Developing a conceptual model for fatigue in children. European Journal of Oncology Nursing 3(1):5–11

Hockenberry-Eaton M, Hinds P, Alcoser P, O'Neill J, Euell K, Howard V, Gattuso J, Taylor J (1998) Fatigue in children and adolescents with cancer. Journal of Paediatric Oncology Nursing 15(3):172–182

Hockenberry MJ, Hinds PS, Barrera P, Bryant R, Adams-McNeill J, Hooke C, Rasco-Baggott C, Patterson-Kelly K, Gattuso JS, Manteuffel B (2003) Three instruments to assess fatigue in children with cancer: the child, parent and staff perspectives. Journal of Pain Symptom Management 25(4):319–328

Hollen P, Hobbie W, Finley S (1997) Cognitive late effect factors related to decision making and risk behaviors of cancer-surviving adolescents. Cancer Nursing 20(5):305–314

Kelly KM, Lange B (1997) Pediatric oncology: oncologic emergencies. Pediatric Clinics of North America 44(4):809–830

Kingma A, Rammeloo LA, van Der Does-van den Berg A, Rekers-Mombarg L, Postma A (2000) Academic career after treatment for acute lymphoblastic leukaemia. Archives of Disease in Childhood 82(5):353–357

Langer T, Martus P, Ottensmeier H, Hertzberg H, Beck JD, Meier W (2002) CNS late-effects after ALL therapy in childhood. Part III: neuropsychological performance in long-term survivors of childhood ALL: impairments of concentration, attention, and memory. Med Pediatr Oncol. 38(5):320–8.

Langeveld N, Ubbink M, Smets E on behalf of the Dutch Late Effects Study Group (2000) "I don't have any energy": the experience of fatigue in young adult survivors of childhood cancer. European Journal of Oncology Nursing 4(1):20–28

Maghnie M (2003) Diabetes insipidus. Hormone Research 59(Suppl 1):42–54

Marrs JA (2006) Nurse, my back hurts: understanding malignant spinal cord compression. Clinical Journal of Oncology Nursing 10(1):114–116

Mittheisz E, Seidl R, Prayer D, Waldenmair M, Neophytou B, Pötschger U, Minkov M, Steiner M, Prosch H, Wnorowski M, Gadner H, Grois N (2007) Central nervous system-related permanent consequences in patients with Langerhans cell histiocytosis. Pediatric Blood Cancer 48(1):50–56

Moore IM, Espy KA, Kaufmann P, Kramer J, Kaemingk K, Miketova P, Mollova N, Kaspar M, Pasvogel A, Schram K, Wara W, Hutter J, Matthay K (2000) Cognitive consequences and central nervous system injury following treatment for childhood leukemia. Seminars in Oncology Nursing 16(4):279–290

Nathan PC, Patel SK, Dilley K, Goldsby R, Harvey J, Jacobsen C, Kadan-Lottick N, McKinley K, Millham AK, Moore I, Okcu MF, Woodman CL, Brouwers P, Armstrong FD, Children's Oncology Group Long-term Follow-up Guidelines Task Force on Neurocognitive/Behavioral Complications After Childhood Cancer (2007) Guidelines for identification of, advocacy for, and intervention in neurocognitive problems in survivors of childhood cancer: a report from the Children's Oncology Group. Archives of Pediatric and Adolescent Medicine 161(8):798–806

Nguyen NP, Sallah S, Ludin A, Salehpour MR, Karlsson U, Files B, Strandjord S (2000) Neuroblastoma producing spinal cord compression: rapid relief with low dose of radiation. Anticancer Research 20(6C):4687–4690

Nicolin G (2002) Emergencies and their management. European Journal of Cancer 38(10):1365–1377

Pollono D, Rey G, Latella A, Rosso D, Chantada G, Braier J (2007) Reactivation and risk of sequelae in Langerhans cell histiocytosis. Pediatric Blood Cancer 48(7):696–699

Precourt S, Robaey P, Lamothe I, Lassonde M, Sauerwein HC, Moghrabi A (2002) Verbal cognitive functioning and learning in girls treated for acute lymphoblastic leukemia by chemotherapy with or without cranial irradiation. Developmental Neuropsychology 21(2):173–195

Ream E, Gibson F, Edwards J, Seption B, Mulhall A, Richardson A (2006) Experience of fatigue in adolescents living with cancer. Cancer Nursing 29(4):317–326

Reimers TS, Mortensen EL, Schmiegelow K (2007) Memory deficits in long-term survivors of childhood brain tumors may primarily reflect general cognitive dysfunctions. Pediatric Blood Cancer 48(2):205–212

Rheingold S, Lange B (2006) Oncologic emergencies. In: Pizzo PA, Poplack DG (eds) Principles and practice of pediatric oncology, 5th edn. Lippincott, Williams and Wilkins, Philadelphia, pp 1202–1230

Smith D, Finucane F, Phillips J, Baylis PH, Finucane J, Tormey W, Thompson CJ (2004) Abnormal regulation of thirst and vasopressin secretion following surgery for craniopharyngioma. Clinical Endocrinology (Oxf) 61(2):273–279

Spencer J (2006) The role of cognitive remediation in childhood cancer survivors experiencing neurocognitive late effects. Journal of Pediatric Oncology Nursing 23(6):321–325

Waber DP, Carpentieri SC, Klar N, Silverman LB, Schwenn M, Hurwitz CA, Mullenix PJ, Tarbell NJ, Sallan SE (2000) Cognitive sequelae in children treated for acute lymphoblastic leukemia with dexamethasone or prednisone. Journal of Pediatric Hematology and Oncology 22(3): 206–213

Walker DA, Perilongo G, Punt J, Taylor R (eds) (2004) Neuropsychological outcome in brain and spinal tumors of childhood. Oxford University Press, New York, pp 213–227

White AM (2001) Clinical applications of research on fatigue in children with cancer. Journal of Pediatric Oncology Nursing 18(2 Suppl 1):1720

Whitsett SF, Gudmundsdottir M, Davies B, McCarthy P, Friedman D (2008) Chemotherapy-related fatigue in childhood cancer: correlates, consequences, and coping strategies. Journal of Pediatric Oncology Nursing 25(2): 86–96

Musculoskeletal System

Deborah Tomlinson • Sue Zupanec

Contents

24.1 **Bone Tumors** 463
- 24.1.1 Limb Salvage Procedures 463
  - 24.1.1.1 Incidence 463
  - 24.1.1.2 Procedure 464
  - 24.1.1.3 Management 464
- 24.1.2 Amputation 464
  - 24.1.2.1 Incidence 464
  - 24.1.2.2 Procedure 464
  - 24.1.2.3 Rotationplasty 467
  - 24.1.2.4 Management 468
- 24.1.3 Comparison of Limb Salvage and Amputation 469
  - 24.1.3.1 Duration of Survival 469
  - 24.1.3.2 Immediate and Ultimate Morbidity 469
  - 24.1.3.3 Function 469
  - 24.1.3.4 Quality of Life 470

24.2 **Altered Bone Mineral Density and Increased Fracture Risk** 470
- 24.2.1 Incidence 470
- 24.2.2 Etiology 471
- 24.2.3 Prevention and Treatment 471
- 24.2.4 Prognosis 472

24.3 **Osteonecrosis** 472
- 24.3.1 Incidence 473
- 24.3.2 Etiology 474
- 24.3.3 Treatment 474
- 24.3.4 Prognosis 475

References 475

24.1 Bone Tumors

The two predominant primary bone tumors in children are osteosarcoma (60%) and Ewing's sarcoma (34%). (Solid tumors are detailed in Chap. 3). Combined, these are the most predominant causes of bone tumors in the lower extremities in children (Nagarajan et al. 2002). Upper- and lower-extremity bone tumors are effectively treated with multimodal treatment, which often involves local control by one of two surgical options:

- Limb-sparing resection
- Amputation

Principles that guide the decision include the following:

1. Reconstruction used should be acceptable to both the child and the parents
2. Risk of short-term and long-term complications should be acceptable
3. Functional and cosmetic outcome should be equal to, or better than, that from amputation (Grimer 2005)

24.1.1 Limb Salvage Procedures

24.1.1.1 Incidence

Limb salvage procedures are feasible in approximately 80–90% of childhood sarcomas (Kumta et al. 2002; Rao and Rodriguez-Galindo 2003). These procedures include custom-made endoprostheses, allografts, and composite-reconstruction (Rao and Rodriguez-Galindo 2003; Hosalkar and Dormans 2004).

24.1.1.2 Procedure

The decision to proceed with limb salvage surgery must consider the following:

- Aggressiveness of the underlying tumor and its stage
- Need to achieve a satisfactorily wide excision of the tumor
- Ability of the reconstructed extremity to be at least as functional as an ablative procedure and prosthesis
- Response to neo-adjuvant therapy (Kumta et al. 2002; Nagarajan et al. 2004; Rao and Rodriguez-Galindo 2003)

Various options are available for skeletal reconstruction, and the type used usually depends on the following:

1. Site of the tumor
2. Patient's age with regard to both skeletal maturity and emotional maturity
3. Patient's prognosis
4. Orthopedic surgeon's expertise

Table 24.1 provides a general outline of the types of limb-sparing reconstructions that are available. However, bones such as ribs, clavicles, digits, scapulae, and fibulae can be removed with adequate margins and with no effect on function.

24.1.1.3 Management

Management is complicated for these patients who face life-threatening illness exacerbated by life-changing surgery. Heightened awareness should be made to psychosocial care. Nursing care encompasses meeting important physical and psychosocial needs. Patients receiving limb-sparing surgery of this nature will often be adolescents, and any change in body image may be detrimental to their psychological well-being. The nursing challenge is to help these children and adolescents balance the limits of their illness and recovery with normal developmental needs.

Postoperative management regarding dressing changes and rehabilitation following limb-sparing surgery is briefly highlighted in Tables 24.2 and 24.3, respectively. Appropriate care includes a multidisciplinary approach to ensure optimal functional outcome (Hosalkar and Dormans 2004). Rehabilitation can take up to 2 years, by which time the patient should have a functioning limb.

24.1.2 Amputation

24.1.2.1 Incidence

Prior to the 1980s, amputation was the main surgical option for malignant bone tumors. This procedure is currently performed in less than 15% of patients, and amputation is reserved for patients with widespread local disease where it is necessary to achieve wide excision. In children, amputation is primarily limited to children with local recurrence not amenable to resection, involvement of neurovascular bundle or bone, or when radiotherapy can result in significant impairment or function (Rao and Rodriguez-Galindo 2003). However, the procedure includes the premise that the resultant limb reconstruction be as functional as possible.

24.1.2.2 Procedure

Amputation in children raises several issues because of the following considerations:

- Etiology
- Expected skeletal growth
- Functional demand on the motor system and prosthesis
- Appositional bone stump overgrowth
- Psychological challenges (Hoalkar and Dormans 2004)

Despite the increased use of limb-sparing procedures, amputation remains a valuable procedure (Grimer 2005). A tumor that extends into an adjacent joint involving blood vessels and nerves would be impossible to remove without contaminating the surgical margins, increasing the risk of local recurrence. Limb function and movement are important, and inadequate surgical intervention may risk long-term survival. Amputation and an artificial limb may offer the best surgical option and function (see Table 24.1).

Table 24.1. Types of limb-sparing reconstruction and amputation (Nagarajan et al. 2002)

Type of reconstruction	Brief description of procedure	Joint or bone commonly affected	Advantages	Disadvantages	Complications
Arthrodesis	Involved resection of the tumor and adjacent joint. Joint is then fixated using plating and autogenous bone or allografts	Knee, shoulder (occasionally wrist and ankle)	Extremely stable and functional reconstruction for a young adult	Physical limitations – inability to bend knee Not sufficient for children with large growth potential	Infection (particularly with allograft bone) Delayed union or nonunion Fracture
Allograft bone	Allograft bones from deceased donors (Removed with ligaments, X-rayed for sizing and frozen). Before use allograft is cultured, placed in antibiotic solution and thawed. Autogenous bone (hip or fibula) may also be used Grafted bone is incorporated over time with native bone	Any without joint involvement Large segment defects usually require allografts over autogenous grafts	Overall allograft survival is good (60–80%) despite complications Can be stable for prolonged time period	May need protracted periods of nonweight-bearing Bracing or casting may be necessary to achieve bone healing High incidence of complications	Nonunion – absence of osseous healing Infection – may require removal of allograft and prolonged use of antibiotics Fracture – usually treated by internal fixation
Endoprosthetic implants	Resection of entire segment of bone involving tumor and replacement with metallic implant used to replace bone and joint. Implant has four components: Metallic stem that anchors prosthesis to remaining femur Metallic distal femur that fills the defect created by resection Prosthetic replacement of proximal tibial articular surface Rotating hinge knee joint	Distal femur	Postoperative rehabilitation Stable joint Immediate weight bearing Rapid functional use of extremity	Survival of prosthesis progressively decreases over time	Infection Aseptic loosening, i.e., loosening of stem within the bone (fibia or femur) Bone resorption Loosening
Composite endo-prosthetic allografts	Attachment of articulating prosthesis to allograft bone that serves as site of attachment to remaining native bone	Proximal femur Proximal tibia Proximal humeral	Stable joint, incorporation of additional bone and allows for attachment of major musculotendinous units	Protracted periods of nonweightbearing	As for endoprostheses and allografts

Table 24.1. (Continued)

Type of reconstruction	Brief description of procedure	Joint or bone commonly affected	Advantages	Disadvantages	Complications
Expanding endoprosthetic implants	Implants inserted as endoprosthetic knee joint. Implant has a mechanism for "active growth" achieved by several interventions from turning of a key within implant to replacement of spacers that increase in size or number as the child grows	Lower extremities	For children with growth potential >4–5 cm. (Bone age of 12 in boys; 10 in girls) Lengthens and provides growth of supporting structures of affected limb while providing ambulation for child Replaced when adult height has been reached	Multiple surgeries may be required Limb lengthening[a] Prosthesis revision Replacement for prosthesis failure Larger prosthesis Aseptic loosening Infections	Aseptic loosening Infection
Amputation	Wide excision of tumor is impossible without complete amputation. Four main types: Transtibial (below-the-knee) Knee disarticulation Transfemoral amputation (above-knee) Hip disarticulation	Majority are transfemoral due to high incidence of bone tumors in distal femur	Provides wide resection for tumors when limb salvage is not possible	May delay chemotherapy Possible greater psychosocial issues	Stump-protheses problems Stump pain Phantom limb pain Bone overgrowth Infection
Rotationplasty	Removing tumor and soft tissues from the back of the thigh, leaving neurovascular bundle and the distal end of tibia and foot. The leg is rotated 180° and tibia reattached to the femur with blood vessels reconnected. The ankle is now at the level of the knee, and the foot now pointing backwards acts as the stump, which can be fitted with an artificial limb at the level of a below-knee amputation. See Fig. 24.1	Majority for tumors of the distal femur (Van Nes rotationplasty)	Impressive functionally Stable reconstruction Useful knee movement Less energy consumption Potentially fewer surgeries No phantom limb pain (Kotz 1997)	Appearance of the limb following reconstruction is less well accepted	Infection Delayed wound healing Disturbances in circulation (particularly thromboses)

[a] An extendable prosthesis is now beginning to be replaced by a noninvasive lengthening device. The extendable prosthesis includes a spring-loaded device, which provides a few millimeters of expansion in approximately 20 seconds using an external electromagnetic field (Rao and Rodriguez-Galindo 2003). Further surgical intervention is not required

Table 24.2. Limb-sparing postoperative management nursing care guidelines for dressing changes. Taken from Gilger et al. (2002)

Dressing changes
First dressing change done by surgical staff 5–7 days following surgery
After this time; dressing changed about every 3 days
Frequency of dressing changes depends on healing

It is important to decide the level of local bone resection to ensure adequate tumor clearance and sufficient tissue availability to ensure skin closure. In the lower extremities, above-knee amputation is the most common level of amputation because of the frequent presentation around the knee joint, and below-knee amputation is done for tumors of the distal tibia. In the upper limb, tumors tend to present more commonly at the proximal humerus. If limb salvage is not possible due to the extent of disease, then disarticulation and forequarter amputation of the shoulder may be required. This level is very disabling, and artificial limbs are often for cosmetic purposes only.

In children, where the aim is to restore function to the limb, it is crucial to consider how much potential skeletal growth they still have before undertaking surgery. The distal epiphyseal plates provide 70% of the potential longitudinal growth of the femur (Nagarajan et al. 2002). Initially, if this plate is lost in surgery, the amputated limb is functional. But as growth occurs, the stump becomes shorter, function becomes limited, and further surgery may be necessary. It is also recognized that in children under the age of 12 years, further bone growth may occur at the ends of long bones, which would also necessitate further surgical intervention.

Prosthetic fitting and rehabilitation should proceed promptly following amputation. However, a child is often fitted for prosthesis during chemotherapy. Fluctuations in body weight and stump size may then necessitate the use of adjustable temporary sockets (Hosalkar and Dormans 2004).

24.1.2.3 Rotationplasty

Rotationplasty is a surgical procedure that is considered a method of amputation because it involves total removal of the tumor and surrounding tissue without reconstruction. The procedure is used to provide the same function of a below-knee-amputation to that of an above-knee-amputation (see Fig. 24.1). A brief outline of the procedure is included in Table 24.1. This surgical option is always discussed in relation to treatment because of its functional outcomes. However, it is a choice rarely made by patients and parents; cosmetic appearance of the limb and the need

Table 24.3. Guidelines for limb-sparing postoperative rehabilitation. Taken from Gilger et al. (2002)

Recovery	Day 1	Day 2	Day 3	Outpatient follow-up
Initiate use of continuous passive motion (CPM) Early mobility: Decreases risk of contractures Facilitates early ambulation May decrease pain	Encourage sitting in bed as much as possible to decrease chances of orthostatic hypotension during transfers Physiotherapy referral Encourage open discussion regarding pain For transfer and while sitting use orthosis to maintain extension to avoid knee flexion contractures	Continue use of CPM when in bed	Ambulate with crutches	Check patient notes and protocol for information regarding use of brace, assistance with ambulation, and use of CPM, etc.

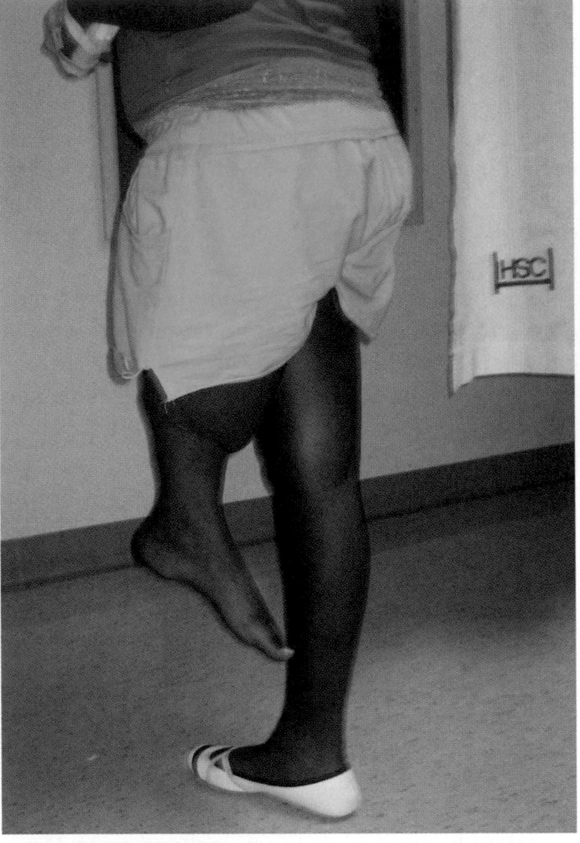

Figure. 24.1

Rotationplasty: 11-year-old girl treated for osteosarcoma of lower leg

for prosthesis are the main issues of this procedure and justifies concern about psychosocial functioning (Hosalkar and Dormans 2004; Ginsberg et al. 2007).

24.1.2.4 Management

Postoperative management regarding dressing changes and rehabilitation of a patient following amputation surgery is briefly highlighted in Tables 24.4 and 24.5, respectively. Phantom limb pain can be a particular problem (described in Chap.30), and appropriate aggressive pain management is required immediately post amputation in an attempt to avoid chronic phantom limb pain.

Table 24.4. Amputation postoperative management nursing care guidelines for dressing changes

Dressing changes
Casts generally applied during surgery
First cast change within 10 days after surgery
Number of changes depends on extent of edema, infection, and muscle involvement

When limb preservation is not possible, patients often view amputation as failure and begin grieving not only the potential loss of the limb but also the belief that life will never be normal again. Restoring individual belief in acquiring some form of normal activity with realistic goals is paramount. Depending on the child's age, preamputation assessment and preparation are offered. The involvement of a play specialist can be beneficial to help prepare children and explain what will happen. The opportunity to visit a local artificial limb center prior to admission has been shown to be not only beneficial preoperatively but appears to help the individual cope better following surgery. Meeting another patient who has had an amputation at the same level, with a positive outcome, can be inspiring, informational, and create a role model as to what can be achieved.

For children who are admitted for amputation, the hospitalization is quite short. Following recovery and with adequate pain management, discharge follows soon after the child is able to transfer and mobilize safely. Function, movement, balance, and safety are part of the physiotherapist's rehabilitation program for working on daily activities. The occupational therapist helps promote independence by providing equipment, advice, and referrals to local services to help patients and their families achieve realistic goals. The patient will be referred back to his or her local artificial limb or physical therapy center for prosthetic rehabilitation.

Younger children may lack or have only limited understanding and will need to be constantly monitored to reinforce the need to exercise to maintain movement. If exercises are not maintained, further problems will develop.

Table 24.5. Guidelines for amputation postoperative rehabilitation. Taken from Gilger et al. (2002)

Day 1	Day 2	Day 3	Outpatient follow-up
Encourage sitting in bed as much as possible to decrease chances of orthostatic hypotension during transfers Physiotherapy referral Encourage discussion about phantom (neuropathic) pain/sensation Do not remove cast – provides protection and controls edema Do not elevate limb after first 24 h unless instructed by physician – prolonged hip flexion can lead to contractures	Continue as per Day 1	Ambulate on crutches	Check patient notes and protocol for information regarding use of brace, assistance with ambulation, and use of CPM, etc.

24.1.3 Comparison of Limb Salvage and Amputation

Many studies have investigated the comparisons between limb salvage and amputation with regard to:

- Duration of survival
- Immediate and ultimate morbidity
- Function
- Quality of life

24.1.3.1 Duration of Survival

Survival rates and local recurrence rates have been comparable in both groups (Sluga et al. 1999; Weis 1999; Bacci et al. 2003). However, some studies of osteosarcoma have shown increased risk of local recurrence in patients undergoing limb salvage surgery, but no increase in mortality (Grimer 2005).

24.1.3.2 Immediate and Ultimate Morbidity

Complications following limb-sparing procedures occur more frequently than in amputation procedures (Nagarajan et al. 2002). Infection remains one of the main complications of all types of limb reconstruction. The overall risk of infection following limb reconstruction surgery is approximately 6–10% (conventional joint replacements have a 0.5% risk of infection). This may be related to the extent and complexity of surgery, immunosuppression in patients on chemotherapy, neutropenia, and central-line infections (Grimer 2005). These complications can directly impact future function and quality of life. However, with new techniques and materials being developed, the outcomes with regard to complications need to be continually evaluated (Nagarajan et al. 2004).

24.1.3.3 Function

Functional outcome is complex and based on more than physical ability (Nagarajan et al. 2002). A commonly used assessment of function is the Musculoskeletal Tumor Society (MSTS) scoring system. This assessment is based on the patient's overall pain, level of activity restriction, emotional acceptance, use of supports, walking, and gait. Another assessment is the self-administered questionnaire of the Toronto Extremity Salvage Score (TESS), which divides functional outcome into:

- Disability, referring to inability or restriction in performing normal activities
- Handicap, referring to the inability to assume, or limitation in assuming, a role that is normal for that person (depending on age, gender, social, and cultural factors) (Davis et al. 1996)

Another reliable and valid tool is the functional mobility assessment (FMA), which consisits of six subcategories:

1. Pain
2. Function with two specific measures, timed up and down stairs (TUDS) time and timed up and go time (TUG). This also measures heart rate and perceived exertion during TUDS and TUG
3. Supports such as crutches, canes, etc.
4. Satisfaction with walking quality
5. Participation in work, school, and sports
6. Endurance measured by the 9 min run–walk (Ginsberg et al. 2007)

The difficulty in determining whether functional differences are notable is the lack of consistency in measurements of function. Generally, observed functional differences tend to be slight (Grimer 2005; Hopyan et al. 2006; Nagarajan et al. 2003); however, there has been indication of significantly improved function with limb-saving surgery when compared with ablative surgery (Renard et al. 2000). Reports of a lack of difference between the two groups may be attributed to "adjustment and accommodation" to their current condition (Nagarajan et al. 2004).However, reports state that functional outcome following rotationplasty is superior to that of amputation (Hillman et al. 2000; Fuchs et al. 2003; Ginsberg et al. 2007).

24.1.3.4 Quality of Life

Definitions of quality of life have changed; therefore, comparison between studies on quality of life (QoL) has been difficult, and reports on differences in quality of life between these patients have varied in their conclusions. Nagarajan et al. (2004) concluded that females reported significantly lower QoL but not more disability. This may reflect gender-related differences in coping styles. Certainly, overall it would appear that there is little difference (Refaat et al. 2002; Lane et al. 2001), despite predictions that the quality of life of patients undergoing limb salvage procedures would be superior to that of patients undergoing amputation. There are little data available regarding quality of life measurements in children following limb salvage or amputation procedures.

Despite the higher complication rate and equivocal improved quality of life, limb-sparing surgery remains current practice at most centers (Nagarajan et al. 2002). This may be due to a perception that saving the limb is of utmost importance.

The management of these patients includes an individualized surgical plan and an awareness of their psychosocial needs after surgery.

24.2 Altered Bone Mineral Density and Increased Fracture Risk

24.2.1 Incidence

Children with malignancy, partcularly ALL, are at risk of developing osteopenia and/or osteoporosis (Wasilewski-Masker et al. 2008). Currently, there is no consensus on the definition of osteopenia and osteoporosis in children (van der Sluis and van den Heuvel-Eibrink 2008); however, osteopenia or osteoporosis has been reported in 45% of surivors of various malignancies (Hesseling et al. 1998). In childhood survivors of brain tumors, the prevalence of osteoporosis was more than 40% of irradiated patients and zero in the non-irriadiated group (Odame et al. 2006). Osteopenia or osteoporosis has been reported in 43–65% of survivors of osteogenic sarcoma or Ewing sarcoma (Hopewell 2003). Pediatric Hodgkin Lymphoma survivors have shown negligible bone mineral deficits (Kaste et al. 2009).

Bone mineral density (BMD) in adulthood is dependent on peak bone mass that is achieved in adolescence or young adulthood. Therefore, in children with cancer, there is a risk of developing a suboptimal peak bone mass (van der Sluis and van den Heuvel-Eibrink 2008). This can result in fractures, kyphosis, and pain (Kaste 2008).

Van der Sluis et al. (2002) have reported a fracture risk six times higher in children with acute lymphoblastic leukemia (ALL) when compared with healthy controls. The risk of fractures increases considerably during treatment and for a period after treatment. Other factors that may play a role in the high fracture risk of children with cancer may include:

- Risk of falling – vincristine-induced neuropathy can cause clumsiness and poorer balance
- Bone quality – reflected in bone resorption rate
- Weight

24.2.2 Etiology

In childhood ALL, skeletal changes are often detected at diagnosis, including osteolysis, sclerosis, osteoporosis, and, occasionally, pathological fractures (van der Sluis and van den Heuvel-Eibrink 2008). These changes are probably caused by the disease process and alterations in mineral homeostasis and bone mass.

In addition, methotrexate, radiotherapy, and corticosteroids are some of the adjuvant antineoplastic treatments currently used and have been described as hindering normal development of bone mass (Nysom et al. 2001; van der Sluis and van den Heuvel-Eibrink 2008; Wasilewski-Masker et al. 2008). Some molecular mechanisms are outlined in Table 24.6.

In the older age group, the bone mass is calculated on the degree of bone loss and the maximum bone mass acquired in the second and third decades of life. If the normal acquisition of bone mass is disrupted during childhood and adolescence, survivors of childhood cancer may develop osteopenia, osteoporosis, and pathological fractures in later life (Azcona et al. 2003; van der Sluis and van den Heuvel-Eibrink 2008). Chemotherapy drugs such as ifosfamide and cisplatinum used in the treatment of bone tumors may interfere with the process of renal calcium and vitamin D metabolism. During treatment for ALL, persistent low levels of bone alkaline phosphatase have indicated a potential flaw in osteoblast differentiation. Azcona et al. (2003) further suggest that many other factors may affect bone mineralization in children with malignancy, including long periods of bed rest, poor diet, growth hormone deficiency (see Chap. 26), and variations in vitamin D metabolism (Azcona et al. 2003; van der Sluis and van den Heuvel-Eibrink 2008). Diagnoses of these anomalies are often made by radiological imaging. However, it is important to be able to recognize potential changes within the skeleton and to be able to differentiate from metastatic disease and recurrence.

24.2.3 Prevention and Treatment

Bone marrow density (BMD) can be assessed using dual-energy X-ray absorptiometry (DEXA).

Therapeutic options are limited. However, simple measures exist such as adequate calcium and vitamin D intake, and stimulating physical activity.

Vitamin D deficiency may occur due to:

- Malabsorption
- Malnutrition
- Lack of sun exposure
- Liver or renal disease

Calcium deficiency may result from reduced intestinal calcium absorption and increased calcium excretion caused by corticosteroids.

Table 24.6. Molecular mechanisms accounting for loss of bone mass (Cohen 2003; van der Sluis and van den Heuvel-Eibrink 2008)

Treatment	Mechanism in bone loss
Methotrexate	Appears to increase bone resorption and excretion (Higher accumulative doses of methotrexate have been associated with greater incidence of osteopenia)
Glucocorticoids	Prevent 1-alpha-hydroxylation of vitamin D in the kidneys to form the active metabolite 1,25-dihydroxy-vitamin D. This leads to impaired intestinal absorption of calcium Inhibit the expression of vitamin D receptor in bone Inhibit production of osteocalcin (principle bone matrix protein) Decrease local production of cytokines, which inhibit bone resorption
Corticosteroids	Decrease osteoblast activity, increase bone resorption, interfere with growth hormone, reduce muscle strength, disturb calcium balance at gut and kidney
Hematopoietic cell transplant	Increase in bone marrow interleukin-6, which may stimulate bone resorption Differentiation of bone marrow stromal cells into osteoblasts is impaired

Dietary advice may include prescription of supplemnts of 500 mg calcium and 400 IU vitamin D/day (van der Sluis and van den Heuvel-Eibrink 2008).

Physical activity is required in children to maintain normal bone density and therefore this should be encouraged to help ensure peak bone mass. High load, short burst, weight bearing exercises stimualte new bone formation.

Established osteoporosis may necessitate treatment with bisphosphonates; e.g., intravenous pamidronate. Bisphosphonates decrease bone resorption by inhibiting bone turnover. Bisphosphonates:

- Inhibit recruitment and function of osteoclasts to produce an inhibitor of osteoclast formation
- Shorten life span of osteoblasts

Future studies may lead to prophylactic treatment with bisphosphonates. Studies are needed to assess the risks and benefits of bisphosphonates in children with osteoporosis (van der Sluis and van den Heuvel-Eibrink 2008).

24.2.4 Prognosis

Bone marrow density does tend to improve, but children have been reported as having low BMD 1 year following cessation of treatment. Follow-up for patients with malignancy should include assessment for osteoporosis. Those at risk should receive early intervention.

24.3 Osteonecrosis

Osteonecrosis, also defined as aseptic or avascular necrosis of bone, is recognized as a major complication of antineoplastic therapy and most specifically ALL and non-Hodgkin's lymphoma (NHL) treatment. Children treated with allogeneic bone marrow transplantation are another group with increased risk of developing osteonecrosis (Mattano 2003). Osteonecrosis is segmental death of one or multiple osseous sites. Osteonecrosis may be asymptomatic but will most often present with one or more of the following symptoms:

- Severe pain
- Joint swelling
- Limited range of motion on exam
- Altered gait, limp, or inability to bear weight

Osteonecrosis in children most commonly affects the weight bearing joints. In children treated for leukemia, the hips are most often affected, followed by the knees, and then less often the ankles. It is common to have bilateral joint involvement and to have mulitarticular involvement. It is important to have high clinical suspicion for osteonecrosis when a pediatric patient on ALL therapy presents with any of the above symptoms. When there is a clinical suspicion, the diagnosis is made using imaging studies. Although imaging studies may include plain X-ray, computed tomography (CT), and magnetic resonance imaging (MRI), MRI is the most sensitive test used to diagnose osteonecrosis (Karimova and Kaste 2007). X-ray is often the first step in the diagnostic process due to the ease, low cost, and availability of this diagnositic test. X-ray findings that are suggestive of osteonecrosis pathology are followed up with MRI to confirm diagnosis. Figure 24.2 demonstrates an X-ray where there is flattening of the femoral epiphysis consistent with osteonecrosis (see Fig. 24.3). MRI studies are able to detect osteonecrosis earlier and more accurately

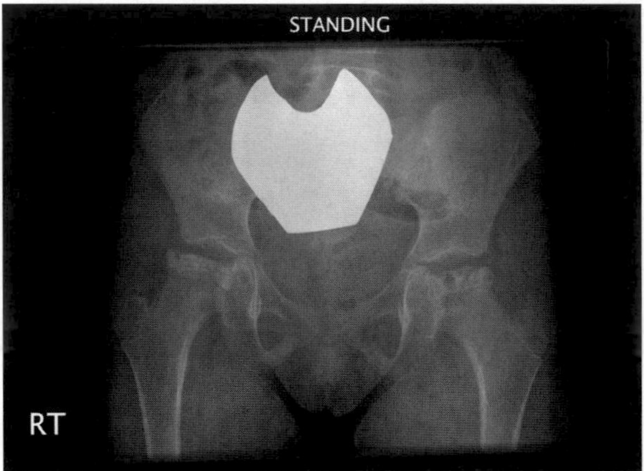

Figure 24.2

X-ray of bilateral osteonecrosis 7 year old child: Flattening of the femoral epiphyses

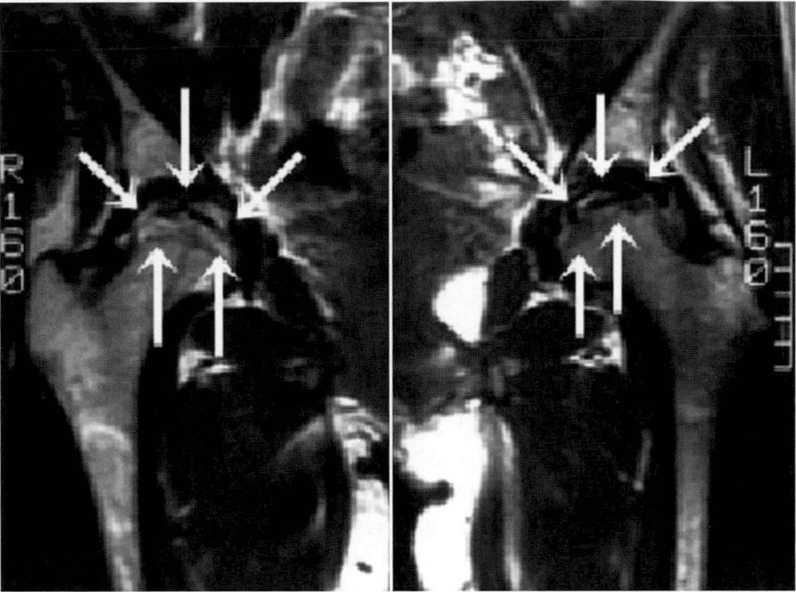

Figure 24.3
MRI bilateral osteonecrosis of the femoral heads

and do not require the use of contrast material (Karimova and Kaste 2007). Osteonecrosis MRI findings will include the appearance of a thin, winding line that clearly defines the interface between living and dead bone, and low-intensity bands on T1-weighted imaging (Marker et al. 2008) (see Fig. 24.4).

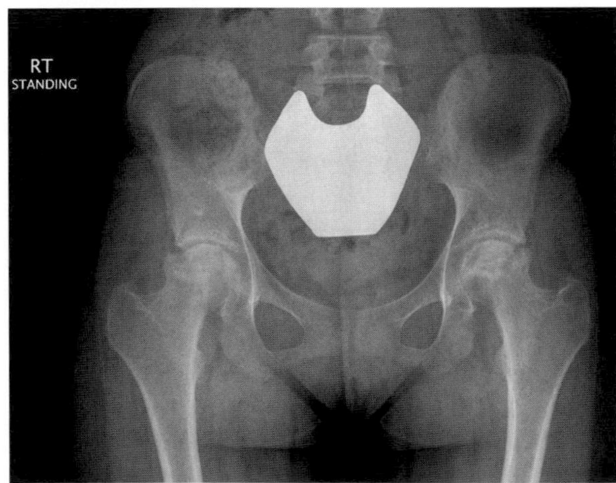

Figure 24.4
X-ray finding of bilateral osteonecrosis in 16 year old young adult

24.3.1 Incidence

The true incidence of osteonecrosis in children treated for cancer is unknown. This is in part because not all children on cancer treatment are routinely screened for osteonecrosis, and osteonecrosis can be asymptomatic, particulary in the early stages.

In pediatric patients who received allogeneic BMT, the reported range for risk of osteonecrosis is 4.3–24.2% (Mattano 2003). Identified risk factors for the development of osteonecrosis associated with allogeneic BMT include:

- Exposure to corticosteroids
- Age greater than 16 years
- Total body irradiation
- Presence of graft versus host disease
- Diagnosis of aplastic anemia (Socie et al. 1994; Fink et al. 1998; Barr and Sala 2008)

Most cases of osteonecrosis associated with ALL treatment occur during the first 3 years on therapy (Stauss et al. 2001). In children receiving treatment for ALL, the reported incidence of osteonecrosis ranges from 1.1 to 9.3% (Mattano et al. 2000). However, when the incidence of osteonecrosis is broken down by risk factors, subgroups of pediatric ALL patients are at greater risk and have higher reported incidence. Age has been identified as a significant risk factor with younger children at a considerably lower risk. For children with ALL less than 10 years of age, the reported risk of osteonecrosis is approximately 1% (Mattano et al. 2000). For children with ALL between ages 10 and 20, the risk of osteonecrosis is much greater and is approximately 14% (Mattano et al. 2000). However, studies have reported osteonecrosis incidences in children and adolescents, greater than 10 years of age, from 61 to 96% (Barr and Sala 2008). Age combined with gender is also predictive of osteonecrosis risk. Researchers have reported that females aged 10–15 have a risk of 19.2% and males aged 16–20 have a 20.7% risk of developing osteonecrosis during ALL therapy (Mattano et al. 2000). Although there is some disagreement about risk factors, some of the reported risk factors for the development of osteonecrosis in pediatric patients treated for ALL include:

- Age greater than 10
- White race
- Female sex
- High BMI
- Higher cumulative dose of dexamethasone (Sala et al. 2007; Niinimake et al. 2007)

In current ALL trials, investigators are evaluating the benefit of intensifying dexamethasone with the aim of improving overall survival (Mattano et al. 2000). If ALL treatments continue to intensify dexamethasone, the incidence of osteonecrosis will need to be closely monitored as improved survival may come with the cost of increased risk of osteonecrosis. Future trials in ALL may consider the inclusion of protective agents to decrease the risk of osteonecrosis, particularly for high-risk subgroups. Prophylaxis treatment for osteonecrosis with statin medications or biphosphonates are being considered and investigated (Sala et al. 2007).

Some genetic polymorphisms have been identified as independent risk factors for developing osteonecrosis. Relling et al. (2004) demonstrated that children on ALL therapy with the thymidylate synthase low activity 2/2 enhancer repeat genotype and the vitamin D receptor Fokl start site CC genotype had an increased risk of osteonecrosis of the hip (Relling et al. 2004). In the future, it will be important to continue to identify subgroups of pediatric patients at higher risk of osteonecrosis using genetic information to consider modifications of therapy such as decreasing steroid dose or providing preventative agents.

24.3.2 Etiology

Although the true pathology of osteonecrosis in children on cancer therapy is unknown, it is agreed that exposure to corticosteroids is a major contributing factor. Other chemotherapy agents have been associated with bone injury and include methotrexate, asparginase, and cyclophosphamide (Sala et al. 2007).

24.3.3 Treatment

Clinical management of osteonecrosis will depend on the severity of the clinical and radiological findings. Observation is considerd acceptable management for small lesions that are asymptomatic (Sala et al. 2007).

For more severe osteonecrosis, initial management will include pain management, discontinuation of physical activity, and avoiding weight bearing (Barr and Sala 2008). Depending on the severity of the pain, the patient will sometimes require admission to hospital for narcotic infusion. Once the diagnosis of osteonecrosis is confirmed, consultation with the orthopedics specialty is recommended to consider potential treatment options. Choice of treatment options will depend on the stage/severity of osteonecrosis. Treatment options include:

- Nonoperative treatment: phamacological therapy, extracorporeal shock-wave therapy, and electromagnetic stimulation
- Operative treatment: core decompression, tantalum implants, bone grafting, osteotomy, total hip arthroplasty (Marker et al. 2008)

In pediatrics, a total hip arthroplasty (total hip replacement) will not be expected to last for the patient's lifetime and therefore other surgical interventions are initially attempted. Core decompression offers an alternative. Core decompression involves drilling either small or large diameter holes into the core of the bone under fluroscopy. These holes are either left open or sometimes are filled in with bone graft. The track of the core decompression relieves bone marrow pressure and induces neovasularization (Marker et al. 2008).

24.3.4 Prognosis

Mild osteonecrosis that is asymptomatic can sometimes heal spontaneously. Small lesions of early stage have the best prognosis (Marker et al. 2008). In the majority of cases, osteonecrosis associated with antineoplastic therapy will progress and require intervention often surgical. Patients with evidence of bone collapse at the time of diagnosis have the worst prognosis and will require joint replacement.

References

Azcona C, Burghard E, Ruza E, Gimeno J, Sierrasesumaga L (2003) Reduced bone mineralization in adolescent survivors of malignant bone tumors: comparison of quantitative ultrasound and dual-energy X-ray absorptiometry. Journal of Paediatric Haematology/Oncology 25(4):297–301

Bacci C, Ferrari S, Longhi A, Donati D, Manfrini M, Giacoma S, Briccoli A, Forni C, Galletti S (2003) Nonmetastatic osteosarcoma of the extremity with pathological fracture at presentation: local and systemic control by amputation or limb salvage after preoperative chemotherapy. Acta Orthopaedica Scandinavica 74(4):449–459

Barr RD, Sala A (2008) Osteonecrosis in children and adolescents with cancer. Pediatric Blood & Cancer 50(2 Suppl): 483–485

Cohen LE (2003) Endocrine late effects of cancer treatment. Current Opinion in Pediatrics 15:3–9

Davis AM, Wright JG, Williams JI, Bombardier C, Griffin A, Bell RS (1996) Development of a measure of physical function for patients with bone and soft tissue sarcoma. Quality of Life Research 5(5):508–516

Fink J, Leisenring W, Sullivan K, Sherrard D, Weiss N (1998) Avascular necrosis following bone marrow transplantation: a case-control study. Bone 22:67–71

Fuchs B, Kotajaravi BR, Kaufman KR, Sim FH (2003) Functional outcome of patients with rotationplasty about the knee. Clinical Orthopaedics and Related Research 415: 52–58

Gilger EA, Groben VJ, Hinds PS (2002) Osteosarcoma nursing care guidelines: a tool to enhance the nursing care of children and adolescents enrolled on a medical research protocol. Journal of Pediatric Oncology Nursing 19(5):172–181

Ginsberg JP, Rai SN, Carlson CA, Meadows AT, Hinds PS, Spearing EM, Zhang L, Callaway L, Neel MD, Rao BN, Marchese VG (2007) A comparative analysis of functional outcomes in adolescents and young adults with lower-extremity bone sarcoma. Pediatric Blood & Cancer 49(7):964–969

Grimer RJ (2005) Surgical options for children with osteosarcoma. The Lancet Oncology 6(2):85–92

Hesseling PB, Hough SF, Nel ED, van Riet FA, Beneke T, Wessels G (1998) Bone mineral density in long-term survivors of childhood cancer. International Journal of Cancer. Supplement 11:44–47

Hillman A, Gosheger G, Hoffman C, Ozaki T, Winkelmann W (2000) Rotationplasty: surgical treatment modality after failed limb salvage procedure. Archives of Orthopaedic and Trauma Surgery 120(10):555–558

Hopewell JW (2003) Radiation-therapy effects on bone density. Medical and Pediatric Oncology 41(3):208–211

Hopyan S, Tan JW, Graham HK, Torode IP (2006) Function and upright time following limb salvage, amputation, and rotationplasty for pediatric sarcoma of bone. Journal of Pediatric Orthopedics 26(3):405–408

Hosalkar HS, Dormans JP (2004) Limb sparing surgery for pediatric musculoskeletal tumors. Pediatric Blood & Cancer 42(4):295–310

Karimova EJ, Kaste S (2007) MR imaging of osteonecrosis of the knee in children with acute lymphoblastic leukemia. Pediatric Radiology 37:1140–1146

Kaste SC (2008) Skeletal toxicities of treatment in children with cancer. Pediatric Blood & Cancer 50(2 Suppl):469–473

Kaste SC, Metzger ML, Minhas A, Xiong Z, Rai SN, Ness KK, Hudson MM (2009) Pediatric Hodgkin lymphoma survivors at negligible risk for significant bone mineral density deficits. Pediatric Blood & Cancer 52(4):516–521

Kotz R (1997) Rotationplasty. Seminars in Surgical Oncology 13(1):34–40

Kumta SM, Cheng JC, Li CK, Griffith JF, Chow LT, Quintos AD (2002) Scope and limitations of limb-sparing surgery in childhood sarcomas. Journal of Pediatric Orthopedics 22 (2):244–248

Lane JM, Christ GH, Khan SN, Backus SI (2001) Rehabilitation for limb salvage patients: kinesiological parameters and psychological assessment. Cancer 92(4):1013–1019

Marker DR, Thornsten M, Seyler M, McGrath S, Delanois R, Ulrich S, Mont M (2008) Treatment of early stage osteonecrosis of the femoral head. The Journal of Bone and Joint Surgery 90(Suppl 4):175–187

Mattano L (2003) The skeletal remains: porosis and necrosis of bone in the marrow transplantation setting. Pediatric Transplantation 7(Suppl 3):71–75

Mattano L, Harland N, Sather M, Trigg M, Nachman J (2000) Osteonecrosis as a complication of treating acute lymphoblastic leukemia in children: a report from the children's cancer group. Journal of Clinical Oncology 18(18):3262–3272

Nagarajan R, Neglia JP, Clohisy DR, Robison LL (2002) Limb salvage and amputation in survivors of paediatric lower-extremity bone tumors: what are the long term implications? Journal of Clinical Oncology 20(20):4493–4501

Nagarajan R, Neglia JP, Clohisy DR, Yasui Y, Greenberg M, Hudson M, Zevon MA, Tersak JM, Ablin A, Robison LL (2003) Education, employment, insurance, and marital status among 694 survivors of pediatric lower extremity bone tumors: a report from the childhood cancer survivor study. Cancer 97(10):2554–2564

Nagarajan R, Clohisy DR, Neglia JP, Yasui Y, Mitby PA, Sklar C, Finklestein JZ, Greenberg M, Reaman GH, Zeltzer L, Robison LL (2004) Function and quality-of-life of survivors of pelvic and lower extremity osteosarcoma and Ewing's sarcoma: the Childhood Cancer Survivor Study. British Journal of Cancer 91(11):1858–1865

Niinimake R, Harila-Saari A, Jartti A, Seuri R, Riikonen P, Paakko P, Mottonen M, Lanning M (2007) High body mass index increases the risk of osteonecrosis in children with acute lymphoblastic leukemia. Journal of Clinical Oncology 25(12):1498–1504

Nysom K, Holm K, Hertz H, Muller J, Fleischer Michaelsen K, Molgaard C (2001) Bone mass after treatment for acute lymphoblastic leukaemia in childhood. Journal of Clinical Oncology 19(11):2970–2971

Odame I, Duckworth J, Talsman D, Beaumont L, Furlong W, Webber C, Barr R (2006) Osteopenia, physical activity and health-related quality of life in survivors of brain tumors treated in childhood. Pediatric Blood & Cancer 46:357–362

Rao BN, Rodriguez-Galindo C (2003) Local control in childhood extremity sarcomas: salvaging limbs and sparing function. Medical and Pediatric Oncology 41(6):584–587

Refaat Y, Gunnoe J, Hornicek FJ, Mankin HJ (2002) Comparison of quality of life after amputation or limb salvage. Clinical Orthopaedics and Related Research 397:298–305

Relling MV, Yang W, Das S, Cook E, Rosner G, Neel M, Scott H, Ribeiro R, Sandlund J, Pui CH, Kaste S (2004) Pharmacogenetic risk factors for osteonecrosis of the hip among children with leukemia. Journal of Clinical Oncology 22(19):3930–3936

Renard AJ, Veth RP, Schreuder HW, van Loon CJ, Koops HS, van Horn JR (2000) Function and complications after ablative and limb-salvage therapy in lower extremity sarcoma of the bone. Journal of Surgical Oncology 73(4):198–205

Sala A, Mattano L, Barr R (2007) Osteonecrosis in children and adolescents with cancer – an adverse effect of systemic therapy. European Journal of Cancer 43:683–689

Sluga M, Windhager R, Lang S, Heinzl H, Bielack S, Kotz R (1999) Local and systemic control after ablative and limb sparing surgery in patients with osteosarcoma. Clinical Orthopaedics and Related Research 358:120–127

Socie G, Selimi F, Sedel L, Frija J, Deverqie A, Esperou Bourdeau H, Ribaud P, Gluckman E (1994) Avascular necrosis of bone after allogeneic bone marrow transplantation: clinical findings, incidence and risk factors. British Journal of Haematology 86:624–628

Stauss A, Su J, Dalton V, Gelber R, Sallan S, Silverman L (2001) Bone morbidity in children treated for acute lymphoblastic leukemia. Journal of Clinical Oncology 19(12):3066–3072

van der Sluis IM, van den Heuvel-Eibrink MM (2008) Osteoporosis in children with cancer. Pediatric Blood & Cancer 50(2 Suppl):474–478

van der Sluis IM, van den Heuvel-Eibrink MM, Hahlen K, Krenning EP, de Muinck Keizer-Schrama SM (2002) Altered bone mineral density and body composition, and increased fracture risk in childhood acute lymphoblastic leukemia. Journal of Pediatrics 141(2):204–240

Wasilewski-Masker K, Kaste SC, Hudson MM, Esiashvili N, Mattano LA, Meacham LR (2008) Bone mineral density deficits in survivors of childhood cancer: long-term follow-up guidelines and review of the literature. Pediatrics 121(3):e705–e713

Weis LD (1999) The success of limb-salvage surgery in the adolescent patient with osteogenic sarcoma. Adolescent Medicine 10(3):451–458, xii

Skin: Cutaneous Toxicities

Martina Nathan • Deborah Tomlinson

Contents

25.1 Alopecia . . . 477
25.1.1 Etiology . . . 477
25.1.3 Treatment . . . 478
25.1.4 Prognosis . . . 479
25.2 Altered Skin Integrity Associated with Radiation Therapy . . . 479
25.2.1 Incidence . . . 479
25.2.2 Etiology . . . 479
25.2.3 Prevention . . . 479
25.2.4 Treatment . . . 480
25.2.5 Prognosis . . . 481
25.3 Radiation Sensitivity and Recall . . . 481
25.3.1 Incidence . . . 481
25.3.2 Etiology . . . 481
25.3.3 Clinical Features . . . 481
25.3.4 Treatment . . . 481
25.3.5 Prognosis . . . 482
25.4 Ultraviolet Recall Reaction/Photosensitivity . . . 482
25.5 Cutaneous Reactions Associated with High-Dose Cytosine Arabinoside . . . 482
25.5.1 Incidence . . . 482
25.5.2 Etiology . . . 482
25.5.3 Prevention and Treatment . . . 482
25.6 Nail Dystrophies . . . 483
25.7 Graft Vs. Host Disease . . . 483
25.7.1 Incidence and Etiology . . . 483
25.7.2 Prevention . . . 485
25.7.3 Treatment . . . 486
25.7.4 Prognosis . . . 486
References . . . 486

25.1 Alopecia

Alopecia is one of the major and frequent toxicities of cytotoxic chemotherapy (Wang et al. 2006). It can vary in degree from sporadic thinning to complete baldness (Batchelor 2001). The degree of this depends on factors such as the type of agents, combination of drugs administered, and their doses (Dougherty 2006). Radiation therapy can also cause alopecia, depending on the area of treatment and the dosage administered to that area. Batchelor (2001) notes that the description of hair loss is frequently under-reported in the literature. Although alopecia is generally reversible, it has been identified as one of the most feared side effects of treatment (Viale 2006). Children on cancer treatment have frequently reported hair loss as a physical problem that created a less satisfying life as a result (Enskär and von Essen 2008; Williams et al. 2006). However, little attention has been given to the management of this side effect .

Table 25.1 describes cytotoxic drugs associated with alopecia in children. The severity of hair loss also depends on the route, dose, and schedule of the drugs. Scalp hair is more severly affected than the slow-growing hair of the eyebrows, eyelashes, or body/pubic hair (Alley et al. 2002).

25.1.1 Etiology

The proliferating hair follicles are inadvertently targeted by cancer treatment, which may produce weak hair or total loss of hair shaft formation (Viale 2006). Upto 90% of all hair follicles are in a phase of rapid growth. Under normal conditions, the growth cycle

Table 25.1. Cytotoxic agents that cause hair loss in children (adapted from Batchelor 2001)

Mild hair loss	Moderate hair loss	Severe hair loss
Bleomycin	Busulfa	Cyclophosphamide
5-Flurouracil	Methotrexate	Daunorubicin
Hydroxyurea	Mitomycin	Doxorubicin (Adriamycin)
Melphalan	Teniposide	Ifosfamide
Cisplatin	Actinomycin	Etoposide
Cytarabine arabinoside	Vincristine	High-dose vincristine
Thioguanine	Vinblastine	
Chlorambucil		
L-asparaginase		
Thiotepa		
Mercaptopurine (6-mp)		

consists of three main phases: anagen, catogen, and telogen. Anagen is the period for the regeneration of the lower, cycling portion of a follicle and the production of the hair shaft (Wang et al. 2006). The hair follicles of skin areas with the most rapid growth, such as the scalp, are affected more than the slower-growing eyebrows, eyelashes, and other body hair. However, repeated treatments with mitotic inhibitor agents can eventually lead to thinning and loss of hair in these areas as well (Alley et al. 2002). Alopecia of this nature is reversible, but the hair that grows back may be different in color or texture. Combination chemotherapy consisting of two or more agents usually produces higher incidence and more severe alopecia compared with single-agent therapy (Wang et al. 2006). Alopecia can be aggravated in the presence of co-existing medical conditions such as malnutrition and other medications associated with alopecia (allopurinol, gentamicin) that may be taken by the child or young person with cancer. The pathobiology of the response of hair follicles to cytotoxic treatment is largely unknown (Botchkarev 2003). It has been indicated that the p53 gene is involved in chemotherapy-induced apoptosis in hair follicles but due to the tumor suppressor nature of the gene, inhibition is restricted (Wang et al. 2006; Botchkarev et al. 2000).

25.1.3 Treatment

Methods to reduce the incidence of chemotherapy-induced alopecia have been studied since the 1970s, with varying evidence for the efficacy of the measures taken. Scalp cooling techniques have proved beneficial as they lead to vasoconstriction, limiting blood flow to the hair follicles and their ability to reduce biochemical activity making hair follicles less susceptible to the cytotoxic effects of chemotherapy (Katsimbri et al. 2000). Dougherty (2006) compared the acceptability and efficacy of homemade scalp cooling systems (gel packs) and commercial cryogel caps (Chemocaps) in female adults with cancer. It was concluded that there was no difference in the efficacy between the systems but the "Chemocap" made by Intermark was more acceptable because of comfort and application. These devices are seldom used in the pediatric and adolescent population, which may be due to the high incidence of hematologic malignancies in this group and the discomfort associated with scalp cooling. However, for adolescents with solid tumors who are greatly affected by the change of body image caused by hair loss, such methods of preserving hair loss could be considered.

A recent study in animal models, examining topical agents such as minoxidil 2% in the prevention of chemotherapy-induced alopecia shows that the severity and duration of alopecia can be reduced but alopecia cannot be prevented (Wang et al. 2006).

Patient reactions to hair loss vary and may be related to the individual's perception of the importance of hair. Hair can have religious connotations; reflect trends of personal expression; and characterize beauty, age, and one's gender (Batchelor 2001). In the pediatric population, adolescents (particularly girls) are generally more likely to be affected by the resulting change in body image caused by hair loss (Wu and Chin 2003). In a study exploring adolescents' perceptions of their body image when faced with cancer and its treatment, Larouche and Chin-Peuckert (2006) found that hair loss was cited as one of the major factors responsible for altering body image. Adolescents described hair loss as being the greatest physical challenge to overcome while being treated for cancer. Parents of younger children may be more distressed than their child about the hair loss, as it confirms the harsh reality of initial treatment (McGrath 2002).

Nurses can play an important role in assisting children, adolescents, and parents to cope with alopecia. Nurses can help prepare for alopecia by providing information on the process and strategies for protecting the skin and eyes following hair loss (Batchelor 2001). Advice regarding applying sunscreens on the scalp in hot weather should be given. Encouraging adolescents to accept body changes by introducing positive coping strategies and appropriate resources, e.g. wigs, hats may be helpful during treatment (Abrams et al. 2007). Shaving the head once hair loss becomes apparent is relatively common and can help with scalp irritation as well as avoiding prolonged hair loss, which may be uncomfortable for the patient.

25.1.4 Prognosis

Alopecia does not present a medical threat to children or adolescents with cancer; however, it may be psychologically devastating, particularly to the adolescent.

25.2 Altered Skin Integrity Associated with Radiation Therapy

25.2.1 Incidence

Radiotherapy is used in the treatment of childhood cancer and is usually provided as an adjuvant treatment to cytotoxic chemotherapy (Felyn and Gardyn 2006). As skin reactions are not always documented, it is difficult to estimate the true incidence of reactions (Wells and MacBride 2003). However, it has been reported that 95% of patients treated with radiation therapy experience a skin reaction (McQuestion 2006). It is unclear whether this incidence includes children, and the severity of the reaction is unreported, but it does include radiation-recall skin reactions.

Advanced planning and delivery techniques of radiotherapy help decrease its effect on the skin, but the radiation invariably affects some of the skin cells.

25.2.2 Etiology

Cells in the basal layer of the epidermis are sensitive to radiotherapy because of their rapid proliferation rate. Cells in the epidermis have a life cycle of 2–3 weeks, and skin reactions often begin around this time.

Factors that influence the onset, duration, and degree of skin reactions include dosage and site of radiation and concurrent cytotoxic chemotherapy. Patient-related issues may include nutritional status and the general health of the patient.

Table 25.2 lists four recognized stages of radiation skin reaction.

25.2.3 Prevention

Preventative measures must be initiated from the time radiotherapy begins. The skin condition of children receiving radiotherapy should be assessed daily. Radiation skin reactions may not be preventable, but general principles of skin care included in skin-care policies may help decrease the severity of reactions (McQuestion 2006). Principles include the following:

1. Ensuring good skin hygiene to prevent increased irritation of the epithelium and to prevent bacteria build-up. Advice should include the need to use mild soap and warm water, pat skin dry, and preserve treatment marks.
2. Washing hair gently, if the head is treated, avoid scrubbing; drying hair on a low setting of a hair dryer if necessary.
3. Avoiding deodorants and perfumes at the radiation site.
4. Preventing dehydration of the skin by applying moisturizing cream or aqueous cream, which helps to retain water and lubricates to reduce friction.
5. Protecting skin from the sun during treatment and for 8 weeks following treatment. High-factor sunscreen should be used for at least 1 year post treatment (and preferably for life).
6. Avoiding hot water bottles and ice packs on the treatment field for 8 weeks.
7. Swimming is allowed, but the irradiated area should be showered gently, with lukewarm water afterwards and an aqueous cream applied.

Table 25.2. Stages of radiation skin damage (Boot-Vickers and Eaton 1999; Hopkins et al. 1999; Wells et al. 2004; MacMillan et al. 2007)

Stage	Reaction	Cause	Treatment
Erythema	Reddening of skin within 1 week of beginning therapy Hot, irritable rash	Dilation of capillaries in response to the damage	Water and mild soap. Water-based moisturizing cream/aqueous cream/sucralfate cream A topical steroid (usually 1% hydrocortisone) to reduce irritation, itching, and soreness *This treatment should be prescribed and used sparingly as it can inhibit healing due to its antiinflammatory properties*
Dry desquamation	Dry, flaky skin usually 2–4 weeks after onset of therapy Peeling skin irritation Often occurring in skin folds	Cell death in the upper layers of skin Decreased ability of epidermal basal cells to replace surface cells Sweat and sebaceous glands are damaged Friction increases damage	As for erythema If damage is due to friction, a self-adhesive, thin, aerated dressing may be applied and left intact until treatment is complete. If used, this dressing needs to be kept dry
Moist desquamation	Skin peeling or denuding with exudate; often white or yellow in color	Damage to the epidermis that exposes the dermis and allows leakage of serous fluid from the tissues Area is at risk from infection and fluid loss *A break in therapy may be necessary to allow repair of tissue*	Wound-healing principles (institutions may vary in treatment policies) Dry dressings/Hydrogel dressing covered with gauze and secured without the use of adhesive tape *Dressing must be removed during radiotherapy treatment as it could alter the dimensions for the penetration of the radiation*
Necrosis	Darkened tissue that eventually turns black	Therapy has exceeded the tolerance dose and causes basal cell death, leading to ulceration and necrosis	Surgery with debridement ± grafting

8. Choosing loose-fitting clothing that will not cause friction or trauma to the treatment site.

Another preventative measure in reducing toxicity is the prescribed use of amifostine (cytoprotective drug) throughout radiotherapy in children with cancer (Phan et al. 2004; Anacak et al. 2007).

25.2.4 Treatment

Treatment for skin damage caused by radiation therapy varies.

Treatment options are included in Table 25.2. The College of Radiographers (2001) recommended the use of aqueous creams to soothe irritated skin, though Wells et al. (2004) found no additional benefit using creams over washing with mild soap and water. Hydrogel dressings continue to be a recognized form of treatment for moist desquamation; however, MacMillan et al. (2007), in a randomized comparison of dry dressings vs. hydrogel, concluded that dry dressings appeared more comfortable and effective. Further research is needed in this area including pediatric patients as these studies did not include children.

25.2.5 Prognosis

Appropriate skin assessment and care should prevent permanent skin damage from radiation therapy. Nurses have a role to routinely perform skin assessment and address concerns regarding altered skin integrity for children and adolescents.

25.3 Radiation Sensitivity and Recall

25.3.1 Incidence

Some cytotoxic drugs can sensitize the skin to radiation (Alley et al. 2002). Radiation recall dermatitis is the development of an inflammation reaction throughout a previously irradiated area, following administration of certain drugs (Ristic 2004). The incidence in the pediatric population is unreported, but drugs that are particularly associated with radiation sensitization and recall are listed in Table 25.3. Radiation recall dermatitis can occur when the precipitating agent is administered within days or even years after radiation (Azria et al. 2005). Radiation recall usually occurs on first exposure to a particular trigger drug (Ristic 2004).

Factors to consider include identifying children and young people at increased risk. Distel et al. (2003) highlight that severe radiotherapy toxicity in pediatric cancer patients may be a result of increased sensitivity due to immunodeficiency syndromes. Ataxia telangiectasia gene mutation and protein kinase deficiency have been associated with such problems (Yeo and Johnson 2000).

Table 25.3. Cytotoxic drugs commonly associated with radiation interactions (adapted from Alley et al. 2002)

Radiation interaction	Drug
Radiation sensitization and recall	Bleomycin Dactinomycin Daunorubicin Etoposide 5-Fluorouracil Hydroxyurea Melphalan Methotrexate Vinblastine
Photosensitivity	5-Fluorouracil Methotrexate Vinblastine

25.3.2 Etiology

The mechanisms of radiation recall sensitivity are undefined. Possibilities include the following:

- Depletion in tissue stem cells within the irradiated field caused by the radiation therapy and subsequent chemotherapy exposure causes a "remembered" reaction by the remaining cells (Yeo and Johnson 2000).
- Radiation induces heritable mutations within surviving cells, producing a group of defective stem cells that are unable to tolerate a second insult with systemic chemotherapy (Indinnimeo et al. 2003).
- A third explanation is based on vascular reactions such as increased permeability (Azria et al. 2005).

Azria et al. (2005) distinguish between radiation recall and radiation enhancement, which refers to an acute skin reaction when chemotherapy is given within a week of radiation.

25.3.3 Clinical Features

Clinical features include erythema, desquamation, edema, vesicle formation, and ulceration. Necrosis and hemorrhage may occur (Ristic 2004). Patients may complain of pain and pruritis. Radiation recall dermatitis may occur in other organs such as mucous membranes, muscles, and gastrointestinal tract (Azria et al. 2005).

25.3.4 Treatment

Radiation recall dermatitis may resolve spontaneously without treatment. Close observation is required if the reaction appears mild (Azria et al. 2005). Corticosteroids and antiinflammatory agents may be prescribed to treat symptoms. The drug therapy causing the reaction may need to be discontinued. These actions should produce an improvement quickly although the time taken for resolution of cutaneous manifestations remains the same with or without steroid or antihistamine treatment (Camidge and Price 2001).

25.3.5 Prognosis

Most of the cutaneous lesions heal with supportive therapy. A decision to continue with the chemotherapeutic agent is usually determined by the severity of the reaction and the chemoresponsiveness of the tumor to the particular agent (Yeo and Johnson 2000).

25.4 Ultraviolet Recall Reaction/Photosensitivity

Ultraviolet reaction, also known as sunburn recall, photo recall, is a rare phenomenon that can occur with chemotherapy or antibiotics (Goldfeder et al. 2007). Patients experience reactivation of a prior sunburn. No specific reports in the pediatric population exist, likely due to the limited years of sun exposure.

There is no reported incidence of photosensitivity in children; however, it is established that ultraviolet radiation (sunlight) can produce effects on the skin of patients previously treated with cytotoxic therapy similar to those seen in radiation recall (Goldfeder et al. 2007). Table 25.3 lists the main drugs used in pediatrics that are likely to cause photosensitivity.

It has also been reported that children and adults previously treated with cytotoxic agents have an increased number of benign melanocytic nevi (moles) (Hughes et al. 1989; Kakrida et al. 2005). Melanocytic nevi, which commonly develop during childhood and adolescence, are identified as risk factors for future development of melanomas. Sunburn and intermittent sun exposure appear to be related to melanoma development (Rager et al. 2005).

Children and caregivers should be educated on the need for adequate sun protection: using sunscreen, seeking shade, wearing sun hats. Interestingly, studies show that the use of sunscreen on its own can often increase the number of sunburn incidences (Davis et al. 2002; Horsley et al. 2003). It may be assumed that sunscreen is offereing more protection than it actually is; people may then be less likely to cover up or seek shade. This finding emphasizes a need for education regarding the proper use of these products and an increased need for protective measures for the entire population.

25.5 Cutaneous Reactions Associated with High-Dose Cytosine Arabinoside

25.5.1 Incidence

Despite a paucity of literature, the incidence of cutaneous toxicity associated with high-dose cytosine arabinoside (HDAC) has been stated to range from 3 to 72% (Richards and Wujcik 1992). A study by Cetkovska et al. (2002) reported the overall incidence of cutaneous reaction to be 53% in 172 patients aged 16–71 treated with HDAC. Whitlock et al. (1997) found that 22% (4 of 18) of children developed cutaneous reactions with HDAC. Only literature in this area.

25.5.2 Etiology

The etiology of toxicity associated with HDAC is unclear. This toxicity can range from erythema to painful swelling, bullae formation, and desquamation. The severity of the reaction appears to be related to the dose and the number of consecutive doses. Erythema of this nature that begins on the palms and soles is known as hand–foot syndrome, or palmar–plantar erythrodysesthesia, and was originally described in patients receiving HDAC (Alley et al. 2002). However, other drugs have been associated with this toxicity, including 5-fluorouracil, doxorubicin, and methotrexate (Alley et al. 2002).

25.5.3 Prevention and Treatment

No therapy has been shown to prevent this condition, but most skin changes clear spontaneously (Cetkovska et al. 2002). Although this side effect is considered manageable, nurses must explore measures that could minimize these complications and reduce their impact on the patient's quality of life.

25.6 Nail Dystrophies

Nail changes associated with chemotherapy can include banding discoloration, oncholysis, and infection (Viale 2006). Although nail changes in patients receiving chemotherapy are reportedly fairly common (Alley et al. 2002), they are unreported as a problem for children. However, transverse ridges may occur (Beau's lines) associated with commonly used agents such as cyclophosphamide, doxorubicin, vincristine, and cytosine arabinoside (Koh et al. 2004). This side effect is temporary and resolves slowly following treatment. Nurses should be aware that nail changes are a possibility, and observe nails for such changes that could have an impact on the patient's physical and psychological well-being (Viale 2006).

25.7 Graft Vs. Host Disease

25.7.1 Incidence and Etiology

Graft vs. host disease (GvHD) occurs when transplanted donor cells recognize and react to recipient histoincompatible cells, causing tissue damage (Fig. 25.1). It remains a major complication after allogeneic hematopoietic stem cell transplantation (SCT), especially shown in adult studies with the increased use of stem cells from unrelated and mismatched donors.

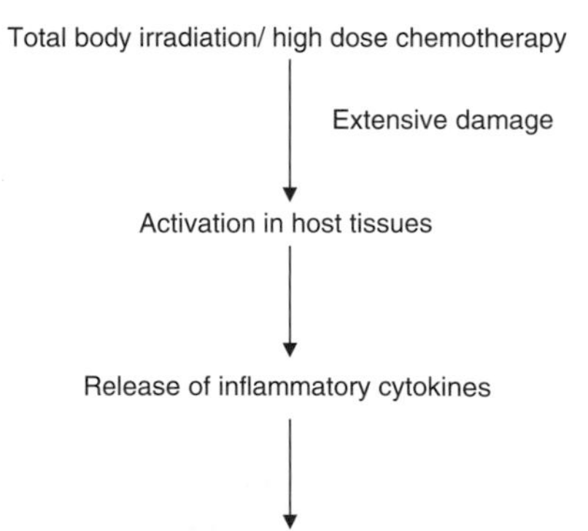

Figure 25.1
Mechanisms involved in phase 1 of GvHD

Patients who receive an allogeneic bone marrow transplant (BMT) fulfill the criteria necessary for the development of GvHD as originally proposed by Billingham (1966):

- Administration of adequate numbers of immunocompetent cells
- Donor and recipient histocompatibility
- Inability of the recipient to destroy the donor cells

Table 25.4 shows a three-phase model that elucidates the major processes that lead to GvHD (Ferrara et al. 1999).

There are few studies regarding this area in relation to children; however, Rembenger and Ringden (2007) demonstrated no difference in incidence of GvHD between peripheral blood stem cells and bone marrow allogeneic transplants. However, the sample size of the study was small and larger scale studies are recommended.

GvHD is classified as acute and chronic, although the distinction between them is not simply chronological. Both result from activation of donor T-cells against host antigens, but acute and chronic GvHD may have distinct pathophysiology (Toubai et al. 2008).

The acute form of GvHD typically develops up to 100 days after allogeneic SCT and is graded according to severity (Table 25.5). Clinically relevant grades II to IV occur in approximately 20–50% of patients who receive stem cells from a human leukocyte antigen (HLA) identical sibling donor and in 50–80%

Table 25.4. Processes leading to GvHD (Goker et al. 2001)

Phase	Processes
Phase 1 (conditioning) *Afferent phase*	Recipient conditioning resulting in damage to the tissues that starts before the infusion of the graft; see Fig. 25.1
Phase 2 (induction and expansion) *Afferent phase*	Recognition of the foreign host antigens by donor T-cells and activation, stimulation, and proliferation of T-cells
Phase 3 *Effector phase* (the cytokine storm)	Direct and indirect damage to host cells

Table 25.5. Clinical grading of acute GvHD

Grade	Skin	Liver Bilirubin (mg/dL)	Gastrointestinal
0	No rash	<2	<500 mL diarrhea/24 h
I	Rash <25% of body surface	2–3	>500 mL diarrhea/24 h
II	Rash 25–50% of body surface	3–6	>1,000 mL diarrhea/24 h
III	Generalized erythrodermia	6–15	>1,500 mL diarrhea/24 h
IV	Desquamation and bullae	>15	Severe abdominal pain ± ileus

Table 25.6. Classification of chronic GvHD

Limited chronic GvHD	Extensive chronic GvHD
Either or both Localized skin involvement Hepatic dysfunction	Either generalized skin involvement or localized skin involvement, with or without hepatic dysfunction, or eye involvement or oral mucosa involvement or any other target organ involvement

whose donor is an HLA-mismatched sibling or HLA-identical unrelated donor (Tabbara et al. 2002). The classically recognized target organs affected by acute GvHD are the skin, liver, and gastrointestinal tract, but other organs may be affected.

Chronic GvHD is a result of a later phase of alloreactivity. It occurs in approximately 30% of patients, typically after the first 100 days but up to years after transplantation. It can follow acute GvHD (progressive); can occur after the resolution of acute GvHD (quiescent); or be de novo, in which case there was no acute GvHD. Clinical manifestations of chronic GvHD are similar to autoimmune collagen vascular diseases. It appears to be a syndrome of immune disturbance resulting in autoimmunity and immunodeficiency (Martin 2008). It may involve various organs including the skin, liver, mouth, and eyes. Chronic GvHD can be classified as either limited or extensive (Table 25.6) in an attempt to determine which patients need treatment.

More recently, to incorporate clinical features of GvHD that sometimes present concomitanatly, the consensus classification of GvHD from the National Institutes of Health (NIH) includes late-onset (after day 100) acute GvHD and an overlap syndrome that has features of both acute and chronic GvHD (Toubai et al. 2008; Pasquini 2008).
Acute GvHD is classified as:

- Acute
- Recurrent
- Persistent
- Late onset (Toubai et al. 2008; Pasquini 2008)

Chronic GvHD is classified, depending on the presence of acute GvHD manifestations, as:

- Classic
- Overlap (Toubai et al. 2008; Pasquini 2008)

Acute GvHD can be rapid and devastating, and may involve the skin, liver, hematopoietic, or intestinal tissue (Berquist and Dvorak 2006). The skin is the most commonly affected system of acute GvHD. It is typically characterized by the following signs and symptoms, but these may also be a consequence of chemotherapy, radiation, or other drugs and are therefore not diagnostic of acute GvHD (Goker et al. 2001).

- A pruritic maculopapular rash involving the face, trunk, palms, and soles of the feet usually marks the onset
- The rash usually occurs at or near the time of engraftment
- The rash may look like a sunburn
- In severe cases, the rash develops into generalized erythroderma, bullous lesions, and desquamation, and may progress to epidermal necrosis

Figure 25.2 illustrates the debilitating consequences of chronic GvHD in a 11-year-old girl following unrelated bone marrow transplant. Chronic GvHD,

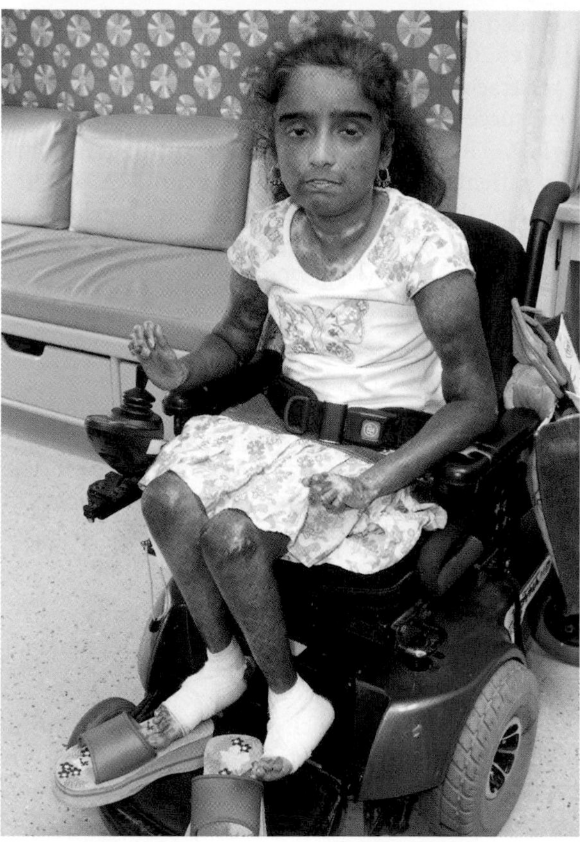

Figure 25.2

An 11-year-old girl, 3 years post unrelated bone marrow transplantation with severe chronic GvHD. Note severe contractures in hands, feet and other joints, skin scarring, and loss of pigmentation. Image courtesy of Dr. Adam Gassas, Hospital for Sick Children, Toronto

long-lasting manifestation of GvHD, can affect multiple organ systems and in contrast to acute GvHD, it is most often characterized by fibrosis of the affected organ (Toubai et al. 2008).

GvHD that affects the liver causes derangement of hepatic function resulting in increased bilirubin, alkaline phosphatase, and aminotransferase levels. In the posttransplant setting, these abnormalities may occur secondary to drug-induced liver toxicity, veno-occlusive disease, or hepatitis. The typical GI GvHD symptons of diarrhea, nausea, anorexia, and vomiting are nonspecific. An efficient and accurate diagnosis of GI GvHD can be established by endoscopic inspection and tissue biopsy specimens for histology and culture. However, endoscopy in this group of children and young people is not without risk (e.g., bleeding, hematoma formation, and risk of infection); therefore, laboratory investigations should be undertaken to outrule infections such as *Clostridium difficile*, cytomegalovirus (CMV), and herpes simplex (Berquist and Dvorak 2006).

For diagnostic purposes, for skin and liver, biopsies may be performed. Liver biopsies are usually performed only when isolated GvHD is suspected. Histologically, the diagnosis is confirmed by lymphocyte infiltration characterized as "satellite cell necrosis" (Langley et al. 1996).

25.7.2 Prevention

The first approach for GvHD prevention is to reduce the risk factors, if possible. Seventy percent of patients receiving HLA-matched transplants develop GvHD (Bron 1994). The most effective approaches to GvHD prevention involve removing T-cells from the graft by lymphocyte depletion. However, these methods increase the risk of graft failure or rejection and relapse as a consequence of a loss of the graft-vs.-leukemia (GvL) effect, which is the attack of immunocompetent cells in the graft against any remaining disease cells in the patient after transplantation (Holler 2006). Pharmacologic GvHD prophylaxis using immunosuppressive drugs is the preferred approach to disrupt the three phases of the GvHD cascade and prevent GvHD. It is aimed at removing or attenuating the activity of donor T-lymphocytes, reducing the risk of graft failure and attempts to maximize the GvL effect (Peters et al. 2000). Immunosuppression with combined drugs; short course of methotrexate and long-term application of cyclosporin appears to have been the gold standard of prophylaxis. Newer pharmacological agents interfering with T-cell activation, such as tacrolimus, are now used frequently in combination with methotrexate. Results are showing significantly lower incidence of GvHD than methotrexate/cyclosporin (Holler 2006). Recently, a new method of BMT where bone marrow (BM) cells are injected direcly into the BM cavity rather than IV, shows less GvHD in animal models (Miyake et al. 2008).

The pathophysiology of chronic GvHD is still not completely understood. This means that it is difficult to design effective prophylactic regimens. However, the prevention of acute GvHD appears to result in a lower incidence of chronic GvHD (Lee and Joachim Deeg 2008). Factors that are associated with a reduced frequency of chronic GvHD include:

- Younger, nonallosensitized donors
- Same-sex donors
- Use of stem cells other than peripheral blood cells mobilized by granulocyte colony-stimulating factors
- Incorporation of thymoglobulin into the conditioning regimen (Lee and Joachim Deeg 2008)

25.7.3 Treatment

GvHD in its most severe forms, affecting especially the gut and liver, is a major cause of treatment-related mortality, and early successful treatment is necessary to allow the patients chance of long-term care (Holler 2006).

Acute GvHD (grades II–IV) is treated by continuing immunosuppression and adding methylprednisolone at 2–2.5 mg/kg/day, with starting doses ranging from 1 to >20 mg/kg/day (Jacobsohn and Vogelsang 2002). Steroids are tapered based on the patient's response rather than a fixed schedule. However, the short- and long-term side effects of methylprednisolone, such as fungal infections, continue to be a cause of concern in such patients.

Immunosuppressive drugs such as steroids, cyclosporin, and tacrolimus are used to treat patients classified as having extensive chronic GvHD. Chronic GvHD may cause significant morbidity, and when mortality occurs it is most often due to infection.

Clinical trials have evaluated various monoclonal antibodies as treatment for GvHD in various settings, especially when refractory to corticosteroids. Infliximab, which blocks the action of tumor necrosis factor (TNF), and daclizumab, which blocks the action of IL-2, have proved effective in the pediatric population (Rodriguez et al. 2007). Rituximab has also shown to be beneficial in chronic GvHD (Holler 2006).

Extracorporeal photochemotherapy (ECP) is a new successful technique used in the treatment of GvHD. This leukapheresis-based process involves the patient's blood being exposed to UVA irradiation and then being returned. This approach limits the risk of infection associated with other treatments (Goyal 2007; Berger et al. 2007).

25.7.4 Prognosis

Although significant improvements have been made in allogeneic SCT, GvHD remains a major complication that can lead to significant morbidity and mortality. The more recent and less damaging approaches to allogeneic SCT may help to reduce GvHD by decreasing the intense conditioning regimen, which

1. Reduces early transplant-related mortality
2. Plays an important role in the development of GvHD

Supportive measures such as symptomatic control, parenteral nutrition, infection prophylaxis, skin care, psychological support, and physical rehabilitation are equally important to minimize further complications and improve quality of life.

References

Abrams A, Hazen E, Penson R (2007) Psychosocial issues in adolescents with cancer. Cancer Treatment Reviews 33(7): 622–630

Alley E, Green R, Schuchter L (2002) Cutaneous toxicities of cancer therapy. Current Opinions in Oncology 14:212–216

Anacak Y, Kamers S, Haydaroglu A (2007) Daily subcutaneous amifostine administration during irradiation of pediatric head and neck cancers. Pediatric Blood and Cancer 48(5):579–581

Azria D, Magne N, Zouhair A, Castadot P, Culine S, Ychou M, Stupp R, Van Houtte P, Dubois JB, Ozsahin M (2005) Radiation recall: a well recognized but neglected phenomenon. Cancer Treatment Reviews 31:555–570

Batchelor D (2001) Hair and cancer chemotherapy: consequence and nursing care–a literature study. European Journal of Cancer Care 10(3):147–163

Berger M, Passolano R, Albianir A, Saflei S, Barat V, Carraro F, Biasin E, Madon E, Fagioli F (2007) Extracorporeal photopheresis for steroid resistant graft versus host disease in pediatric patients. Journal of Pediatric Hematology/Oncology 29(10):678–687

Berquist W, Dvorak C (2006) Optimizing care for GI disorders in children after hematopoietic stem cell transplantation. Gastrointestinal Endoscopy 64(3):386–388

Billingham RE (1966) The biology of graft-vs-host reactions. The Harvey Lectures 62:21–78

Boot-Vickers M, Eaton K (1999) Sin care for patients receiving radiotherapy. Professional Nurse 14(10):706–708

Botchkarev VA (2003) Molecular mechanisms of chemotherapy-induced hair loss. Journal of Investigative Dermatology Symposium Proceedings 8(1):72–75

Botchkarev VA, Komarova EA, Siebenhaar F, Botchkarev NV, Kmarov PG, Maurer M, Gilchrest BA, Gudkov AV (2000) p53 is essential for chemotherapy-induced hair loss. Cancer Research 60(18):5002–5006

Bron D (1994) Graft-versus-host disease. Current Opinions Oncology 6:358–364

Camidge R, Price A (2001) Characterizing the phenomenon of radiation recall dermatitis. Radiotherapy Oncology 59: 237–245

Cetkovska P, Pizinger K, Cetkovsky P (2002) High-dose cytosine arabinoside-induced cutaneous reactions. Journal of the European Academy of Dermatology and Venerology 16 (5):481–485

College of Radiographers (2001) Summary of intervention for acute radiotherapy induced skin reactions in cancer patients; a clinical guideline. College of Radiographers, London

Davis KJ, Cokkinides VE, Weinstock MA, O'Connell MC, Wingo PA (2002) Summer sunburn and sun exposure among US youths ages 11 to 18: national prevalence and associated factors. Pediatrics 110(1 part 1):27–35

Distel L, Neubauer S, Varon R, Holter W, Grabenbauer G (2003) Fatal toxicity following radio- and chemotherapy of medullablastoma in a child with unrecognized Nijmegen breakage syndrome. Medical and Pediatric Oncology 41(1):44–48

Dougherty L (2006) Comparing methods to prevent chemotherapy-induced alopecia. Cancer Nursing Practice 5(6):25–31

Enskär K, von Essen L (2008) Physical problems and psychosocial function in children with cancer. Paediatric Nursing 20(3):37–41

Felyn A, Gardyn S (2006) Radiotherapy for children with cancer from a nursing perspective. European Journal of Oncology 10(3):231

Ferrara JL, Levy R, Chao NJ (1999) Pathophysiologic mechanisms of acute graft-vs-host disease. Biology of Blood and Marrow Transplant 5(6):347–356

Goker H, Ibrahim CH, Chao NJ (2001) Acute graft-vs-host disease: pathophysiology and management. Experimental Hematology 29(3):259–277

Goldfeder K, Levin J, Katz K, Clarke L, Loren A, James W (2007) Ultraviolet recall reaction after total body irradiation, etoposide, and methotrexate therapy. Journal of the American Academy of Dermatology 56(3):494–499

Goyal RK (2007) Refractory graft versus host disease in children: is photopheresis the answer. Journal of Pediatric Hematology/Oncology 29(11):731–732

Holler E (2006) Risk assessment in haematopoietic stem cell transplantation; GVHD prevention and treatment. Best Practice and Research Clinical Haematology 20(2):281–294

Hopkins M, Pownall J, Scott L (1999) Acute and subacute side effects of radiotherapy. In: Gibson F, Evans M (eds) Paediatric oncology: acute nursing care. Whurr, London

Horsley L, Charlton A, Waterman C (2003) Reducing skin cancer mortality by 2010: lessons from children's sunburn. British Journal of Dermatology 148(3):607

Hughes BR, Cunliffe WJ, Bailey CC (1989) Excess benign melanocytic naevi after chemotherapy for malignancy in childhood. British Medical Journal 299(6691):88–91

Indinnimeo M, Cicchini C, Kanakaki S, Larcinese A, Mingazzini PL (2003) Chemotherapy-induced radiation recall myositis. Oncology Reports 10(5):1401–1403

Jacobsohn DA, Vogelsang GB (2002) Novel pharmacotherapeutic approaches to prevention and treatment of GVHD. Drugs 62(6):879–889

Kakrida M, Orengo IF, Markus R (2005) Sudden onset of multiple nevi after administration of 6-mercaptapurine in an adult with Crohn's disease. International Journal of Dermatology 44(4):334–336

Katsimbri P, Bamias A, Pavlidis N (2000) Prevention of chemotherapy-induced alopecia using an effective scalp cooling system. European Journal of Cancer 36(6):766–771

Koh BK, Lee JH, Lee DW, Lee JY, Cho BK (2004) Transverse nail ridging and rough nails after bone marrow transplantation. International Journal of Dermatology 43:77–80

Langley RG, Walsh N, Nevill T, Thomas L, Rowden G (1996) Apoptosis is the mode of keratinocyte death in cutaneous graft-versus-host disease. Journal of the American Academy of Dermatology 35(2 Pt 1):187–190

Larouche S, Chin-Peuckert L (2006) Changes in body image experienced by adolescents with cancer. Journal of Pediatric Oncology Nursing 23(4):200–209

Lee JW, Joachim Deeg H (2008) Prevention of GVHD. Best Practice and Research Clinical Haematology 21(2):259–270

Martin PJ (2008) Biology of chronic GvHD. Implications for a therapeutic approach. Keio Journal of Medicine 57(4):177–183

McGrath P (2002) Beginning treatment for childhood acute lymphoblastic: insights from the parents' perspective. Oncology Nurses Forum 29(6):988–996

MacMillan M, Wells M, MacBride S, Raab G, Munro A, MacDougall H (2007) Randomized Comparison of dry dressings versus hydrogel in management of radiation induced moist desquamation. International Journal of Radiation Oncology, Biology, Physics 68(3):864–872

McQuestion M (2006) Evidence based skin care management in radiation therapy. Seminars in Oncology Nursing 22(3):163–173

Miyake T, Inaba M, Fukui J, Ueda Y, Hosaka N, Kamiyama Y, Ikehara S (2008) Prevention of GVHD by intrabone marrow injection of donor Tcells: involvement of bone marrow stromal cells. Clinical and Experimental Immunology 152(1):153–162

Pasquini MC (2008) Impact of graft-versus-host disease on survival. Best Practice and Research. Clinical Haematology 21(2):193–204

Peters C, Minkov M, Gadner H, Klingebiel T, Vossen J, Locatelli F, Cornish J, Ortega J, Bekasi A, Souillet G, Stary J, Niethammer D; European Group for Blood and Marrow Transplantation (EBMT) Working Party Paediatric Diseases; International BFM Study Group–Subcommittee Bone Marrow Transplantation (IBFM-SG) (2000) Statement of current majority practices in graft-versus-host disease prophylaxis and treatment in children. Bone Marrow Transplant 26(4):405–411

Phan C, Paris K, Josse B et al (2004) Tolerance and practicality of amifostine during radiation of pediatric patients to reduce long term side effects and second malignancies. Radiotherapy Oncology 73:S1–S385

Rager E, Bridgeford E, Ollila D (2005) Cutaneous melanoma; update on prevention, screening, diagnosis, and treatment. American Family Physician 72(2):269–281

Remberger M, Ringden O (2007) Similar Outcome after Unrelated Allogenic Peripheral Blood Stem Transplantation Compared with Bone Marrow in Children and Adolescents. Transplantation 84(4):551–554

Richards C, Wujcik D (1992) Cutaneous toxicity associated with high-dose cytosine arabinoside. Oncology Nurses Forum 19(8):1191–1195

Ristic B (2004) Radiation recall dermatitis. International Journal of Dermatology 43:627–631

Rodriguez V, Anderson P, Trotz B, Arndt C, Allen J, Khan S (2007) Use of infliximab–daclizumab combinations for the treatment of acute and chronic graft versus host disease of the liver and gut. Pediatric Blood and Cancer 49(2): 212–215

Tabbara IA, Zimmerman K, Morgan C, Nahleh Z, Allogeneic hematopoietic stem cell transplantation (2002) Allogeneic hematopoietic stem cell transplantation: complications and results. Archives of Internal Medicine 162(14):1558–1566

Toubai T, Sun Y, Reddy P (2008) GVHD pathophysiology: is acute different from chronic. Best Practice and Research. Clinical Haematology 21(2):101–117

Viale PH (2006) Chemotherapy and cutaneous toxicities: implications for oncology nurses. Seminars in Oncology Nursing 22(3):144–151

Wang J, Lu Z, Au J (2006) Protection against chemotherapy induced alopecia. Pharmaceutical Research 23(11): 2505–2514

Wells M, MacBride S (2003) Radiation Skin Reactions. In: Faithfull S, Wells M (eds) Supportive care in radiotherapy. Churchill Livingstone, Edinburgh

Wells M, MacMillan M, Raab G, MacBride S, Bell N, MacKinnon K, MacDougall H, Samuel L, Munro A (2004) Does aqueous or sucralfate cream affect the severity of erthematous radiation skin reactions? A randomized controlled trial. Radiotherapy and Oncology 73:153–162

Whitlock JA, Wells RJ, Hord JD, Janco RL, Greer JP, Gay JC, Edwards JR, McCurley TL, Lukens JN (1997) High-dose cytosine arabinoside and etoposide: an effective regimen without anthracyclines for refractory childhood acute nonlymphocytic leukemia. Leukemia 11(2):185–189

Williams PD, Schmideskamp J, Ridder EL, Williams AR (2006) Symptom monitoring and dependent care during cancer treatment in children: pilot study. Cancer Nursing 29(3): 188–197

Wu LM, Chin CC (2003) Factors related to satisfaction with body image in children undergoing chemotherapy. Kaohsiung Journal of Medical Science 19(5):217–224

Yeo W, Johnson PJ (2000) Radiation-recall skin disorders associated with the use of antineoplastic drugs: pathogenesis, prevalence, and management. American Journal of Clinical Dermatology 1(2):113–116

Endocrine System

Julie Watson

Contents

26.1 Introduction 489
26.2 Hypothalamic–Pituitary Dysfunction 489
26.2.1 Incidence and Etiology 489
26.3 Growth Hormone Deficiency 491
26.3.1 Treatment 492
26.3.1.1 Investigation 492
26.3.1.2 Growth Hormone Replacement Therapy 492
26.3.2 Prognosis 492
26.4 Hypothalamic–Pituitary–Gonadal Axis 493
26.4.1 Gonadotrophin Deficiency 493
26.4.2 Early or Precocious Puberty 493
26.4.2.1 Treatment 493
26.4.2.2 Prognosis 494
26.5 Thyroid Disorders 494
26.5.1 Treatment 494
26.6 Hypothalamic–Pituitary–Adrenal Axis 495
26.6.1 Treatment 495
26.7 Other Pituitary Hormones 495
26.7.1 Fertility 496
26.7.1.1 Testicular Failure 496
26.7.1.2 Ovarian Failure 496
26.7.2 Treatment 496
26.7.2.1 Assessment of Gonadal Function 496
26.7.2.2 Treatment for Gonadal Dysfunction 496
26.7.3 Prognosis 497
References 499

26.1 Introduction

Endocrine abnormalities following cancer therapy are common, and occur in approximately 40% of childhood cancer survivors at follow-up (Rutter and Rose 2007; Oberfield and Sklar 2002). These include growth hormone, thyrotropin, adrenocorticotropin, and gonadotropin deficiencies, primary hypothyroidism, gonadal failure and obeisity, which negatively impact growth, fertility, quality of life, morbidity, and mortality of cancer survivors (Haller and Schatz 2007). Endocrine disturbances are attributed to the location of the disease, the type and dosage of chemotherapy, the amount and schedule of radiotherapy, and the length of time since treatment (Cohen 2003). A clinical follow-up program for the assessment of late effects of therapy, with prompt recognition and management of endocrine abnormalities, is an essential component of care after the successful treatment of childhood cancer.

26.2 Hypothalamic–Pituitary Dysfunction

Table 26.1. summarizes the physiology of hypothalamic–pituitary function.

26.2.1 Incidence and Etiology

The hypothalamic–pituitary axis is central to the control of the endocrine system (Brougham et al. 2002). Children treated for tumors arising in the region of the hypothalamus and pituitary can develop neuroendocrine dysfunction as a direct result of the tumor or

Table 26.1. Hypothalamic releasing hormones and the pituitary trophic hormones (Drury 1990)

Hypothalamic hormones	Pituitary hormones	Peripheral hormones
Gonadotrophin-releasing hormone (GnRH, LHRH)	Luteinizing hormone (LH) Follicle stimulating hormone (FSH)	Estrogens/androgens
Prolactin inhibiting factor (PIF)	Prolactin	–
Growth hormone-releasing factor (GHRH) Somatostatin (GHRIH)	Growth hormone (GH)	Somatomedin C (insulin-like growth factor) and others
Thyrotropin-releasing hormone (TRH)	Thyroid-stimulating hormone (TSH)	Thyroxine (T_4), triiodothyronine (T_3) Both are present as free and bound forms
Corticotrophin-releasing factor (CRF)	Adrenocorticotrophic hormone	Cortisol
Vasopressin, antidiuretic hormone (ADH)	–	–
Oxytocin	–	–

Table 26.2. Factors related to pituitary hormone deficiencies in pediatric oncology (Cohen 2003; Brougham et al. 2002)

Dependent factor	Effect on hypothalamic–pituitary dysfunction
Radiation dose received	Directly related. GH is the most radiosensitive; caused by doses as low as 18 Gy. Increasing radiation doses cause deficiencies in gonadotrophin, corticotrophin, and thyrotropin secretion
Fractionation schedule	Inversely related, i.e., therapy administered over more fractions will reduce the degree of dysfunction
Interval since completion of therapy	Dysfunction becomes progressively more severe with time since radiation treatment, possibly because of the delayed effects of radiotherapy on the axis, or pituitary dysfunction secondary to earlier damage to the hypothalamus. Evidence indicates that the hypothalamus is more sensitive to radiotherapy than the pituitary
Age at treatment	Younger children are more sensitive to radiation-induced damage of the hypothalamic–pituitary axis compared with older children and adults

surgery required to remove it. More commonly, neuroendocrine problems in childhood cancer survivors are the result of exposure of the hypothalamus to external beam radiation (Sklar 2002). Endocrine dysfunction can occur as a result of:

- Radiation therapy for central nervous system (CNS), orbital, facial, or nasopharyngeal tumors
- Cranial and/or craniospinal radiation for acute lymphoblastic leukemia (ALL)
- Total body irradiation for stem cell transplant (Cohen 2003)

The anterior pituitary hormone deficiencies that result from these treatments depend on several factors, as shown in Table 26.2. The larger the dose of radiation and the longer the time interval since treatment, the greater is the likelihood of injury and development of the associated neuroendocrine problems. The hypothalamus is more radiosensitive and is the primary site of injury with radiation doses less than 50 Gy. Higher doses can damage the anterior pituitary itself, and lead to early, multiple pituitary hormone deficiencies (Gleeson and Shalet 2004). Evidence suggests that the threshold dose of radiation necessary to induce neuroendocrine abnormalities is 18 Gy, given in conventional daily fractions, At this dose, the result is most often isolated growth hormone (GH) deficiency, which may not present until 10 years after treatment. Alteration in gonadotropins (LH/FSH), TSH, and ACTH generally occur only following doses of radiation greater than 30–40 Gy, and may be present within 5 years of treatment, while hypothalamic–pituitary disturbances do not tend to develop until several years after treatment; however, once established, they are often permanent and irreversible (Sklar 2002).

26.3 Growth Hormone Deficiency

Impaired growth and adult short stature occurs frequently in survivors of childhood cancer, especially when individuals are treated at a younger age (Rutter and Rose 2007). A variety of factors, both endocrine and nonendocrine, contribute to impaired growth following cancer therapy, as summarized in Table 26.3.

GH deficiency is the most common endocrine abnormality following cranial radiation. The clinical presentation in children is usually short stature; however, the factors that disrupt normal growth are not dependant on GH alone. Irradiation of skeletal structures (e.g., spine, long bones), glucocorticoids, chemotherapeutic agents, young age at treatment, and other endocrine abnormalities (e.g., early puberty, hypothyroidism) can also contribute to short stature (Rutter and Rose 2007). The incidence and severity of growth failure varies widely because of these confounding factors.

Table 26.3. Factors predictive of short stature in childhood cancer survivors (Sklar 2002)

Clinical variables
Young age at diagnosis/treatment
Female sex
Treatment variables
High-dose radiotherapy (cranial/craniospinal)
Intensive chemotherapy/glucocorticoid therapy
Endocrine abnormalities
Growth hormone deficiency
Early puberty
Hypothyroidism

In addition to linear growth, GH is also responsible for the normal maturation of muscle mass, bone mineral density, fat distribution, cardiac function, and metabolic functions (including glucose and lipid metabolism) (Clayton et al. 2005). Therefore, a deficiency in GH has lifelong health implications, not just the attainment of final height.

Growth can be divided into three stages:

1. Infancy – from birth to 2 years, growth is influenced primarily by nutrition and health status
2. Childhood – GH is the dominant factor, in addition to nutrition and health status
3. Puberty – GH and sex hormones (e.g., estrogen/testosterone) dominate until epiphyseal fusion and growth is complete

Consequently, children treated for cancer at an early age, who subsequently develop GH deficiency prior to completion of growth, are far less likely to achieve their expected final stature, unless they receive GH replacement. In particular, children who are treated before the age of 4 years, and receive greater than 30 Gy of cranial/craniospinal radiation are most effected. Additionally, evidence suggests that females do worse than males, because they are more likely to have early puberty in addition to GH deficiency as a consequence of cancer therapy, as discussed in Sect. 26.4.2 (Armstrong et al. 2007). The effects of glucocorticoids and some chemotherapy agents (6-mercaptopurine, methotrexate) can impair growth due to their effect on osteoclast activity, and other less well-understood mechanisms. However, the effect of these is limited to the time of therapy, and is not sustained after treatment (Gleeson and Shalet 2004).

Diagnosis of GH deficiency can be problematic in this population due to the nature of neurosecretory dysfunction caused by cranial radiation therapy. It is characterized by diminished physiologic secretion of GH in the face of preserved peak responses to provocative testing, such that these tests produce false negative results (Gleeson and Shalet 2004). Over time, however, this discrepancy will diminish, and patients will eventually show diminished peak responses to testing, but they would already demonstrate the effects of GH deficiency. This emphasizes the importance of careful growth monitoring in childhood cancer survivors, in addition to specific hormone testing for early detection of GH deficiency (Clayton et al. 2005).

26.3.1 Treatment

26.3.1.1 Investigation

Children at risk for impaired growth as a result of cancer therapy should be examined regularly, with their growth plotted on the appropiate growth chart. Monitoring should be more frequent from the time of expected onset of puberty through to the fusion of growth plates at full sexual maturation. If there is any decline in growth velocity, or signs of early puberty, formal evaluation for GH deficiency and other endocrine problems should be performed (Oberfield and Sklar 2002). Before establishing any hormone treatment, the following assessments should be made:

1. Accurate measurement of supine length (if under 2 years), standing height, sitting height, and weight
2. Measurement of parents
3. Calculation of decimal age
4. Plotting of growth measurements on appropriate chart
5. Calculation of mid-parental height and target range
6. Calculation of height velocity
7. Pubertal staging
8. Bone age
9. Health/nutritional assessment and appropriate blood tests to screen for other causes of impaired growth (e.g., CBC, LDH, ferritin, TSH, T3, free T4)

A GH stimulation test is performed once GH deficiency is suspected. Laboratory studies can be performed, including clonidine, arginine, and insulin tolerance tests. The gold standard test is the insulin tolerance test (ITT), which is safe and reliable, provided that the test is performed in a pediatric endocrine unit by trained providers who follow a strict procedure of timed blood draws following injection of the insulin bolus (Galloway et al. 2002). The ITT can detect GH deficiency if serum GH levels during the testing period are lower than the expected value in response to stimulation of the anterior pituitary with insulin.

26.3.1.2 Growth Hormone Replacement Therapy

Once it is confirmed that the child is GH-deficient and 2 years have elapsed following cancer treatment, replacement with recombinant GH should be considered.

Somatropin (synthetic human growth hormone) is given in the form of daily subcutaneous injections. Several recent studies have attempted to determine the optimal dosing, and currently, doses of 0.2–0.35 mg/kg/week are routinely used (Gleeson and Shalet 2004). Historically, GH replacement therapy was discontinued at completion of growth and fusion of episeal plates. However, consideration must be given to continuation of GH replacement into adulthood to avoid adverse consequences associated with GH deficiency, such as; reduced muscle mass, increased fat deposition, loss of bone density, cardiovascular effects, and adverse lipid profile (Clayton et al. 2005).

26.3.2 Prognosis

GH replacement therapy appears to be a safe and effective treatment to improve the growth of children who develop GH deficiency as a result of cancer therapy (Dickerman 2007). However, recent studies continue to report reduced final height in many survivors despite GH replacement (Rutter and Rose 2007; Oberfield and Sklar 2002). Poor response to GH therapy is likely related to multiple confounding factors that are both patient-related (e.g., spinal radiation, early puberty) and treatment-related (e.g., suboptimal dosing, late recognition of GH deficiency) (Oberfield and Sklar 2002). Earlier diagnosis of GH deficiency and prompt treatment with GH replacement using contemporary dosing regimes, in addition to increased use of gonadotrophin releasing hormone (GnRH) agonist to delay puberty can improve growth outcomes in these patients (Clayton et al. 2005).

Adverse effects of GH replacement include a risk for benign intracranial hypertension (BIH) and a potential worsening of scoliosis (Haller and Schatz 2007). GH replacement in childhood cancer survivors has not been associated with an increased risk of disease recurrance, despite previous concerns of its mitogenic properties (Gleeson and Shalet 2004). However, it has been suggested that GH therapy could cause an increased risk for second neoplasms in adulthood, and large prospective epidemiologic studies are underway to determine the risk for childhood cancer survivors (Rutter and Rose 2007).

26.4 Hypothalamic–Pituitary–Gonadal Axis

26.4.1 Gonadotrophin Deficiency

Higher doses of cranial irradiation (>50 Gy) for the treatment of childhood cancer can damage the hypothalamic–pituitary–gonadal axis, resulting in gonadotrophin deficiency (Cohen 2003). Paradoxically, lower doses of cranial radiation may result in early puberty, as discussed in Sect. 26.4.2. The incidence and severity of gonadotrophin deficiency is dose-dependent, and the risk increases with the number of years post treatment. It is the second most prevalent anterior pituitary hormone deficiency seen in survivors of CNS tumors in childhood, and occurs in 20–50% of patients (Gleeson and Shalet 2004). Gonadotrophin deficiency presents with decreased serum levels of:

- Follicle stimulating hormone (FSH)
- Luteinizing hormone (LH)

Clinically, gonadotrophin deficiency can exhibit a broad spectrum of severity, from subclinical abnormalities that are detectable by GnRH testing, to a significant reduction in the circulating sex hormones causing delayed puberty, hypogonadism, and impaired growth (Brougham et al. 2002). Exogenous GnRH replacement therapy may restore gonadal function and fertility; however, experience with this treatment is limited to date.

26.4.2 Early or Precocious Puberty

Over the past two decades, studies have provided evidence that cranial radiation is associated with premature activation of the hypothalamic–pituitary–gonadal axis, resulting in early and precocious puberty in children treated for childhood cancer. Low-dose radiation (18–24 Gy) used in ALL is associated with a higher rate of early puberty, predominantly affecting females. High dose radiation (25–50 Gy) used for the treatment of CNS tumors, can cause early puberty in both males and females (Gleeson and Shalet 2004; Sklar 2002). There is a clear linear association between age at treatment, and age at onset of puberty: patients treated at an earlier age will undergo earlier puberty. A higher body mass index (BMI) may also contribute to earlier timing (Sklar 2002). The mechanism for early puberty following cranial irradiation is due to disinhibition of cortical influences on the hypothalamus, causing increased amplitude and frequency of pulsatile GnRH secretion, which stimulates the gonads to produce sex hormones (Brougham et al. 2002).

The majority of patients who experience early puberty will also develop GH insufficiency, compounding the negative effect on growth. Clinical signs of GH deficiency can be masked by early puberty, because the sex hormones cause a pubertal growth spurt, but viewed in the context of their bone age and pubertal status, these children grow at a suboptimal rate and can have significantly reduced final height (Sklar 2002). This further emphasizes the need for specialized follow-up programs for childhood cancer survivors, such that these endocrine disturbances can be identified early and treated appropriately, to produce the best outcome in the patient (Robison et al. 2005).

26.4.2.1 Treatment

Regular clinical assessment of growth and pubertal development in children at risk for early puberty includes:

- Pubertal status (Tanner stage)
- Auxological assessment, including standing and sitting heights

- Biochemical assessment of GH and gonadotrophin secretion
- Radiological assessment of bone age

If either precocious or early puberty is identified and the child is at risk for negative effects (such as reduced final height), puberty can be suppressed using a GnRH analog (GnRHa). This medication is given as an intramuscular (IM) injection either monthly, or every 12 weeks depending on the GnRHa of choice. Combined treatment with GH and GnRHa will improve the final height of the patient, as discussed in Sect. 26.3.2.

26.4.2.2 Prognosis

GnRHa treatment is safe and effective in delaying puberty in both males and females (Dickerman 2007). The most common complication is sterile abcess at the injection site. Despite increased use of GnRHa in childhood cancer survivors treated with cranial radiation, studies continue to document poor growth outcomes, likely due to the multiple confounding factors effecting growth after cancer therapy. Spinal radiation in particular can prevent attainment of expected height despite appropriate hormone replacement (Gleeson & Shalet, 2004). Close monitoring of growth and pubertal development is essential for patients at risk.

26.5 Thyroid Disorders

Thyroid hormones are responsible for the control of our basal metabolic rate, and are essential for normal growth, cellular activity, and tissue repair. The hypothalamus is stimulated by low levels of circulating thyroid hormones (T3, T4), and secretes TRH that causes the pituitary to secrete TSH. This potent stimulus causes the thyroid to secrete T4 and complete its conversion to the active hormones, namely, free-T4 and T3. Disruption of this feedback cycle due to injury at the level of the hypothalamus, pituitary, or thyroid gland itself can cause thyroid hormone abnormalities. Thyroid disorders following treatment for childhood cancer can include: hypothyroidism, both primary and central, hyperthyroidism, and thyroid neoplasms: (Darzy and Shalet 2005). These disorders can be caused by:

1. Radiation therapy to the neck/mantle region for Hodgkin's lymphoma
2. Cranial/craniospinal radiation for CNS tumors or ALL
3. Total body irradiation for stem cell transplant
4. I-131–MIBG monoclonal antibody therapy for neuroblastoma

Primary hypothyroidism is the most common thyroid disorder in this population, and results from direct injury to the thyroid gland from radiation. A 28% incidence in the survivors of Hodgkin's lymphoma, and a 50% risk of developing an underactive thyroid gland after 20 years in survivors who received 45 Gy or more radiation to the thyroid gland has been reported (Sklar 2002). Of note, new cases have been reported as long as 25 years after treatment (Rutter and Rose 2007). Scatter from cranial/craniospinal radiation for CNS can also cause damage, resulting in an incidence of 20–60% in these patients depending on the dose and the time since treatment (Schmeigelow 2003). The effect of adjuvant chemotherapy in not yet clear, but may be associated with increased risk, in addition to female gender (Gleeson and Shalet 2004).

Central hypothyroidism, or TSH deficiency, results from injury to the hypothalamic–pituitary–thyroid axis, as a result of cranial radiation or injury due to tumors in the region and/or their surgical removal. This axis is the least vulnerable to radiation damage, and studies report only a 6% incidence in CNS tumor survivors after 12 years (Gleeson and Shalet 2004).

Thyroid neoplasms, both benign and malignant, occur frequently following radiation of the head and neck. The greatest risk is in patients treated with relatively low-dose radiotherapy (<25 Gy), those treated before 5 years of age, and who are of female gender. Tumors begin to appear 5–10 years after treatment, but the risk of occurance persists for decades (Sklar 2002). Fortunately, these neoplasms are usually well differentiated, and have an excellent prognosis when detected early.

26.5.1 Treatment

Annual clinical assessment of the patient at risk for thyroid dysfunction should include:

1. History/review of systems for signs or symptoms of thyroid dysfunction
2. Physical examination
3. Palpation of thyroid gland
4. Height/weight
5. Serum TSH, T3, Free-T4

A biochemical diagnosis of hypothyroidism relies on the measurement of serum TSH and the active thyroid hormones, T3 and free-T_4. Primary hypothyroidism results in an elevated TSH and a low free-T_4, with or without symptoms of hypothyroidism; compensated hypothyroidism is indicated by an elevated TSH and a normal free-T_4. Diagnosis of central hypothyroidism is often more difficult. However, some authors argue that even when TSH and free-T_4 both fall within the normal range, a more detailed investigation of TSH dynamics, including TRH levels, can confirm the diagnosis of central hypothyroidism (Brougham et al. 2002). The clinical significance of this is in doubt, as is the specificity of TSH/TRH testing in this population (Gleeson and Shalet 2004).

Once the diagnosis of hypothyroidism is made, thyroxine replacement therapy should be initiated. Oral administration of 100 µg/m^2/day is prescribed, to fully suppress the hypothalamus and replace endogenous T4, with bloodwork monitored regularly while on therapy. If patients present with early, compensated primary hypothyroidism, thyroxine replacement should be recommended, because elevated serum TSH can promote growth of thyroid neoplasms.

26.6 Hypothalamic–Pituitary–Adrenal Axis

The hypothalamic–pituitary–adrenal axis appears to be relatively resistant to the effects of radiation therapy, and ACTH deficiency following treatment for childhood cancer is rare. Schmeigelow et al. (2003) reported an incidence of 19% among survivors of CNS tumors that did not involve the hypothalamus/pituitary, after 15 years of follow-up. The effect has a clear dose–response relationship, and only patients treated with high doses of radiation for CNS tumors (>50 Gy) seem to be affected (Brougham et al. 2002). This and other studies suggest that the effects of radiation on this axis present relatively late, often over 10 years after treatment (Gleeson and Shalet 2004). Treatment doses of glucocorticoids may also suppress the hypothalamic–pituitary–adrenal axis, and cause adrenal insufficiency. Dexamethasone at a dosage of 6 mg/m^2/day for 28–42 days can mildly suppress the axis for up to 4–8 weeks following administration (Cohen 2003; Peterson et al. 2003). Aldosterone secretion is usually unaffected because of its dependance on angiotensin II rather than ACTH.

26.6.1 Treatment

Diagnosis of ACTH deficiency can be difficult, and the ITT is the assessment of choice, as with testing for GH. If a diagnosis is made, hormone replacement with mineralocorticoids and/or glucocorticoids may be required, and these individuals need monitoring by an endocrinologist. A hydrocortisone "stress dose" is required during illness or when undergoing surgery in patients whose endogenous hypothalamic–pituitary–adrenal axis is suppressed by hormone replacement therapy (Brougham et al. 2002). Patients at risk need to be educated about the lifetime risk for thyroid disease, and the need for early detection of second neoplasms.

26.7 Other Pituitary Hormones

Prolactin secretion is inhibited by dopamine from the hypothalamus. Damage to the hypothalamus with high-dose cranial radiation (>50 Gy) can disrupt this inhibitory control and result in hyperprolactinemia (Cohen 2003; Brougham et al. 2002). This disorder is seen rarely in childhood cancer survivors, but can be the cause of secondary amenorrhea or galactorrea (Sklar 2002).

Antidiuretic hormone (ADH) deficiency causing diabetes insipidus (DI) has not been attributed to cranial irradiation. However, DI has been associated with intracranial tumors involving the pituitary gland following cranial surgery or secondary to leukemic infiltration. The deficiency in these cases usually persists despite treatment of the underlying malignancy (Brougham et al. 2002), and may require lifelong treatment with exogenous vasopressin.

The syndrome of inappropriate antidiuretic hormone secretion (SIADH), with free water retention and hyponatremia, has been associated with various malignancies and cancer treatments. The associated malignancies are those more commonly seen in adults, including gastrointestinal tumors, breast and prostatic cancers, and primary CNS tumors. However, chemotherapeutic agents commonly used in treatment of childhood cancer which can cause SIADH include: vinca alkaloids (e.g., vincristine, vinblastine), cisplatin, and the alkylating agents; cyclophosphamide and melphalan. Fortunately, SIADH usually resolves with fluid restriction and sodium replacement, and withdrawal of the offending medication, and is rarely a long-term complication (Brougham et al. 2002).

26.7.1 Fertility

Radiotherapy involving the pelvic area and intensive systemic chemotherapy can cause direct damage to the gonadal tissue (testes and ovaries), and reproductive structures. This damage can result in sex hormone deficiencies, subfertility, or infertility in both males and females (Rutter and Rose 2007).

26.7.1.1 Testicular Failure

The adult male testes has two functions:

- Steroidogenesis
- Spermatogenesis

Table 26.4. outlines the physiology of the testes and the effects of radiotherapy and chemotherapy on their function. Damage to germ cells and infertility are common following cancer therapy, and can be induced by both chemotherapeutic agents and irradiation of the testes. However, Leydig cell damage and androgen insufficiency are uncommon, and tend to only occur with higher doses of radiation (Sklar 2002). The mechanism that makes the testes susceptible to the toxic effects of radiation and chemotherapy appears to involve the combination of destruction of the germ cell pool, and when the germ cells survive, inhibition of further differentiation (Thomson et al. 2002).

26.7.1.2 Ovarian Failure

Ovarian function is more complex than the male testes, because of the functional interdependance of the oocyte and sex-hormone producing cells within the follicle. Damage to the germ cells results in loss of both endocrine function and fertility. Fortunately, the young ovary is relatively resistant to chemotherapy-induced damage, and prepubertal/adolescent girls will often recover ovarian function following treatment (Robison et al. 2005). Table 26.5. outlines the main functions and the consequential effects of radiotherapy and chemotherapy.

Additionally, radiotherapy involving the uterus and reproductive structures in childhood is associated with:

- Increased incidence of nulliparity
- Increased rates of spontaneous miscarriage
- Intrauterine growth retardation (IUGR) due to decreased uterine volume and elasticity

It is essential that both survivors and their obstetricians be aware of potential risks, so that pregnancy can be monitored appropriately. Women who have received anthracyclines may also have cardiovascular late effects that create a high-risk situation during childbirth.

26.7.2 Treatment

26.7.2.1 Assessment of Gonadal Function

Table 26.6. summarizes the patient history and investigations necessary when assessing gonadal function in males and females.

26.7.2.2 Treatment for Gonadal Dysfunction

When gonadal failure is diagnosed, Estrogen replacement in girls is started with a small dose of ethinyl oestradiol of 2 μg, increasing in small increments over 2 years until full establishment of puberty. A combined pill of estrogen and progesterone can then be given (e.g., Loestrin 30) for continuation therapy. Boys are started on 100 mg of sustanon every 6 weeks for testosterone replacement, increasing to every 4 weeks until puberty is established. Males who

Table 26.4. Outline of the function of the testes and the associated effects of radiotherapy and chemotherapy

Function	Associated hormones	Target cells	Action	Effects of radiotherapy	Effects of chemotherapy
Steroidogenesis	GnRH released from hypothalamus stimulates luteinizing hormone (LH) from the pituitary	Leydig's cells of somatic cells of testes to produce testosterone	Testosterone acts systemically to produce male secondary sexual characteristics, anabolism, and the maintenance of libido (Testosterone feeds back on hypothalamus/ pituitary to inhibit GnRH secretion)	Leydig's cells are more resistant to damage. Damage occurs at doses of 20 Gy in prepubertal boys and up to 30 Gy in sexually mature males. Secondary sexual characteristics may develop despite impaired spermatogenesis	Similar to radiotherapy effects. Leydig's cells are less sensitive and may be unaffected. Higher doses may cause Leydig cell dysfunction
Spermatogenesis	GnRH released from hypothalamus stimulates follicle stimulating hormone (FSH)	Sertoli's cells in germinal epithelium of the seminiferous tubules	Produces mature sperm (and feedback hormone, inhibin, that appears to feedback on pituitary to decrease FSH secretion) Testosterone also acts locally to aid spermatogenesis	Damage depends on the field of treatment, total dose, and fractionation schedule. Doses as low as 0.1 Gy can affect spermatogenesis with temporary azospermia and oligospermia. Doses over 4 Gy may have a permanent effect	Extent of damage depends on agent administered and dose received[a] Gonadotoxic chemotherapy can cause oligospermia or azoospermia

[a] Gonadotoxic agents include: cis-platin, procarbazine, cytarabine, vinblastine, and alkylating agents such as cyclophosphamide, melphalan, chlorambucil
(Drury 1990; Cohen 2003; Brougham et al. 2002)

have received radiation doses of 24 Gy to the testes or more will likely require lifelong hormone replacement (Sklar 2002).

Patients must be counseled appropriately regarding their fertility status and be advised about the implications for the future. Many adolescent cancer patients may be sexually active during and after treatment, and a lack of information about fertility status and safe sex practices could lead to unplanned pregnancy, sexually transmitted infections, or other complications. Women treated with high doses of gonadotoxic chemotherapy, who are at risk of premature ovarian failure in their 20s and 30s can be advised that their window of opportunity for conception may be limited. Specialized follow-up clinics for childhood cancer survivors can give patients expert advise related to their risk for late effects of therapy.

26.7.3 Prognosis

Concerns that the offspring of patients successfully treated for childhood cancer might have an increased risk of congenital abnormality or increased risk of malignancy have not been substantiated (Thomson et al. 2002). This is with the exception of known genetic or familial cancer syndromes.

Table 26.5. Outline of the function of the ovaries and the associated effects of radiotherapy and chemotherapy (Drury 1990; Cohen 2003; Brougham et al. 2002)

Function	Associated hormones	Target cells	Action	Effects of radiotherapy	Effects of chemotherapy
Estrogen and progesterone production	Pulses of GnRH stimulate release of pituitary LH and FSH	LH stimulates ovarian androgen production (Mid-cycle LH surge induces ovulation) FSH stimulates follicular development and aromatase activity. Follicle differentiates into corpus luteum and secretes progesterone and estradiol during second half of cycle (Aromatase is an enzyme required to convert ovarian androgens to estrogen) FSH stimulates inhibin from ovarian stromal cells (Feedback of inhibin inhibits FSH release)	Estrogen initially, then progesterone, cause uterine endometrial proliferation in preparation for possible implantation; if implantation does not occur, corpus luteum regresses and progesterone secretion falls and menstruation occurs (Pregnancy causes human chorionic gonadotrophin (HCG) production from corpus luteum maintains its function till 10–12 weeks. Placenta then makes sufficient estrogen and progesterone) estrogens induce secondary sexual characteristics	Ovaries may be in the field of pelvic, abdominal, or spinal radiation. Degree of impairment depends on dose, fractionation schedule, and age at the time of treatment The human oocyte is highly sensitive to radiation with 50% death of oocytes at a dose of 4 Gy. The younger the girl at the time of radiotherapy, the larger the oocyte pool and hence, the later onset of premature menopause. Premature menopause can occur in women >40 years of age following treatment dose of 6 Gy (Early menopause has implications for fertility, but also other medical complications including osteoporosis) Doses >20 Gy can cause complete ovarian failure	Prepubertal ovaries appear to be more resistant to cytotoxic agents than postpubertal; possibly because they have more follicles Ovarian function is often retained or recovered with standard doses of chemotherapy High doses of alkylating agents or myeloblative therapy for bone marrow transplant (BMT) is likely to result in permanent ovarian failure

Table 26.6. Assessment of gonadal function

Females: ovarian function	Males: testicular function
Pubertal staging	Pubertal staging
Menstrual history	Testicular volume using prader orchidometer
Basal LH[a] and FSH[b]	Basal LH[a], FSH[b], and inhibin B
Basal estradiol	Basal testosterone
Pelvic ultrasound	Semen analysis

[a] Luteinizing hormone

[b] Follicle-stimulating hormone

Techniques to preserve fertility in patients treated for childhood cancer continue to be investigated. Established options include cryopreservation of spermatozoa (sperm banking) and collection of mature oocytes,and subsequent cryopreservation of embryos. Rates of fertility preservation are often low in the pediatric population, because of the urgency to commence therapy and the developmental stage/maturity required to consider and carry out these options. Experimental strategies are now focusing on the harvesting and storage of gonadal tissue, cryopreservation of immature spermatogenic cells or oocytes, gonadotrophin suppression, and inhibition of follicle apoptosis (Thomson et al. 2002). Following cure, the stored tissue could be autotransplanted or grown in vitro until sufficiently mature for fertilization with assisted reproductive techniques (Brougham et al. 2002). Human primordial follicles survive cryopreservation, and the return of ovarian hormonal activity has been achieved after reimplantation; however, no pregnancies have been reported (Thomson et al. 2002). These developments raise many ethical and legal issues that must be addressed to ensure adequate regulation. Children with cancer must be ensured realistic, safe prospects for fertility in the future, and patients at risk of subfertility require appropriate counseling as part of their routine care.

References

Armstrong GT, Sklar CA, Hudson MM, Robison LL (2007) Long-term health status among survivors of childhood cancer: does sex matter? Journal of Clinical Oncology 25(28):4477–4489

Brougham MFH, Kelnar CJH, Wallace WHB (2002) The late endocrine effects of childhood cancer. Pediatric Rehabilitation 5(4):191–201

Clayton PE, Cuneo RC, Juul A, Monson JP, Shalet SM, Tauber M (2005) Consensus statement on management of the growth hormone-treated adolescent in transition to adult care. European Journal of Endocrinology 152:165–170

Cohen LE (2003) Endocrine late effects of cancer treatment. Current Opinion in Pediatrics 15:3–9

Darzy KH, Shalet SM (2005) Hypopituartism after cranial radiation. Journal of Endocrinology Investigation 25(10 suppl):78–87

Dickerman JD (2007) The late effects of childhood cancer therapy. Pediatrics 119(3):554–568

Drury PL, Drury PL, Drury PL (1990) Endocrinology. In: Kumar PJ, Clark ML (eds) Clinical Medicine 2nd edn. Balliere Tindall, London

Galloway PJ, McNeill E, Paterson WF, Donaldson MDC (2002) Safety of the insulin tolerance test. Archives of Disease in Childhood 87(4):354–356

Gleeson HK, Shalet SM (2004) The impact of therapy on the endocrine system in survivors of childhood brain tumours. Endocrine-Related Cancer 11:589–602

Haller MJ, Schatz DA (2007) Endocrine complications of childhood cancer therapy: evaluation and management. Pediatric Endocrinology Review 4(3):196–204

Oberfield SE, Sklar CA (2002) Endocrine sequelae in survivors of childhood cancer. Adolescent Medicine 13(1):161–169

Petersen KB, Muller J, Rasmussen M, Schmiegelow K (2003) Impaired adrenal function after glucocorticoid therapy in children with acute lymphoblastic leukemia. Medical Pediatric Oncology 41(2):110–114

Robison LL, Green DM, Hudson M, Meadows AT, Mertens AC, Packer RJ, Sklar CA, Strong LC, Yasui Y, Zeltzer LK (2005) Long term outcomes of adult survivors of childhood cancer. Cancer 1(104-11suppl):2557–2564

Rutter MM, Rose SR (2007) Long term endocrine sequelae of childhood cancer. Current Opinions in Pediatrics 19(4):480–487

Schmiegelow M, Feldt-Rasmussen U, rasmussen AK, Poulsen HS, Muller J (2003) A population-based study of thyroid function after radiotherapy and chemotherarpy for a childhood brain tumour. Journal of Clinical Endocrinology and Metabolism 88:136–140

Sklar CA (2002) Endocrine complications of the successful treatment of neoplastic diseases in childhood. Growth Genetics and Hormones 131(6):89–94

Thomson AB, Critchley HOD, Kelnar CJH, Wallace WHB (2002) Late reproductive sequelae following treatment of childhood cancer and options for fertility preservation. Best Practice and Research Clinical Endocrinology and Metabolism 16(2):311–334

Table 27.1. Studies of ototoxic agents in pediatric oncology

Author(s)/patient population	Ototoxic agent	Results	Recommendations
Huang et al. (2002). Patients receiving intensity-modulated radiation therapy (IMRT) vs. conventional radiotherapy	Conventional radiotherapy vs. (IMRT)	Compared with conventional radiotherapy, IMRT delivered 68% of the radiation dose to the auditory apparatus (cochlea) and eighth cranial nerve while still delivering full doses to the desired target volume; 13% of the IMRT group had a grade 3 or 4 hearing loss vs. 64% of the conventional RT group	Larger sample size Further studies Longer follow-ups
Bertolini et al. (2004). Patients (120) treated for neuroblastoma, osteosarcoma, hepatoblastoma, and germ-cell tumors	Cisplatin & carboplatin	Children treated with cumulative cisplatin doses of 400 mg/m^2 necessitate long-term monitoring to avoid missing worsening symptoms Carboplatin (standard dose) alone did not appear to be ototoxic	Hearing loss can progress over time; audiometric testing should occur over an extended amount of time
Li et al. (2004). Children (153) who had completed cisplatin (40–200 mg/m^2/cycle) for germ-cell tumors, hepatoblastoma, neuroblastoma, or osteosarcoma	Cisplatin	Risk of high-frequency hearing loss was related to age at treatment, as well as individual and cumulative doses Children <5 years old were at a greater risk of developing hearing loss than children >15 years old	Importance of audiology monitoring, especially for children <5 years old
Dean et al. (2008). Patients (99) with a variety of malignancies	Carboplatin and cisplatin	Carboplatin when given alone caused ototoxicity in 4% of patients Cisplatin when given alone caused ototoxicity in 57% of patients Carboplatin and cisplatin given together caused 70% ototoxicity in 70% of patients	Findings suggest that patients can receive large doses of carboplatin and still not develop ototoxicity
Lewis et al. (2008). Patients (36) with osteosarcoma; median age 14 years (range: 3–18 years)	Cisplatin	Patients with osteosarcoma who received cisplatin administered as 60 mg/m^2/day for 2 days vs. cisplatin 120 mg/m^2/day for 1 day, resulted in a low incidence of significant hearing loss (12-fold increase)	These results suggest that cisplatin as 120 mg/m^2/day be avoided due to an unacceptable incidence of hearing loss

the outer or middle ear and results in the prevention of sound waves progressing to the inner ear. This type of hearing loss is often temporary because of fluid in the middle ear, an otitis media, or impacted cerumen.

2. Sensorineural hearing loss (SNHL) results from damage to the structures in the inner ear or auditory nerve. For a child with SNHL, sounds are indistinct, and it is often difficult to perceive speech accurately.
3. A mixed hearing loss results from a combination of CHL and SNHL (Mills and Murphy 2007).

Ototoxic agents used for pediatric oncology patients include platinum-based chemotherapeutic agents, aminoglycosides, loop diuretics, and radiation therapy (Brookhouser 2002).

Cisplatin and carboplatin, two platinum-based chemotherapeutic agents, play a critical role in the treatment of a variety of childhood malignancies,

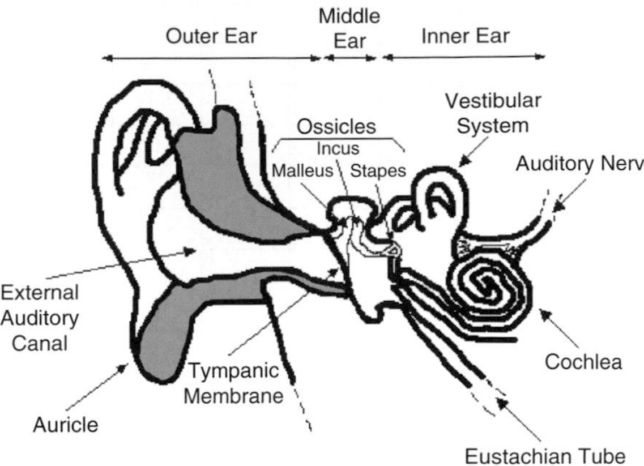

Figure 27.1

Sound waves are funneled through the external auditory canal and hit the tympanic membrane (eardrum). The sound waves hitting the tympanic membrane cause the ossicles of the middle ear to vibrate, setting the oval window (beginning point of the inner ear) in motion. The organ of Corti, located inside the fluid-filled cochlea, is the sensory receptor, which holds the hair cells, or the nerve receptors for hearing. The vibration of the ossicles causes fluid in the cochlea to move, stimulating the hair cells. Specific hair cells react to specific sound frequencies (pitch). Depending on the pitch, specific hair cells are stimulated. Signals from the cochlear hair cells are transmitted into nerve impulses and sent to the brain via the acoustic nerve (Landier 2006). Reprinted from James et al. (2002) with permission from Elsevier

including germ-cell tumors, osteosarcoma, hepatoblastoma, neuroblastoma, retinoblastoma, optic gliomas, and brain tumors. Hearing loss can be a particularly significant side effect of therapy for patients with these types of malignancies, as the average of diagnosis is 4 years or younger. Children who experience hearing loss, even a mild loss, during the first 3 years, can be negatively impacted due to delayed speech and language development (Dean et al. 2008).

Cisplatin initially produces bilateral, irreversible SNHL first in the high-frequency ranges of ≥6,000–8,000 Hz and with continued exposure progresses to the lower frequency ranges. This hearing loss is caused by damage to the inner ear, specifically to hair cells of the organ of Corti, and possibly by damage to the stria vascularis. Damage to the inner ear hair cells should be considered permanent as hair cells do not regenerate. Vestibular toxicity, with ataxia, vertigo, and nystagmus, albeit less common, can also occur. The hearing loss may first be noticed hours to days after the initial dose of cisplatin and may worsen after repeated doses (Bertolini et al. 2004). Li et al. (2004) evaluated 153 children aged 6 months to 18 years who had finished cisplatin therapy (40–200 mg/m^2/cycle) for various germ-cell and solid tumors. It was found that ototoxicity caused by cisplatin in the pediatric population is age and cumulative dose dependent. More specifically, among children ≤5 years receiving a cumulative dose of 400 mg/m^2, there was a 40% chance of developing moderate to severe hearing losses when compared with 5% risk for adolescents aged 15–20 years. Current research suggests that the hearing loss can continue to progress despite the completion of treatment. Ototoxicity remains an irreversible, dose-limiting side effect of cisplatin, requiring identification of those at higher risk and monitoring with frequent hearing assessments making changes in treatment if necessary (Bertolini et al. 2004).

Carboplatin, an analog of cisplatin, introduced in the early 1980s, can also cause a high-frequency hearing loss but when used alone, is much less ototoxic than cisplatin. Higher doses of carboplatin are used in stem cell tranplant conditioning regimens and with hematopoietic growth factors, to increase efficacy of therapy, but the higher doses result in more ototoxicity (Knight et al. 2005). The severity of hearing loss due to carboplatin may be influenced by other factors such as the cumulative dose of carboplatin, prior cisplatin doses, alternate cycles with cisplatin, and radiation therapy (Smits et al. 2006).

The incidence of hearing loss induced by cranial irradiation typically develops within 6–12 months after radiation therapy has been completed and can be seen in up to 50% of patients following doses of 50–60 Gy. Ototoxicity becomes increasingly of concern when radiotherapy is used in combination with cisplatin. The administration of cisplatin after cranial radiation has been reported to increase the ototoxic effects of cisplatin to 60–80% (Jain et al. 2008).

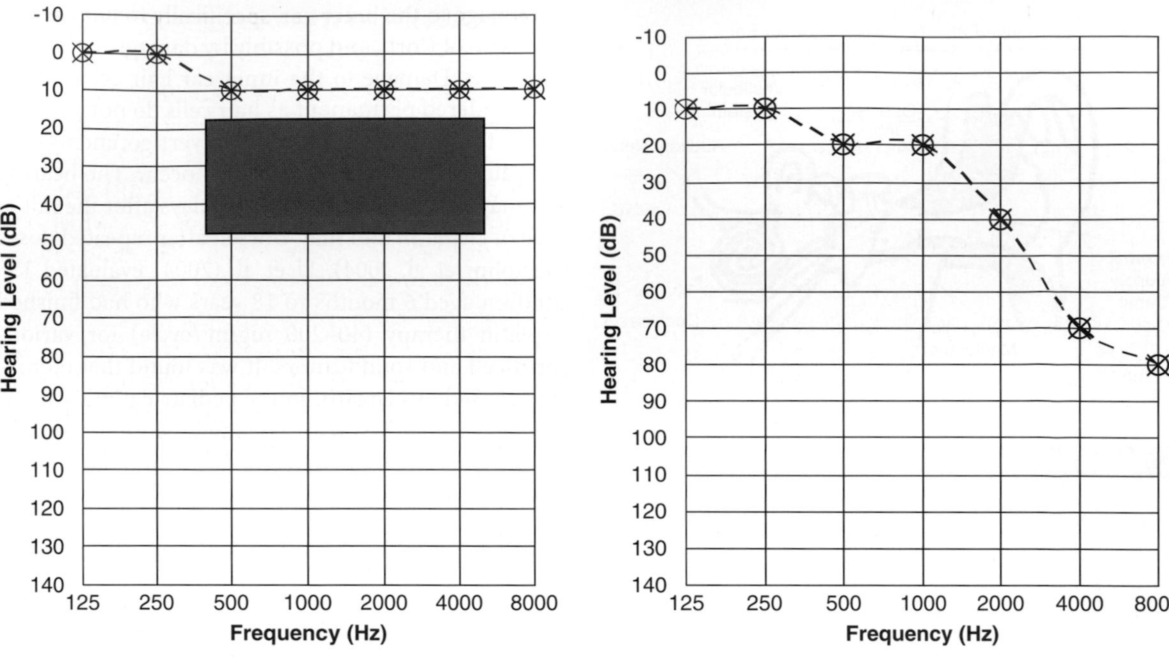

Figure 27.2

Illustration of normal audiogram (air conduction, right ear). Illustration of audiogram showing sensorineural hearing loss (air *dark blue box* = frequency range important for understanding conduction, right ear) speech Courtsey of Brian Filgor

Aminoglycoside antibiotics, used to treat infections caused by aerobic Gram-negative bacteria, such as pneumonia and urinary tract infections, are also known to cause hearing loss. Because of the toxicities of these drugs, the use of these antibiotics in the West has decreased significantly as better alternatives exist. In developing countries, the cost and availablity of these drugs cause them to still be widely used, despite the many side effects that can develop. Ototoxicity due to aminoglycosides is often irreversible. Initially, there is injury to outer hair cell membranes, followed by inner hair cell destruction, with damage most often occurring during prolonged elevated serum trough levels (Landier and Larson-Tuttle 2004; Rybak and Ramkumar 2007).

A synergism exists between aminoglycosides and loop diuretics (furosemide/frusemide). Studies have shown that giving a loop diuretic and then an aminoglycoside antibiotic does not affect hearing more than giving either drug alone. However, when an aminoglycoside is given first, and then the loop diuretic, the organ of Corti is damaged, causing synergistic hearing loss. Ototoxicity caused by a loop diuretic may be due to fluid changes within the inner ear, resulting in problems with nerve transmission. This type of hearing loss typically develops quickly and is reversible (Brookhouser 2002). Furosemide should not be administered as a rapid intravenous infusion (Landier 2008).

Children who are at high risk for hearing loss include those who had:

- Perinatal anoxia or hypoxia
- Low Apgar scores (at 1 or 5 min)
- Hyperbilirubinemia requiring an exchange transfusion
- Mechanical ventilation for more than 10 days
- A history of bacterial meningitis

- Birth weight <1,500 g
- Positive TORCH titer (toxoplasmosis, rubella, cytomegalovirus, syphilis, herpes) while in utero
- Recurrent or persistent otitis media with effusion for at least 3 months
- Prior treatment with ototoxic drugs
- A family history of SNHL (presumably congenital) (Mills and Murphy 2007)

Clinical manifestations during infancy and early toddlerhood that may signify a hearing deficit include lack of a startle, failure to be awakened by loud environmental noises, absence of well-formed syllables ("da," "na," "ya") by 11 months, and monotone and difficult-to-understand speech (Mills and Murphy 2007).

27.2 Prevention and Treatment

Primary prevention or early detection of hearing loss are essential management concerns for pediatric oncology patients receiving ototoxic therapy. Multiple audiologic test options exist for infants and children (Table 27.2). The method used for evaluation is selected based on the child's age, state of health, and their ability to cooperate. Brainstem auditory evoked response (BAER, ABR) is used to evaluate hearing in newborns to 9 months. This electrophysiologic measurement of hearing is recorded from brain wave activity occurring in response to clicks or certain tones obtained in auditory nerves and brainstem pathways. To complete this test, the infant must be asleep, often requiring sedation. For children older than 9 months, pure tone audiometry remains the standard as well as the most common test for hearing evaluation. Testing measures pure-tone thresholds between 250 and 8,000 Hz (Cunningham and Cox 2003; Landier and Larson-Tuttle 2004). Otoacoustic emissions (OAEs) testing can be used for all age patients, but there are limitations. OAE tests the structural integrity of the auditory pathway, but cannot confirm if hearing is normal; therefore, any child undergoing chemotherapy with platinum-based agents or children with an abnormal OAE must undergo further evalution (Landier and Larson-Tuttle 2004). Hearing impairment or sensitivity is measured in decibels (dB), a measurement of loudness or intensity (Mills and Murphy 2007).

- Normal hearing is considered to be in the 0–20 dB range for all frequencies tested in the 125–8,000 Hz (Fig. 27.3).
- Mild hearing loss for a child (20–40 dB) results in the inability to hear soft sounds or a whispered conversation in a quiet room. The child should not have school difficulties, but may benefit from a hearing aid.
- The child with a moderate hearing loss (40–60 dB) will have great difficulty understanding a typical conversation even in a quiet room. This child may need a hearing aid(s) and have difficulties pronouncing some speech sounds.
- A child with moderate to severe hearing loss (60–90 dB) will be able to have a conversation only if he/she is using a hearing aid and the speaker is within 6–12 in. If the hearing loss occurred before age 2, speech and language development will be delayed and will not develop without intervention.
- A child with a profound loss of 90 dB or more may hear only loud sounds and will typically experience sound as a vibration. This child will have great difficulties with speech and language skills (Mills and Murphy 2007).

A child's ability to accurately understand what is being spoken is crucial to language development. High-frequency hearing loss reduces the ability to recognize many of the consonants such as "s," "sh," "f," and "th." Most consonants have a higher pitch than vowels and are more difficult to identify, especially in a noisy environment. Children may also have problems hearing plural forms of words, especially when spoken by other children or women (Knight et al. 2005).

Guidelines from Children's Oncology Group (COG) support the importance of monitoring hearing status throughout all phases of treatment for children receiving ototoxic agents. Based on age, ability to cooperate, and state of health, all children must have baseline testing. All high-risk patients are tested before each chemotherapy cycle using platinum-based agents. All other patients receiving platinum-based therapy should be tested before every other chemotherapy course. It is recommended that all

the drug. Many researchers are cautious, because of the negative effect on antitumor activity (Rybak et al. 2007). Presently, there is one pediatric Phase III randomized study of STS in prevention of ototoxicity in children receiving cisplatin for newly diagnosed germ-cell tumor, hepatoblastoma, medulloblastoma, neuroblastoma, or osteosarcoma being conducted by COG. Patients will be randomized to one of two arms: Arm 1—patients receive STS IV beginning 6 h after completion of each ciplatin infusion and Arm 2—patients do not receive sodium thosulfate (NCI 2009).

Intensity-modulated radiotherapy (IMRT) is another modality being investigated to lessen hearing loss. IMRT has the capability to precisely deliver radiation to the intended site while avoiding surrounding tissues, such as the cochlea and auditory apparatus. This allows for less irradiation of normal tissue, and ultimately dose escalation, providing better disease control while decreasing treatment side effect (Jain et al. 2008).

27.4 Prognosis

The added diagnosis of hearing loss can be difficult for a child and his/her family who is already facing a life-threatening illness. Families need support, education, and guidance with options regarding available communication devices. They may also need assistance navigating the educational system, including understanding the Individuals with Disabilities Education Act and any special interventions the child may be entitled to. Primary prevention and early detection are important in the care and management of the child with an SNHL. A multidisciplinary team needs to be involved to manage the acute and long-term needs of the child with a hearing loss (Landier and Larson-Tuttle 2004).

With the progress in pediatric oncology care, researchers recognize the importance of evaluating the effectiveness of treatment regimens and the impact of overall quality of life for patients and families. Strategies to reach dose intensification and to maximize antineoplastic effects require interventions to minimize the associated side effects. This is particularly important as higher doses of platinum-agents and radiatiion therapy continue to be used in an attempt for cure. The future holds new developments of chemotherapeutic agents, chemoprotectants, and radiologic technology. It is hoped that these new innovative treatments will greatly decrease the incidence of ototoxicity associated with childhood cancer.

References

Bertolini P, Lassalle M, Mercier G, Raquin MA, Izzi G, Corradini N et al (2004) Platinum compound-related ototoxicity in children. Journal of Pediatric Hematology Oncology 26(10):649–655

Brookhouser PE (2002) Diseases of the inner ear and sensorineural hearing. In: Bluestone CD, Casselbrant ML, Stool SE, Dohar JE, Alper CM, Arjmand EM, Yellon RF (eds) Pediatric otolaryngology, 4th edn. Saunders, Philadelphia, pp 798–800

Cunningham M, Cox EO (2003) Hearing assessment in infants and children: recommendation beyond neonatal screening. Pediatrics 111(2):436–440

Dean JB, Hayashi SS, Albert CM, King AA, Karzon R, Hayashi RJ (2008) Hearing loss in pediatric oncology patients receiving carboplatin-containing regimens. Journal of Pediatric Hematology Oncology 30(2):130–134

Fouladi M, Blaney SM, Poussaint TY, Freeman BB, McLendon R, Fuller C et al (2006) Phase II study of oxaliplatin in children with recurrent or refractory medulloblastoma, supratentorial primitive neuroectodermal tumors, and atypical teratoid rhabdoid tumors. Cancer 107(9):2291–2297

Fouladi M, Chintagumpala M, Ashley D, Kellie S, Gururangan S, Hasseall T et al (2008) Amifostine protects against cisplatin-induced ototoxicity in children with average-risk medulloblastoma. Journal of Clinical Oncology 26(22): 3749–3755

Geoerger B, Doz F, Gentet JC, Mayer M, Landman-Parker J, Pichon F et al (2008) Phase I study of weekly Oxaliplatin in relapsed or refractory pediatric solid malignancies. Journal of Clinical Oncology 26(27):4394–4400

Huang E, Teh BS, Strother DR, Davis QG, Chiu JK, Lu HH (2002) Intensity-modulated radiation therapy for pediatric medulloblastoma: Early report on the reduction of ototoxicity. International Journal of Radiation Oncology, Biology, Physics 52(3):599–605

James et al (2002) Nursing care of children–principles and practice. Saunders, Philadelphia

Jain N, Krull KR, Brouwere P, Chintagumpla MM, Woo SY (2008) Neuropsychological outcome following intensity-modulated radiation therapy for pediatric medulloblastoma. Pediatric Blood and Cancer 51:275–279

Kline NE, Bloom D (2003) The child with cognitive, sensory, or communication impairment. In: Hockenberry MJ, Wilson

D, Winkelstein M, Kline NE (eds) Wong's nursing care of infants and children, 7th edn. St. Louis, Mosby, pp 994–997

Knight KR, Kraemer DF, Neuwelt EA (2005) Ototoxicity in children receiving platinum chemotherapy: Underestimating a commonly occurring toxicity that may influence academic and social development. Journal of Clinical Oncology 23(34):8588–8596

Landier W, Larson-Tuttle C (2004) Monitoring and management of ototoxicity. In: Altman AJ (ed) Supportive care of children with cancer: current therapy guidelines from the Children's Oncology Group, 3rd edn. The Johns Hopkins University Press, Baltimore, pp 130–138

Landier W (2006) Hearing loss after treatment for childhood cancer. http://www.survivorshipguidelines.org/pdf/HearingLoss.pdf. Retrieved 11 Feb 2008 from Children's Oncology Group

Landier W (2008) Ototoxicity. In: Kline NE (ed) Essentials of pediatric hematology/oncology nursing. Association of Pediatric Hematology/Oncology Nurses, Glenview, IL, pp 130–131

Lewis M, DuBois S, Fligor B, Li X, Gorin A, Grier H (2008) Ototoxicity in children treated for osteosarcoma. Pediatric Blood and Cancer 52:387–391

Li Y, Womer RB, Silber JH (2004) Predicting cisplatin ototoxicity in children: the influence of age and the cumulative dose. European Journal of Cancer 40:2445–2451

Marina N, Chang KW, Malogolwkin M, London WB, Frazier AL, Womer R et al (2005) Amifostine does not protect against the ototoxicity of high-dose cisplatin combines with etoposide and bleomycin in pediatric germ-cell tumors. Cancer 104(4):841–847

Mills DA, Murphy AC (2007) Sensory alterations. In: Potts NL, Mandleco BL (eds) Pediatric nursing-caring for children and their families, 2nd edn. Delmar Learning, United States, pp 1017–1029

National Cancer Institute (2009) Clinical trials search results. http://www.cancer.gov/search/ResultsClinicalTrialsAdvanced.aspx?protocolsearchid=5406538. Retrieved 25 Feb 2009

Punnett A, Bliss B, Dupuis LL, Abdolell M, Doyle J, Sung L (2004) Ototoxicity following pediatric hematopoietic stem cell transplantation: a prospective cohort study. Pediatric Blood and Cancer 42:598–603

Smits C, Swen SJ, Goverts ST, Moll AC, Imof SM, Schouten-van Meeteren A (2006) Assessment of hearing in very young children receiving Carboplatin for retinoblastoma. European Journal of Cancer 42:492–500

Rybak LP, Ramkumar V (2007) Ototoxicty. Kidney International 72(8):931–935

Rybak LP, Whitworth CA, Mukherjea D, Ramkumar V (2007) Mechanisms of cisplatin-induced ototoxicity and prevention. Hearing Research 226:157–167

Ocular Complications

Martina Nathan • Deborah Tomlinson

Contents

28.1 Ocular Toxicity Associated with High-Dose Cytarabine Arabinoside . . . 511
- 28.1.1 Incidence and Etiology . . . 511
- 28.1.2 Prevention . . . 512
- 28.1.3 Treatment . . . 512
- 28.1.4 Prognosis . . . 512

28.2 Cataracts . . . 513
- 28.2.1 Incidence . . . 513
- 28.2.2 Etiology . . . 513
- 28.2.3 Prevention . . . 513
- 28.2.4 Treatment . . . 513
- 28.2.5 Prognosis . . . 513

References . . . 513

28.1 Ocular Toxicity Associated with High-Dose Cytarabine Arabinoside

28.1.1 Incidence and Etiology

Keratoconjunctivitis is a known side-effect of systemic high-dose cytarabine arabinoside (HDAC). Cytarabine is an antimetabolite that acts within the S phase inhibiting DNA synthesis. It can be administered intravenously or intrathecally. Conjunctivitis is observed in a significant proportion of patients treated with HDAC. The dose of HDAC can be from 2 to 3 g/m2 every 12 h for 2–6 days (Matteucci et al. 2006). Cytarabine penetrates the blood brain barrier after intravenous injection, and may affect the cornea via both the aqueous humor and tears (Hollander and Aldave 2004). Visual symptoms include tearing, photophobia, foreign body sensation, pain, and reduced vision (Schmid et al. 2006; Hollander and Aldave 2004).

The incidence appears to be related to the duration of cytarabine arabinoside (also referred to as cytosine or ara-c) therapy, the intraocular fluid concentration of the drug, the cerebral-spinal fluid (CSF) pharmacokinetics, and the use of corticosteroid eyedrops (Higa et al. 1991):

- Extended periods of administration of HDAC (6–8 days) appear to increase the likelihood of eye problems.
- High levels of cytarabine arabinoside have been found in the CSF, tears, and aqueous humor of patients treated with HDAC. The administration of conventional doses of cytarabine arabinoside (100 mg/m2/24 h) also crosses the blood brain barrier but causes a low concentration in CSF

accounting for the absence of ocular reactions. Any reaction that does occur in conventional dose therapy may be attributed to allergic reaction.

- Cytarabine arabinoside undergoes slower inactivation in the CSF.
- Compared with no therapy, the use of eyedrops can decrease the incidence of ocular symptoms from about 40 to 20% or less (Itoh et al. 1999; Higa et al. 1991).

28.1.2 Prevention

Steroidal eyedrops (prednisolone 1% or dexamethasone 1 mg/mL) currently represent the standard prophylaxis of cytarabine-induced conjunctivitis (Matteucci et al. 2006).

Generally, all treatment schedules that include HDAC also incorporate the administration of corticosteroid eyedrops as routine prophylaxis in the prevention of ocular toxic reactions. The frequency of the administration of eyedrops (prednisolone 1%) would appear to vary from every 2 h to every 8 h (Gococo et al. 1991; Higa et al. 1991). Duration of the eyedrop administration begins before the first dose and usually extends to 48 h following the last dose of HDAC. Results regarding the optimum frequency of eyedrop administration are inconclusive and even 5 min of drug exposure to corneal epithelium has been associated with cell injury (Gococo et al. 1991).

Research involving the use of eyedrops for ocular toxicity associated with HDAC is always subject to small numbers of patients. Higa et al. (1991) and Planer et al. (2004) investigated and compared the efficacy of corticosteroidal eyedrops and artificial tears. The authors suggested that eyedrops decrease ocular toxicity because of dilution of intraocular concentrations of cytarabine arabinoside. This study concluded that artificial tears appeared to be as effective as eyedrops containing corticosteroids if a rigorous administration schedule is employed. However, although glucocoticoid eyedrops should not be used indiscriminately, they are safe and efficacious given over short periods of time (Gococo 1992). The study by Itoh and colleagues (1999) suggested that the incidence could be reduced further with additional eye washing with 0.9% saline and monitoring for proper technique of eyedrop administration (including eye-closure and naso-lacrimal occlusion). These procedures were performed on 34 patients and no ocular toxicity was observed in these cases. The study by Matteucci et al. (2006) compared the incidence, severity, and duration of conjunctivitis in a series of 60 consecutive patients who were randomized to receive either the standard treatment of dexamethasone eyedrops or a combination of dexamethasone and diclofenac eyedrops. Findings demonstrate that the combined administration of dexamethasone and diclofenac significantly reduced the incidence and severity of conjunctivitis compared to dexamethasone alone. Also, the combined drug regime delayed the time of onset, with patients developing conjunctivitis 2–3 days after completion of chemotherapy. It is important to remember that these procedures may be more difficult to adhere to in a young pediatric population.

Interestingly, Mori et al. (2008) found that topical corticosteroids appeared to be ineffective in the reduction of conjunctivitis in adult patients who had received high-dose cytarabine following TBI.

28.1.3 Treatment

Ocular toxicity that occurs despite prophylaxis will usually continue to be treated with corticosteroidal eyedrops. More severe reactions may require referral to an ophthalmologist. Very rarely would the treatment require to be discontinued.

28.1.4 Prognosis

The associated conjunctivitis usually resolves in affected patients within 7 days of the discontinuation of HDAC (Barrios et al. 1987). Glucocorticoid eyedrops will probably remain the prophylactic choice against HDAC-induced keratoconjunctivitis. However, further investigation into a more effective prophylaxis for cytarabine-induced keratoconjunctivitis in this setting may be required (Mori et al. 2008). However, rigorous administration of artificial tears or the addition of nonsteroidal anti-inflammatory drugs (Matteucci et al. 2006) may also decrease the incidence of ocular reaction (Schmid et al. 2006).

28.2 Cataracts

28.2.1 Incidence

The incidence of cataracts in children who received conditioning treatment of TBI prior to bone marrow transplant has been reported as 58–100% (Fahnehjelm et al. 2007; Holstrom et al. 2002). Busulfan has also been related to cataract development, with Holmstrom et al. (2002) reporting an incidence of 21% (5 of 24 children). However, Fahnehjelm et al. (2007) found that children treated with busulfan developed less severe cataracts and did not require cataract surgery.

28.2.2 Etiology

Opacity of the crystalline lens is referred to as a cataract. Several cataractogenic factors involved in cytotoxic therapy include ionizing radiation, corticosteroid treatment, and chemotherapeutic agents. Further factors related to radiation include the total dose, fractionation scheme, and dose rate (Fahnehjelm et al. 2007; van Kempen-Harteveld et al. 2002). Fahnehjelm et al.'s (2007) study demonstrated that there was an increased chance of having cataracts earlier if treated with single-dose TBI compared with fractionated TBI. Autologous BMT patients would appear to have a slower progression of cataract than allogeneic BMT patients (Frisk et al. 2000). This may be due to the reduced need for corticosteroids after autologous BMT (Aristei et al. 2002; van Kempen-Harteveld 2002). However, it has been reported that there was no correlation between prolonged post-transplantation steroid treatment and increased cataract development (Fahnehjelm et al. 2007). Similarly, Stava et al. (2005) found that treatment with corticosteroids was associated with cataracts in only 7% of cases.

28.2.3 Prevention

van Kempen-Harteveld and colleagues (2002) recommend that steroid treatment should be minimized and TBI regimens should include appropriate biologic effective doses to minimize the risk of cataracts (van Kempen-Harteveld et al. 2002). The use of eye shielding during TBI is not performed because the orbit and the central nervous system are potential sites for residual disease.

28.2.4 Treatment

Surgical repair of cataracts is the treatment of choice, including extracapsular cataract extraction and intraocular lens implantation. Patients who undergo surgery may require treatment for secondary cataracts (Fahnehjelm et al. 2007).

28.2.5 Prognosis

Therapy-induced cataract is not considered a severe complication because visual acuity can be restored by surgical treatment without significant complication. However, early diagnosis of cataracts in children is important to prevent the development of amblyopia (Fahnehjelm et al. 2007; Holstrom et al. 2002). Regular evaluation of vision is recommended for children with malignancies whose treatment may be associated with cataracts so that problems may be detected and managed early (Natarajan and Davies 2004; Stava et al. 2005).

References

Aristei C, Alessandro M, Santucci A, Aversa F, Tabillo A, Carotti A, Latini RA, Cagini C, Latini P (2002) Cataracts in patients receiving stem cell transplantation after conditioning with total body irradiation. Bone Marrow Transplant 29(6):503–507

Barrios NJ, Tebbi CK, Freeman AI, Brecher ML (1987) Toxicity of high-dose ara-c in children and adolescents. Cancer 60(2):165–169

Fahnehjelm KT, Törnquist AL, Olsson M, Winiarski J (2007) Visual outcome and cataract development after allogenic stem cell transplantation in children. Acta Opthalmologica Scandinavica 85(7):724–733

Frisk P, Hagberg H, Mandahl A, Soderberg P, Lonnerholm G (2000) Cataracts after autologous bone marrow transplantation in children. Acta Paediatrica 89(7):814–819

Gococo KO, Lazarus HM, Lass JH (1992) The use of prophylactic eye drops during high-dose cytosine arabinoside therapy. Cancer 69(11):2866–2867

Holstrom G, Borstrom B, Calissendorff B (2002) Cataract in children after bone marrow transplantation: relation to conditioning regimen. Acta Opthalmologica Scandinavica 80(2):211–215

29.2 Nutritional Assessment

29.2.1 Hydration Needs

Water comprises a large percentage of a child's body composition, ranging from 45 to 75% of total body weight (Wilson 2007). Pediatric oncology patients are vulnerable to fluid and electrolyte imbalances due to rapid changes in fluid intake/output and fluctuations in electrolytes that can occur during cancer treatment.

- Holliday and Segar created a formula in 1957 that is still commonly used to determine maintenance fluid requirements in children (Table 29.1) (Holliday and Segar 1957).
- Body surface area (BSA) can also be used to calculate fluid requirements; simple equations for calculating BSA are listed in Table 29.2. A patient's maintenance fluid requirement is estimated to be BSA × 1,500–1,600 mL fluid/m^2/day.

However, neither of these formulas takes into consideration the demands of children during times of illness. Fluid requirements are increased in those with fever, gastrointestinal losses (such as diarrhea), dehydration/shock, nephrotoxic medication administration, and during hematopoietic stem cell transplant conditioning. Fluid requirements are decreased in those with congestive heart failure, fluid overload, syndrome of inappropriate secretion of antidiuretic hormone (SIADH), chronic renal failure, and increased intracranial pressure. Hydration needs of ill children must be considered on an individual basis to determine the appropriate provision of fluid and electrolytes.

Table 29.1. Maintenance fluid requirements

Weight (kg)	Daily fluid requirement
0–10	100 mL/kg
11–20	1,000 mL + 50 mL/kg for each kg above 10 kg
>20	1,500 mL + 20 mL/kg for each kg above 20 kg

Table 29.2. Calculating body surface area (m^2)

Mosteller 1987	√[(weight in *kg* × height in *cm*)/3,600]
Reading and Freeman 2005	1/6 × √(weight in *kg* × height in *m*)

29.2.2 Nutrition Needs

Ensuring adequate nutrition for children with cancer presents unique challenges. Pediatric oncology patients often experience decreased oral intake and impaired utilization of nutrients during and after treatment that can lead to malnutrition. Poor intake can result from the disease itself and/or side effects of treatment. Alterations in the metabolism of protein, carbohydrates, fat, vitamins, and minerals can occur in cancer patients resulting in improper utilization of nutrients. Patients at increased nutritional risk are listed in Table 29.3.

Any illness that causes physiological stress and increased catabolism can significantly increase a child's nutritional requirements. There is a lack of research regarding the estimation of energy needs in children with cancer, although some studies have shown that energy needs of patients with cancer may be increased 20–90% over predicted needs (Bechard et al. 2006). Several methods exist for estimating pediatric energy requirements, such as:

- The recommended dietary allowance (RDA)
- The estimated energy requirement (EER)
- The dietary reference intakes (DRI)
- The Harris–Benedict equation

However, these estimates were developed as recommendations for healthy populations, so they may not

Table 29.3. Nutritionally at-risk individuals

Weight loss ≥5% of pre-illness body weight
Weight-for-length or body mass index (BMI) <10th percentile
Voluntary food intake of <70% of estimated requirements for 5 or more days
Anticipated gut dysfunction for >5 days

Table 29.4. Estimating daily calorie needs in children 1 year or older

Step 1: resting energy expenditure (REE) calculations (W = weight in kg)		
Age range (years)	Male (kg)	Female (kg)
1–3	60.9 x W – 54	61 x W – 51
3–10	22.7 x W ÷ 495	22.5 x W ÷ 499
10–18	17.5 x W ÷ 651	12.2 x W ÷ 746
18–30	15.3 x W ÷ 679	14.7 x W ÷ 496
Step 2: multiply REE by an activity/stress factor		
Well-nourished child at bed rest with mild to moderate stress = (REE) × (1.3)		
Very active child with mild to moderate stress = (REE) × (1.5)		
Inactive child with severe stress (trauma, sepsis, cancer, extensive surgery) = (REE) × (1.5)		
Child with minimal activity requiring to catch up growth = (REE) × (1.5)		
Active child requiring catch up growth = (REE) × (1.7)		
Active child with severe stress = (REE) × (1.7)		

World Health Organization 1985 Copyright 1985 by WHO. Adapted with permission

accurately predict the needs of sick children. Estimates of resting energy expenditure (REE) for different age groups have been developed by the World Health Organization (1985). REE can be defined as the amount of energy required to maintain normal homeostatic function during periods of rest. These estimates, multiplied by appropriate activity and/or stress factors (Table 29.4), can be useful to help determine the daily caloric needs of acutely ill children.

Protein requirements may also be elevated in children with cancer, particularly during chemotherapy/radiation and with the use of certain medications (e.g., corticosteroids). Comparatively, as with estimates of energy requirements, there is a lack of research on protein needs in children with cancer. Protein needs in these children are generally estimated to be 1.5–2.5 g/kg body weight or up to twice the RDA for age and gender.

29.2.3 Nutritional History

A complete nutritional history is an important initial step to every assessment. The history should include information about the patient's oral intake and the use of any nutritional support. Information should be obtained from the child, the parent and/or the primary caregiver, and other healthcare providers. Information that will aid in the assessment of fluid status includes the amount and type of fluid intake; the amount of fluid output including urine, stool, emesis, and insensible losses (such as sweat and wound drainage); documentation of rapid weight changes (which can be indicative of fluid retention or depletion); and observation of any physical signs of edema. The consumption of fluids containing sucrose, coffee/tea, sports drinks (such as Gatorade), and any complementary/alternative medicine beverages, especially when a child has electrolyte abnormalities, may be significant. Assessment of nutritional status should include evaluation of physical, psychological, and social factors (Table 29.5). A diet history can be obtained from a 24-hours diet recall or a food diary. A diet recall involves asking the parent or primary caregiver to provide a complete list of all foods and fluids consumed by the child during the past 24 hours. A diet recall is a quick and easy method of obtaining information about oral intake; however, recall bias and under- or over-reporting of intake frequently occur because the list is obtained from memory. A food diary is a more objective

Table 29.5. Pertinent information for a nutritional history

Factors	Assessment
Physical	Oral, enteral, and intravenous nutritional intake
	Weight changes
	Gastrointestinal symptoms
	Alterations in taste and smell
	Oral hygiene
	Food allergies/intolerances
	Fatigue
Psychological	Food preferences
	Food aversion
	Mood: depression, anxiety
	Stress
Social	Food availability
	Preferred method of food preparation
	Cultural diet restrictions

measurement of oral intake, but again the child or parent has to remember to complete the information. Typically, the parent or primary caregiver records the type and amount of the child's food and beverage intake as it occurs for several days. This record generally provides more accurate information than a 24-hours diet recall; however, it also requires diligence on the part of the parent or primary caregiver when recording intake.

29.2.4 Physical Examination

A physical assessment will help the nurse identify subtle clues that a child is at risk for, or currently experiencing, dehydration or malnutrition. Assessment usually begins with an observation of general appearance and activity level. Dehydrated or malnourished children may act lethargic and listless, and may not protest when undergoing medical procedures. Alternatively, they may be irritable or unconsolable.

When a child is dehydrated, extracellular volume decreases. This compromises circulation, resulting in grayish-colored skin, increased capillary refill time, poor skin turgor, decreased saliva and tear production, dry lips and skin, and increased pulse rate. A flat or depressed fontanel can also be noted in infants. Significant fluid losses result in vasoconstriction, which is manifested physically as cool extremities and an increased respiratory rate due to metabolic acidosis. Decreased blood pressure is usually a late sign of dehydration. When a child is overhydrated, extracellular volume increases resulting in edema. Some patients can experience shortness of breath from excessive fluid accumulation in the lungs.

Malnourished children may experience muscle wasting, loss of muscle strength, and depletion of fat stores, which are indicative of a loss of total body energy stores. Some other physical signs of malnutrition, such as hair loss and stomatitis, may be difficult to distinguish from the side effects of cancer treatment. It is important for nurses to monitor pediatric oncology patients for significant and/or unexpected physical changes and consider nutritional etiologies when these changes occur.

29.2.5 Anthropometric Measurements

Anthropometric measurements are important components of a nutritional assessment. Anthropometric measurements include weight, height or length, weight-for-length or body mass index (BMI), and head circumference. These measurements should be plotted on the National Center for Health Statistics growth curves for comparison with the general population. While anthropometric measurements may be quick and convenient, inaccurate readings may be obtained due to improper measuring techniques, inaccurate or uncalibrated equipment, and/or a lack of patient cooperation. Anthropometric measurements are most useful when multiple measurements are obtained by a trained provider over time, as trends are more telling than isolated measurements.

A change in weight may be indicative of an increase or decrease in energy stores; however, a rapid increase or decrease in weight frequently indicates fluid retention or depletion. Therefore, it is important to obtain an accurate baseline weight and closely monitor subsequent changes in weight to accurately assess hydration and nutritional status. It is important for patients to be weighed consistently each time they are weighed (using the same scale, at the same time of the day, and with similar clothing) to maximize the accuracy of measurements. Height/length is another measurement that is useful in the evaluation of nutritional status. Children older than 2 years who can stand upright should be measured standing using a stadiometer to obtain height; children who cannot stand or are younger than two should be measured lying down using a lengthboard to obtain a length. A decrease in linear growth velocity can occur over time in malnourished patients. However, changes in linear growth do not occur as rapidly as weight changes, so this measurement is not as helpful for assessing acute nutritional status. Weight-for-length or BMI ratios reflect body weight in proportion to length/height and are also useful when assessing patients for the presence of acute malnutrition. Weight-for-length should be used when a patient's length is obtained; BMI (weight[kg]/height[m]^2) should be used when height is obtained. Head circumference is used as an indicator of brain growth and correlates with nutritional status until 3 years of age, when head growth slows.

Arm anthropometric measurements are quick, noninvasive, and inexpensive techniques that can help practitioners evaluate body composition. Mid-arm muscle circumference is used as an indicator of muscle mass, while triceps skinfold is used as an indicator of body fat stores. Measurements can be compared to age-specific norms; significant wasting of muscle and/or fat can be an indicator of malnutrition.

29.2.6 Laboratory Evaluation

Laboratory measurements provide additional information that can be utilized to assess a patient's hydration and nutritional status. Measurements of serum electrolytes, osmolality, blood glucose, blood urea nitrogen (BUN), creatinine, and urine electrolytes and osmolality provide useful information in the assessment of a child's hydration and nutritional status. Accurate 24-hours input and output monitoring provides important data regarding fluid imbalances. Intake and output of all fluid must be diligently recorded, including measurements of urine, stool, emesis, and other fluid losses. Diapers and pads soaked with secretions should be carefully weighed to determine the amount of fluid loss.

Plasma levels of protein markers, such as albumin, transferrin, retinol-binding protein (RBP), and prealbumin (also known as transthyretin) are commonly measured to assess nutritional status and evaluate the effectiveness of nutritional interventions. Prealbumin and RBP have the shortest half-lives; changes in levels of these proteins better reflect recent changes in diet or nutrition support. Transferrin and albumin have longer half-lives; low levels of these proteins can be indicative of longer periods of nutritional deficiency. It is important that these measurements be examined critically, as levels can be significantly affected by many nonnutritional factors. Many situations that commonly occur during cancer treatment, such as kidney or liver dysfunction, infection and/or inflammation, fluid overload or dehydration, and the use of corticosteroids can have a significant impact on protein marker levels. Other blood tests, including liver function tests such as alkaline phosphatase, alanine aminotransferase (ALT), aspartate aminotransferase (AST), g-glulamyltransferase (GGT), and bilirubin, should also be performed to aid in the completion of a complete nutritional assessment.

29.3 Principles of Treatment for Dehydration and Malnutrition

29.3.1 Rehydration

Oral rehydration is the treatment of choice for mild to moderate dehydration. Solutions used for oral rehydration should contain high amounts of sodium and moderate levels of sugar (e.g., Pedialyte®, Oralyte®, Infalyte®, Resol®). Children should drink 30–60 mL (1–2 oz) per hour of an oral rehydration solution for the first 24 hours after dehydration has been detected. Restriction of specific foods or administration of the "BRAT" diet (a bland diet consisting of foods such as "bananas, rice, applesauce, and toast") is not recommended.

Severe dehydration requires immediate intravenous fluid administration followed by oral rehydration once the child's condition has stablized. The type of intravenous fluid administration depends on the type of dehydration. Isotonic dehydration is the most common form of dehydration in which electrolyte and water losses are approximately equal. Common causes of isotonic dehydration include diuretic therapy, excessive vomiting, decreased fluid intake, and hemorrhage. This form of dehydration is corrected using isotonic fluids; examples of isotonic fluids include normal saline (NS), lactated Ringer's (LR), and 5%D/0.45%NS. Hypertonic dehydration is the second most common type of dehydration. Hypertonic dehydration occurs when water losses exceed electrolyte losses; this causes fluid to move from cells into the blood stream, which results in decreased cellular size. Treatment of hypertonic dehydration requires the slow administration of free water using appropriate intravenous fluids (usually either 0.45 or 0.9% NS); rapid administration of hypotonic fluid may cause cells to swell, which can lead to severe complications. Hypotonic dehydration occurs when electrolyte losses exceed water losses. Serum sodium levels are typically less than 130 mEq/L in this form of dehydration. Hypertonic fluids (such as 10% dextose or 3% NS) are used to treat hypotonic dehydration.

29.3.2 Oral Nutrition Replacement

Many side effects of cancer treatment (e.g., nausea/vomiting, alterations in taste and smell, mucositis, dry mouth, dysphagia, and early satiety) can affect oral intake. Evaluation by a registered dietitian should be completed once a patient has been diagnosed with cancer. The dietitian can assist the medical team to determine the patient's nutritional requirements, establish nutritional goals, and develop a plan for the nutritional monitoring of the child. The dietitian can also educate the patient and family about strategies for maximizing nutrition intake and the dietary management of side effects of cancer treatment.

Oral nutrition replacement is the treatment of choice for malnutrition, when tolerated. A high-calorie, high-protein diet and oral supplements can help to maximize caloric and protein intake when oral intake declines. Many types of oral supplements are available; supplements vary with regard to flavor, form, and composition. Other strategies for maximizing nutrition intake include: offering small, frequent meals throughout the day; performing oral care before eating; and encouraging the child to participate in food preparation if he/she is able. It is important that an individual approach be taken with each patient and family participation be encouraged for optimal outcomes.

Medical management includes offering medications to help alleviate gastrointestinal side effects, prevent gastroesophageal reflux, and/or stimulate the child's appetite. Commonly used antiemetic medications include ondansetron, granisetron, and promethazine. Lansoprazole and low-dose metoclopramide hydrochloride (0.1–0.2 mg/kg/dose) are common oral medications used to prevent or treat gastroesophageal reflux. Commonly used appetite stimulants include megestrol acetate, dronabinol, and periactin. Most medications are dosed based on the patient's weight or body surface area.

29.3.3 Enteral Nutrition Replacement

When children are unable to meet their nutritional needs orally, nutrition support should be considered. Nutrition support can be used to supplement oral intake or as the primary source of nutrition if oral intake is minimal. It is important for families to be aware that typically children are still allowed to eat, even when receiving nutrition support. Enteral nutrition (i.e., tube feeding) helps prevent gut mucosal atrophy and allows for maintenance of GI flora.

- Nasogastric (NG) tube placement is preferable when short-term nutrition support is anticipated. The following factors should be taken into account when determining whether it is safe to proceed with NG tube placement: oral mucosa status; function of the GI tract; presence of GI side effects such as nausea, vomiting, diarrhea; and adequacy of the patient's platelet count. Generally, a small bore (6–12 French) silicone tube is used and should be replaced every 4–6 weeks.

- When long-term nutrition support is anticipated, or when children are prone to dislodging an NG tube, percutaneous gastrostomy tube (G-tube) placement may be indicated. Gastrostomy tubes are placed by creating a surgical opening through the abdominal wall through which the feeding tube can be inserted directly into the stomach.

Gastric (stomach) feeding is the preferred method for delivering enteral nutrition. Gastric feeding is more natural than postpyloric (intestinal) feeding because the stomach, unlike the intestine, has the ability to dilute hyperosmolar solutions. However, postpyloric feeding may be indicated if the child has upper GI dysfunction, delayed gastric emptying, an intestinal obstruction or fistula, severe gastroesophageal reflux, or is at high risk for aspiration with gastric feeds. Postpyloric feeding can be provided via nasoduodenal (ND)/nasojejunal tube (NJ) or jejunostomy tube. ND/NJ tubes are placed similarly to NG tubes, whereas jejunostomy tubes are surgically placed through the abdominal wall directly into the jejunum. Jejunostomy tubes tend to cause fewer problems than gastrostomy tubes with stomal leakage and skin erosion, nausea/vomiting, and bloating, but increase the patient's risk of diarrhea.

The child's nutritional needs and individual tolerance determine the initiation and progression of tube feedings. Formula can be delivered via a feeding pump or gravity flow. Feeds can be given continuously over a specified number of hours or as boluses throughout the day. Bolus feeding schedules mimic normal feeding patterns and are typically more convenient than continuous feeds. However, continuous infusions may be better tolerated in children who suffer from nausea or reflux. Postpyloric feeds should always be given continuously, as the intestine is not designed to be able to handle large volumes of formula at once. In children who cannot meet their calorie needs with oral intake alone, supplemental continuous feeds can be given nocturnally to allow the child to eat normally during the day. Some children benefit from bolus feeds during the day combined with continuous feeds at night to meet their calorie needs. Feeding schedules should be tailored to meet the child's nutritional requirements and the needs of the family, particularly if feeds are to be administered outside of the hospital setting. Many types of formulas are available for tube feedings. Standard (polymeric) formulas contain mostly intact proteins, fat, and carbohydrate and generally range from 30 to 60 kcal/oz (30 mL). These formulas require an intact GI tract capable of digestion, absorption, and excretion. In patients with malabsorption, maldigestion, or altered GI transit time, a semi-elemental or elemental formula may be needed. Semi-elemental formulas contain hydrolyzed proteins, whereas elemental formulas contain only free amino acids. These formulas vary greatly with regards to nutrient composition and ingredients/additives. A list and description of commonly used formulas is shown in Table 29.6

29.3.4 Total Parenteral Nutrition/ Hyperalimentation

When nutrients are unable to be absorbed by the gastrointestinal tract or when enteral nutrition support is not possible or contraindicated, total parenteral nutrition (TPN) offers an alternative means of nutritional support by infusing nutrients directly into the blood stream. Parenteral nutrition (PN) solutions contain a combination of macronutrients (carbohydrate, protein, fat) and micronutrients (electrolytes, vitamins, minerals). The individual components of TPN are listed in Table 29.7. Peripheral venous catheter administration of parenteral nutrition (PPN) is appropriate when the need for nutrition support is anticipated to be short-term; however, central venous catheter administration is recommended if it is anticipated that TPN will be administered for weeks or months or when nutrient concentrations exceeding that which can be administered peripherally are required. PPN solutions should not be higher than 1,000 mOsm because of the risk of damaging the vein, which generally limits the dextrose concentration to a maximum of 12.5% and the concentration of amino acids to 1.5–2%.

Administration of TPN via central venous access allows for the delivery of higher volumes and an

Table 29.6. Formulas for Infants and Children

Infant formulas (birth–1 year)					
Human breast milk is ideal for infants. If breast milk is unavailable or contraindicated, most infants tolerate standard formula, generally 20 kcal/oz, but can be concentrated to 30 kcal/oz					
Standard	**Premature**	**Soy[a]**	**Semi-elemental[a]**	**Elemental[a]**	**Specialty**
Contain lactose and milk protein	*Specially designed for premies*	*Contain soy instead of milk protein*	*For milk protein allergy or malabsorption*	*For severe allergies or malabsorption*	*For infants with specific needs or disease states*
Enfamil Good start Similac	Enfacare NeoSure	Good start supreme soy Isomil Prosobee	Alimentum Nutramigen Pregestimil	Elecare Neocate Nutramigen AA	Similac PM 60/40 Enfamil AR Similac Sensitive[a]
Pediatric formulas (1–10 years)					
Standard[a]	**With fiber[a]**		**Semi-elemental[a]**	**Elemental[a]**	**Specialty[a]**
Kindercal Nutren Jr Pediasure Boost Kid Essentials	Kindercal w/fiber Nutren Jr w/fiber Pediasure w/fiber Boost Kid Essentials w/fiber		Peptamen Jr Pepdite Jr Vital Jr Peptamen Jr 1.5	Elecare Neocate Jr E028 Splash Vivonex pediatric	Compleat pediatric
Adult formulas (children ≥10 years)					
Standard	**High fiber[a]** **High calorie/high protein[a]**		**Semi-elemental[a]**	**Elemental[a]**	**Specialty[a]**
Boost[a] Carnation instant breakfast Ensure[a] Nutren 1.0[a] Osmolite[a] Resource breeze[a]	Boost w/fiber Boost Plus Boost high protein Ensure Plus Ensure w/fiber Jevity Nutren w/fiber Nutren 1.5 Nutren 2.0 Scandishake		Peptamen Peptamen 1.5 Peptinex DT Vital HN	Elecare Tolerex Vivonex Plus Vivonex TEN	Compleat Nepro NutriHep Portagen Pulmocare Renalcal Suplena

Modular Additives: ***Most modular additives (except for fats) can be added to formula. Modulars can be helpful if the nutrient density needs to be increased without increasing volume. Use caution with infants***					
Carbohydrate[a]	**Protein[a]**	**Fat[a]**	**Fiber[a]**	**Thickeners[a]**	**Human milk fortifiers**
Polycose powder Corn syrup Dextrose Cornstarch (not for infants <6 months)	Beneprotein Casec Promod	MCT oil Microlipid Vegetable oil	Benefiber	Rice cereal Simply thick Thick-it Thicken-up	Enfamil HMF Similac HMF Similac natural care advance
Oral rehydration solutions[a] ***(often used to treat mild or moderate dehydration)***					
Enfalyte, liquilytes, pedialyte, rehydralyte					

[a] Indicates lactose-free, to be used in children who are lactose-intolerant (Rodgers and Gonzalez 2008) Copyright 2008. Adapted with permission

Table 29.7. Components of total parenteral nutrition

Component	Contents
Carbohydrate	Dextrose
Protein	Amino acids
Fat	Lipids
Electrolytes	Sodium, potassium, chloride, calcium, phosphate, magnesium
Trace elements	Copper, zinc, manganese, chromium, selenium
Vitamins	A, C, D, E, K, thiamine, riboflavin, niacin, pantothenic acid, pyridoxine (B6), B12, choline, biotin, folic acid

increased amount of calories. Fluid requirements may be more or less than maintenance estimates depending on the patient's fluid status and clinical condition. Estimates of energy needs should be individually calculated (usually in kilocalories ["kcal"]) based on the patient's diagnosis, activity level, degree of malnutrition (if present), and the goals of nutrition support. Dextrose and amino acids generally provide about 70% of total energy intake, while fat provides the remaining 30%; however, this can vary depending on the patient's tolerance. For TPN calculations, concentrations of dextrose and amino acids are usually expressed in g/dL. Dextrose provides 3.4 kcal/g and amino acids provide 4 kcal/g. Dextrose concentrations generally range from 12.5 to 20%, although some fluid-restricted children may require solutions up to 35% dextrose. Dextrose concentrations may be increased every 24 hours as tolerated until the desired caloric level is attained. Amino acid concentrations may also be increased daily until the goal protein intake (generally 1.5–3 g/kg/day) is achieved. Lipid infusions (intralipids) may be either 10 or 20% solutions, providing 1 and 2 kcal/mL, respectively. Lipid administration can be advanced as tolerated until goal fat intake (typically 1–3 g/kg/day) is attained. Lipid solutions should provide at least 0.5 g fat/kg/day to prevent essential fatty acid deficiency but should not exceed 60% of total kcal, as this can induce ketosis. General electrolyte requirements are listed in Table 29.8, but the amount given in the TPN can vary depending on other intake and losses.

Guidelines for PN formulation are usually institution-specific, and initiation of TPN should involve coordination with a pharmacist, dietitian, and physician or nurse practitioner. A basic approach that can be used when initiating TPN includes the following steps:

1. Assess energy and protein requirements of the patient (see steps 2 and 3)
2. Total daily energy intake (kcal/day) = estimated energy needs (kcal/kg/day) × weight (kg)
3. Total daily protein intake (g/day) = estimated protein needs (g/kg/day) × weight (kg)
4. Determine kcal desired from each component: dextrose, amino acids, lipids
5. Calculate total fluid requirement
6. Subtract other intravenous fluids from total fluid requirement and give remainder of fluid in TPN
7. Determine dextrose and amino acid concentrations based on volume of TPN
8. Determine lipid infusion rate
9. Select electrolyte, mineral, and vitamin concentrations

Children receiving TPN should be monitored for changes in metabolic and fluid status by checking laboratory values, daily weights, and fluid intake/output. Initially, urine should be monitored for glucose with each void but may be decreased to daily monitoring if normal. A baseline serum albumin level should be obtained and then repeated every 3 weeks. It is recommended that prealbumin levels be checked weekly. Triglyceride levels should be obtained 4 hours after the initiation of intralipids and after each rate increase; once stable, monitoring can be decreased to weekly. Serum electrolytes and BUN should be monitored at least 2–3 times per week until the TPN rate is stable; then monitoring may be decreased to weekly. Serum calcium, phosphorus, and magnesium levels should be obtained at least weekly until the TPN rate is stable; then monitoring may be decreased to every other week. Labs may need to be monitored more frequently if levels fluctuate significantly or if the child is not medically stable.

29.4 Special Considerations

29.4.1 Common Hydration Complications

29.4.1.1 Fluid Overload

It is important to continually assess the fluid status of a child receiving treatment for cancer. Most hydration imbalances result from therapy and its associated side effects. Children receiving chemotherapy and blood products are at increased risk of fluid overload. Close monitoring of weight, fluid intake/output, and signs of edema can allow for early interventions to minimize complications from fluid overload, such as restricting fluids and administering diuretic therapy.

29.4.1.2 Electrolyte Abnormalities

Children can develop electrolyte imbalances due to the disease process, treatment side effects, or alterations in fluid status. Routine laboratory evaluations are necessary at the time of diagnosis and throughout therapy. Administration of oral or IV supplements may be needed to maintain normal electrolyte levels (see Table 29.8 for daily electrolyte requirements).

29.4.2 Common Complications of Oral/Enteral Nutritional Supplementation

29.4.2.1 Nausea/Vomiting, Bloating, Reflux, and/or Diarrhea

Nausea/vomiting, bloating, reflux, and/or diarrhea may occur as a result of injury inflicted on the GI tract during cancer treatment. These symptoms can also occur if the rate of enteral feeding is too fast for the child's absorptive capabilities or if the child has an intolerance to the formula being given. One treatment option for intolerance of bolus feeds is decreasing the volume of boluses if gastric residuals are high; however, if bolus feeds are still not tolerated, continuous feeds may be tried. If continuous feeds are not well tolerated, the infusion rate can be slowed. When a particular formula is not well tolerated, a more extensively hydrolyzed formula can be used. Sometimes administering formulas with altered macronutrient composition or at room-temperature may alleviate GI side effects.

29.4.2.2 Gastroparesis

Delayed gastric emptying is a disorder in which the stomach takes an excessive amount of time to empty its contents into the small intestine. Symptoms include abdominal pain, nausea, vomiting of undigested food, and poor appetite. Observable signs include abdominal distention and high gastric residual volume after NG or G-tube feeds. Possible causes include deviated tube placement, rapid tube feedings, GERD, and certain metabolic disorders (such as hypothyroidism). Treatment options include the following: confirming correct tube placement, holding tube feedings if gastric residuals remain high, changing from bolus to continuous feeds, administering prokinetic medications (such as metoclopramide), and elevating the head of the bed at least 30° during and after feedings.

Table 29.8. Electrolyte requirements by patient weight

Electrolyte	<25 kg (mEq/kg)	25–45 kg (mEq/kg)	>45 kg
Sodium	2–6	2–6	60–150 mEq/day
Potassium	2–5	2–5	60–150 mEq/day
Calcium	1–2	1	0.2–0.3 mEq/kg/day
Magnesium	0.5	0.5	0.35–0.45 mEq/kg/day
Phosphate	0.5–1 mmol/kg	0.5–1 mmol/kg	7–10 mmol/1,000 kcal
Chloride	2–3	2–3	2–3 mEq/kg/day

29.4.2.3 Aspiration Pneumonia

Aspiration pneumonia refers to a specific type of pneumonia that develops acutely when gastric contents, food, saliva, or nasal secretions are aspirated into the bronchial tree. This can occur as a result of incorrect feeding tube placement or migration of an NG tube, or due to vomiting or reflux. Aspiration pneumonia most frequently occurs in the lower lobe of the right lung. Signs and symptoms include cough, rales, rhonchi, wheezing, respiratory distress, and fever. Treatment options vary depending on the severity of the pneumonia but usually include administration of antibiotics. Prevention includes assessing NG tube placement before feeding is initiated and elevating the head of the bed at least 30° during and immediately after feedings. If patients exhibit difficulty swallowing, a swallow study should be performed to determine aspiration risk.

29.4.2.4 Skin Irritation

Skin irritation leading to excoriation may occur at the site of NG, gastrostomy, or jejunostomy tubes due to leakage of gastric contents or infection. Local infections and cellulitis are treated with strict skin care; antibiotics may be given as needed.

29.4.2.5 Feeding Tube Obstruction

Tube obstruction can occur due to administration of thick formulas or medications or when the tube is not adequately flushed between formula boluses or medication administration. All tubes should be flushed with water at least every 4 hours during continuous feedings and after all boluses and medication administration. Mixing medications in liquid elixir formulations is recommended.

29.4.3 Common Complications of Total Parenteral Nutrition/Hyperalimintation

29.4.3.1 Electrolyte Abnormalities

Children with malignancies can develop electrolyte imbalances as a consequence of the associated treatment. Routine laboratory evaluations are necessary throughout therapy. Management of electrolytes may be difficult during cancer treatment due to frequent changes in the patient's clinical condition and administration of multiple medications and fluids. Descriptions of common electrolyte imbalances (including causes, symptoms, and treatment) are listed in Table 29.9. Specific formulas for correcting electrolyte abnormalities will depend on the patient's situation; therefore, adjustments should be considered on an individual basis.

29.4.3.2 Hepatic Dysfunction

TPN-related liver dysfunction is typically related to the effects of hyperinsulinemia caused by excessive caloric and/or lipid administration. Children with liver dysfunction may develop fatty liver or cholestatic jaundice. TPN-related liver dysfunction may be detected when significant increases in bilirubin and liver enzymes occur; however, it is frequently difficult to determine the true etiology of liver dysfunction because many medications can also cause elevated liver enzymes. Treatment strategies for TPN-related liver dysfunction include the following: avoiding excessive administration of calories (primarily from carbohydrates and lipids); maintaining an appropriate balance of dextrose, amino acids and lipids; cycling the TPN over fewer hours; and discontinuing the TPN as soon as therapeutically possible.

29.4.3.3 Mechanical Complications

Mechanical complications of TPN are primarily related to the central venous catheter; possible complications include catheter tip migration, obstruction, thrombosis, and infection. Peripheral PN solutions greater than 1,000 mOsm can cause vascular damage. Research has indicated that patients receiving TPN are at increased risk for infections (Beghetto et al. 2005); therefore, aseptic techniques should always be used in venous catheter care. It is essential to ensure that the line is functioning properly prior to every infusion. If catheter displacement or obstruction is suspected, radiologic evaluation should be completed before using the catheter.

Table 29.9. Common electrolyte imbalances in pediatric cancer patients

Electrolyte imbalance	Level	Causes	Symptoms	Treatment
Hypercalcemia	>10.5 mg/dL	Bone malignancies and metastases, excessive concentrations in total parenteral nutrition (TPN), poor dietary intake of phosphorus, renal absorption or excretion, diuretics	Weakness, irritability, lethargy, seizures, coma, abdominal cramping, anorexia, nausea, vomiting, ECG changes	Hydration, hemodialysis, steroids
Hypocalcemia	<8 mg/dL	Decreased intake; vitamin D deficiency, intake, or malabsorption; hypoparathyroidism, pancreatitis	Neuromuscular irritability, weakness, cramping, fatigue, change in level of consciousness, seizures, ECG changes	IV or oral replacement, correct underlying cause
Hyperkalemia	6–7 mEq/L	Renal failure, cellular breakdown, leukocytosis, metabolic acidosis	ECG changes	Kayexalate, insulin, $NaHCO_3$, calcium gluconate
Hypokalemia	<3.5 mEq/L	Decreased intake, increased renal excretion, therapy-induced renal tubular defects, diarrhea, vomiting	Skeletal muscle weakness, dysrhythmias: prolonged Q–T interval, flattened T-waves	Replace with potassium acetate or gluconate
Hyponatremia	<130 mEq/L	Syndrome of inappropriate secretion of antidiuretic hormone (SIADH); ectopic secretion of antidiuretic hormone; renal, adrenal cortical, or cardiac insufficiency; excessive loss secondary to vomiting, diarrhea, or salt-losing nephropathy; neurotoxic effect of cyclophosphamide and vinca alkaloids	Convulsions, shock, lethargy	Fluid restriction, replace losses, treat underlying cause
Hypomagnesemia	<1 mEq/L	Nephrotoxic agents, decreased intake, diarrhea, vomiting, urinary loss	Tetany, seizures, tremors, anorexia, nausea, cardiac abnormalities, weakness, clonus	IV or oral magnesium sulfate, oxide, or gluconate
Hypermagnesemia	>5 mg/dL	Renal dysfunction	Hyporeflexia, respiratory depression, confusion, coma	IV administration of calcium, diuresis
Hypophosphatemia	<3 mg/dL	Poor dietary intake, malabsorption, excessive renal excretion, vitamin D deficiency	Usually not until severe (<1 mg/dL); irritability, paresthesias	IV or oral potassium-phosphate or sodium-phosphate
Hyperphosphatemia	>6 mg/dL	Chemotherapeutic agents, renal insufficiency: glomerular filtration rate <25% normal	Symptoms relative to resulting from hypocalcemia	Restrict intake, phosphorus binders: calcium carbonate, aluminum hydroxide

29.4.4 Common Complications of Enteral and Parenteral Nutritional Supplementation

29.4.4.1 Refeeding Syndrome

Refeeding syndrome describes a combination of metabolic abnormalities, including fluid and electrolyte imbalances, that can occur after nutritional supplementation (oral, enteral, or parenteral) is provided to a severely malnourished patient. Refeeding syndrome is caused by a shift in the body's energy use from stored fat to the newly available carbohydrates; carbohydrate stimulates an increase in insulin production, resulting in intracellular uptake of electrolytes (particularly phosphorus, potassium, and magnesium) that are used in metabolism. This results in acute (and sometimes severe) decreases in serum electrolyte levels, which can cause a multitude of complications, including cardiac arrhythmias/failure, acute respiratory failure, paralysis, muscle necrosis, coma, and death. It is important to identify patients at risk for refeeding syndrome and correct any existing electrolyte abnormalities prior to initiating nutrition support. Refeeding syndrome can be prevented by initiating nutrition support at a reduced caloric rate and increasing feeds slowly toward the goal caloric intake. Strict monitoring of sodium, magnesium, potassium, chloride, bicarbonate, BUN, creatinine, glucose, calcium, and phosphorus is recommended during the first 3–7 days of nutritional rehabilitation. If a patient develops refeeding syndrome, nutritional support should be held until electrolyte abnormalities are corrected.

29.4.4.2 Glycemic Abnormalities

Hyperglycemia and hypoglycemia are common side effects of TPN administration. Hypoglycemia can occur after completion of the TPN infusion and is easily prevented by avoiding abrupt discontinuation of the TPN administration; the administration rate should instead be tapered down as the infusion is being discontinued. Hyperglycemia can occur during the TPN infusion and can be managed by reducing the overall TPN infusion rate, decreasing the dextrose content of the TPN solution, and/or administering insulin as needed. Hyperglycemia can also occur with oral/enteral nutrition in patients under significant physiological stress or on corticosteroids.

29.4.5 Specific Nutritional Concerns of Long-Term Survivors

There is a growing concern regarding the risk of obesity among childhood cancer survivors. Increased incidence of obesity has been noted in children who received treatment for acute lymphoblastic leukemia, brain tumors, and craniopharyngioma (Rogers et al. 2005). Potential factors that may contribute to the increased risk of obesity in childhood cancer survivors include: injury to the hypothalamic–pituitary axis, growth hormone deficiency, excessive caloric intake associated with steroid treatment, and physical inactivity. Children and families should be educated during and after cancer treatment about healthy diet principles and physical activity options for maintaining a healthy weight (Chap. 17).

29.4.6 Specific Nutritional Concerns During Palliative Care

Children receiving palliative care for unresponsive or progressive oncologic diseases have different hydration and nutritional concerns than children receiving treatment. The primary goal of care during this time is alleviating suffering and enhancing the child's quality of life. Families may need education and support to help them understand that reduced nutrient intake will not alter the pathologic process of the disease or shorten the child's life. Because metabolism slows as the body shuts down, a decreased appetite and loss of interest in food are common symptoms as a child nears death. Family members should be strongly encouraged to give the child permission to refuse intake. Forcing a child to consume food will only tire the child and decrease his/her quality of life by causing discomfort in the form of diarrhea, nausea, vomiting, choking, or abdominal distention. Children who remain interested in eating may benefit from small, frequent meals of soft, easily digested foods and by avoiding foods with strong smells to minimize GI discomfort.

Fluid requirements during palliative care are also decreased. Thirst is rare during the final days of life. As with nutrition, there are no data indicating that withholding fluids (orally or intravenously) during the final stage of life is detrimental. Children may be supported with minimal intravenous (IV) fluid administration if intravenous access is available and it is the wish of the child or family. Possible advantages of IV fluid administration include improved oral comfort and bowel function, less delirium, and thinning of secretions. Disadvantages include increases in oral, respiratory, and GI secretions and urine output, which can increase the child's risk of choking, cough, pulmonary congestion, edema (peripheral and pulmonary), vomiting, and urinary incontinence.

References

Bechard L, Adiv O, Jaksic T, Duggan C (2006) Nutritional supportive care. In: Pizzo P, Poplack D (eds) Principles and practice of pediatric oncology. Lippincott Williams & Wilkins, Philadelphia, PA, pp 1330–1347

Beghetto M, Victorino J, Teixeira L, de Azevedo M (2005) Parenteral nutrition as a risk factor for central venous catheter-related infection. Journal of Parenteral and Enteral Nutrition 29(5):367–373

Han-Markey T (2000) Nutritional considerations in pediatric oncology. Seminars in Oncology Nursing 16(2):146–151

Holliday M, Segar W (1957) The maintenance need for water in parenteral fluid therapy. Pediatrics 19(5):823–832

Mosteller R (1987) Simplified calculation of body surface area. New England Journal of Medicine 317(17):1098

Reading B, Freeman B (2005) Simple formula for the surface area of the body and a simple model for anthropometry. Clinical Anatomy 18:126–130

Rodgers C, Gonzalez S (2008) Nutrition support for children with cancer. In: Kline NE (ed) Essentials of pediatric oncology nursing: a core curriculum, 3rd edn. Association of Pediatric Hematology Oncology Nurses, Glenview, IL

Rogers P, Meacham L, Oeffinger K, Henry D, Lange B (2005) Obesity in pediatric oncology. Pediatric Blood and Cancer 45(7):881–891

Wilson D (2007) Balance and imbalance of body fluids. In: Hockenberry M, Wilson D (eds) Wong's nursing care of infants and children. Mosby Elsevier, St. Louis, MO, pp 1140–1179

World Health Organization (1985) Energy and protein requirements (FAO/WHO/UNV Expert Consultation Technical Report Series 724). Geneva, Switzerland

Pain in Children with Cancer

Cara Simon

Contents

30.1 Introduction . . . 529
30.2 Causes of Pain in Childhood Cancer . . . 529
30.3 Assessment . . . 530
30.4 Cultural Issues . . . 536
30.5 Principles of Treatment . . . 536
30.6 Treatment . . . 537
30.6.1 By the Ladder . . . 537
30.6.1.1 Step I: Mild Pain . . . 537
30.6.1.2 Step II: Mild to Moderate Pain . . . 537
30.6.1.3 Step III: Moderate to Severe Pain . . . 538
30.6.1.4 Intractable Pain . . . 538
30.6.2 By the Route . . . 538
30.6.3 By the Clock . . . 538
30.6.4 Opioids . . . 538
30.6.5 Equianalgesia . . . 538
30.6.6 Procedure-Related Pain . . . 540
30.6.7 Patient-Controlled Analgesia (PCA) . . . 540
30.6.8 Adjuvant Medications . . . 542
30.6.9 Nonpharmacologic Treatment . . . 542
Summary . . . 543
References . . . 544

30.1 Introduction

Pain is an unpleasant sensory and emotional experience with actual or potential tissue damage, or described in terms of such damage. It is always subjective and interpreted by the individual. Unrelieved pain in children can lead to mistrust of the medical staff, create fear, and increase anxiety and pain in future procedures. Children may also experience night terrors, flashbacks, sleep disturbances, and eating problems. Long-lasting effects of childhood pain can include posttraumatic stress syndrome, phobic reactions, and depression (World Health Organization 1998).

According to the American Academy of Pediatrics (AAP) and the American Pain Society (APS) (2001), pain in children is often inadequately assessed and undertreated. Uncontrolled or chronic pain in children can leave them victimized, depressed, isolated, and lonely. It can also affect their ability to cope with cancer. The effects of uncontrolled chronic or acute pain are extended to the family and healthcare providers. Parents may experience guilt, anger, and depression. Healthcare providers may have decreased ability to show compassion, may experience feelings of guilt, and may deny that children are, in fact, suffering (World Health Organization 1998). Nurses and other healthcare providers must realize that children feel pain just as adults do (Table 30.1) and that their pain must be treated appropriately.

30.2 Causes of Pain in Childhood Cancer

Almost all children diagnosed with cancer will experience pain at some point in their treatment. Pain in children with cancer can be classified as nociceptive

Table 30.1. Myths and misconceptions about pain control in children

Myth Infants cannot feel pain because their nervous systems are immature	*Fact supported by evidence* Pain pathways are formed before birth. Neonates and infants can remember pain
Myth Some health providers and parents believe that opioids should be administered only as a last resort to avoid drug addiction	*Consequences* Children do not always receive the strong analgesic required to relieve severe pain. Opioid side effects may not be treated as aggressively as they should
Misconception The pharmacology of opioid analgesics, especially their pharmacodynamics and pharmacokinetics, is poorly understood	*Consequence* Health professionals do not select the most appropriate drug, dose, or route of administration for children in pain
Misconception Health professionals do not know how to assess a child's pain level or factors that intensify the pain	*Consequence* Health professional cannot evaluate if changes in drug therapy are effective
Misconception Some health professionals do not know that simple non-drug therapies are effective and can lessen a child's pain	*Consequence* Children and patients are not taught how to use practical cognitive, physical, and behavioral strategies to reduce pain and distress

Adapted from McGrath (1990); World Health Organization (2003)

or neuropathic. Nociceptive pain is usually described as aching or throbbing. Neuropathic pain results from nerve damage or inflammation and is described as burning, tingling, pins and needles, or a piercing sensation. The most common causes of pain can be directly related to the disease itself, to the treatment, or to procedures (Table 30.2). Children often do not convey that they are in pain, but turn inward and become quiet to cope with it.

Neuropathic pain develops in one-third of all patients with cancer. Neuropathic pain responds to opioids but often requires increased doses. Adjuvant medications such as tricyclic antidepressants and anticonvulsants are first-line therapy for neuropathic pain and are used to enhance the analgesic effects of opoids (Table 30.3) (Lucas and Lipman 2002). One example of neuropathic pain is phantom limb pain. Children who undergo limb amputation may develop phantom limb pain, phantom limb sensations, or stump pain. The precise cause of phantom limb pain is unknown. Injury to the nerves during amputation causes changes in the way the central nervous system conducts impulses. The parts of the brain that control the missing limb stay active, causing the illusion of the missing limb even though the amputee knows that the limb is gone.

Phantom limb pain refers to pain felt in an absent limb that was removed because of disease, and is usually experienced in bursts. Very few children have constant pain. The attacks can come frequently or only occasionally. Phantom pain is often described as shooting, stabbing, or burning. The pain is felt at the"end" of the limb, in phantom fingers or toes. In contrast, phantom limb sensations, which are also felt in the absent limb, are not painful. Stump pain is only felt in the stump of the amputated limb. Phantom limb pain is treated with medications (see Table 30.3), stimulation therapy, prosthesis use, and rehabilitation.

30.3 Assessment

Children learn to adapt and may not show visible signs of pain. But it is the health professional's ethical obligation to ask them if they are in pain. Pain assessment is an essential component of the process of pain management in children and is often referred to as the "fifth vital sign."

Table 30.2. Causes of pain in childhood cancer

Type	Clinical presentation	Causes
Bone Skull Vertebrae Pelvis/femur	Aching to sharp, severe pain generally more pronounced with movement Point tenderness common Skull – headaches, blurred vision Spine – tenderness over spinous process Arms/extremities – pain associated with movement or lifting Pelvis/femur – associated with movement; pain with weight bearing and walking	Infiltration of bone Skeletal metastases – irritation and stretching of pain receptors in the periosteum and endosteum Prostaglandins released from bone destruction
Neuropathic Peripheral Plexus Epidural Cord compression	Complaints of pain without any detectable tissue damage Abnormal or unpleasant sensations, generally described as tingling, burning, or stabbing Often a delay in onset Brief, shooting pain Increased intensity of pain with receptive stimuli	Nerve injury caused by tumor infiltration; can also be caused by injury from treatment (i.e., vincristine toxicity) Infiltration or compression of peripheral nerves Surgical interruption of nerves (phantom pain post-amputation)
Visceral Soft tissue Tumors of the bowel Retroperitoneum	Poorly localized Varies in intensity Pressure, deep or aching	Obstruction – bowel, urinary tract, biliary tract Mucosal ulceration Metabolic alteration Nociceptor activation, generally from distension or inflammation of visceral organs
Treatment-related Mucositis Infection Post-lumbar puncture headaches Radiation dermatitis Postsurgical	Difficulty swallowing, pain from lesions in the oropharynx. May extend throughout the entire GI tract Infection may be localized pain from a focused infection or generalized (i.e., tissue infection vs. septicemia) Severe headache following lumbar puncture Skin inflammation causing redness and breakdown Pain related to tissue trauma secondary to surgery	Direct side-effects of Treatment for cancer Chemotherapy Radiation Surgery

From Hockenberry-Eaton (1999) Reprinted with permission

Healthcare providers should specifically assess the presence, severity, location, quality, and intensity of pain in a manner appropriate for the child's cognitive ability. One method is the QUESTT method (Hockenberry et al. 2003):

- Question the child
- Use pain rating scales
- Evaluate behavior
- Secure parents' involvement
- Take cause of pain into account
- Take action and evaluate results

Because pain is subjective, self-reporting is preferred. However, behavioral observations can complement self-reporting or may be used along with physical findings for the preverbal or nonverbal child.

A variety of tools are available to assess pediatric pain. The National Comprehensive Cancer Network (NCCN) Guidelines (2007) recommend use of age appropriate scales to assess pain in pediatrics:

- The FLACC scale can be used in children younger than 3 years or other patients who cannot self-report (Table 30.4). The FLACC scale has been shown to have good reliabilty and validity. Each component of the FLACC scale is scored separately and the summed to determine the FLACC score.

Table 30.3. Co-analgesic agents

Category/drug	Dosage	Indication	Comments
Antidepressants			
Amitriptyline	0.2–0.5 mg/kg p.o. at bedtime Titrate upward by 0.25 mg/kg every 5–7 days as needed Available in 10 and 25 mg tablets Usual starting dose is 10–25 mg	Continuous neuropathic pain with burning, aching, dysthesia with insomnia	Provides analgesia by blocking re-uptake of serotonin and norepinephrine possibly slowing transmissions of pain signals Helps with pain related to insomnia and depression (use nortriptyline if patient is over-sedated) Analgesic effects seen earlier than antidepressant effects Side effects include dry mouth, constipation, urinary retention
Nortriptyline	0.2–1.0 mg/kg p.o. a.m. or b.i.d. Titrate up by 0.5 mg q 5–7 days Maximum: 25 mg/dose	Neuropathic pain as above without insomnia	
Anticonvulsants			
Gabapentin	5 mg/kg p.o. at bedtime Increase to b.i.d. on day 2, t.i.d. on day 3 Maximum: 300 mg/day	Neuropathic pain	Mechanism of action unknown Side effects include sedation, ataxia, nystagmus, dizziness
Carbamazepine	*<6 years* 2.5–5 mg/kg p.o. b.i.d. initially Increase 20 mg/kg/24 h Divide b.i.d. q week prn; Maximum: 100 mg b.i.d. *6–12 years* 5 mg/kg p.o. b.i.d. initially Increase 10 mg/kg/24 h Divide q week prn to usual Maximum: 100 mg/dose b.i.d. *>12 years* 200 mg p.o. b.i.d. initially Increase 200 mg/24 h Divide b.i.d. q week PRN to maximum: 1.6–2.4 g/24 h	Sharp, lancinating neuropathic pain, peripheral neuropathies, phantom limb pain	Similar analgesic effect as amitriptyline Monitor blood levels for toxicity only Side effects include decreased blood counts, ataxia, and GI irritation
Anxiolytics			
Lorazepam	0.03–0.1 mg/kg q4–6 h p.o./i.v.; maximum: 2 mg/dose	Muscle spasm, anxiety	May increase sedation in combination with opioids Can cause depression with prolonged use
Diazepam	0.1–0.3 mg/kg q4–6 h p.o./i.v.; maximum:10 mg/dose		

Table 30.3. (Continued)

Category/drug	Dosage	Indication	Comments
Antidepressants			
Corticosteroids			
Dexamethasone	Dose dependent on clinical situation Higher bolus doses in cord compression then lower daily dose. Try to wean to NSAIDs if pain allows Cerebral edema: 1–2 mg/kg load then 1–1.5 mg/kg/day divided q6 h; maximum: 4 mg/dose Anti-inflammatory: 0.08–0.3 mg/kg/day divided q6–12 h	Pain from increased intracranial pressure Bony metastasis Spinal/nerve compression	Side effects include edema, gastrointestinal irritation, increased weight, acne Use gastroprotectants such as H2 blockers (ranitidine) or proton pump inhibitors such as omeprazole for long-term administration of steroids or NSAIDs in end-stage cancer with bony pain
Others			
Clonidine	2–4 mcg/kg p.o. q4–6 h May also use a 100 mcg Transdermal patch q 7 days for patients >40 kg	Neuropathic pain Lancinating, sharp, electrical, shooting pain Phantom limb pain	Alpha 2 adrenoreceptor agonist modulates ascending pain sensations Routes of administration include oral, transdermal, and spinal Management of withdrawal symptoms Monitor for orthostatic hypertension, bradycardia Sedation common
Mexiletine	2–3 mg/kg/dose p.o. t.i.d may titrate 0.5 mg/kg q2–3 weeks as needed Maximum: 300 mg/dose	Neuropathic pain Lancinating, sharp, electrical, shooting pain Phantom limb pain	Similar to lidocaine, longer acting-Stabilizes sodium conduction in nerve cells, reduces neuronal firing Can enhance action of opioids, antidepressants, anticonvulsants Side effects include dizziness, ataxia, nausea, vomiting May measure blood levels for toxicity

From Hockenberry-Eaton et al. (1999). Reprinted with permission

- The FACES pain rating scale is a well-studied and commonly used method to assess children's pain (Fig. 30.1). Children as young as 3 years old are able to appropriately use this scale. It has been translated into seven different languages and can be correlated with a scale of 0–5 or of 0–10.
- The numeric scale is also a common tool used to assess a child's pain and can be used with children 12 years of age or older; however, it does assume that they have some concept of numbers and their value. It is represented by a line with equal increments from 0 to 5 or 10, with "0" representing no pain and "5" or "10" representing the worst pain imaginable. This tool may be used vertically or horizontally.

When assessing pain in children, it is important to consider that the lack of reporting pain does not equate to the lack of pain itself (Twycross et al. 1998). Behaviors such as watching television, talking on the

Table 30.4. FLACC scale: rating scale to be used in children less than 3 years of age or others who cannot self-report

Categories	Scoring		
	0	1	2
Face	No particular expression or smile	Occasional grimace or frown, withdrawn, disinterested	Frequent to constant quivering chin, clenched jaw
Legs	Normal position or relaxed	Uneasy, restless, tense	Kicking, or legs drawn up
Activity	Lying quietly, normal position, moves easily	Squirming, shifting back and forth, tense	Arched, rigid, or jerking
Cry	No cry (awake or asleep)	Moans or whimpers; occasional complaint	Crying steadily, screams or sobs, frequent complaints
Consolability	Content, relaxed	Reassured by occasional touching, hugging, or being talked to, distractable	Difficult to console or comfort

Each of the five categories *F* face; *L* leg; *A* activity; *C* cry; *C* consolability is scored from 0 to 2, which results in a total score between 0 and 10

From Merkel et al. (1997). Reprinted with Permission

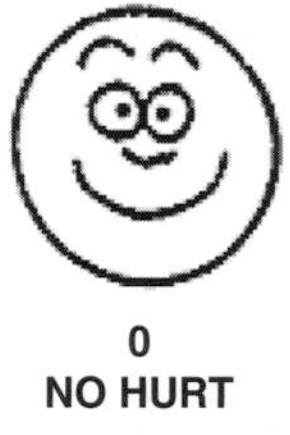
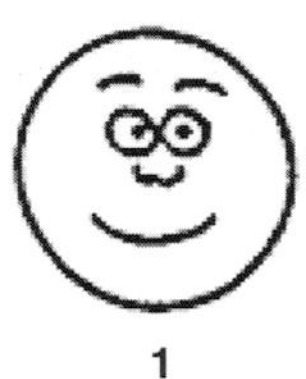
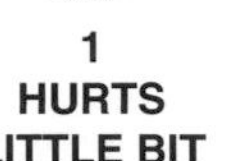
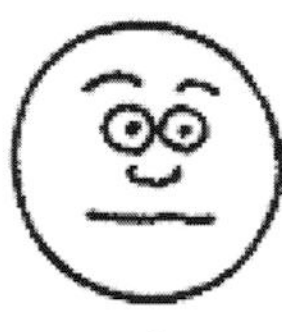
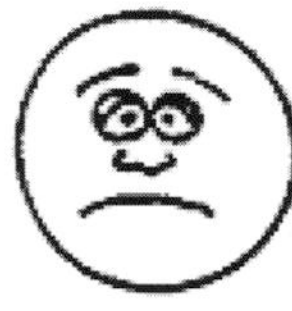
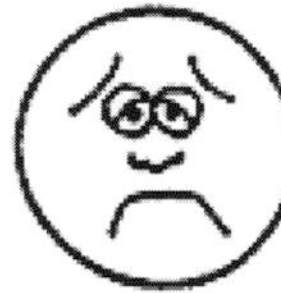
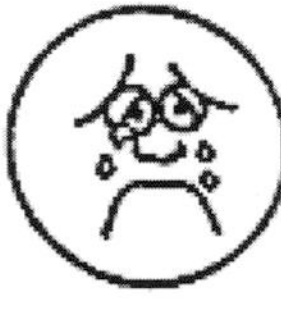
0
NO HURT
1
HURTS
LITTLE BIT
2
HURTS
LITTLE MORE
3
HURTS
EVEN MORE
4
HURTS
WHOLE LOT
5
HURTS
WORST

Fig. 30.1

FACES pain rating scale (from Hockenberry et al. 2005) Original instructions: Explain to the person that each face is for a person who feels happy because he has no pain (hurt) or sad because he has some or a lot of pain. *Face 0* is very happy because it doesn't hurt at all. *Face 1* hurts just a little bit. *Face 2* hurts a little more. *Face 3* hurts even more. *Face 4* hurts a whole lot. *Face 5* hurts as much as you can imagine, although you don't have to be crying to feel this bad. Ask the person to choose the face that best describes how he/she is feeling. Brief word instructions: Point to each face using the words to describe the pain intensity. Ask the child to choose the face that best describes his/her own pain and record the appropriate number. Used with permission. Copyright, Mosby

phone, playing, and sleeping are often distraction methods used to cope with pain but are often misinterpreted by healthcare professionals (Hockenberry-Eaton et al. 1999). Because of the nature of childhood cancer diagnosis and treatment, it is reasonable to expect that all children will need some type of pain management plan, and certainly all children should be assessed for the presence of pain. Physiologic responses to pain from sympathetic involvement include diaphoresis, flushing, pallor, hypertension, tachycardia, tachypnea, and hypoxia. These measures are more commonly observed during acute pain and may dissipate if the pain becomes more chronic in nature.

Table 30.5. Developmental differences in pain expression

Developmental group	Expressions of pain
Infants	May exhibit body rigidity or thrashing, may include arching May exhibit facial expression of pain (brows lowered and drawn together, eyes tightly closed, mouth open and squarish) May cry intensely/loudly May be inconsolable May draw knees to chest May exhibit hypersensitivity or irritability May have poor oral intake May be unable to sleep
Toddlers	May be verbally aggressive, cry intensely May exhibit regressive behavior or withdraw May exhibit physical resistance by pushing painful stimulus away after it is applied May guard painful area of body May be unable to sleep
Preschoolers/young children	May verbalize intensity of pain May see pain as punishment May exhibit thrashing of arms and legs May attempt to push stimulus away before it is applied May be uncooperative May need physical restraint May cling to parent, nurse, or significant other May request emotional support (e.g., hugs, kisses) May understand that there can be secondary gains associated with pain May be unable to sleep
School-age children	May verbalize pain May use an objective measurement of pain May be influenced by cultural beliefs May experience nightmares related to pain May exhibit stalling behaviors (e.g., "Wait a minute" or "I'm not ready") May have muscular rigidity such as clenched fists, white knuckles, gritted teeth, contracted limbs, body stiffness, closed eyes, or wrinkled forehead May include behaviors of preschoolers/young children May be unable to sleep
Adolescents	May localize and verbalize pain May deny pain in presence of peers May have changes in sleep patterns or appetite May be influenced by cultural beliefs May exhibit muscle tension and body control May display regressive behavior in presence of family May be unable to sleep

Hockenberry-Eaton et al. (1999). Reprinted with permission

Manifestations of pain in children differ according to developmental stage (Table 30.5). There are some distinct differences between how infants communicate and react to pain and how children communicate and react to pain. The infant or preverbal child is especially vulnerable to untreated or undertreated pain. Therefore, specific measures have been taken to identify consistent behaviors in infants undergoing painful procedures to quantify cry, oxygen requirements, vital sign parameters, facial expression, and sleep pattern.

30.6.1.3 Step III: Moderate to Severe Pain

To provide pain relief, an opioid for moderate to severe pain should be used, and the dose should be increased until pain is relieved or toxicities occur. If side effects occur, supportive management can be provided (Table 30.8). If appropriate, the nonopioid can be continued. Morphine is the drug of choice. In general, only one medication from each group should be used at the same time.

30.6.1.4 Intractable Pain

Some children with bone metastasis or nerve involvement may have extreme pain unresolved by the previous steps and may require more aggressive treatment. Invasive therapy or procedures may include opioids via epidural catheter, therapeutic nerve block, or cordotomy. These techniques are used as a last resort, with the risk and discomfort of the procedure weighed heavily against the benefit of pain relief. It is also important to note that there is no guarantee that these procedures will provide total or permanent pain relief. If the invasive technique is successful, then one should proceed cautiously when discontinuing previously used opioids, instituting the weaning guidelines as appropriate (Table 30.9).

30.6.2 By the Route

Medications should be administered by the simplest, most effective, least painful route. Oral analgesics are usually available in tablets or elixirs. Intravenous, subcutaneous, and transdermal are also appropriate routes. Intramuscular injections should be avoided because they are painful and may alter the patient's report of pain to avoid more pain. Factors that influence the selection of administration route include severity of pain, type of pain, potency of the analgesic, and the required dosing interval.

30.6.3 By the Clock

When using pharmacologic agents, scheduled or by-the-clock dosing is recommended over "as needed" or prn dosing. Rescue dosing for intermittent or breakthrough pain is also suggested. The dosing interval is determined by the severity of the pain and the duration of the medication used (World Health Organization 1998).

30.6.4 Opioids

There are many considerations when implementing opioid analgesia. First, there is no standard dose. The appropriate dose of an opioid is the dose that provides effective pain relief. Addiction in children with cancer is rare; however, tolerance is common in long-term use and will affect the dose required to maintain analgesia. Tolerance to side effects is also common and beneficial when titrating the dose to achieve desired analgesia. Common side effects include constipation, sedation, pruritus, nausea, and urinary retention (Table 30.8). Physical dependence may occur with prolonged use (longer than 7 days) and is more common than addiction, and opioid weaning is strongly recommended (Table 30.9). Signs and symptoms of withdrawal or physical dependence include diaphoresis, rhinorrhea, lacrimation, irritability, tremors, anorexia, dilated pupils, and goose bumps.

The most common opioid used in treating childhood cancer pain is morphine. Demerol is not recommended because of its short duration of action and toxic metabolite normeperidine, which has been associated with seizures in children. The risk of respiratory depression is still a common barrier to the appropriate dosing of morphine, especially intravenous morphine. This is a rare side effect that is reversible with the administration of naloxone. It occurs more frequently in patients with little or no prior opioid exposure, and is antagonized by pain.

30.6.5 Equianalgesia

Because there are a variety of routes by which to administer opioids, and because patients may need to be switched from one opioid to another, one must consider the equianalgesic conversion factor. For example, when going from an intravenous dose of morphine to an oral dose, the oral dose may need to be larger to achieve the same analgesic effect. This is due largely to the first-pass effect that oral

Table 30.8. Management of opioid side effects

Side effect	Adjuvant drugs	Nonpharmacologic techniques
Constipation	Senna and docusate sodium *Tablet* 2–6 years: 1/2 tablet once a day; maximum: one tablet twice a day 6–12 years: one tablet once a day; maximum: two tablets twice a day >12 years: start two tablets once a day; maximum: four tablets twice a day *Liquid* 1 month to 1 year: 1.25–5 mL q h 1–5 years = 2.5 mL q h 5–15 years = 5–10 mL q h >15 years = 10–25 mL q h Casanthranol and docusate sodium *Liquid*: 5–15 mL q h *Capsules*: 1 p.o. q h Bisacodyl: PO or PR 3–12 years 5 mg/dose/day; >12 years 10–15 mg/dose/day Lactulose: 7.5 mL/day after breakfast *Adult*: 15–30 mL p.o. q day Mineral oil: 1–2 teaspoon p.o./day Magnesium citrate: >6 years = 2–4 mL/kg p.o. once; 6–12 years = 100–150 mL p.o. once; >12 years = 150–300 mL p.o. once Milk of magnesia (MOM) <2 years = 0.5 mL/kg/dose p.o. once; 2–5 years = 5–15 mL p.o. q day; 6–12 years = 15–30 mL p.o. once; >12 years = 30–60 mL p.o. once Polyethylene glycol 0.5–1 packet (17 g) po every day up to t.i.d (mix in 4–8 oz of fluid)	Increase water intake, prune juice, bran cereal, vegetables
Sedation	Caffeine: single dose of 1–1.5 mg p.o. Dextroamphetamine: 2.5–5 mg p.o. in a.m. and early afternoon Methylphenidate: 2.5–5 mg p.o. in a.m. and early afternoon	Caffeinated drinks
Nausea/vomiting	Promethazine: 0.5 mg/kg q4–6 h; maximum: 25 mg/dose (do not use if < 2 years old) Ondansetron: 0.1–0.15 mg/kg i.v. or p.o. q 4 h; maximum: 8 mg/dose Granisetron: 10–40 mcg/kg q 2–4 h; maximum: 1 mg/dose Droperidol: 0.05–0.06 mg/kg i.v. q4–6 h;	Imagery, relaxation Deep, slow breathing
Pruritus	Diphenhydramine: 1 mg/kg i.v./p.o. q4–6 h prn; maximum: 25 mg/dose Hydroxyzine: 0.6 mg/kg dose p.o. q6 h; maximum: 50 mg/dose Naloxone: 0.5 mcg/kg/h continuous infusion(diluted in a solution of 0.1 mg of naloxone per 10 mL of saline) Butorphanol: 0.3–0.5 mg/kg i.v. (use cautiously in opioid tolerant children, may cause withdrawal symptoms); maximum: 2 mg/dose because mixed agonist/antagonist techniques	Oatmeal baths, good hygiene

Table 30.8. (Continued)

Side effect	Adjuvant drugs	Nonpharmacologic techniques
Respiratory depression: mild-moderate	Hold dose of opioid Reduce subsequent doses by 25%	Arouse gently, give O_2, encourage to deep breath
Respiratory depression: severe	Naloxone: *During disease pain management:* 0.5 mcg/kg in 2-min increments until breathing improves Reduce opioid dose if possible *During sedation for procedures:* 5–10 mcg/kg until breathing improves	O_2, bag and mask if indicated
Dysphoria/confusion/ Hallucinations	Haloperidol (Haldol): 0.05–0.15 mg/kg/day divided in 2–3 doses; maximum: 2–4 mg/day	Rule out other physiologic causes
Urinary retention	Oxybutynin: 1 year = 1 mg t.i.d 2–3 years = 3 mg t.i.d >5 years = 5 mg t.i.d 1–2 years = 2 mg t.i.d 4–5 years = 4 mg t.i.d	Rule out other physiologic causes Urinary catheterization

Adapted from Hockenberry-Eaton et al. (1999). Reprinted with permission

Table 30.9. Opioid weaning guidelines

Give 1/2 of previous daily dose for 2 days
Reduce dose by 25% every 2 days
Continue until daily dose equals
0.6 mg/kg/day for child <50 kg
30 mg/day for a child >50 kg (of morphine or equivalent)
After 2 days at this dose (0.6 mg/kg/day), discontinue opioid
[a]Oral methadone may be used to wean as follows Use 1/4 of the equianalgesic dose as initial wean dose, then proceed as stated above

From World Health Organization (1998)

medications undergo in the liver before entering the systemic circulation. Likewise, when switching from one opioid to another, even if it is the same route, the equianalgesia factor still exists. For example, 1 mg of oral hydromorphone is equal to 4 mg of oral morphine. Equianalgesia doses are listed with the opioid doses in Table 30.10.

30.6.6 Procedure-Related Pain

For procedure-related pain, premedication with the appropriate analgesic is warranted (Table 30.11). Nonpharmacologic methods in conjunction with the appropriate analgesia, such as distraction, guided imagery, and relaxation, can be used to successfully relieve this type of pain.

For more invasive procedures, sedation is widely accepted as a standard of care in many centers (Table 30.12). Because of the potential for severe side effects, it is necessary to have appropriately trained staff administer the analgesia and the reversal drug if indicated, monitor the patient at regular intervals, and ensure recovery to baseline neurological and respiratory status on completion of the process. Most centers have instituted protocols to ensure continuity and safety while providing a higher level of analgesia. Included in the protocols are recommendations for NPO status, type and dose of analgesic agents, and their reversals.

30.6.7 Patient-Controlled Analgesia (PCA)

For extended pain control in children with cancer, administration of intravenous morphine and other

Table 30.10. Starting doses for commonly prescribed opioids

Drug	Oral starting doses	Dosage forms	Starting doses IV	IV to PO
Codeine	0.5–1 mg/kg q4 6 h; maximum: 60 mg/dose	Tablet, as sulfate: 30 mg Liquid: 3 mg/mL	N/A	N/A
Paracetamol/acetaminophen w/codeine	0.5–1 mg/kg/dose of codeine q4 6 h; maximum: 2 tablets/dose; 15 mL/dose	Elixir: paracetamol/acetaminophen 24 mg and codeine 2.4 mg/mL with alcohol 7% Suspension: acetaminophen 24 mg and codeine 2.4 mg/mL alcohol free Tablet: 3 paracetamol/acetaminophen 300 mg and codeine 30 mg	N/A	N/A
Hydrocodone and Paracetamol/acetaminophen	3–6 years: 5 mL 3–4 times/day 7–12 years: 10 mL 3–4 times/day >12 years: 1–2 tablets q4–6 h; maximum 8 tablets/day	Tablet: hydrocodone 5 mg and acetaminophen 500 mg Oral solution at: 0.5 mg hydrocodone and 33.4 mg/mL paracetamol/acetaminophen	N/A	N/A
Oxycodone	Instant release: 0.05–0.15 mg/kg/dose up to 5 mg/dose q4–6 h Sustained release: for patients taking >20 mg/day of oxycodone can administer 10 mg q12 h	Instant release: 5 mg Sustained release: 10, 20, 40, 80 mg	N/A	N/A
Morphine	0.3–0.6 mg/kg/dose every 12 h for sustained release 0.2–0.5 mg/kg/dose q4–6 h prn for solution or instant release tablets	Injection: 2, 5 mg/mL Injection, preservative-free: 1 mg/mL Solution: 2 mg/mL Tablet: 15 mg (instant release) Tablet, controlled release: 15, 30, 60, 100, 200 mg	0.1 mg/kg/dose 0.1–0.2 mg/kg/dose q1–4 h; maximum 15 mg/dose	10 mg IV = 30–60 mg PO
Fentanyl	Lozenge: <15 kg: contraindicated >2 years (15–40 kg): 5–15 mcg/kg; maximum dose: 400 mcg >40 kg: 5 mcg/kg; maximum dose of 400 mcg	Lozenge: 100, 200, 300, 400 mcg Transdermal patch: 25, 50, 75, 100 mcg/h Injection: 50 mcg/mL	1–2 mcg/kg/dose; maximum: 50 mcg/dose Continuous i.v. infusion	N/A
Hydromorphone	0.03–0.08 mg/kg/dose p.o. q4–6 h; maximum: 5 mg/dose	Injection: 1, 2, 3 and 4 mg/mL Tablet: 2, 4 mg Syrup: hydromorphone 1 mg and guaifenesin 100 mg/5 mL Suppository: 3 mg	15 mcg/kg i.v. q4–6 h; maximum: 2 mg/dose	1.5 mg IV = 7.5 mg PO
Methadone	0.1–0.2 mg/kg q4–12 h; maximum: 10 mg/dose	Tablet: 5, 10 mg Solution: 1 mg/mL Concentrate: 10 mg/mL	0.1 mg/kg i.v. q 4–12 h; maximum: 10 mg	10 mg IV = 20 mg PO

From Hockenberry-Eaton et al. (1999). Reprinted with permission

Table 30.11. Common procedures in childhood cancer

Procedure	Suggested analgesia
Intravenous catheter, insertion venipuncture	Ice pack, topical lidocaine preparations (e.g., EMLA, ELA-Max), needle free intradermal lidocaine injections (ZIngo™)
Implanted catheter access	Ethyl chloride coolant spray, topical lidocaine preparations (e.g., EMLA, ELA-Max), ionophoretic devices
Lumbar puncture	Topical lidocaine preparations (e.g., EMLA, ELA-Max). Conscious sedation with midazolam, morphine, and/ or fentanyl (see Table 30.6)
Bone marrow aspirate or biopsy	Buffered lidocaine (use in addition to EMLA, ELA-Max, or ethyl chloride coolant spray). Conscious sedation with midazolam, morphine, and/ or fentanyl (see Table 30.6)

Table 30.12. Conscious sedation protocol example

Agent	Dose	Reversal
Midazolam	0.05 mg/kg (maximum 2 mg) IV × 5 doses prn	Flumazenil 0.01 mg/kg IV, maximum. dose 0.2 mg Then 0.005–0.01 mg/kg IV maximum dose 0.2 mg Given q 1 min. Total cumulative dose = 1 mg
Fentanyl	0.6 mcg/kg (maximum 25 mcg) IV × 3 doses prn	Naloxone <20 kg: 0.1 mg/kg/dose i.v. q2–3 min >20 kg or >5 yrs: 2 mg/dose IV q2–3 min

appropriate opioids is often delivered by continuous infusion via a patient-controlled device. Although the opioid of choice is morphine, hydromorphone and fentanyl have also been used. This type of medication delivery is most effective when the parent, caregiver, or child has the ability to understand and implement it. Children who are able to understand and correlate pain relief with pushing the button are appropriate candidates. This method also has the advantage of putting the child in control and prevents the delays that often occur when waiting on a medication to be administered by personnel.

Medications can be delivered in several ways with this method: intermittent boluses, nurse- or parent-administered boluses, and continuous infusion. The delivery device usually has a mechanism for collecting and storing data so that a team member can look at how much medication the patient is receiving, or trying to receive, and correlate that with the level of pain relief. The device also provides the ability to set a maximum amount to be delivered in a given time frame to avoid overdosing. The ability to deliver a constant background infusion helps to achieve and maintain a more steady state of the drug and provide a more constant level of analgesia.

30.6.8 Adjuvant Medications

Medications that are used to provide additional analgesia are known as adjuvant drugs or co-analgesics (Table 30.3). They can aid in providing pain relief by enhancing mood, decreasing anxiety, or by directly providing additional analgesia. They may also be used to treat the side effects of the primary analgesic (Table 30.8).

Adjuvant medications are not routinely prescribed, but are instituted on a per case basis. Ongoing assessment and evaluation of their efficacy is indicated to guide their continued use in the overall plan. It is important to consider that most adjuvant medications also have possible side effects.

30.6.9 Nonpharmacologic Treatment

Nonpharmacologic treatment is indicated as an adjuvant to, not a replacement of, pharmacologic treatment. These treatments are indicated for procedure-related pain as well as for chronic pain.

Cognitive methods are directed at influencing the child's thoughts and/or images. This is also known as distraction and can be very successful with young children because they can be engaged in an activity that interests them, such as music, toys, games, or story telling (Table 30.13). If appropriate, children can be allowed to pick their preferred method.

Imagery is also used to focus the child on a pleasant event, place, or experience that engages all of the senses: sight, sound, taste, smell, touch (Table 30.14). True hypnosis requires specialized training and good cooperation from the child.

Other nonpharmacologic methods include deep breathing, relaxation, cold or warm compresses, and transcutaneous electrical nerve stimulation (TENS). These nonpharmacological methods may be used individually or in combination to enhance the overall pain management plan. Choosing a nonpharmacological technique may depend on the child's age and cognitive ability and the type, severity, and nature of the pain. It may also require the support and participation of the family.

Table 30.14. Favorite imagery scenes for children

Visual imagery
Favorite places
Animals
Flower gardens
TV or movies
Favorite room
Favorite sport
Auditory imagery
Conversations with significant others
Favorite song
Playing a musical instrument
Listening to music
Environmental sound (waves, etc.)
Movement imagery
Flying
Swimming
Skating
Amusement rides

From Hockenberry-Eaton et al. (1999). Reprinted with permission

Summary

Pain in children with cancer can be caused by a number of factors. The cancer mass itself can produce pain by tissue distention or infiltration. Inflammation due to infection, necrosis, or obstruction can also cause pain. Cancer treatment consisting of chemotherapy, radiation therapy, and surgery can cause pain. Nurses must accurately assess the child's pain and intervene appropriately; pain control is of paramount importance (Table 30.15).

Table 30.13. Distraction techniques by age

Age (years)	Methods
0–2	Touching, stroking, patting, rocking, music, mobile over crib
2–4	Puppet play, storytelling, reading books, blowing bubbles
4–6	Breathing, storytelling, puppet play, television, activities
6–11	Music, breathing, counting, eye fixation, television, humor

From Hockenberry-Eaton et al. (1999). Reprinted with permission

Table 30.15. WHO clinical recommendations for pain control in childhood cancer

Severe pain in children with cancer is an emergency and should be dealt with expeditiously
A multidisciplinary approach that offers comprehensive palliative care should be used
Practical cognitive, behavioral, physical, and supportive therapies should be combined with appropriate drug treatment to relieve pain
Pain and the efficacy of pain relief should be assessed at regular intervals throughout the course of treatment
Where possible, the cause of the pain should be determined and treatment of the underlying cause initiated

Procedure pain should be treated aggressively

The WHO "analgesic ladder" should be used for selecting pain relief drugs; that is, there should be a step-wise approach to pain management in which the severity of a child's pain determines the type and dose of analgesics

Oral administration of analgesics should be used whenever possible

Misperceptions regarding opioid addiction and drug abuse should be corrected. Fear of addiction in patients receiving opioids for pain relief is a problem that must be addressed

The appropriate dose of an opioid is the dose that effectively relieves pain

Adequate analgesic doses should be given "by the clock," i.e., at regular times, not on an "as-required" basis

A sufficient analgesic dose should be given to allow children to sleep throughout the night

Side effects should be anticipated and treated aggressively, and the effects of treatment should be regularly assessed

When opioids are to be reduced or stopped, doses should be tapered gradually to avoid causing severe pain flare or withdrawal symptoms

Palliative care for children dying of cancer should be part of a comprehensive approach that addresses their physical symptoms, and their psychological, cultural, and spiritual needs. It should be possible to provide such care in children's own homes, should they so wish

From World Health Organization (1998)

References

American Academy of Pain Medicine, the American Pain Society and the American Society of Addiction Medicine (2001) Definitions related to the use of opioids for the treatment of pain: a consensus document. www.ampainsoc.org. Accessed 11 Oct 2008

American Academy of Pediatrics, American Pain Society (2001) The assessment and management of acute pain in infants, children and adolescents. Pediatrics 108:793–797

Anghelescu D, Oakes L (2002) Working toward better cancer pain management for children. Cancer Practice 1(Suppl 1):S53

Hockenberry-Eaton M, Barrera P, Brown M, Bottomley S, O'Neill J (1999) Pain management in children with cancer handbook. Texas Cancer Council, Austin, TX

Hockenberry M, Wilson D, Winklestein M, Kline N (2003) Family centered care of the child during hospitalization and illness. Wong's nursing care of infants and children, 7th edn. Mosby, St. Louis, pp 1031–1100

Hockenberry MJ, Wilson D, Winklestein ML (2005) Wong's Essentials of Pediatric nursing 7th ed. Mosby, St. Louis, p 1259

Lucas LK, Lipman AG (2002) Recent advances in pharmacology for cancer pain management. Cancer Practice 10(Suppl 1):S14–S20

McGrath PA (1990) Pain in children: nature, assessment and treatment. Guilford, New York

Merkel SI, Voepe-Lewis T, Shayevitz JR, Malviya S (1997) The FLACC: a behavioral scale for scoring postoperative pain in young children. Pediatric Nursing 23(3):293–297

National Comprehensive Cancer Network, Inc. (2007). Pediatric Cancer Pain: NCCN Clinical Practice Guidelines in Oncology (Version 1.2007). Available at http://www.nccn.org. Accessed 11 Oct 2008

Twycross A, Moriarty A, Betts T (1998) Paediatric pain management: a multidisciplinary approach. Radcliffe Medical, Oxon, UK

World Health Organization (1998) Cancer pain relief and palliative care in children. WHO, Geneva

World Health Organization (2003) Pain control in pediatric palliative care. Cancer Pain Release 16 (3,4). http://www.whocancerpain.wisc.edu/eng/16_3-4/myths.html. Accessed 11 Oct 2008

World Health Organization (2008) WHO's pain relief ladder. http://www.who.int/cancer/palliative/painladder/en/. Retrieved on 11 Oct 2008

Blood Transfusion Therapy

Colleen Nixon

Contents

31.1 **Introduction** . . . 546
31.2 **Blood Screening Guidelines** . . . 546
31.3 **Blood Product Processing** . . . 546
31.3.1 Irradiation . . . 547
31.3.2 Washed Red Blood Cells . . . 547
31.4 **Transfusion Complications** . . . 547
31.4.1 Hemolytic Reactions . . . 547
31.4.2 Febrile Nonhemolytic Transfusion Reactions . . . 548
31.4.3 Allergic Reactions . . . 548
31.4.4 Transfusion Associated Graft vs. Host Disease . . . 549
31.4.5 Circulatory Overload . . . 549
31.4.6 Bacterial Contamination . . . 549
31.4.7 Transfusion-Acquired Infections . . . 550
31.4.7.1 Cytomegalovirus . . . 550
31.4.7.2 Transfusion-Related Acute Lung Injury . . . 550
31.4.8 Iron Overload from Chronic Transfusion . . . 551
31.5 **Red Blood Cell Transfusion** . . . 551
31.5.1 Packed Red Blood Cells . . . 551
31.5.1.1 Indications . . . 551
31.5.1.2 Dosing/Transfusion Guidelines . . . 551
31.5.1.3 Crossmatching . . . 551
31.5.1.4 Nursing Implications . . . 552
31.5.2 Whole Blood . . . 552
31.5.2.1 Indications . . . 552
31.5.2.2 Dosing/Transfusion Guidelines . . . 552
31.5.2.3 Crossmatching . . . 552
31.5.2.4 Nursing Implications . . . 552
31.5.3 Exchange Transfusion . . . 552
31.6 **Platelet Transfusion** . . . 552
31.6.1 Indications . . . 552
31.6.2 Procurement . . . 553
31.6.3 Dosing/Transfusion Guidelines . . . 553
31.6.4 Crossmatching . . . 553
31.6.5 Nursing Implications . . . 553
31.7 **Granulocyte Transfusion** . . . 553
31.7.1 Indications . . . 554
31.7.2 Dosing/Transfusion Guidelines . . . 554
31.7.3 Crosssmatching . . . 554
31.7.4 Nursing Implications . . . 554
31.8 **Albumin (5 or 25% solution) and Plasma Protein Fraction (5% solution)** . . . 554
31.8.1 Indications . . . 554
31.8.2 Dosing/Transfusion Guidelines . . . 554
31.8.3 Crossmatching . . . 555
31.8.4 Nursing Implications . . . 555
31.9 **Fresh Frozen Plasma** . . . 555
31.9.1 Indications . . . 555
31.9.2 Dosing/Transfusion Guidelines . . . 555
31.9.3 Crossmatching . . . 555
31.9.4 Nursing Implications . . . 555
31.10 **Cryoprecipitate** . . . 555
31.10.1 Indications . . . 555
31.10.2 Dosing Guidelines . . . 556
31.10.3 Crossmatching . . . 556
31.10.4 Nursing Implications . . . 556
31.11 **Intravenous Immunoglobulin** . . . 556
31.11.1 Indications . . . 556
31.11.2 Dosing/Transfusion Guidelines . . . 556
31.11.3 Crossmatching . . . 556
31.11.4 Nursing Implications . . . 556
31.12 **Erythropoietin** . . . 556
31.13 **Indications** . . . 557
31.14 **Dosing Guidelines** . . . 557
31.15 **Nursing Implications** . . . 557
31.16 **Palliative Care Issues for Transfusion Therapy** . . . 557
31.16.1 Anemia and Thrombocytopenia . . . 557
References . . . 557

31.1 Introduction

Transfusion therapy is an essential component of supportive treatment for patients with cancer, hematologic disorders and those requiring hematopoietic stem cell transplant. Children with malignancy or who are undergoing immunosuppressive treatment often experience myelosuppression that requires the necessary, and sometimes emergent, transfusion of blood and blood products. The United States' blood supply is safer now than ever, but transfusions still carry potential risks to the receipient. These risks include ABO incompatibility due to human error, infectious complications (hepatitis B and C, syphilis and human immunodeficiency virus) and transfusion reactions (febrile and hemolytic). Blood and blood components should be administered judiciously due to cost and supply chain issues. The decision to order blood products must be based on careful assessment of clinical and laboratory indications that a transfusion is necessary. As well, the patient and family need to be well educated about the risks and benefits of transfusions.

31.2 Blood Screening Guidelines

The differences in human blood are due to the presence or absence of certain protein molecules called antigens and antibodies. Antigens are located on the surface of the red blood cell (RBC) membrane and are inherited from parents. Antibodies are proteins in the blood plasma. Each individual has a specific ABO red cell antigen (agglutinogen) and a corresponding serum antibody (isoagglutin) (Table 31.1). ABO incompatibilities occur when RBC antigens and antibodies between the donor and the recipient are mismatched. This will initiate a series of immune responses that can result in the destruction of the cell. The rhesus (Rh) (D) antigen (agglutinogen) is carried on the RBC surface of approximately 85% of the population. The other 15% of individuals are considered to be Rh-negative as they do not carry the Rh (D) antigen, and will develop antibodies if they receive Rh-positive blood. Despite numerous identified blood-type antigens, the ABO and Rh system are the only groups regularly tested before blood transfusion. RBCs have further antibody screening completed using the direct Coombs' test. This test is useful in tracing the presence of antibodies (indirect Coombs') that are bound to the surface of the RBCs, and also helps determining whether a patient may potentially have a reaction to a blood transfusion.

31.3 Blood Product Processing

RBCs are composed of erythrocytes, and can be removed from the whole blood by centrifugation or sedimentation. RBCs are anticoagulated with citrate and may be preserved by the addition of preservatives like adsol or citrate phosphate dextrose adenine (CPDA-1). The addition of adsol extends the storage life of RBCs to 42 days. A unit of cells preserved with adsol contains approximately 350 mL and has a lower hematocrit (55–60%) because of the addition of 100 mL of adenine saline solution. CPDA-1 contains citrate, an anticoagulant that binds to calcium, inhibiting coagulation pathways. The shelf life of cells processed with CPDA-1 is 35 days. Each unit of blood preserved with CPDA contains on average 200 mL of RBCs and 50 mL

Table 31.1. Blood type compatibility

Blood type	Erythrocyte antigens (agglutinogens)	Serum antibodies (isoagglutins)	Compatible RBC type	Can receive blood from
AB	A and B	None	AB	AB, A, B, O
A	A	B	A and AB	A and O
B	B	A	B and AB	B and O
O	None	A and B	AB, A, B, O	O

of plasma, and has a hematocrit of approximately 65–80%. Irradiated PRBCs have a shelf life of 28 days (Barnard and Rogers 2004; Hastings et al. 2006).

Leukoreduction: All blood components (RBC, platelets, and plasma) contain large numbers of leukocytes. During blood product processing, white blood cells (WBCs) distribute themselves throughout the cellular components and are implicated as the cause of more than 90% transfusion-related reactions. Leukoreduction decreases the risk of transfusion-associated reactions such as febrile nonhemolytic reactions, bacterial and viral transmission, cytomegalovirus (CMV) transmission, and platelet alloimmunization. All patients receiving chemotherapy, and frequent blood and platelet transfusions must be ordered for leukoreduced blood products (Conte 2008). Leukocyte reduction is performed at the time of collection or at the bedside. Presently, the American Association of Blood Banks (AABB) and United States Food and Drug Administration (FDA) guidelines specify residual leukocyte counts of less than five million cells per unit of blood or platelets while maintaining at least 85% of the therapeutic component (Anglebeck and Ortolano 2005; Hastings et al. 2006). Many countries have instituted universal leukocyte reduction (URL) at collection, in an effort to eliminate transfusion reactions. The United States is likely to implement this policy in the future (Hastings et al. 2006; Lockwood 2009). It is recommended that patients who are or may be hematopoietic stem cell tranplant receipients, premature infants of CMV-negative mothers, and patients with immune deficiencies receive CMV seronegative, leukoreduced blood products (Hastings et al. 2006).

31.3.1 Irradiation

Irradiation of blood products causes a depletion of T-lymphocytes resulting in prevention of transfusion-associated graft vs. host disease (TA-GvHD). Graft vs. host disease (GvHD) develops when donor T-lymphocytes replicate and engraft in an immunocompromised recipient. These donor lymphocytes proliferate and damage the target organs, especially the bone marrow, skin, liver, and gastrointestinal tract, which although rare, can be fatal. Clinically, GvHD symptoms include fever, vomiting, watery diarrhea, maculopapular skin rash, pancytopenia, and liver dysfunction. These symptoms can be severe and life-threatening, and if left untreated, may have a mortality approaching 90%. Those at risk of TA-GvHD include hematopoietic stem cell transplant patients, premature infants, patients with acquired and congenital immunodeficiencies, patients with hematological malignancies, and patients with solid tumors receiving high-dose cytotoxic and/or immunosuppressive therapy. Measures to prevent TA-GvHD include irradiation of the cellular products and fresh plasma at a radiation dose of 2,500 cGy and leukoreduction. These two measures are the most effective in terms of safety and cost, in the prevention of TA-GvHD (Conte 2008; Hastings et al. 2006).

31.3.2 Washed Red Blood Cells

RBCs are washed using normal saline to remove WBCs, platelets, and plasma proteins, including antibodies. This is a rarely needed intervention, but is indicated for patients who have experienced severe allergic or anaphylactic transfusion reactions. Washed RBCs have a shelf life of no more than 24 h (Conte 2008; Hastings et al. 2006).

31.4 Transfusion Complications

Any transfusion can potentially result in an adverse reaction ranging from a low-grade fever to a life-threatening emergency such as shock. It is important to quickly identify the symptoms that can signal potentially serious reactions that may appear relatively benign, such as fever or nausea and vomiting. Acute reactions are defined as occuring within the first 24 h after a transfusion, and a delayed reaction occurs after 24 h (Hastings et al. 2006; Lanzkowsky 2007).

31.4.1 Hemolytic Reactions

Hemolytic transfusion reactions, in which the transfused RBC are destroyed, are either acute or delayed. Most acute reactions result from inadvertent ABO incompatibility between the patient and the donor during blood cell component transfusion. Reports approximate that more than 90% of hemolytic reactions are the result of human error during collection (mislabeled specimen, wrong specimen in the tube), processing, or administration of the transfusion (Lockwood 2009).

The signs and symptoms of acute hemolytic transfusion reaction will generally appear within the first 5–15 min after the transfusion is started, but can occur at any time during the transfusion. They generally consist of:

- Temperature increase of more than 1 °C or 2 °F
- Hemoglobinuria
- Chills
- Hypotension
- Severe low back pain or chest pain
- Anuria
- Nausea and vomiting
- Dyspnea, wheezing
- Anxiety, impending sense of doom
- Diaphoresis
- Generalized bleeding
- Disseminated intravascular coagulation (DIC)

Laboratory findings include hemoglobinemia, hemoglobinuria, and positive direct Coomb's test.

Management includes:

- Stopping transfusion
- Assessing the airway, breathing, circulation
- Notifying the physican, nurse in charge and blood bank
- Maintain patent IV line
- Assessing the patient's conditions
  - Checking full set of vital signs
  - Rechecking the blood bag for compatibility and patient identification
  - Returning untransfused blood and IV tubing to the blood bank for further evaluation
- Administering oxygen, broad spectrum antibiotics, antihistimines and vigorous hydration as ordered

The onset of a delayed hemolytic transfusion reaction is approximately 2-14 days after the transfusion and presents with signs and symptoms of unexplained fever, jaundice, positive Coomb's test, a hemoglobiin lower than expected and possibly increased lactic dehydrogenase (LDH) and bilirubin levels (American Association of Blood Banks, 2002; Hastings, et al., 2006).

31.4.2 Febrile Nonhemolytic Transfusion Reactions

The most common type of transfusion reaction is a febrile nonhemolytic transfusion reaction (FNHTR), which accounts for approximately 30% of all transfusion reactions (RBC: 1% and platelets: 20%). FNHTR should be considered as a diagnosis for any transfusion in which a patient has a fever spike of more than 1°C (1.8 F) not associated with any other cause. The cause of FNHTR with RBC transfusion may possibly be due to the result of human leukocyte antigen (HLA) alloimmunization. Leukoreduction by filtration or automation can decrease the incidence of this type of reaction. FNHTR with platelet transfusion is thought to be caused by inflammatory cytokine release from WBCs during platelet storage. Leukocyte depletion before platelet storage and post-storage plasma removal can effectively decrease the incidence of FNHTRs.

Fever with chills and rigors most often occurring within the first 30 min of the transfusion is uncomfortable for the patient, but is not usually life-threatening. Any fever during a transfusion needs to be investigated, as it may be the result of infection or due to contaminated or incompatible blood (Domen 2007).

Management includes: See management for hemolytic reactions

Patients with two or more febrile reactions to blood products or who are chronically transfused benefi t from receiving leukocyte-reduced products and premedication with acetaminophen before the transfusion (Hastings et al. 2006) .

31.4.3 Allergic Reactions

Allergens found in the donor's plasma may cause allergic transfusion reactions. If the recipient is sensitive to these, antibodies will be produced. Allergic reactions occur in 1–5% of transfusions, more often occurring with platelets or plasma. There are no laboratory tests to predict who may experience an allergic reaction.

Clinical signs include:

- Urticaria
- Pruritis
- Swollen lips
- Vomiting
- Hypotension
- Wheezing
- Laryngeal edema
- Anxiety
- Irritability
- Progression to anaphylaxis

Allergic reactions to blood transfusions can vary in severity. Mild reactions typically begin during the first hour of the infusion and anaphylaxis occurs during the first few minutes. With complaints of itch or rash, the transfusion must be stopped immediately, IV status maintained, and an antihistamine administered. In the absence of fever and resolution of symptoms, the infusion can be completed within 4 h. Systemic symptoms indicate a more serious allergic reaction and the transfusion should not be restarted. Respiratory symptoms including wheezing, cough, and chest tightness. A beta-2 agonist such as an albuterol nebulizer may be required to relieve the symptoms. Emergency management including oxygen, epinephrine, steroids, or fluid boluses may be needed if life-threatening symptoms develop (Hastings et al. 2006).

31.4.4 Transfusion Associated Graft vs. Host Disease

TA-GvHD occurs when transfused lymphocytes are not recognized by the immunocompromised patient, resulting in engraftment of the transfused cells that mount an attack against the host. Blood-relative donors with similar HLA haplotypes may increase the risk of occurrence. Symptoms may present 3–30 days after transfusion and include:

- Erythematous maculopapular dermatitis
- High fever
- Liver dysfunction
- Severe gastrointestinal symptoms (anorexia, diarrhea, vomiting)
- Pancytopenia

Prevention of this phenomenon includes administering only irradiated cellular components (RBCs and platelets) and plasma.

31.4.5 Circulatory Overload

Circulatory overload may occur during transfusion of any blood product, but typically RBCs, plasma products, and 25% albumin are associated with this side effect. Patients who are chronically transfused or have a hemoglobin (Hgb) level of less than 5 g/dL, infants, young children, and older adults (especially with pre-existing cardiac or pulmonary comorbidities) are at greatest risk for developing this complication. Transfusion volumes and rates must be closely monitored. Symptoms such as dyspnea, cough, tachycardia (or gallop), hypertension (>50 mm rise in BP), and severe headache can occur suddenly and quickly. Early recognition of these symptoms and close monioring of at-risk patients is imperative to treat circulatory overload. If symptoms do occur, the transfusion is immediately stopped, the patient is made to sit upright, and oxygen is provided.

31.4.6 Bacterial Contamination

Blood components contaminated with bacteria is rare, although there are opportunites for this to occur anytime during the donation process, through blood storage and the peri-transfusion time period. The decreased frequency in bacterial contamination can be attributed to requirements that the Ammerican Association of Blood Banks (AABB) have put into effect. Since 2004, all AABB accredited collection facilities and hospital transfusion services have processes to limit and identify bacterial contamination in blood components. The use of the blood diversion pouch has also helped to eliminate the risk of bacterial contamination during blood donation. During the blood collection process, the product is designed to divert the initial 10–20 mL of blood (potentially, the source of bacteria from the venipucture) before filling the remainder of the collection bag. The result of this practice change has been a 50% decrease in the contamination of whole blood products (Lockwood 2009). Platelets and fresh frozen plasma (FFP) are both associated more often with bacterial contamination, because platelets are stored at room temperature (20–24°) for up to 5 days and FFP requires thawing (Navid and Santana 2006).

The clinical presentation of a patient transfused with a contaminated blood product typically starts within the first 30 min of the transfusion and includes: fever, chills, rigors, vomiting, and hypotension leading to shock. Late signs of transfusion-transmitted bacterial contamination are DIC, acute renal failure, and hemoglobinuria.

Management includes: should be the same steps as hemolytic reactions and febrile nonhemolytic transfusion reactions

31.4.7 Transfusion-Acquired Infections

Fears regarding the safety of our blood supply have resulted in a donor screening process that is the foundation for the prevention of transmission-associated infections. The process includes: voluntary self-exclusion, confidential self-exclusion (donor asks that blood be discarded), and testing for certain infections in every donor. Each allogeneic donation is tested by the FDA-licensed test and is ensured to be negative for antibodies to HIV, hepatitis C virus, human lymhotropic virus, and hepatitis B core antigen, and nonreactive for hepatititis B surface antigen, as well as syphillis, West Nile virus, and Chagas disease (American Association of Blood Banks 2002; Lockwood 2009; Navid and Santana 2006).

The risk of transfusion-transmitted diseases per unit of transfused blood (Lockwood 2009) is given below:

HIV	1:2,135,000
Hepatitis B	1:205,000
Hepatitis C	1:1,935,000
HTLV	1:2,993,000
Other (Yersinia, Malaria, Babesiosis, Chagas)	1:1,000,000

31.4.7.1 Cytomegalovirus

Infection with CMV is common among the general population, with as many as 80% of blood donors having CMV antibodies. For immunocompetent individuals, the acute infection is typically asymptomatic. The consequences of CMV infection in the pediatric oncology patient is uncertain. If CMV is transmitted to severely immunocompromised patients, including low-birth weight premature infants with mothers who are CMV-seronegative, patients infected with HIV, and hematopoietic stem cell tranplant receipients, serious infections and death can occur. Leukocyte reduction and the transfusion of CMV-serognegative blood products to these high-risk patient populations have reduced the risk of CMV transmission (Conte 2008; Navid and Santana 2006).

31.4.7.2 Transfusion-Related Acute Lung Injury

Transfusion-related acute lung injury (TRALI) is a potentially life-threatening blood transfusion complication characterized by the acute onset of noncardiogenic pulmonary edema with hypoxemia (<90% oxygen saturation), dyspnea, tachypnea, fever, and hypotension. TRALI typically develops within 1–6 h following transfusion of blood or blood products causing microvascular permeability, resulting in fluid and protein to leaking into the lungs. Radiologic films show bilateral patchy interstitial and alveolar infiltrates without evidence of circulatory overload (Barnard and Rogers 2004; Hastings et al. 2006).

The spectrum of symptoms can range from mild to severe. As with many of the transfusion complications, recognition of the symptoms and prompt management is key, as TRALI is one of the most common causes of transfusion-related morbidities and mortalities. It is estimated that TRALI is fatal in 5–10% of known cases (Joyce 2007). The specific mechanism of TRALI is unclear, although it is postulated to begin when antibodies from the donor plasma react with the receipient's WBCs, causing them to infiltrate and damage the pulmonary endothelium. This damage results in microvascular permeability, causing pulmonary edema. If TRALI is suspected during the transfusion, the transfusion must be immediately stopped. Patients typically require supplemental oxygen and often ventilatory support. The patient's hypotension will have little or no response to fluid rescuscitaiton, and diuretics should not be administered. Most patients who develop TRALI recover completely within 48–96 h. There are no tests or predictors to show who will develop TRALI, and it is often a diagnosis of exclusion made primarily on clinical and radiological findings (Barnard and Rogers 2004; Hastings et al. 2006; Joyce 2007).

31.4.8 Iron Overload from Chronic Transfusion

Transfusion-related iron overload is a long-term complication in children requiring multiple RBC transfusions. Each unit of blood contains approximately 250 mg of iron and our total body iron stores are about 3–5 g; thus, patients who receive repeated transfusions are at risk for iron overload. Monitoring the patient's ferritin, serum iron, and transferrin saturation blood levels can give a sense of total body iron stores, but only a liver biopsy or testing using total body iron scan with a superconducting quantum interference device (SQUID) can give accurate results (American Association of Blood Banks (2002; Hastings et al. 2006).

Signs of iron overload do not generally appear for many years, and if left untreated, the organs most affected are the liver, heart, and endocrine system. Iron overload coupled with late effects related to cancer therapy can have a profound effect on organ toxicity. Chronic iron overload due to multiple transfusions is treated with deferoxamine, most commonly by IV infusion (15 mg/kg/h) or subcutaneous infusion via a portable, controlled infusion device over 8–24 h (Lexi-Comp 2009). Regular follow-up is recommended to evaluate the treatment response (Abetz et al. 2006).

31.5 Red Blood Cell Transfusion

31.5.1 Packed Red Blood Cells

31.5.1.1 Indications

Pediatric oncology patients undergoing chemotherapy and radiation experience anemia, and require RBC transfusion support due to:

- Decreased RBC production (impaired erythropoiesis, infiltration of marrow by disease)
- Increased RBC loss (gastrointestinal bleeding, surgery, repetitive blood sampling, epistaxis)
- Increased RBC destruction (hemolysis, infection, shortened survival due to treatment)

RBC transfusions are indicated for symptomatic anemia to improve tissue oxygenation and correcting the anemia without significantly increasing the volume (Table 31.2).

31.5.1.2 Dosing/Transfusion Guidelines

- Pediatric dosing: 10–15 mL/kg over 2–4 h (2–5 mL/kg/h) and completed within 4 h.
  - Expected Hgb level increase is approximately 2.5–3 g/dL for each 10 mL/kg transfused
  - Irradiated, Leukocyte reduced
  - Infuse using a filter
- Adult dosing: 1–2 U over 2–4 h (completed within 4 h)
  - Expected Hgb level increase of approximately 1 g/dL (hematocrit by 3%) for each unit transfused
  - Irradiated, Leukocyte reduced
  - Infuse using a filter

31.5.1.3 Crossmatching

- The patient and donor's blood must be ABO and Rh compatible
  - Crossmatching must occur within 72 h of transfusion and with every RBC transfusion

Table 31.2. Disease and treatment transfusion guidelines based on hemoglobin

Indication	Hemoglobin
Prior to a course of chemotherapy	<8 g/L
Receiving radiation therapy	<10 g/L
Recovering from therapy-induced bone marrow suppression	<7–8 g/L and low reticulocyte count
Signs and symptoms of anemia	<7–8/L
Active bleeding	<8 g/L or acute blood loss of >10% total blood volume

Adapted from (Barnard and Rogers 2004; Conte 2008)

31.5.1.4 Nursing Implications

- Monitor clinical signs and symptoms of symptomatic anemia (tachycardia, tachypnea, pallor, headache, lethargy, hypotension, and dizziness)
- Evaluate the above-mentioned signs and symptoms closely before making a decision to transfuse the patient
- Assess for signs and symptoms of transfusion reaction (fever, chills, back pain) and fluid overload (cough, edema, dyspnea, and tachycardia)
- Monitor for congestive heart failure due to RBC being infused too quickly in any patient who is chronically transfused or has a Hgb level of less than 5 g/dL
- Maintain the Hgb level above 10 g/dL during radiation, as oxygenated tissues and tumors respond better to radiation
- Provide appropriate patient and family education

31.5.2 Whole Blood

31.5.2.1 Indications

- Rarely administered, but may be used for emergencies, such as hypovolemia and signs of cardiovascular insufficiency as when massive blood loss has occurred

31.5.2.2 Dosing/Transfusion Guidelines

- 8 mL/kg increases Hgb by 1 g/dL
- Infuse using a filter

31.5.2.3 Crossmatching

- The patient and donor's blood must be ABO and Rh compatible

31.5.2.4 Nursing Implications

- Refer to packed red blood cells (PRBC) nursing interventions

31.5.3 Exchange Transfusion

- Replaces the recipient's RBC and plasma with compatible donor components
  - Process involves withdrawing the patient's blood and administering PRBCs in small increments of 10–50 mL, determined by the patient's weight
- May be indicated for patients with hyperleukocytosis (>100,000/mm^3) with associated hyperuricemia or tumor lysis syndrome
- Patients with hyperleukocytosis should not have a HgB level of more than 10 g/dL, as this can result in increased morbidity and mortality
- Platelets can be transfused, as this does not affect viscosity

31.6 Platelet Transfusion

31.6.1 Indications

Pediatric oncology patients undergoing chemotherapy and/or hematopoietic stem cell transplant rely heavily on the use of platelet support due to extended periods of thrombocytopenia (Table 31.3). These children experience thrombocytopenia due to:

- Decreased platelet production (tumor progression and/or myelosuppressive chemotherapy)
- Increased platelet destruction (sepsis, DIC)
- Hypersplenism
- Platelet consumption due to bleeding and transfusion (antiplatelet antibodies cause platelet destruction)

Table 31.3. Disease/treatment-specific platelet transfusion guidelines

Disease/treatment	Platelet count
Thrombocytopenia due to chemotherapy, radiation or bone marrow failure	10,000
Diagnostic/Routine LP to administer chemotherapy	50,000
Requiring surgery	>50,000–100,000/mm^3
	>10,000/mm^3 for neurosurgery

Adapted from (Brunetti and Cohen 2005; Navid and Santana 2006, Slichter, et al., 2007)

Platelet count, clinical manifestations and the child's diagnosis and therapy schedule should guide the decision to transfuse platelets for treatment and/or prophylaxis. Specific guidelines for platelet transfusion continue to vary and to be disputed widely (Slichter, 2007).

31.6.2 Procurement

Platelets are either removed from a unit of whole blood or collected by apheresis and suspended in a small amount of plasma, and stored at room temperature on an agitator for up to 5 days (function and viability decrease with storage).

Platelets can be prepared as follows:

- Random-donor platelets that combine 4–8 U from different donors and are pooled together for a transfusion product
- Single-donor platelets (apheresis-platelet product) - through an apheresis machine, 4–8 U of platelets are removed from the donor, while at the same time the donor's RBCs and plasma are returned
  - Lower risk of infection and decreased antigen exposure
- HLA-matched platelet, collected by apheresis from a donor with HLA antigens common with the recipient
  - 50–60% of patients who are refractory to platelets will respond to HLA-matched platelets

The lifespan of a normal platelet is approximately 9–10 days, and a transfused platelet is about half of that (Domen 2007).

31.6.3 Dosing/Transfusion Guidelines

- 0.5–1 U of platelets/10 kg
- Infuse rapidly (20–60 min) through 170-mm diameter filter
- Irradiated, leukocyte reduced
- 60-min posttransfusion, 1 U of platelets should increase a patient's platelet count by 10,000 cell/mm^3

31.6.4 Crossmatching

- ABO-compatible platelets should be administered whenever possible, as this can also enhance platelet recovery and survival
- Platelets should be Rh compatible
  - Whenever possible, administer platelets from Rh-negative donors to Rh-negative females with childbearing potential
  - Administration of Rh (D) immunoglobulin should be considered when Rh-positive platelets must be transfused to Rh-negative patients

31.6.5 Nursing Implications

- Monitor and document patient's vital signs per institutional blood-monitoring standard
- Platelet counts greater than or equal to 10,000/mm^3 are considered safe in a stable pediatric oncology patient
- For the patient who is refractory to platelets, partially or fully HLA-matched platelets from family members may be sufficient to overcome this. However, direct donation of HLA-matched platelets from family members should be avoided for patients who may undergo a hematopoietic stem cell transplant in the future.
- For patients who are platelet refractory and exhibit bleeding, using random pooled platelets has proven to be useful in controlling the bleeding
- Provide appropriate patient and family education
- The possibility of platelet refractoriness should be considered if the posttransfusion platelet count indicates a poor response to transfusion (Chap. 19; Sect. 19.4.4)

31.7 Granulocyte Transfusion

Granulocyte transfusions may be used in patients with an expected period of prolonged neutropenia (absolute neutrophil count <500 cells/mm) and with serious bacterial and/or fungal infections that do not respond to antimicrobial medications. Bacterial infections appear to be more responsive to granulocyte transfusions than fungal infections. Previous studies on profoundly neutropenic, septic patients led to differing views on the efficacy of granulocyte transfusions, as the yield of functional donor granulocytes was often inadequate. Evidence now exists that with the administration of granulocyte colony-stimulating factor (GCSF), and in certain circumstances with corticosteroids to donors before leukopheresis, large numbers of neutrophils are able to be transfused into these patients. The success of the granulocyte transfusion is dependent on the dose of granulocytes infused (Conte 2008; Domen 2007; Hastings et al. 2006; Lanzkowsky 2007; Navid and Santana 2006; Strauss 2007).

31.7.1 Indications

- Profoundly neutropenic patients with septicemia (particularly gram-negative) or fungal infection with positive blood cultures (>48 h), unresponsive to the appropriate antibacterial or antifungal therapy
- Absolute neutrophil count (ANC) less than 500 with expected recovery of more than several days
- Patient is expected to survive if the infection is controlled
- Patient with granulocyte dysfunction who has an overwhelming infection

31.7.2 Dosing/Transfusion Guidelines

Presently, there are no clear guidelines on the optimal dose, frequency, and duration of granulocyte transfusion. The literature suggests:

- Large infants and children require a minimum dose of $1–2 \times 10^{10}$/kg neutrophils per granulocyte transfusion
- Adolescent dosing is $5–8 \times 10^{10}$ neutrophils per granulocyte transfusion
- Typically administered over 2–4 h
- Treatment should occur daily from 4 to 7 days, and the patient's condition improves and neutrophil count recovery is evident

31.7.3 Crosssmatching

- ABO and Rh-compatible
- Irradiate granulocytes to prevent GvHD
- HLA matching for all alloimmunized patients

31.7.4 Nursing Implications

- Do not administer using a leukocyte-depleting filter
- Administer through a standard blood set 170-μm filter
- Granulocytes are obtained via apheresis for a specific patient and administered within 24 h (ideally within 8 h of collection), as granulocyte function decreases with storage.
- Assess for granulocyte reactions
  - Chills, febrile reactions, rash, GvHD (granulocytes should always be irradiated), fluid overload
- Administration of amphotericin B and granulocytes should be administered at least 4 hours apart to decrease the risk of severe pulmonary reactions.
- Premedicate with anti-inflammatory medication, antihistamines, and possibly corticosteroids before granulocytes administration
- Monitor and document the patient's vital signs per institutional blood transfusion standard, as anaphylaxis can occur
- Provide appropriate patient and family education

31.8 Albumin (5 or 25% solution) and Plasma Protein Fraction (5% solution)

Plasma volume expanders include albumin (96% albumin and 4% globulins) and plasma protein fraction (PPF) (83% albumin and 17% globulins). Albumin is available as 5 and 25% solutions, and PPF as a 5% solution.

31.8.1 Indications

- Volume expansion
- Hypoproteinemia
- Fluid replacement during plasma exchange

31.8.2 Dosing/Transfusion Guidelines

- 5% albumin is administered at 1 g/kg equaling 20 mL/kg, administered at a rate of 1–2 mL/min (faster if the patient is in shock)

- Twenty-five percent albumin is administered at 1 g/kg equaling 4 mL/kg at a rate of 0.2–0.4 mL/min
- PPF is dosed at 10–15 m/kg administered at a rate of 5–10 mL/min

31.8.3 Crossmatching

- ABO and Rh not required

31.8.4 Nursing Implications

- Assess for signs and symptoms of fluid overload, nausea, vomiting, chills, fever, and urticaria
- Monitor for sudden drop in blood pressure during administration
- Viruses cannot be transmitted as the process used to prepare the products destroys the viruses
- Monitor and document the patient's vital signs according to the institutional blood transfusion standard, as anaphylaxis can occur
- Provide appropriate patient and family education

31.9 Fresh Frozen Plasma

After RBCs are removed from whole blood, the clear fluid that remains is the plasma. FFP is obtained from a single donor and is frozen within 6 h of collection, and stored at −18°C or colder. FFP contains plasma proteins, fibrinogen, Factor IX, Factor V, and Factor VIII.

31.9.1 Indications

- Coagulation-factor deficiencies in bleeding patients, DIC, liver failure, and dilutional coagulopathy
- Signifcantly prolonged prothrombin time (PT) or partical thromboplastin time (PTT)
- Antithrombin III (AT-III) deficiency, protein C or S deficiency requiring surgery
- Vitamin K deficiency with bleeding
- Thrombocytic thrombocytopenia purpura (TTP)
- FFP should not be used when the coagulopathy can be corrected with other therapy (Vitamin K or Factor Concentrates).

31.9.2 Dosing/Transfusion Guidelines

- Dose is determined by the patient's size and clinical condition, typically 10–20 mL/kg
- Infuse over 30-60 minutes as long as patient can tolerate the amount of fluid; infuse within 6–24 h of thawing
- Infuse using a filter

31.9.3 Crossmatching

- Plasma products must be ABO compatible and leukocyte reduced
- Crossmatching and Rh compatibility are not required for plasma product transfusions

31.9.4 Nursing Implications

- Monitor for signs and symptoms of allergic reaction
- Monitor PT and PTT levels
- Coagulation factors typically increase by 15–20%
- Plasma carries the same risk of disease transmission (except CMV) as whole blood
  - If only volume expansion is required, use saline or colloids (albumin)
- Monitor and document patient's vital signs according to the institutional blood transfusion standard
- Provide appropriate patient and family education

31.10 Cryoprecipitate

Cryoprecipitate is the portion of plasma that precipitates when FFP is thawed at 1–6°C, and is used to replace fibrinogen and clotting-factor deficiences (Miller, et al. 2007).

31.10.1 Indications

- Administration of cryoprecipitate allows for more rapid correction of Factors VIII, XIII, fibrinogen, and von Willebrand factor at a reduced volume compared with FFP
- Treatment of bleeding due to hypofibrinogenemia

- DIC where both fibrinogen and Factor VIII may be depleted
- Prophylaxis or treatment of significant Factor XIII deficiency
- Patients with von Willebrand's disease (vWD) and Hemophilia A have been treated with cryoprecipitate

31.10.2 Dosing Guidelines

- 10–15 mL (1 U)/6–10 kg of body weight
- Transfuse within 6 h from the time plasma is thawed
- Doses typically repeated every 8–12 h, until the desired Factor VIII level is achieved or the bleeding stops
- Infuse using a filter

31.10.3 Crossmatching

- Crossmatching and Rh compatibility are not required for plasma product transfusions
- ABO compatibility is suggested
- CMV testing and leukoreduction are not necessary

31.10.4 Nursing Implications

- Assess for signs and symptoms of bleeding
- An assessment of the cause of bleeding should be made before continuing therapy
- Cryoprecipitate should not be used in the treatment of Hemophilia B (Factor IX deficiency, Christmas disease)
- Monitor and document the patient's vital signs according to the institutional blood transfusion standard
- Provide appropriate patient and family education

31.11 Intravenous Immunoglobulin

31.11.1 Indications

Intravenous immunoglobulin (IVIG) provides passive immune protection and is used for the treatment of hypogammaglobulinemia. The FDA has approved IVIG for the following conditions: primary immunodeficiencies (congenital, inherited, or acquired, in which the condition causes an absent or inadequate immune system), B-cell chronic lymphocytic leukemia, hematopoietic stem cell transplant, idiopathic thrombocytopenic purpura (ITP), Kawasaki disease, and HIV infection. Many other diseases are being treated with off-label IVIG therapy. IVIG is a preparation of immune globulins (95% IgG with small amounts of IgA, IgM, IgG, and IgE) obtained from pooled plasma of at least 1,000 donors (Kirmse 2009).

31.11.2 Dosing/Transfusion Guidelines

The dose of immunoglobulin is 200–400 mg/kg every 3–4 weeks, infused over 2–4 h. The infusion rate is started slowly and titrated until the maximum rate is obtained. The infusion rates differ among brands, because of the differences in the concentration of the immunoglobulin.

31.11.3 Crossmatching

- Crossmatching is not required

31.11.4 Nursing Implications

- IVIG is considered a blood product and should be monitored according to the institutional blood monitoring standard, as anaphylaxis can occur
- IVIG should only be administered IV using a filter supplied with the product
- Infusion should begin within 2 h of reconstitution
- Monitor for side effects, such as flushing, headache, chills, tachycardia, back and abdominal pain, and fluid retention
- Reactions can often be managed by slowing the rate of the infusion or stopping for a short time
- Premedication with antihistamines and/or corticosteroids is often needed
- Provide appropriate patient and family education

31.12 Erythropoietin

Erythropoietin (epo) is a glycoprotein that controls RBC production in the body, and is mainly produced in the kidney.The production of epo is induced by hypoxia and a decreased Hgb, which in turn stimulates the hematopoietic progenitors in the bone marrow and stimulates RBCs to mature. The use of epo has been studied in multiple randomized controlled trials in adults undergoing chemotherapy and radiotherapy. Subjects receiving epo have demonstrated an increase in Hgb, decrease in transfusion needs, and reported improved quality of life due to diminished fatigue. Few trials have evaluated the role of epo in the pediatric population and further investigation is needed (Hastings et al. 2006; Navid and Santana 2006).

31.13 Indications

- Erythropoiesis-Stimulating Agents (ESAs) are only appropriate in the treatment of anemia in cancer patients due to concomitant chemotherapy, and therapy should be discontinued following completion of chemotherapy
- Patients whose cultural and religious beliefs prohibit the use of RBC transfusions

31.14 Dosing Guidelines

- epo of 100–300 units/kg/dose subcutaneous injection; three times a week, or 600–900 U/kg/dose once weekly.
- Darbopoietin of 1.5–4.5 µg/kg/dose subcutaneous injection every 2–4 weeks

Both dosing parameters should increase the Hgb by 1–2 g/dL (Barnard and Rogers 2004).

31.15 Nursing Implications

- Monitor complete blood count (CBC) regularly
- Monitor the ferritin level prior to starting the therapy; if low, the patient should be on iron supplementation
- Monitor for hypertension, pain at injection site, headache, fever, diarrhea
- Provide appropriate patient and family education

31.16 Palliative Care Issues for Transfusion Therapy

Children at the end of life, particularly patients with hematologic malignancies as well as those with solid tumors and metastatic disease affecting the bone marrow, suffer from the side effects of anemia and thrombocytopenia. Discussion with the patient and family must take place to plan how the symptoms related to anemia and thrombocytopenia will be handled to align with the family goals (Wolfe and Sourkes 2006).

31.16.1 Anemia and Thrombocytopenia

Transfusion of RBCs is an appropriate palliative care intervention, especially if the patient has symptomatic anemia, such as dizziness, shortness of breath, and tachycardia or signs of continued blood loss. Platelet transfusion support should be discussed with the patient and family, if there is a concern that the child will be thrombocytopenic and may bleed or hemorrhage. Depending on the family's wishes, blood sampling should be kept to a minimum. On the other hand, interventions should be based on the patient's symptoms, as transfusions of blood components must occur at a clinic or hospital. Families need to be supported by their healthcare providers in the decisions that they make about transfusions at the end-of-life stage (Wolfe and Sourkes 2006).

References

Abetz L, Baladi JF, Jones P, Rofail D (2006) The impact of iron overload and its treatment on quality of life: results from a literature review. Health and Quality of Life Outcomes 4:73

American Association of Blood Banks, American Red Cross and Community Blood Center (July 2002). Circular of Information for the use of human blood and blood components. Arlington, VA: retrieved on 10 April 2009 from http://www.aabb.org/Documents/About_Blood/Circulars_of_Information/coi0702.pdf

Anglebeck JH, Ortolano GA (2005) Universal leukocyte reduction. Journal of Infusion Nursing 28(4):273–281.

Barnard DR, Rogers ZR (2004) Blood component therapy. In: Altman AJ (ed) Supportive care of children with cancer: currenttherapy and guidelines from the Children's Oncology Group. Johns Hopkins University Press, Baltimore

Brunetti M, Cohen J (2005) In: Robertson J, Shillkofski N (eds) The harriet lane handbook: a manual for pediatric house officers, 17th edn. Mosby, St Louis, pp. 335–361

Conte TM (2008) Blood product support. In: Kline NE (ed) Essentials of pediatric hematology/oncology nursing, 3rd edn. Association of Pediatric Hematology/Oncology Nurses, Glenview, IL, pp 178–182

Domen RE (2007) Blood product transfusions in the hematological malignancies. In: Sekeres MA, Kalaycio ME, Bolwell BJ (eds) Clinical malignant hematology. McGraw Hill, New York, NY, pp 1127–1138

Hastings CA, Lubin B, Feusner J (2006) Hematologic supportive care and hematopoietic cytokines. In: Pizzo P (ed) Principles and practice of pediatric oncology, 5th edn. Lippincott-Williams & Wilkins Publishers, Philadelphia, pp 1231–1286

Joyce JA (2007) Transfusion-related acute lung injury. American Association of Nurse Anesthetists 75(6):437–444

Kirmse J (2009) The nurse's role in administration of intravenous immunoglobulin. Home Healthcare Nurse 27(22): 104–111

Lanzkowsky, P (2007). Supportive care and management of oncologic emergencies. In: Manual of pediatric hematology and oncology, 4th edn. Elsevier, Amsterdam, pp 717–726

Lexi-Comp ONLINE (2009). Deferoxamine. Retrieved 16 April 2009 from http://online.lexi.com/crlsql/servlet/crlonline

Lockwood WB (2009) Transfusion medicine today: mission accomplished? Medical Laboratory Observer 41:12–16

Miller Y, Bachowski G, Benjamin R, Eklund DK, Hibbard AJ, Lightfoot T et al (2007) Practice guidelines for blood transfusion: a compilation from recent peer-reviewed literature, 2nd edn. American Red Cross, Washington, DC

Navid F, Santana VM (2006) Hematological supportive care. In: Ching-Hon Pui (ed) Childhood leukemias, 2nd edn. Cambridge University Press, Cambridge, pp 829–849

Slichter SJ (2007) Evidence-based platelet transfusion guidelines. Hematology 2007:172–178

Strauss RG (2007) Red blood cell transfusion and erythropoietin therapy. In: Kliegman RM, Jenson HB, Behrman RE, Stanton BF (eds) Nelson textbook of pediatrics, 18th edn. Saunders, Philadelphia, pp 2055–2060

Wolfe J, Sourkes B (2006) Palliative care for the child with advanced cancer. In: Pizzo P (ed) Principles and practice of pediatric oncology, 5th edn. Lippincott-Williams & Wilkins Publishers, Philadelphia, pp 1531–1555

Cytokines

Linda D'Andrea

Contents

32.1 Principles of Treatment 559
32.2 Future Perspectives 563
References 564

32.1 Principles of Treatment

Cytokines are biological response modifiers in the form of non-antibody proteins that when released from a cell interact with receptors on another cell, essentially acting as a messenger between them and resulting in a response. These immunoregulators are produced throughout the body from cells of diverse origin and are quite versatile in their function, stimulating humoral and cellular immune responses as well as the activation of phagocytic cells (Durum 2000). The list of cytokines in the following tables as well as their descriptions are intended neither to be comprehensive nor complete, but rather an overview at those which are more commonly known and their principal activities as they related to pediatric oncology.

Cytokines that are secreted by lymphocytes are termed lymphokines, whereas those secreted by monocytes or macrophages are termed monokines. The three main classes of cytokines are Interferons (INF), interleukins (IL), and hematopoietic growth factors (Fig. 32.1).

1. INF activate natural killer (NK) cells and macrophages and are further divided into three classes: alpha, beta, and gamma. Generally, they are produced in response to the presense of a viral illness and have direct antiviral properties as well as an antiproliferation effect on tumor cells (McCune 2008).
2. IL are termed as such because they are not only secreted by leukocytes but are also able to affect the cellular responses of leukocytes, targeting cells of hematopoietic origin (Table 32.1). The list of identified IL grows continuously, and they are named

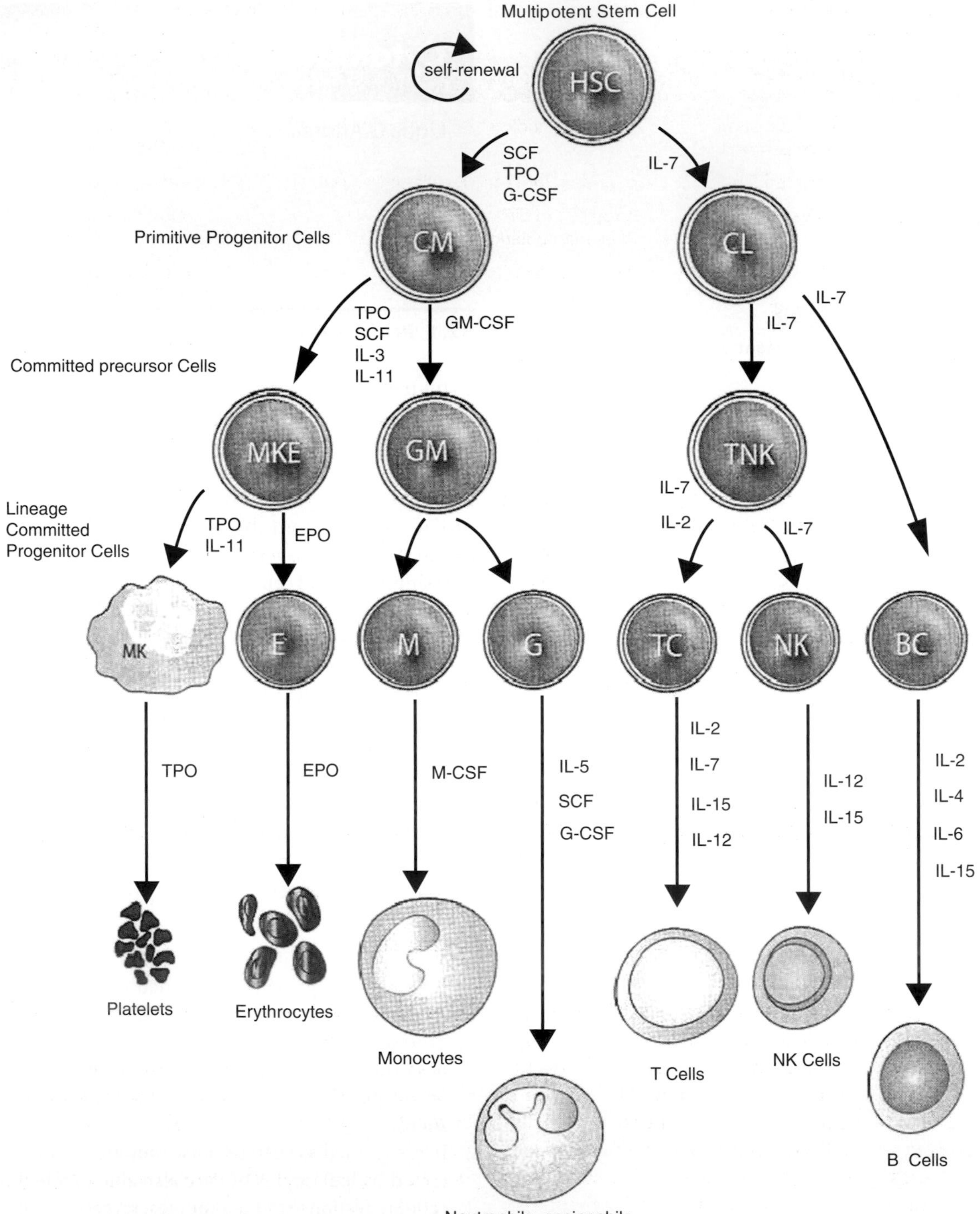

Figure 32.1

The Hematopoietic Cascade (Wadhwa and Thorpe 2009)

Table 32.1. Source and activity of selected interleukins and interferons (adapted from Wadhwa and Thorpe 2008; Jinushi and Dranoff 2005)

Cytokine	Primary source	Primary activity	Commercial product
IL1-α and β	Monocytes and macrophages	Direct and indirect stimulation of hematopoiesis	No product approved due to severity of toxicity
IL-2	Activated T-cells	Activation of T- and B-cells and NK cells	Not available commercially
IL-3	Activated T-cells	Growth and differentiation of hematopoietic progenitor cells	Not available commercially
IL-4	Activated T-cells	B-cell proliferation and differentiation	No product due to limited effectiveness
IL-6	Monocytes and macrophages	B-cell proliferation and differentiation, synergistic hematopoietic and thrombopoiesis	No product due to limited effectiveness
IL-9	T-cells	Hematopoietic and thymopoietic effects	
IL-11	Stromal cells	Synergistic hematopoietic and thrombopoietic effects	Yes, Neumega (Oprelvekin)
IL-12	Monocytes and macrophages	Activates and mediates a proliferation of cytotoxic T-cells and NK cells	No product approved due to severity of toxicity
INF-α and -β	Macrophages, neutrophils, and some somatic cells	Antiviral effects, induction of class I MHC on all somatic cells, activation of NK cells and macrophages	
INF-γ	Activated TH1 and NK cells	Activates macrophages, neutrophils, NK cells, promotes cell-mediated immunity, antiviral effects, tumor suppression	

based on the order in which they are discovered. Currently, several IL are being used and studied as an adjunct therapy, assisting in the recovery from cytotoxic therapy, and in combination with other treatment modalities in the treatment of some pediatric cancers.

IL-2 has a potent effect on the activation and mediation of T-cells, enhancing their anti-neuplastic properties, as well as the activation of NK cells. In one capacity, it is currently used in conjunction with GM-CSF and a monocloncal antibody, 14.18, which recognizes the GD2 disialoganglioside, in the treatment of high-risk neuroblastoma (Osenga et al. 2006). The treatment was able to be administered safely with the toxicity reversible, and the combination shows promise moving forward with the idea of targeted single agent or combination immunotherapy being a mainstay in many cancer treatments.

Placebo-controlled clinical trials of recombinant human interleukin-11 (rhIL-11, also known as oprelvekin [Neumega, Wyeth]) in patients with nonmyeloid malignancies have demonstrated significant efficacy in preventing post-chemotherapy platelet nadirs ≤20,000/mL, and reduced the need for platelet transfusions while allowing chemotherapy to continue without dose reductions. The FDA-recommended pediatric dose of rhIL-11 is 75 mcg/kg subcutaneously (SQ) once daily, beginning 6–24 h after the administration of chemotherapy until a post-nadir platelet count ≥50,000/μL is reached (Reynolds 2000). Laboratory studies including a complete blood count (CBC) should be done twice or three times weekly while the child is receiving IL-11. With limited data in children, general use in pediatric oncology patients is not yet recommended.

3. Hematopoietic growth factors, some of which are also referred to as colonly-stimulating factors (CSFs), are necessary for the proliferation and differentiation of blood cells. It is the cloning of these factors that has had a signigicant impact on the way in which cytotoxic therapies are carried out as well as a critical function in promoting patient recovery from such therapies (Table 32.2). Granulocyte-CSF (G-CSF) has specific proliferative effects on the cells of the granulocyte lineage and also increases the activity of erythropoietin. In contast, granulocyte-macrophage-CSF (GM-CSF) has proliferative effects on both classes of lymphoid cells. They have been used to treat myelosuppression since the 1990s, shortening the duration of febrile neutropenia, effectively mobilizing hematopoietic stem cells for transplantation, and enhancing neutrophil engraftment after hematopoietic stem cell transplantation (Levine and Boxer 2002). Studies have shown that there is no statistically significant difference between G-CSF and GM-CSF in terms of duration of neutropenia; however, GM-CSF has a greater incidence of local reactions at injection sites (Hastings et al. 2006). Laboratory monitoring is needed to determine when therapy can be discontinued (Table 32.3).

When the chemical polyethylene glycol (PEG) was added to G-CSF (filgrastim), the result was a new drug with slowed renal clearance and increased half-life, pegfilgrastim. This allowed for the administration of one injection of pegfilgrastim per cycle vs. daily injections of filgrastim with comparable days of neutropenia, thereby minimizing trauma in adults (Green et al. 2003). Although the sample size was small, this was confirmed in a study involving pediatric patients with Ewing sarcoma with a pegfilgrastim dose of 100 mcg/kg/dose (Wendelin et al. 2005).

Table 32.2. Growth factors (adapted from Hastings et al. 2006; Levine and Boxer 2002; Spielberger et al. 2004; Wadhwa and Thorpe 2008; Wolff et al. 2001)

Factor	Commercial product	Principal source	Indication	Primary activity
Erythropoietin	Epoetin-alpha (Epogen, Amgen); (Procrit, Ortho-Biotech)	Kidney	Anemia related to chronic renal failure, zidovudine-treated HIV infection, cancer chemotherapy	Promotes proliferation and differentiation of erythrocytes
G-CSF	Filgrastim (Neupogen, Amgen)	Monocytes, macrophages	Neutropenia related to cancer chemotherapy; stem cell mobilization for collection in anticipation of hematopoietic transplantation	Promotes growth of granulocytes, primarily neutrophils
GM-CSF	Sargramostim (Leukine, Immunex)	B- and T-cell, macrophages	Neutropenia related to cancer chemotherapy	Promotes growth of granulocytes and macrophages; regulates neutrophils
Keratinocyte growth factor	Palifermin	Fibrinoblasts	Mucositis	Stimulates epithelial cell growth
Thrombopoietin		*E. coli*	Thrombocytopenia (not approved by FDA for use)	Stimulates the production and maturation of megakaryocytes

Table 32.3. Doses of selected growth factors (adapted from Hastings et al. 2006; Spielberger et al. 2004, Wendelin et al. 2005)

Factor	Dose	Laboratory monitoring
Erythropoietin	Cancer chemotherapy: 150 units/kg IV or SQ three times weekly	CBC and reticulocyte count at least weekly; check iron level and endogenous serum erythropoietin levels at baseline
G-CSF	Neutropenia: 5 mcg/kg/dose SQ or IV daily until post-nadir ANC ≥ 10,000 cells/mm^3. Studies now show that stopping when the ANC reached 1,500 may be adequate. First dose administered 24 h after last dose of chemotherapy or up to day +5 without significant difference in the duration of neutropenia	CBC two to three times per week
	PBSC mobilization: 10–15 mcg/kg/day SQ for at least 4 days prior to leukopheresis	
GM-CSF	Neutropenia: 250 mcg/m^2/day for 3 weeks or until post-nadir ANC ≥1,500 cells/mm^3 for 3 consecutive days	CBC two to three times per week
	PBSC mobilization: 250 mcg/m^2/day IV over 24 h, or SQ daily	
Palifermin	60 mcg/kg/day	
Pegfilgrastim	100 mcg/kg/dose	CBC two to three times per week

Human keratinocyte growth factor, although not a hematopoietic growth factor, is worth mentioning for its impact on the care of pediatric patients who develop mucositis as a complication of treatment. With its stimulation of epithelial cell growth, palifermin has dramatically improved the recovery of children suffering from mucositis by reducing both its severity and duration (Spielberger et al. 2004).

Erythropoietin (Epo) is a growth factor that is synthesized primarily by the kidney in response to the amount of oxygen available to the tissues and renal cells and is the primary regulator of erythropoiesis. It was the first hematopoietic growth factor to be identified as an important regulatory factor in erythropoiesis. Epo stimulates the proliferation and differentiation of immature erythrocytes; it also stimulates the growth of erythroid progenitor cells (e.g., erythrocyte burst-forming and colony-forming units), and induces the differentiation of erythrocyte colony-forming units into proerythroblasts (Wadhwa and Thorpe 2008). It is used in the treatment of anemia associated with chronic kidney disease and cancer, as well as chemotherapy-induced anemia. However, in two recent studies, some alarming patterns have emerged including an increase in disease recurrence and mortality associated with the factor (Hastings et al. 2006).

Thrombopoietin (TPO) is a factor that is primarily produced by the liver and stimulates the production of blood cells, especially platelets. TPO was thought to be useful in shortening the time for platelet recovery after chemotherapy. However, results have been discouraging and it has yet to become approved for routine use regardless of being cloned over 15 years ago, owing to issues with toxicity and the report of thrombocytopenia in healthy human subjects (Wadhwa and Thorpe 2008) (Table 32.4).

32.2 Future Perspectives

Immunotherapy, including cytokines, is at the forefront of new treatment modalities in many pediatric

Table 32.4. Potential side effects (adapted from Hastings et al. 2006; Spielberger et al. 2004; Wadhwa and Thorpe 2008)

Factor	Reported side effects
Erythropoietin	High blood pressure, skin rash, headaches, flu-like symptoms, bone pain, seizures; recent trials have demonstrated an increase in disease recurrence and mortality associated with the factor
G-CSF	Headache, fever, chills, nausea, vomiting, diarrhea, fatigue, weakness, decreased appetite, thrombosis, flushing, muscle and bone pain, local reaction at site of injection, rashes, decreased kidney, and liver function
GM-CSF	Redness at the injection site, low-grade fever, muscle aches, fatigue, rash, headache, nausea, dizziness
Palifermin	Rash, pruritus, erythema, cough, edema, taste alteration, arthralgia, rhinitis, perianal pain, paresthesia numbness
Thrombopoietin	Thrombocytosis, thrombosis, marrow fibrosis, veno-occlusive disease, interactions with other growth factors

cancers as researchers push forward with the challenge of minimizing the toxicity while maximizing the effectiveness of the mentioned agents. For example, we know that IL-3 is capable of stimulating multipotential hematopoietic stem cells to differentiate and may have an impact on future treatment options. The activation and mediation of NK cells have become of increasing intrest and several studies are in their early stages.

In the last two decades, we have made great progress in the cloning and utilization of growth factors, but there is more work to be done. Recombinant human TPO has not had the success that was hoped for. The need to develop a more effective platelet growth factor remains critical for the treatment of treatment-related thrombocytopenia, especially in myelodysplasia, idiopathic thrombocytopenic purpura (ITP), and lymphoproliferative disorders. This type of growth factor would also improve the yield of platelet donations, thus perhaps decreasing the number of donors needed.

References

Durum SK (2000) Interleukins: overview. In: Rosenberg S (ed) Principles and practices of the biologic therapy of cancer, 3rd edn. Lippincott Williams & Wilkins, Philadelphia, PA, pp 3–31

Green MD, Koelbl H, Baselga J et al (2003) A randomized double-blind multicenter phase III study of fixed-dose single-administration pegfilgrastim versus daily filgrastim in patients receiving myelosuppressive chemotherapy. Annals of Oncology 14:29–35

Hastings CA, Lubin BH, Feusner J (2006) Hematologic supportive care for children with cancer. In: Pizzo P, Poplack D (eds) Principles and practice of pediatric oncology, 5th edn. Lippincott Williams & Wilkins, Philadelphia, PA, pp 1231–1268

Jinushi M, Dranoff G (2005) Immunosurveillance: Innate and adaptive antitumor immunity. In: Prendergast G, Jaffee E (eds) Cancer immunotherapy: immune suppression and tumor growth. Elsevier, Amsterdam, pp 29–41

Levine JE, Boxer LA (2002) Clinical applications of hematopoietic growth factors in pediatric oncology. Current Opinion in Hematology 9:222–227

McCune R (2008) Biologic response modifiers. In: Kline N (ed) Essentials in pediatric hematology/oncology nursing: a core curriculum, 3rd edn. Association of Pediatric Hematology Oncology Nurses, Glenview, IL, pp 108–112

Osenga KL, Hank JA, Albertini MR et al (2006) A phase I clinical trial of the hu14.18-IL2 (EMD 273063) as a treatment for children with refractory or recurrent neuroblastoma and melanoma: a study of the Children's Olcology Group. Clinical Cancer Research 12:1750–1759

Reynolds CH (2000) Clinical efficacy of rhIL-11. Oncology 14(9 Suppl 8):32–40

Spielberger R, Stiff P, Bensinger W et al (2004) Palifermin for oral mucositis after intersive therapy for hematologic cancers. The New England Journal of Medicine 351:2590–2598

Wadhwa M, Thorpe R (2008) Haematopoietic growth factors and their therapeutic use. Thrombosis and Haemostasis 99:863–873

Wadhwa M, Thorpe R (2009) Haematopoietic growth factors and their therapeutic use. Thromb Haemost 99:864

Wendelin G, Herwig L, Schwinger W, Sovinz P, Urban C (2005) Once-per-cycle pegfilgrastim versus daily filgrastim in pediatric patients with Ewing sarcoma. Journal of Pediatric Hematology/Oncology 27:449–451

Wolff SN, Herzig R, Lynch J et al (2001) Recombinant human thrombopoietin (rhTPO) after autologous bone marrow transplantation: a phase I pharmacokinetic and pharmacodynamic study. Bone Marrow Transplantation 27:261–268

Care of the Dying Child and the Family

Angela M. Ethier

Contents

33.1 Children's Understanding of Death 565
33.1.1 Infants (0–12 Months) and Toddlers (12–24 Months) 565
33.1.2 Preschool Children (3–5 Years) 566
33.1.3 School-Age Children (6–11 Years) 567
33.1.4 Adolescents (12–19 Years) 567
33.2 Explaining Death to Children 567
33.3 Pediatric Palliative Care 568
33.3.1 Principles 568
33.3.2 Locations of Care 568
33.4 Grief 569
33.4.1 Principles 569
33.4.2 Assessment of Child and Family. 569
33.4.3 Interventions. 571
33.5 Cultural and Spiritual Care 571
33.5.1 Principles 571
33.5.2 Assessment of Child and Family. 571
33.5.3 Interventions. 571
33.6 Nearing Death 573
33.6.1 Physical Symptoms Near the End of Life 573
33.6.2 Death-Related Sensory Experiences . . . 574
33.7 Care Following the Child's Death 575
33.7.1 Interventions Immediately Following the Child's Death 575
33.7.2 Bereavement Interventions 575
33.8 Resources. 575
33.8.1 Resources for Children 575
33.8.2 Resources for Adults 576
References 576

33.1 Children's Understanding of Death

Death is a complex concept made up of the following sub-concepts: (a) universality, all living things die; (b) inevitability, death is unavoidable; (c) unpredictability, it is unknown when one will die; (d) irreversibility, death is final, you cannot come back to life; (c) non-functionality, all life-defining capabilities cease; (d) causality, there are external (e.g., car accident) and internal (e.g., illness) causes of death; (e) noncorporeal continuation, there is some form of personal continuation after the physical death of the body (e.g., ascension of soul to heaven, reincarnation, legacy) (Schoen et al. 2004; Slaughter 2005; Speece and Brent 1996). Understanding death is a process that begins in childhood.

Children's concept of death has been shown to be influenced by their: (a) age/cognitive development, (b) nationality, (c) religion, (d) life-limiting illness, (d) personal experiences with death, and (e) family members' explanations and attitudes surrounding death (Silverman 2000; Speece and Brent 1996; Spinetta 1974). A child's understanding of death generally seems to follow their cognitive development (Slaughter 2005; Speece and Brent 1996) and matures as they ages (Grollman 1990). Nurses can assist parents in their children's age-specific understanding of, and reactions to, death (Ethier 2008) (Table 33.1).

33.1.1 Infants (0–12 Months) and Toddlers (12–24 Months)

It is unknown how preverbal children view death, but it is believed that they have no concept of it. Older toddlers may perceive death as temporary and

Table 33.1. Children's general understanding of and reactions to death. Modified from Hellsten et al. (2000); Silverman (2000)

Understanding of death	Characteristic behaviors alternating with playing
Ages 0–1 years	
Unknown	Altered sleeping patterns
Ages 1–2 years	
Perceives death as temporary and reversible	Searching behaviors
Aware of constant activity in the house	Irritable
Aware of family members grief reactions	Protests changes in routine
Aware that someone in the home is missing	Regresses
Ages 3–5 years	
Perceives death as a state of being less alive	Concerned about own well-being
Begins to perceive irreversibility	Emotional outbursts
May feel responsible as a result of magical thinking	Intensification of normal fears
Interprets euphemisms literally	Regresses
Ages 6–11 years	
Begins to understand the concept of death	May play death games
May ask many questions about death	Worries that other important people will die
Personifies death	Concerned with being viewed as different from peers
May be morbidly interested in skeletons, gruesome details of violent deaths	May express and demonstrate range of emotions
Ages 12–19 years	
Perceives death much like an adult	Expresses intense emotions
Questions existence of an afterlife	May exhibit reckless behaviors
Develops strong philosophical view	Boys may be less likely to talk about their feelings as a result of cultural norms

reversible, expecting the deceased person to return before accomodating themselves to the absence after several months. Infants and toddlers are affected by their family members' emotional and physical state and respond to the emotions of those around them. They react to separation from caregivers and to alterations in routine and surroundings. Behavioral responses can include crying, fussiness, agitation, clinging, biting, hitting, turning away, withdrawal, regression in speech, toileting, eating, and drinking, and physical illness. Toddlers move between grieving and playing, which may be misunderstood as not experiencing grief (Ethier 2008; Silverman 2000).

33.1.2 Preschool Children (3–5 Years)

Preschoolers have a limited understanding of death. They perceive death as a state of being less alive, comparable to the state of someone who is sleeping or who goes away on a trip. They view death as reversible and temporary. At around 4–5 years of age, some preschoolers may begin to have a limited understanding of the irreversibility of death. While they may acknowledge that the deceased person cannot come back to life, they may rationalize this as the deceased person cannot get out of the coffin (Silverman 2000). Preschoolers' magical thinking can lead them to believe that their misdeeds or thoughts have caused their illness or the illness of family members. As a result, they might feel guilty and responsible for having caused someone's illness or death. Preschoolers hear the literal meaning of words (Ethier 2008). Therefore, euphemisms regarding death (e.g., "pass away," "lost") should not be used (Grollman 1990). Children at this age who hear death as "gone to sleep" may fear going to sleep for fear of dying. Their greatest fear about death is being separated from their parents. Children of this age often hear, see, and understand more than adults are aware that they can. Their ideas and feelings of death are strongly influenced by their parents' reactions. The terminally ill preschooler's greatest fear may be dying alone without their parents' presence (Silverman 2000). Because of their limited coping strategies for dealing with loss, they may appear to be indifferent, being unable to tolerate feelings of grief for long. Playing can provide them with relief and an alternative method of coping. Behavioral responses among preschoolers can include asking repeated questions, complaining about physical symptoms (stomachaches, headaches), showing signs of regression, displaying intensification of their normal fears, having emotional outbursts, displaying irritability, and undergoing disturbances in their eating and sleeping patterns (Ethier 2008).

33.1.3 School-Age Children (6–11 Years)

School-age children have a deeper understanding of death, with 6-year olds generally tending to understand the death sub-concepts of universality and irreversibility and comprehending non-functionality and causality around the age of 7 years (Slaughter 2005). Some studies suggest that children with cancer gain a more mature, biological understanding of death at an earlier age than their healthy peers (Silverman 2000; Slaughter 2005). School-age children tend to ask more questions about life and death than younger children do, including questions about what happens to the body after death. Remnants of magical thinking may persist through the age of 9 years, creating feelings of punishment, guilt, and fear. They frequently personify death as someone who comes in the night, dressed in black. Dying is viewed as a threat to the school-age child's security. They may experience teasing from peers for being different (e.g., experiencing a loss). Behavioral responses too may include difficulties in eating and sleeping, physical symptoms (e.g., stomache, headache), fearing abandonment, worrying about the health and safety of other family members, difficulty in concentrating, problems in school, and emotional outbursts. At times, the school-age child's reactions to death may seem less emotional and more matter-of-fact (Ethier 2008; Silverman 2000).

33.1.4 Adolescents (12–19 Years)

Adolescents understand death much as adults do, although they tend to think they will not die as a young person, but rather in old age. They ask about dying and death and search for the spiritual meaning of what follows it. Their immediate concerns may relate to their physical appearance and to being different from their peers. Isolation from their peers and increased dependence on their families are difficult for adolescents. They often display intense emotional reactions toward dying and death, and their behavioral responses can include anger, withdrawal, an intensified fear of death, and risk-taking behaviors, such as reckless driving, drug use, and sexual activity (Ethier 2008; Silverman 2000).

33.2 Explaining Death to Children

Talking about death with children is often avoided by parents and healthcare providers who may aim to protect children or do not have the energy or knowledge to help children (Bluebond-Langner 1978; Heiney et al. 1995; Kirwin and Hamrin 2005; Vianello and Lucamante 2001). Parents who have talked with their dying child about death have not regretted doing so, while some parents who did not talk with their child about dying regretted it (Kreicbergs et al. 2004). Avoidance can lead to fear, guilt, misconceptions, the pain of grieving alone, and experiencing psychiatric sequela as a child and into adulthood for surviving siblings (Kirwin and Hamrin 2005; Schoen et al. 2004).

Healthcare providers may provide information and/or assistance to parents about children's general developmental understanding of and reactions to death and how to explain death in a developmentally appropriate manner for their child(ren). Parents are encouraged to approach the discussion of death with a child gently. "*What* is said is significant, but *how* you say it will have a greater bearing on whether youngsters develop morbid fears or will be able to accept, within their capacity, the reality of death" (Grollman 1990, p. 1). Grollman (1990) advises beginning the discussion of death with a child by using a nonthreatening example such as trees and leaves and how long they live. Speak on the child's developmental level, providing basic information slowly, directly, and honestly (CPACFH 2000; Fochtman 2002). Allow the child's questions to guide the discussion, avoiding unnecessary or unwarranted information. Clarify misconceptions and let the child know they did not cause the cancer/death. Avoid the use of euphemisms ("pass away," "lost"). Use simple, concrete, age appropriate words including "die" and "dead." Consider the developmental age of each child participating in the discussion (Ethier in press a). Allow the child to express his or her feelings, while accepting whatever emotions the child expresses. Provide warmth and support during the discussion, and speak with a calm and reassuring voice. Ask the child to repeat what has been discussed in order to clarify any misconceptions (Hellsten et al. 2000). Books, such as *The Fall of Freddie the Leaf* by Leo Buscaglia or movies can be used to encourage discussion (CPACFH 2000; Ethier 2005a; Fochtman 2002). Play, art, and music can facilitate the child's expression of feelings (Rollins and Riccio 2002). Encourage family members to discuss the child's impending death openly and honestly with the child and other family members, including siblings (Ethier 2008).

33.3 Pediatric Palliative Care

33.3.1 Principles

"Palliative care for children is the active total care of the child's body, mind, and spirit, and also involves giving support to the family. It begins when illness is diagnosed, and continues regardless of whether or not a child receives treatment directed at the disease" (World Health Organization 2008).

The goal of palliative care is to attain the best quality of life for the dying child. Care may be transitioned from curative to palliative, with a focus on managing symptoms to promote comfort (Johnston et al. 2008). Pediatric palliative care encompasses the child and family as the center of care that addresses their physical, psychological, spiritual, cultural, and social needs. An interdisciplinary team is utilized to build systems and mechanisms of support. It involves continuity of team members and shared decision-making consisting of open communication and respect for the goals, preferences, and choices of the child and family to guide the child's medical care (Last Acts 2002). Palliative care affirms life and views death as a normal process. It does not hasten or postpone death. Bereavement care is provided to family members following the child's death (Fochtman 2002).

33.3.2 Locations of Care

It is important to determine the child's and family's preference for the location of palliative care. Pediatric palliative care can be provided in the hospital or home, or sometimes in the hospice setting. Often, the child and family will move among the various settings. Care in the hospital can be provided amongst familiar staff and surroundings, with consistent interdisciplinary team members providing care. The hospital setting affords immediate access to medications for pain and symptom management. Home care provides the necessary supplies, medications, and periodic nursing visits to allow the child to receive care at home, and hospice provides supportive care to the dying child and family members in the child's home (Ferrell and Coyle 2002). Respite care is sometimes available in an inpatient hospital or hospice setting. Unfortunately, only a limited number of hospitals and hospices in the United States (US) provide palliative/end-of-life care for children (Fowler, et al. 2006; Johnston et al. 2008). Although most parents prefer a home death for their child with cancer, most childen in the US and Germany die in the hospital, whereas home is the most common location of death in the United Kingdom (UK), Canada, and Brazil (Fowler et al. 2006; Kurashima et al. 2005; Vickers et al. 2007; Widger et al. 2007). Dussel et al. (2008) identified that parents whose children received home care and honest, open, end-of-life communication from the pediatric oncologist were more likely to plan the location of their child's death, the home, and report favorable outcomes.

33.4 Grief

33.4.1 Principles

Grief may be defined as the physical, psychological, behavioral, and spiritual responses to loss (Table 33.2) (DeSpelder and Strickland 2005) and is exhibited by both children and adults. Grief is a natural and expected reaction to the potential or actual loss of a loved one and many secondary losses (e.g., the family unit as it once was, care and support of grief-stricken parents or spouse, support of deceased child's healthcare providers and environment). There is no right way to grieve. Everyone grieves in their own way and on their own timeline.

Although some grief reactions of children are similar to adults (e.g., crying, withdrawal, sadness, anger, sleep disturbances), some are unique to children of specific developmental ages (e.g., regression, guilt due to magical thinking, feelings of abandonment) (Baker and Sedney 1996) (Table 33.1). Children process their grief over a longer duration of time than adults due to their limited life experiences and coping abilities (Ethier 2009b). Expressing their grief less intensely at first, children gradually rework their experiences of loss and grief as they mature and achieve developmental milestones (Ethier 2008; Stahlman 1996). Uninformed adults may misinterpret a child's distinctive grief reactions as indifference or simply that children do not grieve. Children's grief process and expressions of loss may be influenced by their: developmental age; previous losses; circumstances surrounding illness, treatment, and death; ability and opportunities to express grief and ask questions; family and other significant individuals' knowledge of children's understanding of death and grief reactions; family communication style; child's role in the family; and sibling's relationship with the ill/deceased child (Stahlman 1996). Children process grief through play, art activities, conversation, introspection, and written expressions (Ethier 2008).

The grief process for parents whose children died from cancer is described by Rando (1983) in three phases: (1) acceptance, acknowledging the death of their child; (2) confrontation, expressing grief for their deceased child; and (3) accommodation, readjusting to a life without the physical presence of the deceased child (Aho et al. 2006). Parental grief seems to decrease for some about 7 years following their child's death to cancer (Kreicbergs et al. 2007). Adults work through grief through verbal, written, physical, and creative expressions. Sharing grief is often therapeutic (Hellsten et al. 2000).

Grief behaviors, as shown in Table 33.3, persisting over several months may necessitate referral to a mental healthcare provider (CPACFH 2000; Field and Behrman 2003). Suicidal thoughts or actions and expressions to inflict hurt on another require immediate professional care (Hellsten et al. 2000).

33.4.2 Assessment of Child and Family

A grief assessment includes the child, family members, (e.g., parents, siblings, grandparents), and significant others. Assessment begins at diagnosis and is ongoing throughout the child's care and following death during the bereavement period (American Association of Colleges of Nursing and City of Hope National Medical Center 2003; Ethier 2009b). Assessing a child's coping with death can lead to interventions facilitating the child's expressions of grief and supporting positive coping strategies (Schoen et al. 2004). Assessment of a child may include eliciting their feelings and behavioral expressions of grief using art, play, or an age-appropriate book. Assessment of adult family members may include eliciting their feelings and behavioral expressions of grief and determining their: desire to talk with the ill child and sibling(s) with or without healthcare providers and others present, knowledge of the general grief process among children, perceptions of the ill child's anticipatory grief expressions, perceptions of the sibling(s)'s grief expressions, a communication style (e.g., closed, open) as a family. Cultural and spiritual

Table 33.2. Normal grief symptoms

Physical/behavioral	Guilt feelings
Accident proneness	Indecisiveness
Allergies/asthma	Irritability
Appetite changes	Isolation
Constipation/diarrhea	Jealousy
Dizziness/dry mouth	Lack of initiative
Heartache	Loneliness
High blood pressure	Loss of interest in living
Hives/rashes/itching	Moodiness
Indigestion	Nightmares
Insomnia/oversleeping	Rumination
Loss of appetite/overeating	Sadness
Low energy	Suspiciousness
Low resistance to infection	Thoughts of own death
Migraine headaches	Withdrawal from relationships
Muscle tightness	*Intellectual*
Pounding, rapid heartbeat	Confusion
Recurrent nausea	Difficulty in concentrating
Restlessness	Disbelief/denial
Sexual disinterest or difficulty	Errors in language usage
Sleep disturbances	Forgetfulness
Stomachache	Inattention
Tearfulness	Lack of attention to detail
Weakness in legs	Lack of awareness of external events
Emotional/social	Loss of creativity
Agitation	Loss of productivity
Anger	Memory loss
Angry outbursts	Overachievement
Anxiousness	Past-oriented
Complacency	*Spiritual*
Critical of self	Anger at God
Difficulty in relationships	Feelings of abandonment
Exaggerated positive behaviors	Search for meaning (e.g., "why" questions)
Fear of groups or crowds	

Table 33.3. Warning signs of complicated grief

Absence of grief
Separation anxiety
Persistent blame or guilt
Aggressive, antisocial, or destructive acts
Suicidal thoughts or actions
Persistent unhappiness
Eating disorder
Unwillingness to speak about the deceased or expression of only positive or only negative feelings about the deceased
Persistent disrupted sleep
Prolonged dysfunction in work
Decline in school performance
Physical symptoms of the deceased child
Exhibiting proneness to accidents
Engaging in addictive behaviors (e.g., drugs, food)

Adapted from Ethier (2008). Copyright by the Association of Pediatric Oncology Nurses and Committee on Psychosocial Aspects of Child and Family Health (CPACFH) (2000)

beliefs are considered for each individual since these influence grief (CPACFH 2000; Ethier 2009b).

33.4.3 Interventions

Interventions for the child (Table 33.4) and family (Table 33.5) include educating them about the grief process; encouraging mutual participation among family members, including siblings, in caring for the child; providing the child and family with a safe and nonjudgmental environment in which to express their grief while supporting them with expressions of acceptance, patience, and respect; facilitating honest, open communication among the child, parents, siblings, and the healthcare team; avoiding euphemisms and trite expressions; assisting the child and siblings to express their feelings (Robinson et al. 2006) through the use of play and creative activities (e.g., providing art supplies, musical instruments, puppets, toy figures) (Rollins and Riccio 2002); educating the family about their child's age-specific understanding of death; answering all questions, avoiding unnecessary or unwarranted information; and sharing personal feelings of grief, which demonstrates that sadness, tears, anger, disbelief, and guilt are acceptable (CPACFH 2000; Ethier 2008). Comfort care measures are provided to enhance the child's sense of security and include distraction techniques (such as music, video games, movies, books), pets, familiar toys, therapeutic touch or massage, and visits from friends and family members.

33.5 Cultural and Spiritual Care

33.5.1 Principles

Culture is a system of socially acquired beliefs, values, and rules of conduct for a particular group (Hellsten et al. 2000). Race is only one aspect of an individual's culture. Culture is multifaceted (Table 33.6), frequently changes, and is often transmitted unconsciously (American Association of Colleges of Nursing and City of Hope National Medical Center 2003).

Spirituality involves finding the meaning of one's life, connecting with a higher power or others, and developing the ability to live with uncertainty (Mazanec and Tyler 2003). Spirituality may or may not involve participation in organized religion.

33.5.2 Assessment of Child and Family

Assessing the cultural and spiritual needs of the child and family are particularly imperative at the end of life (Robinson et al. 2006). Components of cultural and spiritual assessment (Table 33.7) include identifying the child and family's beliefs, concerns, wishes related to their culture, and wishes related to their religious, spiritual, or existential issues.

33.5.3 Interventions

Providing culturally competent care includes being flexible, displaying empathy, portraying a nonjudgmental approach, and facilitating communication (American Association of Colleges of Nursing and City of Hope National Medical Center 2003). Cultural sensitivity involves knowledge, attitudes, attributes,

Table 33.4. Grief interventions for children. From Hellsten et al. (2000). Reprinted with permission

Ages 0–2 years	Maintain routines but allow for flexibility
	Choose familiar and supportive caregivers
	Assign a support person for each child during funeral, burial, and other rituals
	Acknowledge all feelings of child and adult by naming feelings and giving permission to express anger and sadness in developmentally appropriate ways
	Give hugs when needed to help child feel secure
Ages 3–5 years	**Reinforce that when people are sad, they cry; crying is natural**
	Read stories
	Provide materials for child to draw pictures
	Encourage dialog among family members
	Expect misbehavior as child struggles with confusing feelings
	Offer play with themes of death while providing supportive guidance
	Preschool and school-age kids may benefit from knowing that the person is no longer breathing, unable to talk, or other physical indicators that a person is not alive
Ages 6–9 years	**Listen to determine what information the child is seeking**
	Increase physical activity while role-modeling stress-reducing behaviors
	Work on identifying more sophisticated feelings (i.e., frustration, confusion)
	Encourage creative outlets for feelings (i.e., drawing, painting, clay, blank books)
	Preschool and school-age kids may benefit from knowing that the person is no longer breathing, unable to talk, or other physical indicators that a person is not alive
Ages 10–12 years	**Encourage creative expressions of feelings**
	Explore support group/peer-to-peer connection
	Establish family traditions and memorials
	Incorporate children into rituals, not just at time of death, but at important anniversaries (e.g., taking balloons to the cemetery; creating a special Christmas tree ornament, which is always hung first; having birthday dinners and memory nights)
Ages 13–19 years	**Allow for informed participation**
	Encourage peer support
	Suggest individualized and group expressions of grief
	Recommend creative outlets, (i.e., writing, art, and music)

and skills (American Association of Colleges of Nursing and City of Hope National Medical Center 2003). Communication with the child and family who speak a different language from the nurse involves an interpreter (Table 33.8). If possible, family members are not used as translators for the child and family. Conversational style, personal space, eye contact, touch, time orientation, view of healthcare providers,

Table 33.5. Grief interventions for parents and siblings

Parents can be	Siblings can be
Encouraged to spend time with all of their children	Informed about dying sibling's situation
Encouraged to maintain normal activities	Allowed to talk and ask questions
Encouraged to take time for themselves	Comforted and supported regardless of expressions
Encouraged to share their feelings with spouse/significant other	Involved in activities with dying sibling
Encouraged to seek respite care as needed	Encouraged to see and say good-bye after sibling dies, but not forced
Encouraged to show emotions without overwhelming their children	Encouraged to attend funeral or memorial services, but not forced
Encouraged to model healthy coping behaviors (e.g., crying, participation (not forced) in the funeral and other rituals, using the name of the deceased child, remembering the deceased child)	
Encouraged to return to routines as soon as possible following the ill child's death to enhance the sibling(s)'s sense of security and stability	

Table 33.6. Components within culture

Ethnic identity
Gender
Age
Differing abilities
Sexual orientation
Religion and spirituality
Financial status
Place of residency
Child's role
Educational level

Adapted from American Association of Colleges of Nursing and City of Hope National Medical Center (2003). Copyright 2003 by the American Association of Colleges of Nursing and City of Hope National Medical Center

and auditory versus visual learning styles are considered when communicating with the child and family (American Association of Colleges of Nursing and City of Hope National Medical Center 2003). Respect is shown for the child and family's cultural and spiritual beliefs and traditions.

33.6 Nearing Death

33.6.1 Physical Symptoms Near the End of Life

Children with cancer are reported to experience multiple distressing symptoms during the last month of their life. Frequently reported symptoms near the end of life for children with cancer include pain, decreased appetite, fatigue, changes in breathing, nausea, changes in bowel and bladder habits, altered sleeping, and decreased mobility (Hongo et al. 2003; Jalmsell et al. 2006; Lavy 2007; Pritchard et al. 2008). Interventions focus on managing the child's distressing symptoms and providing comfort care. Creating a comfortable environment with child and family input that may include changing sensory stimuli (e.g., turning down, turning off, or removing unnecessary medical equipment; changing the room lighting or temperature), assisting in the presence or absence of individuals present in the room, providing soothing music, providing familiar comfort objects, and assisting in meeting the child and family's needs related to cultural and spiritual beliefs and rituals. Physical care measures (e.g., mouthcare, hygiene. positioning) are provided

Table 33.7. Components of cultural and spiritual assessment

How does the child identify him/herself?
Where were the child and family/caregivers born?
If immigrants, how long have they lived in this country? How old were they when they came to this country? Where were their grandparents born?
What is the child and family's ethnic affiliation and how strong is the ethnic identity?
Who are the child's and family's major support people: family members, friends? Does the patient live in an ethnic community?
How does the child and family's culture affect decisions regarding their medical treatment? Who makes decisions? What are the gender issues in the child's culture and in their family structure? Is the decision-making a shared responsibility?
What are the primary and secondary languages, speaking and reading ability, and educational level?
How would you characterize the nonverbal communication styles of the child and family?
What is their religion, its importance in daily life, and current practices? Is religion or spirituality an important source of support and comfort? What are other aspects of spirituality?
What are the food preferences and prohibitions?
What is the economic situation, and is the income adequate to meet the needs of the child and family? What healthcare coverage is available?
What are the health and illness beliefs and practices?
What are the customs and beliefs around the transitions of illness and death? What are their past experiences regarding death and bereavement? How much do the child and family wish to know about the disease and prognosis? What are their beliefs about the afterlife and miracles? What are their beliefs about hope?
What are their beliefs about pain and suffering?

Adapted from American Association of Colleges of Nursing and City of Hope National Medical Center (2003). Copyright 2003 by the American Association of Colleges of Nursing and City of Hope National Medical Center

Table 33.8. Communicating with the use of translators

Assess the translator's comfort with the topic to be discussed before the conversation
Explain the purpose of the meeting to the translator
Ask the translator to meet with the child and family before the discussion to establish trust
Speak to the child and family, not the interpreter, using simple language and avoiding medical jargon, pausing between sentences to allow the interpreter to translate every word
Ask the child and family to repeat what you've discussed to verify comprehension
Encourage the same translator to continue working with the same family throughout care

Adapted from American Association of Colleges of Nursing and City of Hope National Medical Center (2003). Copyright 2003 by the American Association of Colleges of Nursing and City of Hope National Medical Center

in a manner and frequency that is non-disruptive to the child and family. Family members are encouraged to participate in care measures as desired. Anticipatory guidance may lessen the distress experienced by the dying child and family members. This may include information about the body slowing down, increasing periods of sleep, decreasing desire for food and beverage, decreasing frequency and amount of urination, loss of bowel and bladder control, decreasing movement of extremeties, changes in breathing and breath sounds, mottled and cool skin, and decreasing level of consciousness (Hellsten et al. 2000).

33.6.2 Death-Related Sensory Experiences

Some children report death-related sensory experiences (DRSEs), seeing or hearing someone or something others cannot related to dying (Ethier 2005b). DRSEs may be expressed months, weeks, days, hours, and/or minutes before death by both children who have and have not been told they are going to die from their disease. The experiences for the child frequently include the sight of known and unknown deceased individuals (e.g., grandparent, child who underwent cancer treatment) and spiritual beings (e.g., angels, God). An awareness of their own death seems to be conveyed in children's DRSEs, which often result in a lack of fear about dying. Providing anticipatory guidance about DRSEs and validation after their occurrence may facilitate communication among child and parent. Parents have reported the experiences to be comforting, easing their grief following the child's death (Ethier 2005b).

Table 33.9. Facilitating bereavement

Allow children and adults who are grieving to complete process, which includes these steps
Tell story of their loved one
Identify and express emotions
Find meaning from experience and loss
Make transition from their relationship with the physical presence of the deceased child/sibling to development of a relationship based on the history, memories, and the notion of who the child/sibling would have been

Adapted from Hockenberry-Eaton (1998). Copyright 1998 by the Association of Pediatric Oncology Nurses

33.7 Care Following the Child's Death

33.7.1 Interventions Immediately Following the Child's Death

Appropriate healthcare providers (e.g., hospital, home care, and/or hospice) are notified of the child's death. Tubing and other medical devices are removed from the child's body, if possible, and the family is encouraged to hold the child, if desired. Privacy is offered and the family is allowed to remain with the child's body as long as needed. Additional interventions immediately after the child's death include allowing the parents and siblings to participate, as desired, in preparing the child's body; supporting the family's cultural and spiritual preferences; and assisting with notification of the child's death if requested (Hellsten et al. 2000; Pitorak 2003). Removal of the child's body is discussed. When death occurs in the hospital setting, parents are reassured that the healthcare provider will remain with the child's body when they leave and the family is walked to their car (Pitorak 2003). Funeral or memorial arrangements of the deceased child are communicated to the healthcare team who are encouraged to attend the services.

33.7.2 Bereavement Interventions

Facilitating bereavement (Table 33.9) assists family members through the grief process. Helping the family to find healthy ways to remember the child may include storytelling, developing rituals, and creating a memory book. Family members should be referred to other healthcare providers (e.g., social workers, psychologists, psychiatrists, counselors, marriage and family therapists, pastoral counselors, and/or school-based guidance counselors) as indicated. Complicated grief symptoms may necessitate referral to a mental healthcare provider. Suicidal thoughts or actions and expressions to inflict hurt on another require immediate professional care (Hellsten et al. 2000).

33.8 Resources

33.8.1 Resources for Children

Preschool to age 8

Klaus B (2000) Laura's star. Little Tiger Press, London

Hickman M (1984) Last week my brother Anthony died. Abingdon Press, Nashville, TN

Lawrence M (1987) For everyone I love. Children's Hospice International, Alexandria, VA

Mellonie B, Ingpen R (1983) Lifetimes. Bantam Books, New York

Joy S (2004) The day great grandma moved house: a story explaining death and bereavement to young children. Kevin Mayhew

Stickney D (2002) Waterbugs and dragonflies. Continuum International Publishing Group, Academi

Susan V (1997) Badger's parting gifts. HarperCollins, London

Williams M (1971) The velveteen rabbit. Doubleday, Garden City, NY

Ages 8–11

Buck P (1947) The big wave. John Day, New York

Buscaglia L (1982) The fall of Freddie the leaf. Holt, Rinehart and Winston, New York

Center for Attitudinal Healing (1979) There is a rainbow behind every dark cloud. Celestial Arts, Berkeley, CA

Coutant H (1974) First snow. Knopf, New York

Brown KL, Brown M (1996) When dinosaurs die: a guide to understanding death. Time Warner Trade Publishing, New York

Susan V (1997) Badger's parting gifts. HarperCollins, London. (Or younger age group)

White EB (1952) Charlotte's web. Harper & Row, New York

Ages 12 and Up

Agee J (1959) A death in the family. Avon, New York

Coerr E (1977) Sadako and the thousand paper cranes. Putnam, New York

Craven M (1973) I heard the owl call my name. Doubleday, Garden City, NY

Grollman S (1988) Shira: a legacy of courage. Doubleday, New York

Klein N (1974) Sunshine. Avon, New York

Rofes E (1985) The kids' book about death and dying. Little Brown, Boston

33.8.2 Resources for Adults

Books

Buckman R (1996) "I don't know what to say...": how to help and support someone who is dying, 2nd edn. Key Porter Books, Toronto

Farrant A (1998) Sibling bereavement: helping children cope with loss. Continuum International Publishing Group, Academi

Fitzgerald H (1992) The grieving child: a parent's guide. Simon & Schuster, New York

Grollman EA (1990) Talking about death to children: a dialogue between parent and child. Beacon, Boston

Kübler-Ross E (1983) On children and death: how children and their parents can and do cope with death. Simon & Schuster, New York

Lintermans G, Stolzman G (2006). The healing power of grief: the journey through loss to life and laughter. Champion Press, Belgium, WI

Kerstin P (1996) What do we tell the children?: books to use with children affected by illness and bereavement. Barnardo's, London

Tedeschi R (2004). Helping bereaved parents: a clinicians guide. Brunner-Routledge, Houve, East Sussex

Organizations

Center for Loss and Grief Therapy, 10400 Connecticut Avenue, Suite 514, Kensington, MD 20985, USA (+1-301-942-6440)

Children's Hospice International, 2202 Mt. Vernon Avenue, Suite 3C, Alexandria, VA 22301, USA, (+1-800-703-684-0300; www.chionline.org)

Christian Lewis Trust, Cancer Care for Children, Tel.: (01792) 480500 Fax (01792) 480700, enquiries@christianlewistrust.org, (http://www.christianlewistrust.org)

CLIC Sargent (Cancer and Leukaemia in Childhood), Head office, Abbey Wood Business Park Filton, Bristol, BS34 7JU; Tel.: 0800 197 0068, Email: helpline@clicsargent.org.uk (http://www.clicsargent.org.uk)

The Candelighter's Childhood Cancer, Foundation, 7910 Woodmont Avenue, Suite 240, Bethesda, MD 20814, USA, (+1-800-366-2223; www.candlelighters.org)

Web sites

Children's Cancer Web: http://www.cancerindex.org/ccw/

End-of-Life Care for Children: www.childendoflifecare.org

Last Acts: www.lastacts.org

Macmillan Cancer Relief: http://www.cancerlink.org

References

Aho AL, Tarkka MT, Astedt-Kurki P, Kaunonen M (2006) Father's grief after the death of a child. Issues in Mental Health Nursing 27(6):647–663

American Association of Colleges of Nursing and City of Hope National Medical Center (2003) ELNEC/End-of-Life

Nursing Education Consortium/Pediatric Palliative Care Faculty Guide

Baker JE, Sedney MA (1996) How bereaved children cope with loss: an overview. In: Corr CA, Corr DM (eds) Handbook of childhood death and bereavement. Springer, New York, pp 109–129

Bluebond-Langner M (1978) The private worlds of dying children Princeton. Princeton University Press, NJ

Committee on Psychosocial Aspects of Child and Family Health (CPACFH) (2000) The pediatrician and childhood bereavement. Pediatrics 105:445–447

DeSpelder LA, Strickland AL (2005) Survivors: understanding the experience of loss. The last dance: encountering death and dying, 7th edn. McGraw Hill, Boston, pp 267–307

Dussel V, Kreicbergs U, Hilden JM, Watterson J, Moore C, Turner BG, Weeks JC, Wolfe J (2008) Looking beyond where children die: determinants and effects of planning a child's location of death. Journal of Pain and Symptom Management 37(1):33–43

Ethier AM (2008) Children and death. In: Kline N (ed) Essentials of pediatric hematology/oncology nursing: a core curriculum, 2nd edn. Association of Pediatric Oncology Nurses, Glenview, IL, pp 228–229

Ethier AM (2009a) Children and death. In: Ethier AM, Rollins J, Stewart J (eds) Pediatric Oncology Palliative Care Resources. Association of Pediatric Hematology Oncology Nurses, Glenview, IL

Ethier AM (2009b) Children's grief and mourning. In: Ethier AM, Rollins J, Stewart J (eds) Pediatric Oncology Palliative Care Resources. Association of Pediatric Hematology Oncology Nurses, Glenview, IL

Ethier AM (2005a) Book review: Fall of Freddie the leaf: A story of life for all ages. Journal of Pediatric Oncology Nursing 22(2):112–113

Ethier AM (2005b) Death related sensory experiences. Journal of Pediatric Oncology Nursing 22(2):104–111

Ferrell BR, Coyle N (2002) An overview of palliative nursing care. American Journal of Nursing 102(5):26–31

Field MJ, Behrman RE (eds) (2003) When children die: improving palliative care for children and their families. National Academies Press, Washington, D.C

Fochtman D (2002) Palliative care. In: Baggott CR, Kelly KP, Fochtman D, Foley GV (eds) Nursing care of children and adolescents with cancer, 3rd edn. Saunders, Philadelphia, pp 400–425

Fowler K, Poehling K, Billheimer D, Hamilton R, Wu H, Mulder J, Frangoul H (2006) Hospice referral practices for children with cancer: a survey of pediatric oncologists. Journal of Clinical Oncology 24(7):1099–1104

Grollman EA (1990) Talking about death to children: a dialogue between parent and child. Beacon Press, Boston

Hellsten MB, Hockenberry-Eaton M, Lamb D, Kline N, Bottomley S (2000) End-of-life care for children. Texas Cancer Council, Austin, TX

Heiney SP, Dunaway C, Webster J (1995) Good grieving – An intervention program for grieving children. Oncology Nursing Forum 22(4):649–655

Hockenberry-Eaton MJ (1998) Essentials of pediatric oncology nursing: a core curriculum. Association of Pediatric Oncology Nurses, Glenview, IL, p 230

Hongo T, Watanabe C, Okada S, Inoue N, Yajima S, Fujii Y, Ohzeki T (2003) Analysis of the circumstances at the end of life in children with cancer: symptoms, suffering, and acceptance. Pediatrics International 45:60–64

Jalmsell L, Kreicbergs U, Onelöv E, Steineck G, Henter J (2006) Symptoms affecting children with malignancies during the last month of life: a nationwide follow-up. Pediatrics 117(4):1314–1320

Johnston DL, Nagel K, Friedman DL, Meza JL, Hurwitz CA, Friebert S (2008) Availability and use of palliative care and end-of-life services for pediatric oncology patients. Journal of Clinical Oncology 26(28):4646–4650

Kirwin KM, Hamrin V (2005) Decreasing the risk of complicated bereavement and future psychiatric disorders in children. Journal of Child and Adolescent Psychiatric Nursing 18(1):62–78

Kreicbergs U, Lannen P, Onelov E, Wolfe J (2007) Parental grief after losing a child to cancer: impact of professional and social support on long-term outcomes. Journal of Clinical Oncology 25(22):3307–3312

Kreicbergs U, Valdimarsdottir U, Onelov E, Henter JI, Steineck G (2004) Talking about death with children who have severe malignant diseases. The New England Journal of Medicine 351(12):1175–1186

Kurashima AY, Latorre Mdo R, Teixeira SA, De Camargo B (2005) Factors associated with location of death of children with cancer in palliative care. Palliative & Supportive Care 3(2):115–119

Last Acts (2002) Precepts of palliative care for children/adolescents and their families. http://www.apon.org//files/public/last_acts_precepts.pdf. Retrieved 30 Nov 2002

Lavy V (2007) Presenting symptoms and signs in children referred for palliative care in Malawi. Palliative Medicine 21:333–339

Mazanec P, Tyler MK (2003) Cultural considerations in end-of-life care. American Journal of Nursing 103(3):50–58

Pitorak EF (2003) Care at the time of death. American Journal of Nursing 103(7):42–52

Pritchard M, Burghen E, Srivastava DK, Okuma J, Anderson L, Powell B, Furman WL, Hinds PS (2008) Cancer-related symptoms most concerning to parents during the last week and last day of their child's life. Pediatrics 121: e1301–e1309

Rando TA (1983) Grief, dying, and death: clinical interventions for caregivers. Research Press, Champagne, IL

Robinson MR, Thiel MM, Backus MM, Meyer EC (2006) Matters of spirituality at the end of life in the pediatric intensive care unit. Pediatrics 118:e719–e729

Rollins JA, Riccio LL (2002) ART is the heART : a palette of possibilities for hospice care. Pediatric Nursing 28(4):355–363

Schoen AA, Burgoyne M, Schoen SF (2004) Are the developmental needs of children in America adequately addressed during the grief process? Journal of Instructional Psychology 31(2):143–148

Silverman PR (2000) Grieving and psychological development, Never too young to know: death in children's lives. Oxford University Press, New York, pp 41–59

Slaughter V (2005) Young children's understanding of death. Australian Psychologist 40(3):179–186

Speece M, Brent S (1996) The acquisition of a mature understanding of three components of the concept of death. In: Corr CA, Corr DM (eds) Handbook of childhood death and bereavement. Springer, New York, pp 29–50

Spinetta JJ (1974) The dying child's awareness of death: a review. Psychological Bulletin 81(4):256–260

Stahlman SD (1996) Children and the death of a sibling. In: Corr CA, Corr DM (eds) Handbook of childhood death and bereavement. Springer, New York, pp 149–164

Vianello R, Lucamante M (2001) Children's understanding of death according to parents and pediatricians. The Journal of Genetic Psychology 149(3):305–316

Vickers J, Thompson A, Collins GS, Childs M, Hain R, Paediatric Oncology Nurses' Forum/United Kingdom Children's Cancer Study Group Palliative Care Working Group (2007) Place and provision of palliative care for children with progressive cancer: a study by the Paediatric Oncology Nurses' Forum/United Kingdom Children's Cancer Study Group Palliative Care Working Group. Journal of Clinical Oncology 25(28):4472–4476

Widger K, Davies D, Drouin DJ, Beaune L, Daoust L, Farran RP, Humbert N, Nalewajek F, Rattray M, Rugg M, Bishop M (2007) Pediatric patients receiving palliative care in Canada: results of a multicenter review. Archives of Pediatrics and Adolescent Medicine 161(6):597–602

World Health Organization (2008) WHO definition of palliative care. http://www.who.int/cancer/palliative/definition/en/. Retrieved on 24 Aug 2008

Subject Index

506U78 (nelarabine) 13
5-HT3 360

A

ABO blood group 249, 251
– incompatibility 547
– mismatch 249–251
Absolute neutrophil count 173, 381
Acrolein 434
Acquired anemia 145
Acupuncture 296–297
Acute chest syndrome 154–155
Acute lymphoblastic leukemia 3–19
Acute myeloid leukemia 19–25
Acute promyelocytic leukemia (APL) 20–24
Adaptive immune response 284
Adenosine deaminase deficiency 277
Adenovirus 280
Adiposity rebound 340
Adolescents 16, 567
Adrenocorticol carcinoma 116–117
Adrenocorticotrophic hormone 490
Adsol 546
Agent orange 20
Airway 407–408
Alkalization 344, 345
Alkylating agents 216–217
Allogenic HSCT 244–245
Allopurinol 221, 344
All-transretinoic acid (ATRA) 23, 24
Alopecia 477–479
Alpha feto protein (AFP) 73, 74
Alveolar rhabdomyosarcoma 101
Amifostine 221
Aminocaprioc acid 193, 200
Amputation 69, 464–470
Analgesia 537, 538
Anaphylaxis 230
Anaplastic large cell lymphoma (ALCL) 44, 45
Androgen 490
Anemia 380–381
Angiogenesis 283, 286, 290, 292
Ann Arbor classification - HL 38
Anorexia 338
Anthracycline antibiotics 218
Anthropometric measures 518–519
Antiangiogenic inhibitors 86, 92, 221
Antibiotics 383–385
Anticipatory nausea 361–362
Anti-diuretic hormone (ADH) 460, 490, 495
Antiemetics 363, 368
Antifibrinolytic medication 193
Antigen - Cluster-of-differentiation (CD) 11
Antigens 546
Antimetabolites 216
Antithymocyte globulin 252
Antitumor antibiotics 217–218
Aplastic anemia 167–170
Aplastic crisis 152–153
Arginine vasopressin 460, 492
Aromatherapy 301–302
Ascites 448
Aspergillus 384, 386, 396
Aspiration pneumonia 525
Assent 311
Astrocytoma 129, 133–134
Ataxia-telangiectasia 4, 45, 72
Atovaquone 386
Audiogram 504, 506
Audiometry 506
Auditory evoked response 505
Autoimmune hemolytic anemia 36, 145
Autologous HSCT 243, 245
Autosomal dominant gene transfer 196
Autosomal recessive gene transfer 197
Auxological assessment 493

B

Bacteremia 385, 393, 396
Basal metabolic rate (BMR)
Basophils 3
Beckwith-Weideman syndrome (BWS) 72, 73, 87, 101
Belmont report 309
Bereavement 575
– resources 575–576
bevacizumab 65
BFM (Berlin-Frankfurt-Munster 313
Biological response modifiers 283
Biological therapy 288
Biotherapy 284
Blast cells 2, 8
Blood banks 551
Blood coagulation (see coagulation) 394
Blood group 546
Blood values, normal 380
Bloom syndrome 4, 66
Body mass index (BMI) 339, 518
Body surface area (BSA) 516
Bone age 494
Bone infarcts 66
Bone marrow stem cells 244–246
Bone mineral density 470–472
Bowel obstruction 271
Brachytherapy 237
Brain stem glioma 129
Buffy coat 249
Burkitt's lymphoma 44, 45

C

C. difficile 369
Cachexia 337–339
Cadherin 66
Calorie requirements 517
Campath 252
Camptothecan analogs 218
Cancer Immunome Database 292
Cancer vaccines 292
Candida albicans 357
Candida albicans 384, 385
Candidemia 384
Capizzi Methotrexate 15

Cardiac toxicity 441–447
Cardiomegaly 450
Cardiomyopathy 441–447
  and Anthracyclines 445–446
Cataracts 513
Catecholamines 80
CD34 selection 249
Cell cycle 204–205
Central venous catheters 273
Central venous devices 384, 385
Cerebellar astrocytoma 129
Chagas disease 550
Chelation 161
Chemoreceptor trigger zone 360
Children's Cancer and Leukemia Group (CCLG) 315
Choriocarcinomas rhabdomyosarcoma 113
Christmas disease 187
Chromosomes 6, 7, 20, 21, 45, 46, 72, 204
– translocations 11, 12, 45, 87
– Philadelphia 12, 25, 26, 220, 290
– trisomy 10, 20, 72
Chronic myeloid leukemia 25–26
Circulatory overload (see Fluid overload)
Citrate phosphate dextrose adenine (CPDA) 546
Clear cell sarcoma of kidney 86
Clinical Research Associate 324–329
Clinical research nurse 328–329
Clinical trials 207–208, 307–324
Clotting 448
Central nervous system (CNS) shunts 384
Coagulation 396, 546
Cobalt machine 234
Code of Federal Regulations 310
Codman's angle/triangle 67
COG (Children's Oncology Group) 313
Cognitive deficits 458–459
Colony stimulating factors 286, 388–389
– Granulocyte colony stimulating factor (G-CSF) 246
– Granulocyte Macrophage colony stimulating factor(GMCSF) 561
Complimentary therapy 295–304
Conformal radiotherapy 235
Congenital mesoblastic nephroma 86
Conscious sedation 542
Consent 310
Constipation 364–366
Cooley anemia (see Thalassemia, beta)
Coomb's test 548
Cord blood banking 247
Corticotrophin-releasing factor (CRF) 490
Cortisol 490
Costello syndrome 101
Co-trimoxazole (see Sulfamethoxazole-trimethoprim)
Craniopharyngiomas 129, 136
Cross matching 555, 556
Cryptorchidism 412
Cultural care 571–573
Cushing syndrome 116
Cystic fibrosis 277
Cytokines 285, 290, 338, 559, 563
Cytomegalovirus (CMV) 249, 356, 387, 392, 547, 550
Cytotoxic T-lymphocytes 279

D

Dapsone 388
Darbopoetin 381
DDAVP (see Desmopressin)
Death related sensory experience 574–575
Death, understanding of 565–567
Dehydration 519–523
Dental caries 358–359
Denys Drash syndrome 87, 412
Deoxyribonucleic acid (DNA) 6
Desferrioxamine 161
Desmopressin (DDAVP) 192, 199
Desquamation 480
Dexrazoxane 221
Diabetes insipidus 459–460
Diabetes mellitus 348
Diamond-Blackfan anemia 4, 145
Diaphoresis 548
Diarrhea 366–369
DIC 550, 555
Dietary reference intake (DRI) 516
Diffuse large B-cell lymphoma (DLBCL) 44
Digitized karyotype imaging/multicolor spectral karyotyping 7
Dimethyl sulfoxide (DMSO) 245, 250
Disseminated intravascular coagulation 20, 393–395
Distraction 543
DMSO (See Dimethyl sulfoxide)
Donor stem cells 252
Donor volunteers 246
Down syndrome (trisomy 21) 4, 19, 21, 24
Drug - excretion 417–425
– dose modification 420–424
– interaction 420, 423
– safe handling 424–425
Drug resistance 206
Drug-resistant genes 278
Dumbbell tumors 79
Dyskeratosis congenital 4

E

Electrolyte imbalance 524, 526
Electrolytes 525
embryonal carcinoma 113
Embryonal rhabdomyosarcoma 101
Emetics 362
End of life 573–574
Energy therapy 303
Engraftment 249
Enteral nutrition 520–521
Enterocolitis 384
Enucleation 97
Eosinophils 3
Ependymoma 129, 135, 136
Epidermal growth factor receptor 220
Epidermis 479
Epstein Barr Virus 34, 45, 49, 279, 356
Equianalgesia 538–540
Erythema 482
Erythrocytes 3, 546
Erythropoietin 148–149, 381, 556–557, 563, 564
Estimated energy requirement (EER) 516
Estrogen 491, 496, 498
Ethics 308–310
European Union Directive 310
EURO-WING 64
Ewing's sarcoma 60
Exchange transfusion 552
External beam radiation 235–237
Extracellular protein 2
Extragonadal germinomas 113
Extravasation 227–229
Ezrin 66

F

FAB (French-American- British) 10, 21, 22
Faces scale 533–534
Factor VIII 187, 188, 190–193
– recombinant 191
Factor IX 187, 188, 190, 191
Familial adenomatous polyposis (FAP) 72, 73
Fanconi Anemia 4, 72, 145, 244
Fatigue 454–457
Febrile neutropenia 383
FEIBA 193
Fentanyl 542

Fertility 496
Fever (pyrexia) 382
Fibrosis (see Pulmonary fibrosis)
Fibrous dysplasia 66
FLACC 534
Flexner-Winterstein rosettes 96
Flow cytometry for immunophenotyping 7
Fluid overload (circulatory overload) 250, 251, 524, 549
Fluid requirements 516
Fluorescence in situ hybridization (FISH) 7
Follicle stimulating hormone (FSH) 490, 497
Follicle stimulating hormone (FSH) 493
Food and Drug Administration (FDA) 307, 311
Fractionated radiation 238
Fracture risk 470–472
Fusion proteins 286–287

G

Gallium scan 37
Gastroparesis 524
GCSF 554
Gemtuzamab ozogamicin (GMTZ) 25
Gene therapy 71
Genes 278
Gene marking 279
Gene therapy 279
Genetic deficit repair 278
Germ cell tumors 110–116, 129
Germinoma 136–138
Glaucoma 95
Gleevec 13
Glioma 129, 132–135
– Diffuse pontine glioma 135
– visual pathway 137
Glomerular filtration rate 417
Glucose tolerance 348–349
Glucose-6-phosphate dehydrogenase 165–167
Gonadal function 496
Gonadotrophin 494
Gonadotrophin-releasing hormone (GnRH, LHRH) 490
Good Clinical Practice 309, 325
Gorlin basal cell nevus syndrome 101
Graft versus host
– skin 284–286
– transfusion associated 391–392, 547, 549
– gastrointestinal 372–374
Graft versus leukemia (GVL) 251, 289
Granulocyte transfusion 390–391
Grief 569–571
Growth hormone (GH) 491–493
Growth hormone-releasing factor (GHRH) 490

H

Haematopoesis 2
Hair loss (see alopecia)
Hand-foot syndrome 482
Haplo-type 248
Harris-Benedict equation 516
Hearing loss 501
Helsinki, Declaration of 309
Hematopoiesis 380, 561
Hematopoietic growth factors 562
Hemoglobin SC 144
Hemoglobinuria 548
Hemolytic anemia 162–167
– autoimmune 164–165
Hemolytic oxidants 166
Hemophilia 187–194
Hemorrhagic cystitis 217, 432–437
Hemosiderosis 160
HEPA filter 389
Hepatitis 374–375
– Hepatitis C 550
Hepatoblastoma 72–77
Hepatocellular carcinoma (HCC) 72
Hepatomegaly 445, 448
Hereditary multiple exostoses 66
Herpes simplex HSV 387
High-dose cytarabine arabinoside
– effect on skin 482
– effect on eyes 513
Histiocytes 28
Hodgkin lymphoma 33–44
Homer-Wright rosettes 62
– pseudorosettes 81
Homovanillic acid (HVA) 80, 81
Human Genome Project 292
Human immunodeficiency virus (HIV) 34, 49, 550
Human leucocyte antigen (HLA) 248, 252, 390, 393
Humate-P 199
Hydrocephalus 130–131
Hydroxyurea (HU) 157–158
Hygiene hypothesis 4
Hyperbilirubinemia 448
Hypercalcemia 347–348, 526
Hyperdiploidy 11
Hyperglycemia 527
Hyperkalemia 341, 346, 432, 526
Hyperleukocytosis 8, 20, 21, 389
Hypermagnesemia 432, 526
Hypernatremia 432
Hyperphosphatemia 341, 346, 432, 526
Hypersensitivity 230
Hyperuricemia 341, 346
Hypocalcemia 341, 346, 432
Hypodiploidy 11, 18
Hypoglycemia 527
Hypogonadism 493
Hypokalemia 432, 526
Hypomagnesemia 526
Hyponatremia 432, 526
Hypospadias 412
Hypothalamic-pituitary axis 489
Hypothalamic-pituitary-adrenal axis 465
Hypothalamic-pituitary-gonadal axis 493–494
Hypothyroidism 491, 494

I

Idiopathic thrombocytopenic purpura (ITP) 36, 180, 181
Imagery 543
Immune suppression 396–398
Immune tolerance 193
Immunomodulators 292
Immunotherapy 279
Infratentorial tumor 130
Innate immune response 284
Insulin tolerance test (ITT) 492
Intensity modulated radiation therapy (IMRT) 63, 235
Interferon 285–286, 561
Interleukin 286, 287, 338, 559, 561
Intracranial pressure 130
Intravenous immunoglobulin 556
Intracranial hemorrhage 180
Ionizing radiation 233
Iron deficiency anemia 145–149

J

Jaundice 375, 548
Juvenile myelomonocytic leukemia 26–27

K

Karyotype 6, 11
Keratinocyte growth factor 562

Keratoconjunctivitis 511
Kerley B lines 450
Kernohan grading 133
Kinlen's theory 4
Klinefelter syndrome 4
Knudson 94
Kostmann severe congentila neutropenia 4

L

Lactate dehydrogenase (LDH) 62
Lactic dehydrogenase 548
Laminar air flow 389
Langerhans cells histiocytosis 27, 28, 29
Large cell lymphoma 44, 45
L-asparaginase 13, 14, 220
Lead poisoning 144
Leucocytes 3
Leucovorin calcium 221
Leukemia
– environmental links 5
– twins 4, 6
– standard risk 9, 10, 12
– high risk 10, 16, 18
– very high risk (VHR) 10
– markers 11
– T-cell 7, 18
– B-cell 7, 18
– transient 24
Leukemogenesis 4, 17
Leukocoria 94, 95
Leukocyte depletion 548, 554
– filters 558
Leukocytes 396
Leukopheresis 8
Leukoreduction 547
Leutinizing hormone (LH) 490, 498
Li-Fraumeni syndrome 4, 66, 72
Limb-salvage 463–464, 469–470
Linear accelerator 235
Liver transplantation 75
Ludwig Institute of Cancer Research 292
Lupus 180
Luteinizing hormone (LH) 493
Lymphoblastic lymphoma 44, 46
Lymphocytes 3, 397–398
Lymphokine-activated killer cells 3

M

Massage 298, 302–303, 320
Medullablastoma 130, 132
Melanoma 117
Meningoencephalitis 47
Menstruation 498
Mesna 221
Meta-iodobenzylguanidine (MIBG) 237
– MIBG scan 80
– MIBG therapy 84, 86, 237, 238
Microarray profiling 7
Midazolam 542
Mind-body therapy 298–300
Minimal residual disease (MRD) 10, 16, 17, 19, 23
Monoclonal antibodies 11, 258, 285, 287–288,
Monocytes 3
Movement therapy 300–301
MTP-PE 69
Mucositis 354–358
Mustard gas 204, 217
Mycoplasma 404
Myelodysplastic syndrome (MDS) 22
Myelomonocytic leukemia 26
Myocytes 445

N

Nadir 380
Nail dystrophies 483
Nasogastric tube 521
Nasopharyngeal carcinoma 118
National Cancer Institute (NCI) 9
National Cancer Research Institute (NCRI) 315
Natural killer (NK) cells 3, 559
Nausea 261–265
Near-haploid 11
Necrosis, skin 480
Nephrectomy 412–417
Nephrotic syndrome 412
Nephrotoxicity 425–432
Neuroblastoma 77–86
Neuroectodermal tumor (PNET) 129, 132
Neurofibromatosis 4
Neurofibromatosis 101
Neuron specific enolase 80
Neuro-opthalmological testing 138
Neutropenia 173–178, 381–389
Neutrophil 3, 381
Nijmegen/Berlin breakage syndrome 4
Non-Hodgkin lymphoma 44–55
Non- rhabdomyosarcomatous soft tissue sarcomas 107–110
Noonan syndrome 101
Novoseven (See Recombinant factor VIIa) 193
NSAID (non-steroidal anti inflammatory drugs) 537
Null cells 3
Nuremberg code 309

O

Obesity 339–341
Omaya reservoirs 384
Oncogene 6, 107, 278
Ondansetron 361
Opioids 541
Opsoclonus-myoclonus ataxia 79
Oral mucositis 356
Oral mucositis assessment scale 355
Osteochondroma 66
Osteomyelitis 66
Osteonecrosis 472–475
Osteopenia 470, 471
Osteoporosis 470–472
Osteosarcoma 65–71
Otoacoustic emissions testing 505, 506
Ovarian dysgerminomas 113
Oxytocin 490

P

Paget's disease 66
Palfermin 222, 357, 562, 563
Palmar-plantar erythrodysesthesia 482
Pancreatitis 272, 375
Paranchymal lung lesions 35
Particle radiation 233
Patient controlled analgesia (PCA) 540–542
Pegfilgrastim 562
Pentamidine 386, 388, 402
Periodic-acid Schiff 10
Peripheral stem cells 249
Peripherally inserted central venous catheters (PICC) 273
Perirectal cellulitis 371–372
Peristalsis 364
p-glycoprotein 66
Phagocytic cells 559
Pharmacodynamics 206–207
Pharmacogenomics 206–207
Pharmacokinetics 206–207
Pharmacokinetics 417–418
Pheresis 246
Plant derivatives 218
Plasma volume expanders 554
Plasmid vectors 280

Platelet refractoriness 392–393
Platelet transfusions 389–390
Pleomorphic rhabdomyosarcoma 101, 102
Pleural effusions 450
Pleuropulmonary blastoma 118–119
Pneumocystis jiroveci pneumonia (PCP) 14, 386, 401
Pneumonitis 404–406
Pneumothorax 272
Podophyllotoxins 218
Polymerase chain reaction (PCR) 6, 7
Port-a-catheter 273
Positron emission tomography (PET) 37, 62
Post transplant lymphoproliferative disorder (PTLD) 44, 45
Precocious puberty 73
Pregnancy 497
PRETEXT 74
Progesterone 498
Prolactin 490
Prolactin inhibiting factor (PIF) 490
Proteasomes 295
Prothrombin 191
Protooncogenes 6, 45
Pruritus 539
Puberty 491, 493–494, 497
– precocious 493–494
Pulmonary fibrosis 406
Pyrexia and neutropenia (see febrile neutropenia)

Q

Quality of life 319–320

R

Radiation-recall skin reactions 479, 481
Radioiodine I-131 237
Randomised control trial (RCT) 308
Recombinant factor VIIa (Novoseven) 191
Recombinant tissue plasminogen activator 274
Recommended daily allowance (RDA) 516
Red blood count values 142
Reed Sternberg cells 35, 37, 38
Refeeding syndrome 527
Refractoriness to platelets 553
Rehydration 519–520
Relapsed acute lymphoblastic leukemia 17–19
Renal cell carcinoma 86
Renal failure 425–431
Renal failure 550
Retcam 96
Reticuloendothelial system 398
Retinal detachment 95
Retinoblastoma 93–100
Retinoic acid syndrome (RAS) 23
Retinoids 86
Reverse isolation/barrier nursing 389
Rhabdoid tumor of the kidney 86
Rhabdomyosarcoma 100–107
Rhesus (Rh) 546
Rituximab 165
Rotationplasty 69, 70, 467–468
Rothmund-Thomson syndrome 66
Rubinstein-Taybi syndrome 101

S

Saccrococcygeal germ cell tumors 114
Sealed radiation sources 237
Secondary malignancy 17, 93
Septic shock 395–396
Severe combined immunodeficiency (SCID) 244, 277
Shwachman-Diamond syndrome 4
SIADH (syndrome of inappropriate antidiuretic hormone secretion) 496
Sickle cell 144, 145, 149–158, 244
Simulation, CT 234
Soft tissue sarcomas 107–110
Somatomedin C 490
Somatostatin (GHRIH) 490
Southern blotting 7
Spermatogenesis 497
Spherocytosis 145, 162
Spinal cord compression 453–454
Spinal tumor 138
Spiritual care 571–573
Spleen 398
Splenectomy 165, 183
Splenic sequestration 152
Splenomegaly 345
St Jude staging for NHL 51
Stem cell collection 244–247
Stereotactic radiotherapy 235
Steroidogenesis 497
Stimate 192, 199
Strabismus 94
Sulfamethoxazole-trimethoprim 388, 403
Superior vena cava syndrome 47
Supratentorial tumor 130
Survival trends 314
Syngeneic HSCT 244
Syphilis 550

T

Tanner stage 493
Taxanes 218
T-cell depletion 249, 251
Testicular seminomas 113
Thalassemia 144,145, 158
– alpha 158
– beta 159–160
Thalidomide 290
Thiopurine purine methyltransferase (TPMT) 15
Three dimensional radiotherapy 235
Thrombocytes 3
Thrombocytic thrombocytopenia purpura 555
Thrombocytopenia 179–184, 389–390
Thrombopoietin 562, 564
Thyroid carcinoma 119
Thyroid gland 494
Thyroid-stimulating hormone (TSH) 490, 494
Thyrotropin-releasing hormone (TRH) 490
Tissue typing 247–248
T-lymphocyte infusion 252, 279
Topoisomerase 218
Total body irradiation 237
Total parenteral nutrition 521–523
Typhylitis 272, 369–371
Tranexamic acid 193, 200
Transfusion 380–381
– packed red cell 551–552
– whole blood 552
– platelet 552–553
– exchange 552
– granulocyte 553–554
– albumin 554–555
– fresh frozen plasma 555
– cryoprecipitate 555–556
Transient myeloproliferative disorder (TMD) 24
Translators 574
Trimethoprim 388
Trisomy syndrome 4
Tumor cell lysis 52, 341–343
Tumor lysis syndrome 52
Tumor necrosis factor 285
Tumor suppressor gene 66, 77, 87
– p53 12, 66, 278
– RB1 66, 94

Two-hit theory 94
Typhylitis 369–371
Tyrosine kinase 220
Tyrosine kinase inhibitors 86

U

UKCCSG (United Kingdom Childhood Cancer Study Group) 313
Ultraviolet reaction 482
Umbilical cord blood 246–247
Unsealed radiation sources 237
Uric acid metabolism 343
Uricolytic agents 52

V

Vanillymandelic acid (VMA) 80, 81
Varicella zoster 356, 387
Vasoactive intestinal peptide 79
Vasopressin 490, 495
Vectors 280
Veno-occlusive disease 447–450
– Hepatic 447–449
– Pulmonary 449–450
Venous occlusive event (VOE) 156
Ventriculoperitoneal shunting 131
Ventriculostomy 131
Vinca-alkaloids 219
Viral-mediated gene transfer 278
Viral vectors 280
Vitamin K 555
Vomiting 359–364
Vomiting centre 359
Von Willebrand 191, 194–200

W

WAGR 87
Waldeyer's ring 47
WHO classification
– AML 22
– HL 38
WHO pain relief ladder 537
– clinical recommendations for pain control 543
Wilm's tumor 86–93, 413–415
Wiscott-Aldrich syndrome 45

X

Xanthine 343
Xerostomia 359
X-linked disease 188

Y

Yolk sac tumors 112, 113
Yondelis 65

Z

Zoledronic acid 71

Printing and Binding: Stürtz GmbH, Würzburg